Dyslexia: A Global Issue

NATO ASI Series

Advanced Science Institutes Series

A Series presenting the results of activities sponsored by the NATO Science Committee, which aims at the dissemination of advanced scientific and technological knowledge, with a view to strengthening links between scientific communities

The Series is published by an international board of publishers in conjunction with the NATO Scientific Affairs Division

A	Life Sciences	Plenum Publishing Corporation
B	Physics	London and New York
C	Mathematical and Physical Sciences	D. Reidel Publishing Company Dordrecht and Boston
D	Behavioural and Social Sciences	Martinus Nijhoff Publishers The Hague/Boston/Lancaster
E	Applied Sciences	
F	Computer and Systems Sciences	Springer-Verlag Berlin/Heidelberg/New York
G	Ecological Sciences	

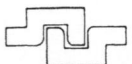

Series D: Behavioural and Social Sciences – No. 18

Dyslexia: A Global Issue

edited by

R.N. Malatesha

Director, Reading Program
Fayetteville State University
Fayetteville, North Carolina 28301, USA

and

H.A. Whitaker

Department of Hearing and Speech Sciences
University of Maryland
College Park, Maryland 20741, USA

1984 **Martinus Nijhoff Publishers**
The Hague / Boston / Lancaster
Published in cooperation with NATO Scientific Affairs Division

Proceedings of the NATO Advanced Study Institute on Dyslexia: A Global Issue, Maratea, Italy, October 10–22, 1982

Library of Congress Cataloging in Publication Data

NATO Advanced Study Institute on Dyslexia: a Global
    Issue (1982 : Maratea, Italy)
    Dyslexia : a global issue.

    (NATO ASI series. Series D, Behavioural and social
sciences ; no. 18)
    "Proceedings of the NATO Advanced Study Institute on
Dyslexia: a Global Issue, Maratea, Italy, October 10–22,
1982"--T.p. verso.
    1. Dyslexia--Congresses. I. Malatesha, R. N.
II. Whitaker, Harry A. III. North Atlantic Treaty
Organization. Scientific Affairs Division. IV. Title.
V. Series.
RJ496.A5N38 1982   616.85'53   83-23787

ISBN-13: 978-94-009-6931-5   e-ISBN-13: 978-94-009-6929-2
DOI: 10.1007/ 978-94-009-6929-2

Distributors for the United States and Canada: Kluwer Boston, Inc., 190 Old Derby Street, Hingham, MA 02043, USA

Distributors for all other countries: Kluwer Academic Publishers Group, Distribution Center, P.O. Box 322, 3300 AH Dordrecht, The Netherlands

PREFACE

Reading is one of the highest forms of acquired cognitive functions. It comes as no surprise, therefore, that the study of reading has attracted numerous investigators who, in spite of their diverse background, have been motivated by one ultimate goal -- to understand how we read and how we learn to read. A substantial proportion of these investigators have attempted to gain knowledge about the neuropsychological processes that underlie the reading process by studying individuals who fail to acquire reading skill (developmental dyslexia) and individuals who acquire a reading deficit as a result of brain pathology (alexia; acquired dyslexia). Over the years, these two sources, using different techniques and methods, have yielded a good deal of information. Unfortunately, the empirical findings that have been obtained under these two circumstances have, to a large extent, failed to influence the other. Bringing these two approaches (developmental dyslexia and acquired alexia) together, therefore, remains a top priority.

With a view towards bringing these two disciplines together, the Scientific Affairs Division of the North Atlantic Treaty Organization (NATO) awarded us a grant to conduct an Advanced Study Institute (ASI) in Maratea, Italy, from October 10-22, 1982. This volume is the result of that Institute.

The book is divided into four parts: developmental reading and spelling disorders, acquired alexia, diagnosis and remediation, and research implications. In the first two parts, the nature and etiology of reading and spelling disorders are discussed from the perspectives of neuropsychology, linguistics, psychology, and education. Different diagnostic and remedial procedures are dealt with in Part Three, and Part Four focuses on research implications for the study of dyslexia and alexia. The present volume stresses the importance of distinguishing various subtypes of reading and spelling disorders and will be useful to neuropsychologists, educators, and linguists.

We thank NATO Scientific Affairs Division for their support of the Institute. The participants of the Institute are recognized scholars, and we thank them for their contribution. We also wish to thank Mr. A. Guzzardi and the entire staff of Hotel Villa del Mare for their help in making this Institute a success.

We wish to express our gratitude to Dr. Craig Sinclair, NATO Scientific Affairs Division; Dr Tilo Kester and Mrs. Barbara Kester; International Transfer of Science and Technology; Mrs. G.P. Rekha; and Mrs. Henny Hoogervorst, of Martinus Nijhoff Publishers, for their help in various aspects of the Institute and of this book.

R.N. Malatesha
H.A. Whitaker

TABLE OF CONTENTS

PART FOUR

THE THREE PHASES OF DEVELOPMENTAL DYSLEXIA[1]

P. G. Aaron   Tom Bommarito   Cathy Baker

Dept. of Educational and School   Educational Opportunites
Psychology   Program
Indiana State University   Indiana State University
Terre Haute, Indiana   Terre Haute, Indiana

INTRODUCTION

Developmental dyslexia, or specific reading disability, is not
an isolated unitary symptom but is one aspect of a much larger syndrome that can manifest itself in different forms. In addition to
the poor oral reading and comprehension skills, the dyslexia syndrome includes diminished ability to process certain linguistic inputs
(Byrne & Shea, 1979; Liberman, Shankweiler, Liberman, Fowler, & Fischer, 1977) syntactic deficits in language output (Fry, Johnson, &
Muehl, 1970; Loban, 1963; Semel & Wigg, 1975), and poor spelling ability (Boder & Jerrico, 1982; Nelson, 1980). Our own research carried
out with young adults (mostly college students) over the past 5 years
confirms the co-occurrence of these symptoms (Aaron & Baker, 1982).
Two previous studies that involved more than 20 dyslexic subjects
(Aaron, Hickox, & Baker, 1982; Aaron, Lucenti, & Baxter, 1980) found
all the subjects to be poor in spelling. The misspelled words ranged
from 14 to 35 when they were required to reproduce by writing a list
of 36 orally presented words. The list included common words such as
"sit" and relatively uncommon words such as "pessimistic". In addition, at least one subgroup of dyslexic subjects was found to be poor
in syntactic aspects of expressive and receptive language as measured
by NSST (Lee, 1969). Similar errors were found in their written sentences as well. In a recent series of experiments, we tested four
reading disabled college students. Our findings further confirm the

---

1. Research reported in this chapter was supported by a grant from
the Research Committee, Indiana State University, Terre Haute,
Indiana.

observation made earlier that dyslexia is a syndrome that manifests itself in more than one form. Samples of their written sentences which contain syntactic errors are shown in Table 1. Even though a majority of the sentences written by these four subjects were grammatically correct, the fact that subjects who have reached college do occasionally produce such garbled sentences reflects a basic syntactical difficulty experienced by these subjects.

TABLE 1. Agrammatic Sentences Written by RD Subjects

C. K. :   She improvised away in which to complete the job quickly.
          I am a typed letter to Steve and was sent back.

B. G. :   I crave cocolet cack sinda.
          The accountant was amiable to the fact.

T. M. :   The paper became unfolded and scattered over the yard.
          She wanted a 280 Z when though she wanted a V. W.

S. A. :   We saw a movie about the disaster of the earth dying.
          The dog heard a noise and cocked then leaped up for the door.

This brief review of dyslexic symptoms reiterates the fact that developmental dyslexia is indeed a collection of symptoms. In addition, it also indicates that the underlying causal mechanism affects both input (reading and comprehension of written language) and output (spelling and written language) aspects of verbal information processing. Any viable theory of dyslexia should, therefore, be comprehensive enough to account for all these deficits. The study reported in this chapter was designed to develop a hypothesis that will attempt to accomplish this broad objective.

The proposition that the different varieties of developmental dyslexias are analogous to alexias is not accepted universally (Baddeley, Ellis, Miles, and Lewis, 1982; Ellis, 1969 a). Nevertheless, our past investigations reveal a striking similarity between the three major forms of alexia and the subtypes of dyslexia. Even if the existence of similarities between the two forms of reading disorders is proven beyond any reasonable doubt, the neuropsychological model of reading disorders will turn out to be of limited practical value. This is so because understanding of the reading process has to go beyond establishing simple correlations between reading dysfunction and the anatomical locale of the impaired function. The precise nature of the processes which are mediated by regions of the brain that make reading possible would still remain to be elucidated. In order to develop an operational and testable hypothesis that will explain reading disability, we therefore, resorted to models of information processing. The one we selected is the traditional model, namely, the paradigm that considers information to be processed through three stages: iconic, short-term (STM), and long-term memory (LTM). The iconic stage is sometimes referred to as sensory storage and STM as working memory. The procedure adopted was to see if reading disability could be associated with processes in any one or more of these stages and further to examine if such a deficit in information processing ability could account for all the symptoms of developmental dyslexia mentioned earlier.

SUBJECTS

Five students attending college served as subjects of the reading disabled group during the entire course of the study. Out of these, four subjects (3 males and 1 female) had a substantially higher performance IQ than verbal IQ and were, therefore, considered as belonging to one subgroup of developmental dyslexia. The case of the fifth student, whom we suspect of belonging to another subgroup, is discussed at the end of the chapter. The discussion that follows is based on the performance of these four reading disabled subjects (hereafter referred to as RD group) in various tests and tasks. Another group of four college students with no reading deficits was used as a control group. The performance of all the subjects on the WAIS test and the Stanford Diagnostic Reading Test are shown in Tables 2 and 3. The tests and tasks that are described in this paper were administered in the course of nearly twenty sessions which lasted for more than six months.

EXPERIMENTAL PROCEDURES AND RESULTS
  Apparatus

Whenever exposure time was one of the experimental variables, a Gerbrands projection tachistoscope was used. The set-up involved two Kodak carousal projectors with two electronically operated shutters mounted on the projection lens. The image was projected on a rearview screen with the subject being seated about 40 centimeters away from the screen. The projected image spanned a distance of 1.25 centimeters horizantally and 3.2 centimeters vertically. One experimenter was seated on the side opposite the subject behind the screen and operated the tachistoscope. When the subject had to respond orally and the response has to be recorded, another experimenter sat beside the subject and recorded the subject's responses on specially prepared recording sheets. Before every experiment, the subject was given a few trials.

The experimental procedures and findings are discussed under three sub-headings: iconic memory, short-term memory, and long-term memory.

TABLE 2. WAIS - R Scores of Subjects

	VIQ	PIQ	FIQ	DIGIT* SPAN	BLOCK* DESIGN
R. D. Group					
C. K.	98	121	108	8	13
B. G.	100	110	103	4	10
T. M.	107	120	113	13	13
S. A.	108	120	114	13	14
$\bar{X}$	103.25	117.75	109.50	9.50	12.50
Control Group					
B. H.	105	100	103	10	9
A. C.	118	108	114	9	11
D. R.	126	125	129	14	13
P. S.	108	120	114	12	15
$\bar{X}$	114.25	113.25	115.00	11.25	12.00

* Scaled scores

ICONIC MEMORY

Experiment 1

Two experiments were designed and carried out in order to assess the span of immediate memory (channel capacity) of the subjects.
A 4 X 3 (4 rows, 3 columns) matrix of consonants typed in lower case letters was presented for a period of 200 msecs+ and the subject
was asked to report, without delay, as many consonants as he could
recall from the entire matrix. Each subject was given 10 practice
trials and was tested on 20 matrices. The second experimenter recorded the subject's responses.

+. Sperling (1960) has shown that exposure duration over a wide range was not an important parameter.

TABLE 3. Performance of Subjects on Stanford Diagnostic Reading
          Test*

	Reading rate	Vocabulary	Decoding	Comprehension
R. D. Group				
C. K.	4.7	13.0	9.3	7.8
B. G.	4.0	13.0	4.3	9.0
T. M.	5.6	13.0	11.0	6.8
S. A.	7.1	10.7	11.5	8.3
Control Group				
B. H.	13.0	13.0	13.0	13.0
A. C.	13.0	13.0	13.0	13.0
D. R.	11.7	13.0	13.0	13.0
P. S.	12.0	11.8	12.1	12.1

* Grade equivalent

Results

From the data shown in Table 4 and Figure 1, it can be seen that the performance of the RD group does not differ appreciably from
that of the control group.   Two reading disabled subjects reported
as many consonants as two control subjects did, while the other two
RD subjects reported fewer consonants than any of the control subjects.

Experiment 2

The "partial report" paradigm devised by Sperling (1960) was
adopted, with some minor modifications, for this experiment.   The
stimuli were similar to the ones used in Experiment 1.   The subject
was, however, required to report only the row that was indicated by
a probe which was visually presented in the form of an arrow[+].   The
probe appeared on the screen 100 msecs after the stimulus had disappeared.   The exposure duration of the matrix was 200 msecs and 20
matrices were presented to each subject.

[+]. The arrow was placed sufficiently away from the consonants so as
to avoid any masking effect.

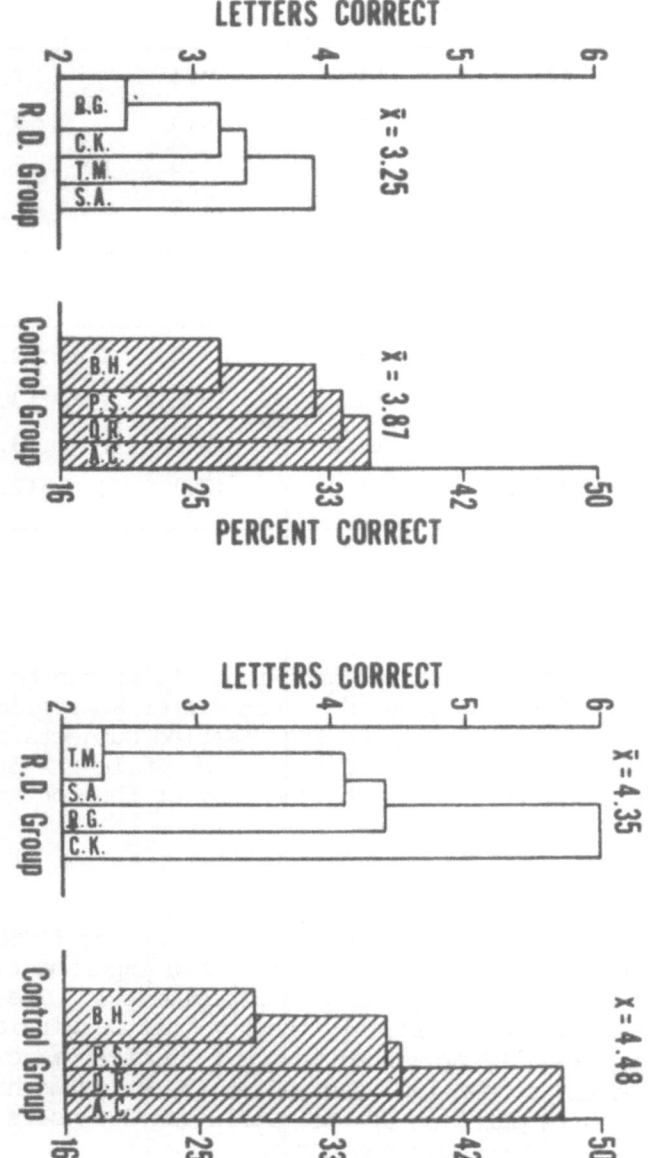

FIGURE 1. Number of consonants reported in Sperling-type tasks.
(Left graphs: Whole report; Right graphs: Partial report).

TABLE 4. Channel Capacity for Consonants in Sperling-Type Task*

	Number of consonants recalled	
	Whole report	Partial report**
R. D. Group		
C. K.	3.2	6.0
B. G.	2.5	4.4
T. M.	3.4	2.6
S. A.	3.9	4.4
$\bar{X}$	3.25	4.35
Control Group		
B. H.	3.2	3.4
A. C.	4.3	5.7
D. R.	4.1	4.4
P. S.	3.9	4.4
$\bar{X}$	3.87	4.48

* Exposure duration 200 msecs; ISI 100 msecs; no masking.

** Number of letters actually reported was multiplied by 3.

Results

The number of consonants reported by subjects from both groups is shown in Table 4 & Figure 1. The two groups did not differ from each other in any striking manner as far as the number of consonants they reported under partial report conditions. In fact, the highest number of consonants reported was by C. K. from the R. D. group. Three RD subjects had higher scores than one of the normal readers. Even though we failed to replicate Sperling's findings under "partial report" conditions, the results could be taken to indicate that the two groups did not differ from each other in their channel capacity at the initial stages of visual processing.

Experiments 3 & 4

These two experiments were designed to assess the duration for which the stimulus stayed on in the iconic store. A backward masking paradigm was used, the mask being made up of fragmented printed material. The two experiments differed in the type of stimuli used, with Experiment 3 using consonants and Experiment 4 employing photographic slides of human faces. The stimulus was presented for 50 msecs and was followed by the mask at varying ISI. The ascending method of limits was used, starting with an ISI of 10 msecs and terminating when the subject reported 5 consecutive consonants correctly. In Experiment 4, the same procedure was followed except that the subject, after every presentation, had to choose, from an array of 4 faces, the one he had seen before. This experiment, by using pictures of human faces, obviated the need for any verbalization.

Results

Table 5 shows the data obtained from Experiments 4 and 5. Data show a great deal of overlap in the performance of subjects. If any conclusion could be drawn, it is that the RD group retained stimuli at the iconic storage for a shorter duration than the control group. Further, the observation that there was a substantial degree of variation within each group suggests that iconic storage duration may not be a contributing factor to reading disability.

Experiment 5

Whether letters within a word are processed in parallel or in a serial fashion from left to right has continued to be a controversial issue in information processing psychology. Since longer words take relatively longer time to report than shorter words, Gough (1972) and Gough and Hillinger (1980) have argued that words are processed serially. Other studies, however, indicate that letters within a word are processed simultaneously, in parallel (Massaro, 1975; Sperling, 1970). It is quite possible that skilled readers use both strategies as the situation demands. Nevertheless, if good readers process verbal stimuli in one fashion and poor readers process the same stimuli in another fashion, we may suspect that processing style is a significant variable that affects the reading process. Experiment 5 was utilized to detect differences between the two groups in processing styles during the initial stages of information processing. The basic design of the experiment was similar to the one employed by Sperling in his "partial report" paradigm. An array of 5 consonants was exposed for a duration of 200 msecs. After an ISI of 100 msecs, a probe arrow pointed to one of the five consonant positions. The arrow pointed in a top down direction and, during the entire experiment, appeared randomly a total of 75 times. Thus, the consonant occupying each of the 5 positions had to be reported 15 times. The subject reported the letter he thought was in the position the arrow pointed to. The response was recorded by the second experimenter.

TABLE 5. Duration of Iconic Store for Letters and Faces*

	Letters	Faces
R. D. Group		
C. K.	80.0	40.0
B. G.	100.0	80.0
T. M.	80.0	80.0
S. A.	100.0	40.0
$\bar{X}$	90.0	60.0
Control Group		
B. H.	80.0	120.0
A. C.	160.0	80.0
D. R.	60.0	100.0
P. S.	100.0	120.0
$\bar{X}$	100.0	105.0

* Exposure duration 50 msecs; all data in msecs.

Results

    The findings are shown both in graphic (Figure 2) and numerical
formats (Table 6). Again, the variation within the groups exceeded
the variation obtained between groups. The highest number of consonants was reported by S. A. from the RD group. Inspection of Figure
2 shows that subjects in both groups tend to recall more consonants
from the initial and final positions of the array than from the in-
between positions.

Discussion

    The results of the first five experiments are summarized brief-
ly. The first two experiments which assessed the channel capacity
of the two groups show that there is not much difference between the
two groups in their ability to process verbal information at the iconic stage. The channel capacity of both groups appears to be betwe-
en 3 and 4 bits. This approximates the figure of 3.7 reported by
Pennington and Luezaz (1975) for normal college students. The

P. G. Aaron, T. Bommarito, and C. Baker

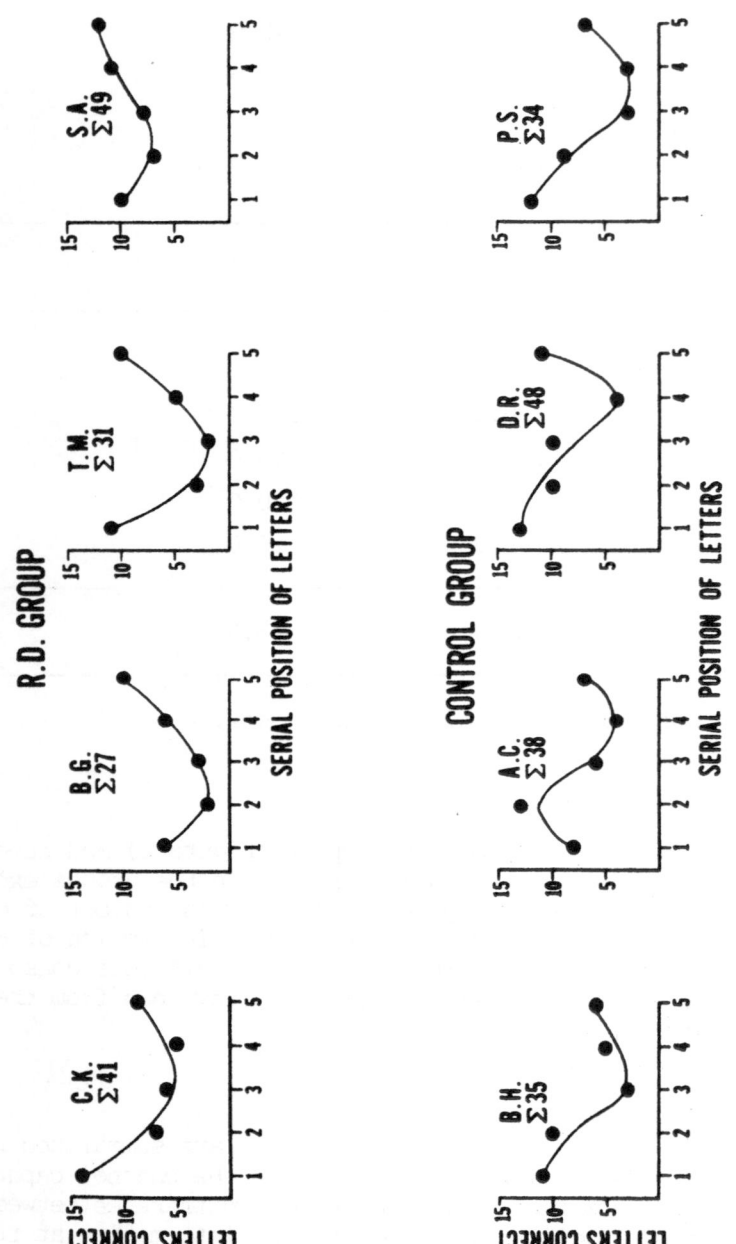

FIGURE 2. Processing style with reference to serial position of consonants.

TABLE 6. Performance of Subjects in Various STM Experiments

	No. of letters correctly reported from an array of consonants	No. of faces correctly recognized
R. D. Group		
C. K.	41	19
B. G.	27	18
T. M.	31	12
S. A.	49	27
$\bar{X}$	37.25	19.0
Control Group		
B. H.	35	16
A. C.	38	17
D. R.	48	22
P. S.	34	18
$\bar{X}$	38.75	18.25

experiments that used backward masking indicate that the speed of information processing is also very similar for these two groups. This statement applies to both verbal and nonverbal stimuli. Further, the two groups appear to be similar in their style of processing an array of consonants and probably they do so in parallel. The first experiment which measured channel capacity and the remaining four experiments which specifically assessed the iconic store capabilities show that the two groups are essentially similar to each other in their capacity to process information and the style with which such processing is accomplished at the iconic stage.

There is, therefore, insufficient evidence to implicate some factor at the iconic storage stage in dyslexia. Even though Stanley and Hall (1973) and Lovegrove and Brown (1978), using backward masking techniques and different stimuli, have reported positive findings, others have failed to find such differences between normal and

poor readers. In fact, Fisher and Frankfurter (1977), who used a backward masking letter identification and a localization task, found
reading disabled children to perform better than normal readers. This finding, is, therefore, in conflict with those of Stanley and Hall
and Lovegrove and Brown. Ellis and Miles (1981), who have reviewed
some of the studies that investigated iconic storage processing in
reading disabled children, also conclude that there is not enough evidence that a disorder at the level of iconic storage could account
for the large differences observed between dyslexic and control children in their reading abilities.

     An iconic storage deficit hypothesis of reading disability could
be rejected on rational grounds as well. It is well-documented that
dyslexic children's difficulties are limited to verbal and other abstract materials alone and not to stimuli such as objects and pictures which they encounter in their immediate everyday environment.
If this were not so, these children might see the world as a blurr-
ed streak or as a mosaic of bits and pieces depending on whether they are pathologically fast or slow in processing information at the
iconic stage. In addition, an iconic stage deficit cannot account
for output deficits such as erratic spelling and faulty linguistic
constructions commonly reported for these children.

     Previous research shows that when the stimulus material to be
reported is in the form of an array of letters, the beginning and
end letters are reported more accurately with the center letter falling in between (Averback & Coriell, 1961; Pennington & Luezaz, 1975).
Even though we failed to obtain such a W shaped curve reported by
these investigators, the overall patterns of response shown by both
groups were similar in that both groups reported more letters at both ends of the array than in any other position. Thus, we have no
strong reason to suspect processing style at the iconic stage to be
a contributing factor to reading disorder.

     In summary, the results of these five experiments provide no
substantial evidence to suspect that reading disabled subjects differ from normal readers in their sensory register capacity, processing speed, or in the strategy they use in the uptake of printed verbal material.

SHORT-TERM MEMORY

     There exists sufficient evidence to show that, at the STM sta-
ge, auditory and visual inputs are kept in temporary storage by two
independent mechanisms. Baddeley (1980) has labeled these as articulatory loop and visuo-spatial scratch pad. We will call them as
phonological and visual STM, respectively. It is generally believed
that phonological working memory operates through a process of rehearsal. The disruptive effects of Peterson-Peterson type interference tasks on verbal recall, as well as the confusions caused during

recall by words which sound alike, but do not look similar to the stimulus words provide evidence for the existence of such rehearsal.
In addition, the need on the part of the listener to maintain in temporary storage the sequence of word strings he hears from a speaker,
in order to extract meaning of a sentence mandates, the existence of
a phonological short-term memory system.

The mechanism by which visual information is retained in the
STM is much less clear, even though a number of studies show that a
visual STM does exist (Kroll, Park, Parkinson, Bieber, and Johnson,
1970; Kroll, 1975; Wickelgren, 1979). Further, studies carried out
under the Posner-Keele paradigm indicate that letters could be represented either by their names or by some kind of visual code and that
single letters could be rehearsed via visual imagery. The study by
Kroll (1975) in which shadowing was used as a distractor task found
that acoustic stimuli do not disrupt visual memory for letters. Phillips and Baddeley (1971) found that subjects could successfully identify two successively presented nonverbalizable stimuli up to 9
secs ISI. These studies suggest that the existence of a visual STM
cannot be seriously doubted.

The STM deficit theory of dyslexia has been in vogue for a number of years. Some investigators such as Jorm (1979) attribute reading deficits to an inability to keep several codes or chunks of information simultaneously in STM. Others, (Bakker & Schroots, 1981;
Doehring, 1968) have implicated an inability of STM to maintain input items (such as those in WISC digit span) in the correct order of
sequence as a major source of reading disability. It has to be recognized that short-term memory deficit, as far as reading is concerned, could occur at two locations: (a) at the point of entry where
information is coded into the STM and (b) at the retention phase where such information is kept in storage temporarily. In the former
condition, STM for input material suffers because the information
is not packaged into a rehearsable, or otherwise, retainable, form,
and in the latter condition, it is due to the incapacity of the STM
to retain, for an optimal duration, information that has already be-
en received. This distinction is one of the many aspects of STM that needs to be given important consideration. As Carr (1981) put
it, STM is a broad and malleable enough concept to potentially sub-
sume a very large and diverse collection of individual phenomena.
In the present context it, therefore, became imperative that the experiments, which investigated STM with reference to reading behavior
maintain the distinction between these two factors, namely, the encoding process of STM and the storage capacity of STM.

The next series of experiments was designed to seek answers to
the following questions:

(1) Do RD and control groups differ from each other in their
information processing abilities at the STM stage?

(2) If so, does such a deficit exist at the encoding or storage level?

(3) Does the deficit, if it exists, encompass both phonological and visual STM or is it limited to one of the two systems?

Experiment 6

A number of mini-experiments were conducted to find answers to these questions. Since all these experiments were based on essentially similar design, they are grouped together and described under Experiment 6. The Gerbrands projection tachistocope was used to present all the stimuli on a rearview screen. Two different kinds of stimuli were used: verbal and nonverbal. There were five categories of verbal stimuli: concrete nouns, function words, high frequency pronounceable non-words, low frequency pronounceable nonwords, and nonpronounceable trigrams. The nonverbal stimuli used were of two kinds: drawings of objects and transparent slides of human faces. Three kinds of responses were required of the subjects: oral, written, and recognition. The responses were made under two conditions: immediate and delayed. All the verbal materials were presented for a duration of 500 msecs and the nonverbal materials for 200 msecs. Under delayed conditions, the subject was required to wait for 2 secs and, upon seeing a signal, to respond. The 2 seconds interval was not filled with any activity.

Stimuli

Eighty trigram nouns of common objects were typed on cards and were made into projection slides. Each slide had four words arranged one below the other. Similarly, 80 three-letter function words and high frequency and low frequency pronounceable nonwords (Rumelhart, 1977) and nonpronounceable trigrams (CCC) were photographed and made into slides. Thus, there were 20 slides in each of the five categories of stimuli. Examples of each of the stimulus categories are shown in Table 7.

Procedure

Depending upon the nature of response required, the stimuli were presented at three different sessions separated by at least a week. During the first session, the subject was required to make an oral report of as many stimuli as he could recall after each slide was presented (immediate recall). During the second session, a 2 secs delay was interposed between presentations and oral reports (delayed recall). In the final session, the subject was asked to write down as many stimuli as he could remember (written response). The exposure duration was 500 msecs for all three conditions.

TABLE 7.   Sample of Stimuli Used in The Study

Concrete nouns	Function words	High Freq. pronounceable nonwords	Low freq. pronounceable nonwords	Nonpronounceable trigrams
hat	too	wil	fub	dpv
sea	for	rey	kob	kqw
car	off	lex	jeb	lrx
bed	why	ein	eph	htn

Results

Data obtained from Experiment 6 are shown in Tables 8 and 9. Figure 3 presents the data in graphic form. It can be seen that both groups recalled more concrete and function words than any other category of stimuli. ANOVA with repeated measures yielded the following results. As could be expected, the group factor was significant (F = 30.51, df = 1,6 p < .001). The main effect of words (stimuli) was also significant (F = 170.0, df = 4,24, p < .001). There was, in addition, significant interaction between Words by Response by Group (F = 2.19, df = 8,48, p < .04). The response factor by itself was not significant. Further, t test comparisons of scores obtained in the immediate and delayed response conditions showed that none of the differences was significant. Mere visual analysis of the data will confirm this conclusion (see Tables 10 and 11 and Figure 4). In fact, there is a slight increase in the number of stimuli recalled under the delayed conditions. This increase, however, could be attributed to practice effect. Written responses, which usually take longer time to execute than oral responses, were also not significantly different from immediate and delayed oral recalls (see Tables 12 and 13 and Figure 5). These analyses show that there was no decline in recall scores as a result of delay or response mode.

Further analysis of the stimuli effect with the aid of t tests showed that in immediate recall the RD and control groups differed from each other in the number of (a) function words (b) high frequency pronounceable nonwords, and (c) low frequency pronounceable nonwords recalled correctly (t = 5.01, df = 3, p < .01; t = 5.03, df = 3, p < .01; t = 3.21, df = 3, p < .05) recalled. Interestingly, the difference between the RD and control groups' recall scores of nonpronounceable trigrams was small and turned out to be statistically non-significant (t = 2.26, df = 3, p > .05). The difference between the number of concrete words reported by the two groups also turned

TABLE 8.   Mean Number of Trigrams Correct - Immediate Recall*

	Concrete words	Function words	Pronounce-able high freq. non-words	Pronounce-able low freq. non-words	Nonpronoun-able tri-grams
R. D. Group					
C. K.	2.6	2.0	0.9	0.8	1.0
B. G.	1.9	1.8	1.0	1.0	0.7
T. M.	2.1	1.8	1.8	1.1	1.0
S. A.	2.1	2.0	1.0	1.2	0.8
X̄	2.18	1.90	1.20	1.02	0.88
Control Group					
B. H.	3.2	3.3	2.1	2.1	1.1
A. C.	3.0	2.9	2.8	2.2	1.2
D. R.	3.2	3.3	2.9	2.7	1.7
P. S.	2.6	3.5	2.1	1.8	1.1
X̄	3.00	3.38	2.50	2.20	1.28

* Exposure duration 500 msecs.

Main interaction effect for Words by Group significant. F = 15.51,
p < .001
Main interaction effect for Words by Response by Group significant.
F = 2.19, p < .05

out to be small and non-significant (t = 1.79, df = 3, p > .05).
The data did not show any ceiling effects.

Discussion

We conclude from these experiments that there is no loss in recall as a result of short periods of delay. The poor performance of
RD subjects in processing pronounceable nonwords and function words
could not, therefore, be attributed to a failure to retain information

TABLE 9. Percent Total Trigrams Correct - Immediate Recall

	Concrete words	Function words	Pronounceable high freq. nonwords	Pronounceable low freq. nonwords	Nonpronounceable trigrams
R. D. Group					
C. K.	65.0	50.0	21.2	20.0	23.8
B. G.	46.5	45.5	25.0	23.8	17.5
T. M.	51.3	43.8	32.5	26.3	23.8
S. A.	51.3	48.8	25.0	30.0	20.0
$\bar{X}$	53.5	47.0	25.8	25.0	21.3
Control Group					
B. H.	78.8	81.3	52.5	51.0	27.5
A. C.	75.0	72.5	60.0	55.0	26.3
D. R.	78.8	93.8	71.3	66.3	42.5
P. S.	65.0	86.3	51.0	43.8	27.5
$\bar{X}$	74.4	83.4	58.7	54.0	30.9

Main effect for Groups significant: $F = 30.51$, $p < .001$
Main effect for Words significant : $F = 170.0$, $p < .001$

---

t test results were not significant for the following:
Oral report of concrete words, between groups: $t = 1.79$, $p > .05$
Oral report of Nonpronounceable trigrams between groups: $t = 2.26$,
$p > .05$

---

t test results were significant for the following:
Oral report of function words between groups: $t = 5.01$, $p < .01$
Oral report of high freq. pronounceable nonwords between groups:
$t = 5.03$, $p < .01$
Oral report of low freq. pronounceable nonwords between groups:
$t = 3.21$, $p < .05$

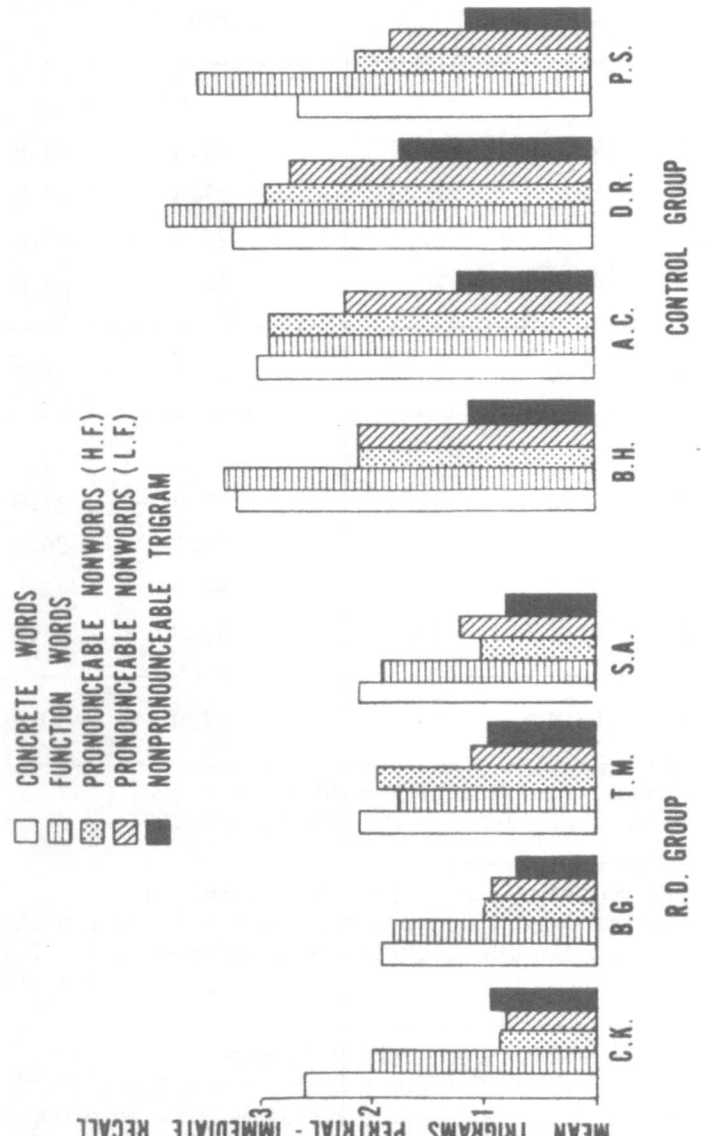

FIGURE 3. Mean number of stimuli recalled during immediate recall.

TABLE 10. Percent Words Correct - Immediate And Delayed Recall

	Concrete words		Function words	
	Imm. recall	Del. recall	Imm. recall	Del. recall
R. D. Group				
C. K.	65.0	48.7	50.0	41.3
B. G.	46.5	51.0	45.5	56.3
T. M.	51.3	55.0	43.8	58.7
S. A.	51.3	70.0	48.8	61.2
$\bar{X}$	53.5	56.2	47.0	54.4
Control Group				
B. H.	78.8	76.3	81.3	88.8
A. C.	75.0	75.0	72.5	87.5
D. R.	78.8	83.8	93.8	92.5
P. S.	65.0	53.8	86.3	68.8
$\bar{X}$	74.4	72.4	83.4	84.4

Main interaction effect for Words by Response by Group significant:
$$F = 2.19, \ p < .05$$
No t test comparison of mode of response within any group is significant.

in STM. Since the number of concrete words and nonpronounceable trigrams recalled by the RD group was almost as high as those of the control group, their STM capacity also may not be suspect. The groups, however, differed from each other in their recall of function words and pronounceable nonwords. What can we attribute this difference to? It cannot be due to familiarity alone since nonpronounceable trigrams are novel items and the groups did not differ from each other significantly in this respect. One important characteristic which is common to the three groups of words, that is, function words, high frequency pronounceable nonwords, and low frequency pronounceable nonwords is that they could be encoded only through a phonological transformational process. Thus, pronounceability emerges as an important operation that separates the two groups. Concrete words are amenable to direct visual lexical access and the groups do not differ a great deal from each other in recalling them. Where

TABLE 11.   Percent Trigrams Correct - Immediate And Delayed Recall

	Pronounceable high frequency nonwords		Pronounceable low frequency nonwords		Nonpronounceable trigrams	
	Imm. recall	Del. recall	Imm. recall	Del. recall	Imm. recall	Del. recall
R. D. Group						
C. K.	21.2	21.2	20.0	20.0	23.8	21.3
B. G.	25.0	30.0	23.8	21.3	17.5	22.5
T. M.	32.5	40.0	26.3	26.3	23.8	16.3
S. A.	25.0	35.0	30.0	32.5	20.0	25.0
$\bar{X}$	25.8	31.6	25.0	25.1	21.3	21.3
Control Group						
B. H.	52.5	67.5	51.0	60.0	27.5	43.8
A. C.	60.0	62.5	55.0	62.5	26.3	27.5
D. R.	71.3	75.0	66.3	65.0	42.5	43.8
P. S.	51.0	50.0	43.8	52.5	27.5	31.3
$\bar{X}$	58.7	63.8	54.0	60.0	30.9	36.3

Results of t test comparisons:

Control group

High freq. pronounceable nonwords vs. trigrams: $t = 6.56$, $p = < .01$
(significant)

Low freq. pronounceable nonwords vs. trigrams: $t = 6.81$, $p = < .01$
(significant)

R. D. Group

High freq. pronounceable nonwords vs. trigrams: $t = 1.37$, $p = > .05$
(not significant)

Low freq. pronounceable nonwords vs. trigrams : $t = 1.16$, $p = > .05$
(not significant)

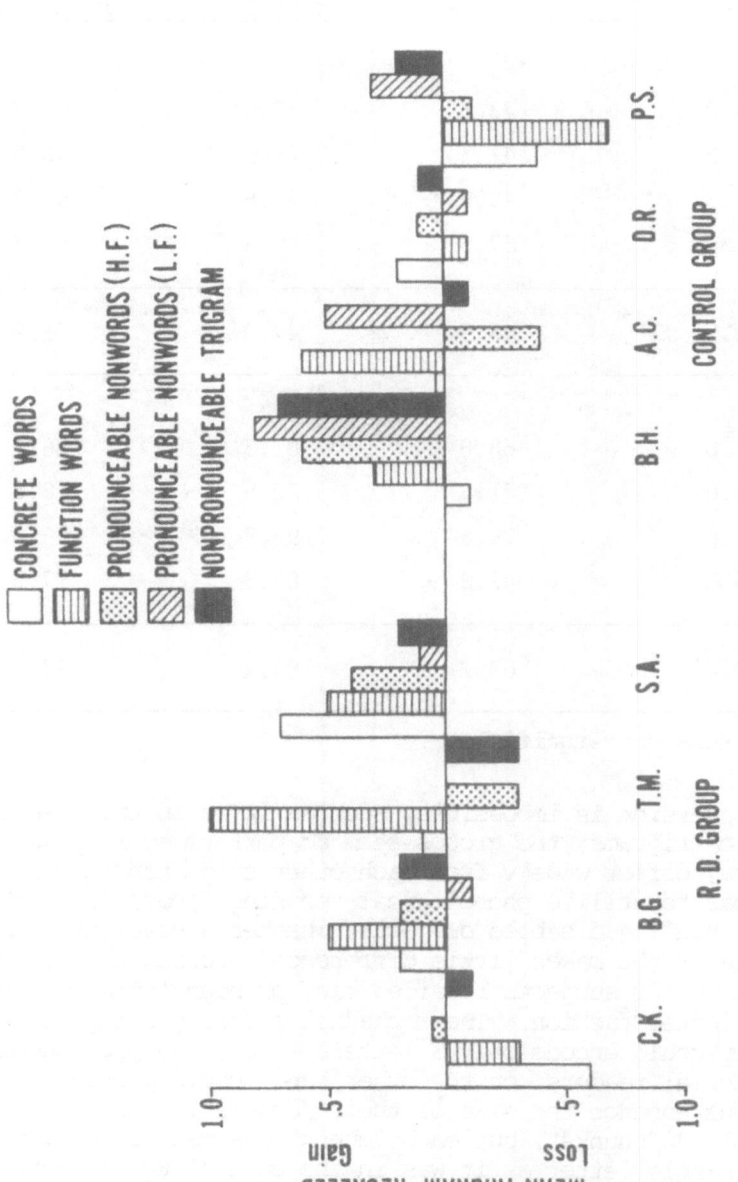

FIGURE 4. Mean number of stimuli recalled during 2 secs. delay condition shown as gain or loss with reference to immediate recall.

TABLE 12.   Percent Words Correct - Recall And Written Response

	Concrete words		Function words	
	Immediate recall	Written response	Immediate recall	Written response
R. D. Group				
C. K.	65.0	43.8	50.0	53.8
B. G.	46.5	41.3	45.5	46.3
T. M.	51.3	45.0	43.8	55.0
S. A.	51.3	57.5	48.8	52.5
$\bar{X}$	53.5	46.9	47.0	51.9
Control Group				
B. H.	78.8	68.8	81.3	86.3
A. C.	75.0	71.3	72.5	78.8
D. R.	78.8	78.8	93.8	96.3
P. S.	65.0	42.0	86.3	77.5
$\bar{X}$	74.4	65.2	83.4	84.7

t test comparisons not significant.

phonological conversion is impossible, such as it is in the case of nonpronounceable trigrams, the groups seem to perform equally well. The groups, thus, differ widely from each other only when information processing has to utilize phonological recoding. Data from Table 8 show that for reading disabled subjects, whether a novel trigram is pronounceable or not makes little difference. During the study, we noticed that the RD subjects recalled many pronounceable nonwords in a letter by letter fashion. Their channel capacity being about 3 "chunks", they could encode only 3 letters (i.e., one pronounceable nonword). Normal readers, on the other hand, could pronounce 3 nonwords and thus enhance the size of their "chunks". They, too, could encode only 3 "chunks", but each "chunk" was made up of a trigram and not a single letter as it was in the case of RD subjects. These findings suggest that the deficiency of RD subjects occurs at the point where the stimuli are encoded and not at the retention phase. Our findings are in general agreement with those reported by other investigators. For instance, Seymour and Porpodas (1979) found that when reading orthographically regular nonwords, the four

TABLE 13.   Percent Trigrams Correct - Recall And Written Response

	Pronounceable high frequency nonwords		Pronounceable low frequency nonwords		Nonpronounceable trigrams	
	Immediate recall	Written response	Immediate recall	Written response	Immediate recall	Written response
R. D. Group						
C. K.	21.2	41.3	20.0	27.5	23.8	23.7
B. G.	25.0	28.8	23.8	17.5	17.5	25.0
T. M.	32.5	37.5	26.3	32.5	23.8	23.7
S. A.	25.0	35.0	30.0	37.5	20.0	21.3
$\bar{X}$	25.8	35.7	25.0	28.8	21.3	23.4
Control Group						
B. H.	52.5	56.3	51.0	57.5	27.5	30.0
A. C.	60.0	51.3	55.0	47.5	26.3	22.5
D. R.	71.3	76.3	66.3	62.5	42.5	38.8
P. S.	51.0	53.8	43.8	45.0	27.5	28.8
$\bar{X}$	58.7	59.4	54.0	53.1	30.9	30.0

t test comparisons not significant.

dyslexic boys they had studied were found to be slower than a matched control group of normal readers. They concluded that dyslexic
children rely on a defective operation of grapheme-phoneme conversion while reading. Snowling (1980) compared the reading performance
of dyslexic children with that of normal readers by administering a
recognition memory task for pronounceable nonwords. She presented
the nonwords to either visual or auditory modality and required the
subject to recognize them immediately from the converse modality.
Snowling observed that the grapheme-phoneme correspondence skill increased with reading age and concluded that dyslexics have a specific difficulty in grapheme-phoneme conversion. Similarly, Perfetti
and Hogaboam (1975) tested vocalization latencies of skilled and less skilled readers. They found that children who were classified as
skilled readers showed only small differences among known words, unknown words, and pseudowords, whereas unskilled readers took a much
longer time to report pseudowords than known words. These authors

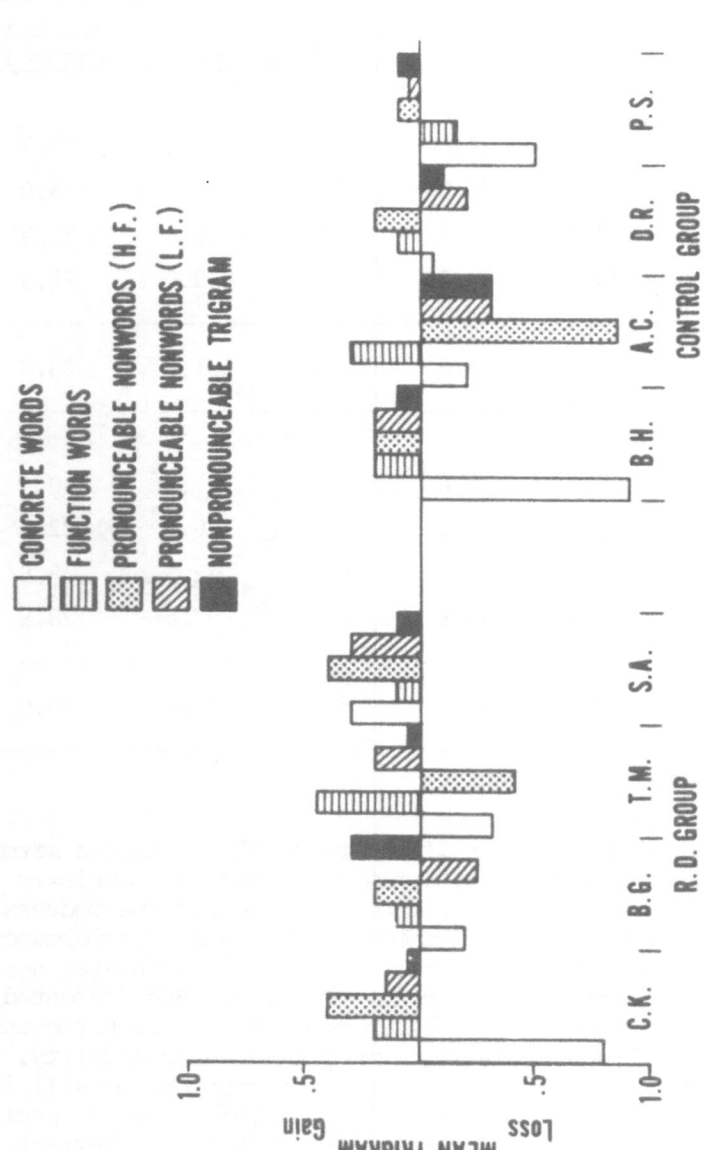

FIGURE 5. Mean number of stimuli reproduced through writing shown as gain or loss with reference to immediate oral recall.

interpreted their findings to indicate that less skilled readers may have less well-developed, less automatic, decoding skills. In addition, Katz and Wicklund (1972) have reported that good and poor readers do not differ in their processing rates for single letters but are differentially sensitive to letter patterns.

The study by Snowling found that for the dyslexics, increase in reading age was attributable mainly to an increase in sight vocabulary. Possibly, acquisition of sight vocabulary depends more on visual features of the word such as concreteness and imageability than on its phonemic features. Richardson (1975), for example, found that free recall of word lists were affected by concreteness and imageability and that these factors are independent. Jorm (1977) reports that poor readers found high imagery words easier to read than low imagery words and that good readers, in addition to imagery, were also influenced by the frequency of the word occurrence. Data presented in Tables 8 and 9 show that concreteness as well as frequency plays a role, albeit a minor one, in the recall of words. The almost "normal" number of concrete nouns recalled by RD subjects may be due to the "concreteness" factor which facilitated STM visual processing of these words. The RD subjects, in the present study, reported fewer function words than concrete words. The opposite trend is seen in the case of normal readers. It appears, then, that concreteness is an important factor on which the poor reader seems to rely. Jorm interprets the findings of his previously described study in terms of differential effect of word imagery on the strategy the readers use: phonics by good readers and whole word reading by poor readers.

If concreteness is a crutch the RD subjects depend upon, then they should be expected to do as well or better than normal readers on tasks that employ concrete nonverbal stimuli such as pictures which need not be phonologically recoded. The next experiment was designed to test this possibility.

Experiment 7

Two types of stimuli were used in this experiment: line drawings of familiar objects and photographs of human faces. For the line drawings twenty-two slides were made. Each slide had eight line drawings which were arranged in the form of a 2 x 4 matrix (2 rows and 4 columns). Each slide was exposed for 200 msecs. The subject was asked to recall as many names of objects as he could remember after presenting each slide. In order to test the possibility that oral verbalization could turn out to be an important factor, a second, nonverbal response condition was introduced. Under this condition, the subject was asked to point to the pictures of objects he had seen, in a 16 x 16 display which contained all the pictures used in the experiment.

The second class of stimuli was made up of pictures of human

faces, which under ordinary circumstances, are resistant to verbal
labeling. In this respect, the face differs from line drawings of
familiar objects. Forty-one slides, each containing 4 closely matched faces, were prepared. Pictures were chosen with care so as not
to include cues such as necktie or fancy hairstyles. Each slide was
exposed for 200 msecs, and was immediately followed by a test slide
which had one of the 4 faces the subject previously had seen. The
subject had to indicate which position the test face had occupied in
the previous display. In order to test "longer term" retention of
nonverbal stimuli, another series of 41 photographs of faces which
were mounted on an album was used. All photographs were shown con-
secutively without interruption for about 5 seconds each. After all
the 41 faces had been shown, the subject was tested on a multiple-
choice test. Each test item had an array of 4 faces one of which
was a stimulus the subject had seen before. The subject had to indicate the photograph he had seen before.

Results

The results are shown in Tables 14 and 15. The performance of
the two groups in the recall and recognition of line drawings did
not differ in any significant manner. The RD group, in fact, did
slightly better than the control group in immediate recall of names
of drawings. The depressed score obtained by both groups in picture
recognition task is partly due to the search time required to locate
the correct drawings in the 16 x 16 display. It may be noted that
the channel capacity of both groups for this nonverbal stimulus hov-
ers around the magic number 3. The two groups did equally well on
both the tests of memory for faces. In the "longer term" retention
of memory for faces, one subject from the RD group secured a perfect
score.

Experiment 8

This test was designed to assess the ability of poor readers to
perform mental rotation tasks. Such tests involve the utilization
of some dynamic process and cannot be carried out at the iconic level. The test material consisted of 24 drawings of clock faces.
Each clock face had the hour 12 written at the bottom of the face
in an inverted fashion. No other number appeared on the clock face
and hours were indicated by points. The two hands were drawn to show the time. Each clock face was shown in the inverted position for
200 msecs and the subject had to draw the hands to indicate the correct time on a test sheet which showed the numbers on a clock face
in the upright position. In a few test items, the minute hand showed the full hour, while in others it pointed to half and quarter hours.

TABLE 14. Picture Recall and Recognition Scores

| | Pictures recalled | | Pictures recalled | |
	Percent total	Mean per exposure	Percent total	Mean per exposure
R. D. Group				
C. K.	43.2	3.5	28.9	2.3
B. G.	36.4	2.9	33.5	2.7
T. M.	37.5	3.0	23.9	1.9
S. A.	32.9	2.6	25.0	2.0
$\bar{X}$	37.5	3.0	27.8	2.2
Control Group				
B. H.	35.8	2.9	29.0	2.3
A. C.	36.4	2.9	30.1	2.4
D. R.	21.0	3.1	26.1	2.1
P. S.	27.8	2.2	22.7	1.8
$\bar{X}$	30.3	2.8	27.0	2.2

Results

The results of the clock rotation task showed that the RD subjects' performance was as good as that of the normal readers. It
may be concluded that the poor readers are not deficient in "mental
rotation" operation.

Discussion

The performance of the RD group is equal to or better than that
of the control group in tasks that require no verbal transformation
of the stimuli. The drawings of objects require the association of
a verbal label, but do not require an additional transformation operation. It may be concluded that disabled readers encounter no difficulty with nonverbal stimuli such as the ones used in these experiments. In addition, the RD subjects appear to be competent in all
aspects of processing information at the visual STM level. These
include input retention and other manipulative skills such as "image"
rotation.

TABLE 15.   Performance of Subjects on Face Recognition Tasks*

	Delayed recognition after 41 consecutive presentations (exposure duration: 5 secs per face)	Immediate recognition after simultaneous presentation of 4 faces (exposure duration: 200 msecs)	Delayed recognition 2 secs after simultaneous presentation of 4 faces (exposure duration: 200 msecs)
R. D. Group			
C. K.	100.0	46.3	61.0
B. G.	73.1	43.9	39.0
T. M.	90.2	29.2	36.6
S. A.	80.3	65.9	63.4
$\bar{X}$	85.9	46.3	50.0
Control Group			
B. H.	71.0	39.0	53.7
A. C.	78.0	41.4	53.7
D. R.	75.6	53.7	63.4
P. S.	85.3	43.9	39.0
$\bar{X}$	77.5	44.5	52.4

* All scores in percent

LONG-TERM MEMORY

Miles and Ellis (1981) have described lexicon as "an internal dictionary which provides standards against which incoming stimuli can be matched" (p. 217). Coltheart (1978) has proposed that each word the reader knows is represented in this internal lexicon as a lexical entry which contains information about the word's meaning, pronounciation, and spelling. Further, he has discussed a "radical possibility" that the internal lexicon is not a unified body of knowledge concerning the meanings, spellings, and pronounciations of words and that we could, instead, distinguish between a phonological lexicon and a semantic lexicon. He, however, is not in favor of such a proposition in explaining the reading aloud of nonwords because phonological lexicon would make possible the pronounciation of all known words but no nonwords since such neologisms do not have lexical entries. It is quite possible, however, that alternate strategies might be used to pronounce nonwords. Pronouncing by analogy may be one such strategy. Besides, a phonological lexicon may be viewed as containing rules for pronounciation of words rather than pronounciation of each word itself. Thus, in this section, when reference is made to a phonological lexicon, it implies a rule-based lexicon. Cases of deep dyslexics (Marshall & Newcombe, 1973), developmental dyslexic subjects who can understand the meaning of a word but come up with a different pronounciation, as well as hyperlexic children who can pronounce words but do not comprehend their meaning (Healy, 1982), suggest that phonemic and semantic aspects of morphemes are not bound together and can be affected independently.

Some writers have suggested that reading disability is due to either an impoverished lexicon or deficiency in lexical encoding strategies (Ellis & Miles, 1981). These two concepts, that is, the content of the lexicon and the encoding process which accesses the lexicon, however, are two independent variables.

Experiments 1 and 2 have shown that there is no substantial difference between the RD and control groups in the number of consonants named. It has, therefore, to be concluded that the difficulty encountered by RD subjects does not reside in accessing the name code for individual consonants, which do not have meaning by themselves. The reading deficit, however, could involve the semantic lexicon which contains meanings for words. This possibility is discussed in the next section.

Procedure and Results

Estimates of the size of the putative semantic lexicon were obtained by extracting data from language and reading tests. It is assumed that the size of the subject's vocabulary would provide a crude measure of the size of his semantic lexicon. The vocabulary scores obtained by subjects on the Test of Adolescent Language and on the Stanford Diagnostic Reading Test are shown in Table 16.

If vocabulary size is taken as a measure of the size of semantic lexicon, then all the subjects in the RD group fall within the average range. Additional support for this conclusion could be derived form the findings of Experiment 6 which showed that reading disabled subjects are able to encode and recall almost as many concrete words as normal readers do. This indicates that RD subjects can access the semantic lexicon almost as efficiently as normal readers do provided the words have a rich semantic loading. Since function words do not have much of a semantic loading, they cannot be accessed in the same way as concrete words. The statement that

P. G. Aaron, T. Bommarito, and C. Baker

TABLE 16. Vocabulary Size of Subjects

	Test of Adolescent Language*		Stanford Diag. Reading Test**
	Listening vocabulary	Reading vocabulary	Reading vocabulary
R. D. Group			
C. K.	11	11	13.0
B. G.	14	8	13.0
T. M.	8	7	13.0
S. A.	8	11	10.7
X̄	10.25	9.25	12.4
Control Group			
B. H.	13	13	13.0
A. C.	11	10	13.0
D. R.	12	12	13.0
P. S.	8	12	11.8
X̄	11.0	11.75	12.5

* Scaled Scores, maximum possible, 20.
** Grade Equivalents

dyslexic individuals have deficiency at the lexical level, therefore, needs to be modified. It appears that reading disabled individuals, at least the ones described in this paper, do not have an impoverished semantic lexicon.

Discussion

    Ellis and Miles (1981), after reviewing some of the related experiments, conclude that "in the case of dyslexic subjects.....the linguistic deficiency is not one of articulatory encoding but is rather at the 'lexical level'; that is, it affects those functions which involve access to the lexicon and the retrieval of appropriate lexical codes" (p. 191). Data from the present study support the latter part of the statement but not the former. In fact, the present series of studies shows that reading disabled individuals are deficient in the strategies that are used in accessing the lexicon and not in the semantic lexicon itself. Even this deficit is actually a carry-over from the STM entry point. The studies by Snowling (1980) and by Perfetti and Hogaboam (1975) show that dyslexic children do have phonetic encoding difficulties. In support of their position that encoding is relatively unimportant, Ellis and Miles cite their own study in which dyslexic children were found not to be affected as much by articulation suppression as normal readers were. These findings are in conflict with those of a study reported by Lieberman et al. (1980) who found that normal readers were more affected by phonological confusion than dyslexic children were.

The proposition that RD subjects have deficits in phonological encoding ability is clearly evident in the experiments which used pronounceable nonwords as stimuli. Since these stimuli cannot be retrieved "directly" by accessing the semantic lexicon, their processing depends on the application of the grapheme phoneme correspondence (GPC) rules or syllabic segmentation or phonetic parsing. This is so because nonwords have no entries in the semantic lexicon. This is likely to be true in the case of function words as well since they do not possess meaning by themselves. This view is borne out by studies of aphasic patients which indicate "the existence of a syntactic mechanism that is independent of lexically based heuristic strategies for assigning meaning and that focal brain damage can cause selective disruption of these two components" (Caramazza & Berndt, 1978, p. 898). The difficulty encountered by Broca's aphasics and deep dyslexic patients in the usage of function words indicates that the syntactic lexical system is different from the semantic lexical system.

Coltheart (1978), after reviewing a number of studies, has concluded that, for the printed word, two routes of entries are available to the internal lexicon; the "direct route" which uses a visual representation of the word, and the "indirect route" which uses a phonological representation of the word. The present experimental findings suggest that phonological conversion seems to be the only method available for encoding verbal stimuli which is devoid of semantic content. Since the RD subjects show adequate encoding ability for concrete words that have semantic lexical entries and relatively poor skill in the encoding of function and nonwords, it can be concluded that, in these subjects, it is not the semantic lexicon per se, but the phonological encoding strategy that is deficient.

READING ERROR ANALYSIS

Analyzing the nature of errors committed by the disabled reader during the process of reading connected prose is an ecologically valid method which provides some insight into the nature of the underlying operations that are responsible for generating such errors.

Our experience with dyslexic subjects shows that the reading errors they commit fall into characteristic patterns and differ from the errors produced by nondyslexic reading retarded subjects. Consequently, reading error analysis is a useful tool in differential diagnosis.

Procedure

Subjects were asked to read aloud three passages from the Stanford Diagnostic Reading Test and this was audio-taped. The tapes were later played back, transcribed, and analyzed for errors.

Results

The Four RD subjects committed a large number of reading errors, even though the subjects' errors differed from each other quantitatively but not qualitatively. Subjects in the control group committed few or no errors. Analysis of errors committed by the RD group showed that these subjects tended to omit, substitute, or add many function words. Their errors involved more function words than content words. When content words were misread, the errors were primarily due to misapplication of the GPC rules. Misreading of many content words revealed that all three types of paralexic errors, that is, visual (origin -> organ), derivational (courage -> courageous), and semantic (dream -> sleep) (Patterson & Marcel, 1977), were committed by these subjects. Semantic paralexic errors, however, were not as numerous as the other two types of errors.* Only two RD subjects committed such errors (C. K.: adults -> people; B. G.: London -> England). In spite of their small number, these errors assume significance since they are committed by mature, healthy individuals. The reading of these RD subjects, however, contained few neologisms. Such errors were committed by R. R. whose case is discussed briefly at the end of the section and whom we consider to belong to a different subgroup of dyslexia.

A typical sample of misreading by the RD subject is shown in Table 17. One cannot fail to appreciate the similarity between the reading errors committed by these subjects and the ones committed by the deep dyslexic patients described by Marshall and Newcombe (1973).

---

* Once in a rare while semantic paralexic errors occur in spelling as well (e. g., relief -> Rolaid).

TABLE 17. Errors Committed by B. G. and T. M. in Oral Reading

---

Text: As a one way city, London is practically impenetrable.
B. G.: As a one way city England is particularly impenetrable.

Text: for the stranger.
B. G.: for the stranger.

Text: Ways, mews   streets and places run
B. G.: ways (I don't know) streets and places run

Text: at weird angles, and squares go clockwise,
B. G.: at wide angles, and square goes clockwise,

Text: with seemingly no visible way out.
B. G.: with seemingly no visible way out.

Text: Places run at weird angles............
T. M.: Places run as weird angles............

Text: With the one way streets done in four colors........
T. M.: With _____ one way streets done in four colors.....

Text: For quick reference...........
T. M.: For quick references..........

Text: The east border is green.......
T. M.: _____east border is green......

Text: According to the publisher's managing director.........
T. M.: According to the publisher_ managing director......

Text: It is available in book stores and in airports.
T. M.: It is available in book stores and _____ airports.

GENERAL DISCUSSION AND CONCLUSIONS

It might be appropriate at this point to summarize the major findings of the series of experiments.

1. Difficulties are encountered by RD subjects when phonological recoding is the major operation to be used for processing printed verbal material.
2. The two groups do not differ from each other in their STM capacity as judged by the subjects' ability to recall consonants, non-pronounceable nonwords, and names of drawings of objects. These

observations indicate that the dyslexics do not have a capacity deficit at the STM stage.
3. In processing stimuli that are not amenable to phonological encoding, RD and control subjects do not differ from each other.
4. The information process deficit appears to be limited to phonological recoding ability and seems to spare visual encoding as well as
visual image manipulation abilities.
5. Information that is recoded is not lost during short intervals.
6. Concrete words that have a high level of semantic content are processed by RD subjects almost as well as by normal readers. Stimuli
with little or no semantic content such as function words and pronounceable nonwords, are inefficiently processed by RD subjects. Normal readers are affected in neither the same fashion nor to the same
extent by this semantic content factor.
7. The processing difficulty is limited to pronounceable stimuli
and not necessarily to "nameable" stimuli. It appears then, that
the deficit is limited to a transformation process which involves coding and does not include the associative process.

A number of studies indicate that visual and phonological encoding strategies are the two major processes involved in the reading
process. Byrne and Shea [1979] who used a task in which good and po-
or readers were asked to indicate whether a word in a continuous list
of items had occurred before, found that good readers encoded both
semantic and surface phonological aspects of words whereas poor readers were relatively insensitive to the surface features of language.
Considering the importance of their roles in reading, these two processes, visual coding and phonological coding, merit further discussion.

Visual coding and reading

Visual coding involves the conversion of a sequence of letters
into a single semantic unit which enables the direct accessing of
meaning. The independence of visual coding from phonological coding
is demonstrated by studies that have introduced modality-specific
interference in verbal learning tasks. (Murray & Newman, 1973; Salzberg et al., 1971). The fact that scripts such as Chinese which are
written in the ideographic form could be read and understood illustrates that reading could be accomplished with the aid of visual coding alone without recourse to a phonological conversion of the script. The visual code, however, has its own liabilities. It appears to utilize an analog process (Paivio, 1975), which could explain
why semantic accessing of the lexicon is faster than phonological
accessing of the lexicon which uses a sequential process. Conversely, the visual imagery, being spatial and simultaneous in nature,
may not be suitable for the processing sequentially, stimuli such as
multi-syllabic abstract words. In addition to this, the visual code
is also less suitable for the processing of verbal stimuli such as
function words and CVC trigrams, which have little or no semantic

content. In a language such as English where order of words acts as syntactic marker, the phonological code assumes much importance. The direct accessing of the semantic content by the visual process may also put an undue amount of burden on the memory system and this may be one of the reasons why the ideographic script is considered as a major impediment for the attainment of full literacy in China. Utilizing the visual code for processing the printed word when it is not efficient to do so, therefore, results in impaired reading comprehension and causes typical reading errors.

The number of human faces and drawings of figures processed by RD subjects falls between 2 and 3 units and they do not differ from control subjects in this respect. The few semantic paralexic errors committed by two RD subjects while reading as well as their phonetic misspellings suggest that RD subjects do use visual coding mechanism for reading. In fact, it is quite possible that they are overly dependent upon this strategy for reading.

Phonological Coding and Reading

There is substantial amount of evidence to show that reading involves phonological recoding of the print (Baddeley, 1966; Barron, 1980; Conrad, 1964; Kleiman, 1975). It appears that under certain conditions, phonemic recoding appears to be a more efficient strategy for the processing of the printed word than visual coding. These conditions may involve circumstances where input has to be maintained over a period of time, where order of items in STM is important for comprehension, and where input is not readily amenable to visual coding (Allport, 1979; Baddeley, 1979). Neuropsychological observations also support such a contention. For example, Martin and Caramazza (1982), who investigated an aphasic patient with deficit in phonological coding ability, conclude that "if the order of the words which must be retained is important and if these words include function words.......then phonemic memory code would be more advantageous than a visual code" (p. 67). It may be inferred that failure to utilize phonological coding when it is advantageous to do so could result in syntactical and spelling errors as well as misreading of function words. Thus, the syntactical errors found in the writing of the RD subjects, the spelling errors, and the misreading of function words, could all be attributed to a deficiency in phonemic recoding. It appears that the same processes that underlie the spelling of a word also are responsible for the production of a sentence. In this sense, a word is a miniature sentence or, conversely, a sentence is an expanded version of a word. This statement, of course, is limited to the alphabetical script. The correct spelling of a word depends on the correct sequential placement of the letters that make up the word; the correct production of a sentence also depends upon the accurate syntactical ordering of words within the sentence. Certain letters in a word bear more phonetic marking than others (e.g., vowel vs. consonant) and certain words in a sentence bear more syntactic marking than others (e.g., function vs. content words). It is quite possible, therefore, that any process (or lack of it) which is responsible for the production of spelling errors is also responsible for the production of syntactic errors. If we identify this process as phonological coding, then we can explain spelling errors and written syntactic errors at the sentence level as well as oral reading errors all at once. Ellis (1979 b) has suggested that there is an equivalence between auditory-verbal STM and the response buffer used for preplanning sequences of speech, and that both may depend on phonemic codes for their respective operations as well as for retaining order information. Furthermore, semantic and syntactic aspects of a sentence may be processed separately. This has been demonstrated by Mehler (1963) who, using a prompted method of recall of sentences, found that subjects analyze sentences into a kernel or semantic component plus the syntactic transformation. Since phonological coding also plays an important role in the maintenance of the order of input stimuli, as well as retention of them through rehearsal, we can expect reading comprehension defects to accompany phonological coding deficits as well.

Phonological coding as an information reducing strategy

Why does phonological coding turn out to be so important in cognitive tasks such as reading and language usage? Phonological coding appears to be the most effective strategy for reducing information and thus, keeping the cognitive load within bounds. This, in turn, enhances the efficiency of STM. As mentioned earlier, specific reading disability appears not to be an STM capacity limitation but a process limitation. Daneman and Carpenter (1980) who tested their subjects under conditions of heavy demands of information storage and processing arrived at a similar conclusion. Subjects in this study read aloud a series of sentences and then recalled the final word of each sentence. The reading span, or the number of final words recalled, correlated quite highly with comprehension measures. Results led the authors to conclude that individual differences in reading comprehension may reflect differences in working memory. According to these investigators, the good reader's chunks should be richer and he might capitalize on his chunking efficiency in the comprehension and working memory span tasks.

In cognitive psychology concepts such as coding and chunking are used to describe processes wherein information is reorganized into a condensed format.* Such a reduction in information may be

---

* This is not to deny the role played by factors such as word length (Baddeley, 1975), even though in the present context, monosyllabic words of similar length were used.

accomplished with the aid of both visual and phonological processes. The possibility that visual encoding is used as an information reducing strategy is documented by a number of studies. Egan and Schwartz (1979) who explored memory for symbolic circuit drawings using skilled and unskilled electronics technicians found that the former recalled more information than the latter and that organization of functional concepts into chunks contributed to such a difference. Similar chunking has been reported for the remembering of chess positions by chess masters (Chase and Simon, 1973). Visual chunking, however, may have its own limitations, chief among them being that the material to be organized has to be concrete and rich in semantic loading.

Phonological chunking was recognized even during the early days when the concept was introduced . Miller (1956) observed that phonemes could be considered as bits and words as chunks. It is also believed that the capacity of STM measured in terms of chunks is independent of the material of which those chunks are made (Simon, 1974). Our experimental findings support this assertion since it was found that both RD and control subjects had an STM capacity in the range of 3 to 4 chunks regardless of whether the chunks were consonants, syllables, or drawings of objects. This figure is in agreement with evidence provided by Johnson (1972), which indicates that the optimum chunk size is about 3. The only way to increase the STM capacity is to build larger and larger chunks by increasing the number of bits each chunk can hold. In the reading process, visual modality seems to be adapted to conceptual or semantic chunking (as in remembering positions of chess pieces). Such a chunking is basically associative in nature. The phonological STM, however, seems to be capable of transformational chunking by converting bits of syllables, graphemic units or vocalic centre groups, into phonological chunks. The RD subjects do not seem to be in possession of a strategy to accomplish this transformational organization. Put another way, they do not have a code to effect this transformation.

A code could be viewed as a rule or algorithm that is stored in memory and is used both for transforming the input information and for elaborating the out-put information. Unlike the associational visual chunking strategy where individual associations have to be learned anew, the phonological code could be used again and again in a recurrent fashion in different contexts. The phonological chunking which is code based, therefore, turns out to be an efficient information reducing device.

Whether the phonological code operates through the application of GPC rules, segmentation of words into syllables, or the VCG parsing of the word is uncertain, Coltheart (1978), who has discussed this issue, is in favor of the phonological unit that permits GPC conversion, whereas Rozin and Gleitman (1977) argue that the syllable is the basic unit of the phonetic processing. Liberman et al.

(1977) found that knowledge of syllabication units was better developed in children than knowledge of phonetic parsing units. It is
possible that all these codes are used by the skilled reader as the
occassion demands.

In addition to information reduction, phonological chunking appears to preserve order information as well. Johnson (1972), for
example, states that "if subjects encounter a task in which they are
required to learn the pattern of encoding for a sequence, but are
not required to learn the items or their order, the item and order
information would be learned as completely and as efficiently as if
the task required such learning" (p. 156). According to this view,
sequential order information is an integral part of phonological chunking and the two are welded together. Subjects deficient in phonetic chunking will, therefore, be deficient in retaining sequence
information as well. It should be noted that sequential ordering
skill is a prerequisite to spelling correctly as well as for producing syntactically acceptable sentences.

Finally, Posner and Warren (1972), on the basis of their studies, conclude that successive codes can be laid down and maintained
in parallel. One code does not replace another, but they remain and
compete for the limited rehearsal capacity of the subject. Coltheart (1978) expresses a similar view in somewhat different language.
According to him, reading is sometimes visual and sometimes phonological and may vary from person to person and from occasion to occasion. It may be added that since certain stimuli such as function
words and "unknown" words are not easily amenable to semantic or visual coding, the phonological coding is essential for processing these stimuli. We would, therefore, state that reading of a sentence
is simultaneously visual and phonological and that not being able
to use one or the other can impede the reading process. The existence of such parallel processes has been recognized by other researchers (e.g., Allport, 1977), even though whether the processes are
competitive or cooperative with each other is not clear yet.

Information reduction and other subtypes of dyslexia

The attention of this paper was focused on one subtype of dyslexia which is characterized by a deficiency in phonological coding.
Our experience shows that subjects falling into this category are
far more numerous than subjects belonging to the other subtypes.
Theoretically, it is possible that two other subtypes, namely, subjects who are deficient in visual semantic coding ability and subjects who have an impoverished semantic lexicon, could also exist.
The fifth RD subject mentioned in the beginning of the section seems
to be deficient in visual coding skill. Some pertinent data regarding this subject are shown in Table 18.

As can be seen she exhibited poor visual memory for nonverbali-

TABLE 18. Performance of R. R. on Some Selected Tests

VIQ	PIQ	FIQ	Digit Span	Memory for faces	Memory for consonants	Memory* for pictures	Verbal Stimuli (immed. recall)**			
							Concrete words	Function words	Non-words	Tri-grams
90	85	90	10	2 S. D. below mean	3.2	2.4	49	56	34	16

* Maximum possible = 8

**Maximum possible = 80

zable stimuli. She recalled more function words than the 4 RD subjects described earlier. The reading errors she committed while reading continuous text showed that such errors did not involve function words but rather centered around "unknown" words, suggesting that she has very poor sight vocabulary. She did plod through unknown
words phoneme by phoneme, thus, putting a great deal of load on her
memory which reduced her comprehension to about the level of 7th grade. Her oral reading contained numerous neologisms.

Summary

     A failure to reduce input information effectively increases the
load STM has to carry which, in turn, affects its efficiency. One
way to reduce printed verbal information is to use phonological recoding strategy. This requires the utilization of a code which may
chunk individual letters in a word by applying GPC rules or syllabic
segmentation of the word or by parsing vocalic center groups. Such
a code works as a "gate keeper" in the sense that it organizes the
input information into chunks and elaborates the outgoing information into bits. Inability to use the code, therefore, will adversely
affect receptive skills such as reading comprehension, and expressive skills such as spelling and oral reading. Further, sequential
order information appears to be an integral component of phonological recoding. Consequently, when phonological recoding is defective, verbal material (such as syntax and spelling), which is critically dependent upon correct ordering of elements suffers. While the
phonological code can handle semantically empty words, visual encoding can mediate only semantically rich stimuli. It can, however,
perform this encoding at a faster rate than the speed with which
phonological encoding is accomplished. Skilled reading requires
the deployment of both codes more or less simultaneously. Inability
to do so results in dyslexic syndrome. The information reduction
explanation of developmental dyslexia could, therefore, account for
all the symptoms encountered within the dyslexia syndrome.

REFERENCES

Aaron, P. G., Baxter, C. F., & Lucenti, J. Developmental dyslexia
     and acquired alexia: Two sides of the same coin? Brain and
     Language, 1980, 11, 1-11.
Aaron, P. G., Baker, C., & Hickox, G. In search of the third dysle-
     xia. Neuropsychologia, 1982, 20, (2), 203-208.
Aaron, P. G., & Baker, C. The neuropsychology of dyslexia in colle-
     ge students. In R. N. Malatesha and L. C. Hartlage (Eds.),
     Neuropsychology and Cognition (Vol. 1). Martinus Nijhoff,
     The Hague, 1982.
Averbach. E., & Coriell, A. S. Short-term memory in vision. Bell
     System Technical Journal, 1961, 40, 309-328.

Allport, D. A. On knowing the meaning of words we are unable to report: the effects of visual masking. In S. Dornic (Ed.) Attention and Performance VI. Hillsdale, N. J. Lawrance Erlbaum, 1977.

Allport, D. A. Word recognition in reading. In P. A. Kolers, M. G. Wrolstad, & H. Bouma (Eds.). Processing of Visible Language, N. Y. Plenum, 1979.

Baddeley, A. D. Short-term memory for word sequences as a function of acoustic, semantic and formal similarity. Quarterly Journal of Experimental Psychology, 1966, 18, 362-365.

Baddeley, A. D., Thomson, N., & Buchanan, M. Word length and the structure of short term memory. Journal of Verbal Learning and Verbal Memory, 1975, 14, 575-589.

Baddeley, A. D. Working memory and reading. In P. A. Kolers, M. E. Wrolstad, & H. Bouma (Eds.). Processing of Visible Language, N. Y. Plenum, 1979.

Baddeley, A. D. The concept of working memory: A view of its current state and probable future development. Cognition, 1981, 10, 17-23.

Baddeley, A. D., Ellis, N. C., Miles, T. R., & Lewis, V. J. Developmental and acquired dyslexia: A comparison. Cognition, 1982, 11, 185-199.

Bakker, D. J. & Schroots, H. J. Temporal order in normal and disturbed reading. In D. T. Pavlidis, & T. R. Miles (Eds). Dyslexia Research and its applications to education. N. Y. John Wiley, 1981.

Barron, R. W. Visual and phonological strategies in reading and spelling. In U. Frith (Ed). Cognitive Processes in Spelling, N. Y.: Academic Press, 1980.

Boder, E., & Jarrico, S. The Boder Test of Reading-Spelling Patterns. New York: Grune & Stratton, 1982.

Byrne, B., & Shea, P. Semantic and phonetic memory codes in beginning readers. Memory and Cognition, 1979, 7, (5), 333-338.

Caramazza, A., & Berndt, R. S. Semantic and Syntactic processes in aphasia: A review of the literature. Psychological Bulletin, 1978, 85, 898-918.

Carr, T. H. Building theories of reading ability: on the relation between individual differences in cognitive skills and reading comprehension. Cognition, 1981, 9, 73-114.

Chase, W. G., & Simon, H. A. Perception in chess. Cognitive Psychology, 1973, 4, 55-81.

Coltheart, M. Lexical access in simple reading tasks. In G. Underwood (Ed). Strategies of Information Processing, N. Y.: Academic Press, 1978.

Conrad, R. Acoustic confusion in immediate memory. British Journal of Psychology, 1964, 55, 75-84.

Daneman, M., & Carpenter, P. A. Individual differences in working memory and reading. Journal of Verbal Learning and Verbal Behavior, 1980, 19, 450-466.

Doehring, D. Patterns of Impairment in Specific Reading Disability.
    Bloomington, Indiana University Press, 1968.
Egan, D. E., & Schwartz, B. J. Chunking and recall of symbolic draw-
    ings. Memory and Cognition, 1979, 7, (2), 149-158.
Ellis, A. W. Developmental and acquired dyslexia: Some observations
    on Jorm. Cognition, 1979, 7, 413-420 (a).
Ellis, A. W. Speech production and short term memory. In J. Norton
    & J. C. Marshall (Eds.). Psycholinguistic Series, Vol. 2: Stru-
    cture and Processes. Cambridge, MA: MIT Press, 1979 (b).
Ellis, N. C., & Miles, T. R. A lexical encoding deficiency: Experi-
    mental evidence. In G. T. Pavlidis & T. R. Miles (Eds.).
    Dyslexia Research and its Application to Education. N. Y. John
    Wiley & Sons, 1981.
Fisher, P. F., & Frankfurter, A. Normal and disabled readers can
    locate and identify letters: Where's the perceptual deficit?
    Journal of Reading Behavior, 1977, 9, 31-43.
Fry, M. A., Johnson, C. S., & Muehl, S. Oral language production in
    relation to reading achievement among select second graders.
    In D. J. Bakker & P. Satz (eds.). Specific Reading Disability:
    Advances in Theory and Method, Rotterdam: Rotterdam University
    Press, 1970.
Gough, P. B. One second reading. In J. F. Kavanah & I. G. Matting-
    ly (Eds.). Language by Ear and by Eye, Cambridge, Mass.: MIT
    Press, 1972.
Gough, B. P., & Hillinger, L. M. Learning to read: an unnatural act.
    Bulletin of the Orton Society, 1980, 179-196.
Healy, J. M. The enigma of hyperlexia. Reading Research Quarterly,
    1982, 17, (3), 319-338.
Johnson, N. F. Organization and the concept of a memory code. In
    A. W. Melton & E. Martin (Eds.). Coding Processes in Human
    Memory, Washington D. C., V. H. Winston & Sons., 1972.
Jorm, A. F. Effect of word imagery on reading performance as a fun-
    ction of reader ability. Journal of Educational Psychology,
    1977, 69, 1, 46-54.
Jorm, A. F. The cognitive and neurological basis of developmental
    dyslexia: A theoretical framework and review. Cognition, 1979,
    7, 19-34.
Katz, L., & Wickland, D. A. Letter scanning rate for good and poor
    readers in grades two and six. Journal of Educational Psycho-
    logy, 1972, 63, 363-367.
Kleiman, G. M. Speech recoding in reading. Journal of Verbal lear-
    ning and Verbal Behavior, 1975, 14, 323-330
Kroll, N. E., Parks, T., Parkinson, S., Bieber, S. L., & Johnson,
    A. L. Short-term memory while shadowing: recall of visually
    and of aurally presented letters. Journal of Experimental Psy-
    chology, 1970, 85, 220-224.
Kroll, N. E. Visual short-term memory. In D. Deutsch & J. A. Deut-
    sch (Eds.). Short Term Memory. N. Y.: Academic Press, 1975.
Lee, L. Northwestern Syntax Screening Test. Evanston, IL: North-
    western University Press, 1969.

Loban, W. The language of elementary school children. NCTE Research Report No. 1; Urbana, IL. National Council of Teachers of
English, 1963.

Lovegrave, W., & Brown, C. Development of information processing in
normal and disabled readers. Perceptual and Motor Skills, 1978,
46, 1047-1054.

Liberman, I. Y., Liberman, A. M., Mattingly, I. Y., & Shankweiler,
D. Orthography and the beginning reader. In J. F. Kavanaugh
& R. L. Vanezky (Eds.). Orthography, Reading and Dyslexia,
Baltimore, MD: University Park Press, 1980.

Liberman, I. Y., Shankweiler, D., Liberman, A. M., Fowler, C., &
Fischer, F. W. Phonetic segmentation and recoding in the beginning reader. In A. S. Reber & D. L. Scarborough (Eds.).
Toward a Psychology of Reading. Hillsdale, NJ: Lawrence Erlbaum Associates, 1977.

Marshall, J. C., & Newcombe, F. Patterns of paralexia: a psycholinguistic approach. Journal of Psycholinguistic Research, 1973,
175-199.

Martin, R. C., & Caramazza, A. Short-term memory performance in the
absence of phonological coding. Brain and Cognition, 1982, 1,
50-70.

Massaro, D. W. Primary and secondary recognition in reading. In
D. W. Massaro (Ed). Understanding Language, New York: Academic
Press, 1975.

Mehler, J. Some effects of grammatical transformations on the recall of English sentences. Journal of Verbal Learning and Verbal
Behavior, 1963, 2, 346-351.

Miller, G. A. The magical number seven, plus or minus two: Some limits on our capacity for processing information. Psychological
Review, 1956, 63, 81-97.

Miles, T. R., & Ellis, N. C. A Lexical encoding deficiency: clini-
cal observations. In G. T. Pavlidis & T. R. Miles (Eds.).
Dyslexia Research: Its Application to Education. New York:
John Wiley & Sons, 1981.

Murray, D. J., & Newman, F. M. Visual and Verbal Coding in Short-
term Memory. Journal of Experimental Psychology, 1973, 100,
58-62.

Nelson, H. E. Analysis of Spelling errors in normal and dyslexic
children. In U. Frith (Ed). Cognitive Processes in Spelling.
New York: Academic Press, 1980.

Paivio, A. Imagery and Long-term memory. In A. Kennedy & A. Wilk-
es (Eds.). Long Term Memory, New York: John Wiley & Sons, 1975.

Patterson, K. E., & Marcel, A. J. Aphasia, dyslexia, and the phonological coding of written words. Quarterly Journal of Experimental Psychology, 1977, 29, 307-318.

Pennington, F. M., & Luezaz, M. A. Some functional properties of
iconic storage in retarded and nonretarded subjects. Memory
and Cognition, 1975, 3, 295-301.

Perfetti, C. A., & Hogaboam, T. Relationship between single word
decoding and reading comprehension skill. Journal of Educatio-

nal Psychology, 1975, 67, 461-469.

Phillips, W. A., & Baddeley, A. D.   Reaction time and short term visual memory. Psychonomic Science, 1971, 22, 73-74.

Posner, M. I., Boies, S. J., Eichelman, W. H., & Taylor, R. L. Retention of Visual and name codes of single letters. Journal of Experimental Psychology, 1969, 79, 1-16.

Posner, M. I., & Warren, R. E.   Traces, concepts, and conscious con- structions. In A. W. Melton & E. Martin (Eds.). Coding Proce- ss in Human Memory. Washington, D. C.: Winston & Sons, 1972.

Richardson, J. E.   Imagery, concreteness, and lexical complexity. Quarterly Journal of Experimental Psychology, 1975, 27, 211-223.

Rumelhart, D. E.   Toward an interactive model of reading. In S. Dor- nic (Ed.). Attention and Performance VI, Hillsdale, NJ: Law- rance Erlbaum Associates, 1977.

Salzberg, P. M., Parks, T. E., Kroll, N. E., & Parkinson, S. R. Retroactive effects of phonemic similarity on short-term recall of visual and auditory stimuli. Journal of Experimental Psy- chology, 1971, 91, (1), 43-46.

Semel, E. M., & Wiig, E. H.   Comprehension of Syntactic structures and critical verbal elements by children with learning disabi- lities. Journal of Learning Disabilities, 1975, 8, 1, 53-58.

Seymour, P. H. K., & Porpodas, C. D.   Lexical and non-lexical proce- ssing of spelling in developmental dyslexia. In U. Frith (Ed.). Cognitive Processes in Spelling. London: Academic Press, 1979,

Simon, H. How big is a chunk. Science, 1974, 183, 482-488.

Snowling, M. J.   The development of grapheme-phoneme correspondence in normal and dyslexic readers. Journal of Experimental Child Psychology, 1980, 29, 294-305.

Sperling, G.   The information available in brief visual presentati- ons. Psychological Monographs, 1960, 74, (11), pp. 1-29.

Sperling, G.   Short-term memory, long-term memory, and scanning in the processing of visual information. In F. A. Young & D. B. Lindsley. Early Experience and Visual Information Processing in Perceptional and Reading Disorders. Washington, D. C.: National Academy of Sciences, 1970.

Stanley, G. & Hall, R.   Short-term visual information processing. Child Development, 1973, 44, 841-844.

Weber, R. J., & Harnish, R. R. Visual imagery for words: the Hebb test. Journal of Experimental Psychology, 1974, 102, 409-414.

Wickelgren, W. A. Cognitive Psychology, Englewood Cliffs, NJ: Pre- ntice Hall, 1979.

TOWARD A RATIONAL TAXONOMY OF THE DEVELOPMENTAL DYSLEXIAS

John C. Marshall
Neuropsychology Unit
Neuroscience Group
The Radcliffe Infirmary
Oxford

In societies where the educational system aims to produce
100 per cent literacy, a substantial minority of children experience great difficulty in learning to read and many never achieve a
fluent command of visual language skills. How is this population
to be further characterized ? It has sometimes been argued that
reading retardation is <u>always</u> subsiduary to some more general disability (low intelligence, lack of motivation, sensory-motor impairment, or a cross-modal learning deficit, for example). Such a
view is now almost impossible to uphold (Benton and Pearl, 1978).
At the other extreme, the World Federation of Neurology has postulated a unitary syndrome of 'specific developmental dyslexia' that
was defined as "a disorder manifested by difficulty in learning to
read despite conventional instruction, adequate intelligence and
socio-cultural opportunity. It is dependent upon fundamental cognitive disabilities which are frequently of constitutional origin"
(Benton and Pearl, 1978). This definition has been justifiably
savaged by Benton (1975) and by Rutter (1978), although these scholars do not, of course, deny that one can find a group (or, better,
groups) of dyslexic children for whom reading failure is, in some
sense, 'unexpected'.

It is now generally accepted that children with developmental
dyslexia do not constitute a homogenous population. Current work
has convincingly undermined the notion that developmental dyslexia
is a simple, single-component syndrome, and many recent studies have accordingly attempted to define distinct patterns of deficit <u>wi-
thin</u> the global diagnosis of specific reading impairment (Decker
and DeFries, 1981). Mattis, French and Rapin (1975) have isolated
three subgroups of dyslexic children and adolescents: Reading disorder in association with articulatory and graphomotor

dyscoordination; reading disorder in association with visuo-spatial
perceptual impairment; and reading disorder with more general language disorder. A similar taxonomy is presented by Denckla (1979), who
adds to the classification reading problems in the context of sequencing difficulty and of verbal learning and recall deficits. The
gross distinction between developmental dyslexia with visuo-spatial
processing deficits and with audio-verbal deficits has been related
to differences in the development of hemispheric organization; Fried,
Tanguay, Boder, Doubleday and Greensite (1981) have reported electrophysiological evidence that supports this clinical subtyping.

Although many current investigations of the developmental dyslexias are often markedly eclectic, much work in effect recapitulates
early approaches to the acquired dyslexias. In particular, there has
been conceptual recapitulation of nineteenth century studies in which
the primary classification is based not on the character of the reading impairment per se but rather on the presence of associated agraphia, aphasia, acalculia, agnosia, apraxia etc. (De Massary, 1932;
Nielsen, 1946). Thus the most notable characteristic of the developmental taxonomies reviewed in Benton and Pearl (1978) is that they
are not systematic analyses and classifications of reading impairment. Rather they comprise groupings of children with a reading disorder, where the grouping is determined by the associated symptomatology. Such taxonomies typically fail to specify in any detail the
precise nature of the reading disorder that the children manifest;
they also fail to establish whether the associated deficits constitute necessary and/or sufficient conditions for the emergence of reading impairment. Such group studies are severely limited in terms of
both the theoretical insight that they generate and the practical value of whatever therapeutic measures they may suggest. By contrast,
"the detailed investigation of individuals who are backward readers
often helps to clarify the relation between ..... different specific
weaknesses and to explain the way in which they may operate singly
or together in causing severe reading difficulties" (Bradley, Hulme
and Bryant, 1979).

Although occasional case-reports of developmental dyslexia can
be found, there is in general a serious paucity of such studies in
the literature. And there is an even more acute lack of intelligible
frameworks within which the results of such studies could be interpreted. Our own approach to this problem has been somewhat extreme.
I shall assume (I hope uncontroversally) that the syndromes of developmental dyslexia must be defined over a functional architecture of
visible language processing. But I shall further speculate that the
relevant functional architecture is the one that correctly characte-
rizes the normal, fluent, adult reading system. The syndromes of
developmental dyslexia will accordingly be interpreted as consequent
upon the selective failure of a particular adult component (or components) to develop appropriately, with relatively intact, normal
(adult) functioning of the remaining components. In effect, this is

to adopt a highly modular, 'preformist' approach to the development of the reading system. The paradigm explicitly denies that developmental failure distorts the architecture of the system as a whole; it also, of course, denies that the <u>normal</u> development of reading skill changes in a 'stage-wise' manner whereby the character of reading mechanisms at stage <u>n</u> is qualitatively distinct from their character at stage <u>n</u> + 1. To the extent that these presuppositions are true, taxonomies of the acquired dyslexias should map in a one-to-one fashion onto taxonomies of the developmental dyslexias. If the presuppositions are false - and both the acquisition of normal reading and the description of developmental pathology require an 'epigenetic' interpretation - then the syndromes of developmental dyslexia will fail to match the syndromes of acquired dyslexia.

THE ARCHITECTURE OF THE NORMAL READING SYSTEM:

If the program outlined above is to be carried out, we must first propose an architecture for the normal, adult reading system. The model that I currently favor is diagrammed in Figure I.

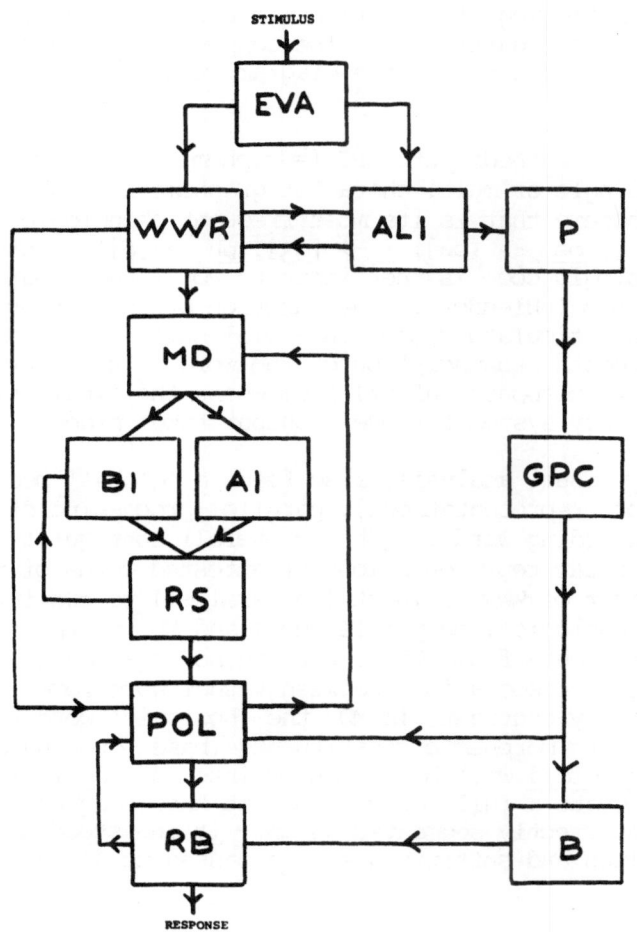

The interpretation of the diagram is as follows:
EVA = Early visual analysis. This component extracts local and global visual features from the stimulus array. Local features (i.e.
those that support individual letter recognition) are fed to ALI
(= Abstract letter identities) where explicit but abstract (e.g. ca-
se-indiscriminate) letter identities are assigned. Multi-letter strings are assumed to be explicitly segmented into their component
letters (e.g. C + A + T). ALI feeds into P (= Graphemic Parser).
The function of component P is to re-segment (where necessary) the
output of ALI into regular graphemic 'chunks'. A graphemic chunk
is a letter or letter-sequence that maps onto a single phoneme in
words that contain the relevant segment. The representation of
C + A + T will not require further re-segmentation, but sequences
such as C + O + A + L must be reanalysed as C + OA + L. That is,
oa is (normally) a vowel diagraph with the pronunciation [ou]. It
is, of course, not a diagraph in boa or oasis. Such graphemic 'exception' words will be mis-parsed by P. The component must cope with
vowel, diphthong, and consonant n-graphs that correspond to a single
phoneme in output phonology; the 'window size' of the parser must,
in the normal case, be set at $n \geq 4$ (cf. augh, eigh, eau, ch, ng).
The form and functioning of the graphemic parser is outlined in Venezky (1970) and Coltheart (1978); the component must have access to
a knowledge-base (not shown in the diagram) that lists the n-graphs
of the language.

    The output of P feeds into GPC (=Grapheme/Phoneme correspondence
rules). Each single or multi-character grapheme is associated with
the (single) phoneme that is its most frequent phonologic realization
(e.g. ea -> [i:]; oe -> [ou]; j -> [dʒ]; ph -> [f]). This regular,
segmented phonologic code is then input to POL (=Phonological output
lexicon), and to B (=Blender). The function of the latter mechanism
is to assign an articulatory code that will suffice to instruct the
vocal tract's smooth pronunciation of the word. This representation
is input to RB (= Response Buffer) from where the final triggering
of the articulatory system for overt output takes place.

    EVA (Early visual analysis) also feeds a 'global' mechanism,
WWR (= Whole word representations); parallel-processing of stimulus
information, including word-length and overall configuration, serves
to locate the visual representations of attested words of the language. The output of WWR is input (in parallel) to two further devices, POL (=Phonological output lexicon) and MD (=Morphemic decomposition). The route from WWR to POL can be regarded as a set of
direct, unanalysed associations between visual word-forms and their
pronunciations. By contrast, in MD, the 'holistic' word form is
decomposed into its morphemic constituents (base form and affixes).
For example, undecided will be segmented into un + decid + ed. MD
does not incorporate a full lexico-semantic knowledge-base; hence
unit will be incorrectly segmented as un + it and steed as ste + ed.
Potential prefixes and suffixes are then passed to AI (= Affix

interpretation) and stems to BI (=Base interpretation). In these
components, the segmented forms receive a full syntactico-semantic
interpretation. The output of BI and AI is forwarded to RS (=Re-syn-
thesis) where the combined form is checked for lexical consistency.
Thus recent will have been segmented (by MD) into re + cent; both
prefix and stem are attested lexical entries (and interpreted as such
by BI and AI). Output is blocked, however, by RS, which has access
to a knowledge-base that contains no entry for the multimorphemic interpretation of recent. The word will accordingly be recirculated as
a whole to BI where an entry will be found. This entry is then passed back to RS and on to POL, from whence the phonological realization
of the word can be placed in the Response Buffer for eventual output.

Six major varieties of acquired dyslexia can, to a first approximation, be defined over a functional architecture of the type outlined in Figure I.

SYNDROMES OF ACQUIRED DYSLEXIA:

The acquired syndromes I shall consider here are: Attentional
Dyslexia (Shallice and Warrington, 1977); Visual Dyslexia (Marshall
and Newcombe, 1973); Surface Dyslexia (Marshall and Newcombe, 1973);
Direct Dyslexia (Schwartz, Saffran and Marin, 1980); Phonological Dyslexia (Beauvois and Derouesne, 1979); and Deep Dyslexia (Marshall
and Newcombe, 1973).

1: In attentional dyslexia, individual letters can be recognized
and named with reasonable accuracy; similarly, individual words are
read quite well. Patients are impaired when required to name the
letters of an individually presented word or letter-string. Given
that singly-presented letters can be named, this latter deficit is
obviously not consequent upon "a nominal difficulty specific to letter names" (Shallice and Warrington, 1977). It must rather be the
case that the route from EVA to ALI malfunctions when Early visual
analysis must cope with a multi-character string. The deficit cannot
be purely sensory or visual, for Shallice and Warrington (1977) report that flanking letters with numbers does not impair performance
to the same extent as when a letter is flanked by other letters.
The phenomenon is thus in some sense 'categorial'; Shallice (1981)
accordingly speaks of a material-specific 'Filter control system"
that mediates between early visual processing and the analysis of
letter-form. Failure of this system leads to "later systems being
flooded by information from irrelevant parts of the visual field"
(Shallice, 1981).

2: In visual dyslexia (sometimes known as 'agnosic' dyslexia), the
primary malfunction is with the component labelled 'Whole Word Representations'. Let us assume (with Morton, 1979) that stimulus features feed, in parallel, all words (visual input logogens) that contain these features until the threshold of one logogen is exceeded.

If brain-damage selectively perturbs these thresholds, errors should arise in which the responses are all words and share many visual characteristics with the stimulus word; one might furthermore expect that the direct count word frequency of the false responses will, on average, be higher than that of the stimuli presented. Patients with visual dyslexia can have reasonably intact individual letter naming and can often sequentially name the letters of words that they misread; in these patients it is important to distinguish carefully between visual dyslexia and letter-by-letter reading (Patterson and Kay, 1982). Thus M. B. (Newcombe and Marshall, 1973) made visual errors to words (e.g. mow -> "now"; rid -> "rib"; beg -> "big") at a time when a sequential letter naming strategy was no longer adopted. The deficit, then, can be specific to whole word recognition, although when letter-identification is intact there must be a further deficit that prevents the operation of the 'phonic' route from ALI to P and GPC.

3: In surface dyslexia, 'sight' vocabulary is seriously impaired; the route from EVA to WWR is, for the most part, unavailable. The patients accordingly read by parsing the output of ALI into graphemic constituents and then applying grapheme-phoneme correspondence rules in order to obtain an internal phonological representation. In reading aloud, this representation is output via the response buffer; in reading for meaning, it is the phonologic representation (right or wrong) that determines the patient's semantic interpretation (Newcombe and Marshall, 1981). 'Regularization' errors (e.g. of -> "off"] arise by virtue of the normal mode of GPC functioning.

4: In direct dyslexia, the central 'linguistic' core of the reading system (from MD to RS) is functionally disconnected from WWR. Patients will be able to read aloud nonsense-syllables by the 'phonic' route implicated in surface dyslexia; regularly-written words will be read by either (or both) the phonic route or (and) the system of direct associations between WWR and POL; presented with words where the relationship between orthography and pronunciation is irregular, the latter route (visual input lexicon to phonological output lexicon) will be operative when performance is correct. These patients may show excellent reading aloud of both regular and irregular words with little or no comprehension as assessed by a wide variety of semantic categorization and picture-making tasks (Schwartz, Saffran and Marin, 1980).

5: In phonological dyslexia, non-word reading is significantly worse than word reading, indicating that the phonic route from EVA to ALI, P, and GPC is functionally impaired. The reading of lexical stems (i.e. words without derivational or inflectional morphology) both aloud and for meaning can be almost intact (although some visual errors may be made). With multi-morphemic words, however, numerous errors are made in which closed-class prefixes and suffixes are added, dropped, or substituted. Typical examples (from Patterson,

1982) include think -> "thinking"; disposal -> "dispose"; ineradi-
cable -> "eradicate"; solve -> "absolve". In some, but not all,
patients, function word omissions and substitutions are found in single word reading or, more often, in text reading. The patients do
not make either 'regularization' errors or semantic errors. In Figure I, the 'derivational' errors that characterize the syndrome must
arise somewhere within the route MD to AI and RS. Neither the 'phonic' route nor the direct input/output (WWR to POL) route are sufficiently intact to 'block' these derivational errors at the phonological output lexicon.

6:    In deep dyslexia, the phonic route is functionally unavailable
(nonsense words cannot be read); when words are read aloud their
meaning is (at least approximately) known, indicating that WWR->POL
plays little or no role in performance. As in phonological dyslexia,
'derivational' errors are very common, and in addition (contrary to
the case in phonological dyslexia), frank semantic substitutions are
found on single word reading. There must accordingly be both impairment of the route MD -> AI -> RS (a malfunctioning that is responsible for derivational errors) and of the route MD -> BI -> RS (a malfunctioning that is responsible for semantic paralexias). It is not
yet known whether these two overt deficits could be functionally
unified by postulating a singular malfunction at RS. Patients with
deep dyslexia show a very strong part-of-speech effect such that
performance on concrete nouns is better than on adjectives, verbs,
and abstract nouns; 'function-words' are almost never read correctly.
It is possible that the function-word deficit might, in some way,
be assimilated to the problems with affixes; both could be represented in a specialized closed-class dictionary (see Kean, 1982, for
some thoughts on this problem with respect to Broca's aphasia).

SYNDROMES OF DEVELOPMENTAL DYSLEXIA:

      To what extent, then, is there evidence that developmental dis-
orders of reading can be sensibly partitioned into reasonably close
analogues of the varieties of acquired dyslexia? I shall look in
turn at putative developmental parallels for each of the six syndromes described in the previous section.

1:    Developmental attention dyselxia? As far as I know there are
no reports of single-case studies that contrast children and adults
on the dimensions relevant to attentional dyslexia. Nonetheless,
there is circumstantial evidence that makes it plausible to speculate that a developmental analogue may exist. Differences between
letter and word recogntion are in part controlled by the trade-off
between the effects of lateral masking and orthographic redundancy
(Massaro and Klitzke, 1979). Lateral masking between adjacent letters will tend to impair word perception vis-a-vis single letter
perception; orthographic structure, plus such global features of
the stimulus array as whole word length and shape, will tend to

J. C. Marshall

augment the recognition of words vis-a-vis individual letters. In
experiments on normal adults, Massaro and Klitzke (1979) have compared letter and word recognition in a paradigm in which the test items
were followed, at variable intervals, by a mask of random letter-
fragments. At short interstimulus intervals, words were recognized
better than individual letters; at long intervals the opposite effect
was found. This at least suggests that, in some conditions, accurate
letter-perception is not a prerequisite for accurate word-perception.

     It is well known that the effects of lateral inhibition are stro-
ngest towards the fovea (Woodworth, 1938: Bouma, 1973). Thus with
(roughly) central fixation, the medial letters of words will suffer
a further disadvantage over and above the fact that initial and final
letters are only masked on one side. Bouma and Legein (1977) have
compared groups of normal and dyslexic children and shown that this
adverse interaction towards the fovea is strongest in dyslexic children, despite the two groups scoring equally well on the recogntion
of isolated letters. The study does not indicate whether every child
within the dyslexic group has an extreme sensitivity to lateral masking. However, Bouma and Legein's finding does not make it reasonable
to expect that some dyslexic children with good individual letter-
naming ability but poor spelling may be able to recognize words without being able to name the letters that comprise the words.

2:     Developmental visual dyslexia? Once again I am aware of no published studies in which developmental analogues of visual dyslexia
have been sought. I do not, of course, mean to imply by this that
no one has noticed that some dyslexic children make 'visual' errors.
From the earliest days of systematic study of children with reading
disorders, attention has been focused on 'reversal' errors on letters.
(e.g. b -> "d"; p ->"b") and 'order' errors on words (e.g. dog ->
"god"; tar -> "rat"). Similarly, some previous taxonomies (e. g.
Boder, 1973) lay considerable stress upon the differential occurrence
of visual errors in different varieties of developmental dyslexia.
Boder (1973) gives such typical examples as house -> "horse",
money -> 'monkey", and step -> "stop", examples that we have previously noted are not easily distinguished from the errors of patients
with acquired visual dyslexia (Marshall, Newcombe and Hiorns, 1975).
The issue here then is simply whether or not reasonably 'pure' cases
of developmental visual dyslexia can be found, that is, cases in
which visual confusions constitute the sole error type. If such
cases do exist, one would want to investigate in much more detail the
precise mechanisms that underly the occurrence of visual errors in
children and adults. We have previously noted (Marshall, Newcombe
and Holmes, 1975) that, in normal children learning to read there is
a reliable effect of part-of-speech upon the accuracy of single-word
reading. If such effects were found in reading-impaired children
with (presumptive) visual dyslexia, the phenomenon would not require
one to postulate a deficit that referred to part-of-speech. Nonetheless, 'pure' developmental visual dyslexia (if it exists) could, in

principle, be a syndrome in which 'lingusitc' factors enter into the
overt symptomatology in addition to visual confusions that are defined over purely visual parameters.

3.   Developmental surface dyslexia? Here we are on somewhat safer
ground. Holmes (1973; 1978) was the first to report on the very close
similarity of patients with acquired surface dyslexia (Marshall and
Newcombe, 1973) and some children with developmental reading disorder.
She noted that the 'context-sensitive' nature of English orthography
was the main stumbling block for children who experienced difficulty
in acquiring an extensive sight vocabulary. The children accordingly
experienced great difficulty when attempting to read words that contained complex consonant clusters, highly 'ambiguous' letters, such
as s, f, c, g, P and r whose phonic value depends heavily upon the
graphemic context, silent consonants, 'rule of e' (c. f. pin versus
pine), and vowel digraphs. Typical errors from the boys reported by
Holmes (1973) include: bathe -> "bath", ceiling -> "selling", and
gorge -> "George"; substantial numbers of neologistic errors are made,
as when ch is realized as [tʃ], rather than [k] in such words as anchor,
character, or monarch; homonym confusions are in evidence as when
mare is interpreted as the mayor of a town. Subsequent work has confirmed and extended Holmes' findings (see Coltheart, Masterson, Byng,
Prior, and Riddoch, 1983, for an intensive contrastive analysis of
two cases of surface dyslexia, one developmental and one acquired);
there is now little doubt that a close developmental analogue to
surface dyslexia exists, although there is, of course, still considerable controversy concerning the precise mechanisms responsible (see
Marcel, 1980).

4.   Developmental direct dyselxia? In 1967, Silberberg and Silberberg described a group of 28 children whose ability to read words
aloud was dramatically better than their comprehension of written words, and indeed better than their oral langue functioning in general.
The intelligence levels of the children varied from mentally defective
to above average. Silberberg and Silberberg proposed the expression
'hyperlexia' for these children, and a number of subsequent reports
have confirmed their existence in populations as diverse as the mentally retarded, the autistic, 'idiot savants', and (otherwise) basically normal children (see Healy, 1982, for an excellent review of
this literature).

These children obviously have either failed to acquire the central syntactico-semantic component of the lexicon or have grossly
impaired access to that lexicon in the visual modality. Granted that
deficit, however, their relatively successful reading aloud could be
mediated either by the system of grapheme/phoneme correspondence rules (in which case the children would be analogous to adults with
acquired surface dyslexia) or by the direct 'holistic' visual input/
phonological output route (in which case they would be analogous to
adults with acquired direct dyslexia). The early literature on hyper-

lexia suggested that some of these children had advanced 'word-call-
ing' skills that extended to complex, irregular words. The first
serious study of this issue, however, comes from Aram, Rose and Horwitz (this volume). Their patient, MD, is a developmental hyperlexic
now in his late 30s. MD has good grapheme-phoneme correspondence
skills as witnessed by his excellent performance when reading nonsense words; in addition, he must "have established a considerable
store of word-specific print to sound associations" (Aram, Rose, Horwitz, this volume), for his ability to read aloud irregular 'exception' words is also very good. Yet oral reading appears to bypass
the lexico-semantic system; the patient is thus very similar to the
case of acquired direct dyslexia reported by Schwartz, Saffran, and
Marin (1980). Further evidence that word recognition is, in some
sense, 'holistic' in hyperlexia is provided by Cobrinik (1982). The
hyperlexic children in this study were significantly better than normal controls in a task where "'incomplete words', in which letter-
identifying cues were made ambiguous through deletion" had to be recognized.

5:    Developmental phonological dyslexia? Temple and Marshall (1983)
have reported on a seventeen year old girl, H. M., who is at least
of average intelligence and has an above average oral vocabulary.
She is grossly impaired at non-word reading in comparison to word
reading; her responses to non-words are frequently real words that
bear a fairly close visual similarity to the stimulus. When reading
words, a very substantial proportion of her errors are either visual
or derivational paralexias. H. M. makes no semantic errors, no regu-
larizations of the type seen in surface dyslexia, and very few of her
responses are neologisms. Overall, this developmental case is very
similar indeed to the case of acquired phonological dyslexia reported
by Patterson (1982). Further details of H. M.'s performance (and
that of another English case of developmental phonological dyslexia
can be found in Temple (this volume). Sartori and Job (1982) have
reported the existence of developmental phonological dyslexia in Italian. Their case, a 12 year old boy of above average intelligence,
showed relatively accurate word reading (especially for nouns) with
poor reading aloud of non-words. There can be little doubt that, to
a first approximation at least, phonological dyslexia exists in both
an acquired and a developmental form.

6:    Developmental deep dyslexia? Despite very intensive search, a
truly convincing developmental analogue to deep dyslexia has not yet
been found. Papers in which semantic paralexias are reported in children with severe reading problems have not been explicit about whether errors occurred in single-word reading or only when reading text
(cf. Boder, 1973). If these errors occur solely in sentence reading,
they are not diagnostic of deep dyslexia. Normal adults make semantic substitutions when reading text aloud under time pressure (Morton,
1964), and it has often been argued that in children it is the good
readers who make maximum use of linguistic redundancy and are thus

inclined to 'guess' (predict) words that make syntactic and semantic sense in the context. Goodman (1969) has reported such extreme examples as The lady's wig was . . . .   -> "The lady's fake hair was . . .". And he remarks, that "it appears likely that a reader who requires perfection in his reading will be a rather inefficient reader." However, the search for a genuine developmental analogue continues unabated, and experienced clinicians do report having seen developmental dyslexics who make semantic paralexias on single word reading (M. Newton, personal communication: E. Boder, personal communication). In thus far unpublished papers, Linda Siegel (McMaster University) and Rhona Johnston (University of St. Andrews) have reported on children who make a few semantic errors on single words, but it is not currently clear whether the full symptom-complex of deep dyslexia can be found in developmental cases. Nonethelss, it would not be irrational on the current evidence to predict that a convincing developmental analogue will eventually be discovered.

CONCLUSIONS:

     The approach to the acquired dyslexias that I have taken here is only one decade old. With the exception of Holmes' pioneering work (Holmes, 1973), the history of systematic efforts to describe the developmental dyslexias in terms of the functional architecture (and hence taxonomic classes) implied by the acquired dyslexias is even briefer. Given these temporal constraints, it is somewhat surprising to find that, at least superficially, the study of developmental dyslelxia has even now revealed considerable communality with partitionings derived from the investigation of acquired dyslexia. To the extent that strict analogies hold between the two conditions (and available evidence suggests that this is indeed the case) the 'preformist' paradigm outlined in the introduction is upheld.

     More seriously, however, I want to conclude with a point about reserach paradigms in the study of the dyslexias. Intuitively, I feel that it is really quite unlikely that the acquired and develop mental dyslexias will be interpretable over a single, static functional architecture. There should, I suspect, be some qualitative changes in functional architecture that arise both in the course of the normal growth of reading skill and in consequence of developmental impairments. To this extent, an epigenetic framework will be required. But I believe very strongly that the best way to discover that framework is (for the time being) to uphold the current preformist paradigm. If we continue to look for detailed similarities between the two conditions we will be able to see more clearly just where the analogy breaks down.

REFERENCES

Beauvois, M. F. and Derouesne, J. Phonological alexia: Three dissociations. Journal of Neurology, Neurosurgery and Psychiatry,
1979, 42, 115-1124.
Benton, A. L. Developmental dyslexia: Neurological aspects. In
W. J. Friedlander (Ed.), Advances in Neurology, Vol. 7. New
York: Raven Press, 1975.
Benton, A. L. and Pearl, D. (Eds.): Dyslexia: An appraisal of current knolwdege. New York: Oxford University Press, 1978.
Boder, E. Developmental dyslexia: A diagnostic approach based on
three atypical reading-spelling patters. Developmental Medicine
and Child Neurology, 1973, 15, 663-687.
Bouma, H. Visual interference in the parafoveal recognition of initial and final letters of words. Vision Research, 1973, 13,
767-782.
Bouma, H. and Legein, Ch. P. Foveal and parafoveal recognition of
letters and words by dyslexics and by average readers. Neuropsychologia, 1977, 15, 69-80.
Bradley, L., Hulme, C. and Bryant, P. E. The connection between different verbal difficulties in a backward reader. Developmental
Medicine and Child Neurology, 1979, 21, 790-795.
Cobrinik, L. The performance of hyperlexic children on an "incom-
plete words" task. Neuropsychologia, 1982, 20, 569-577.
Coltheart, M. Lexical access in simple reading tasks. In G. Under-
wood (Ed.), Strategies in Information Processing. London:
Academic Press, 1978.
Coltheart, M., Masterson, J., Byng, S., Prior, M. and Riddoch, J.
Surface dyslexia. Quarterly Journal of Experimental Psychology,
In Press.
De Massary, J. L'Alexie. Encephale, 1932, 1, 53-78.
Decker, S. N and DeFries, J. C. Cognitive ability profiles in fami-
lies of reading-disabled children. Developmental Medicine and
Child Neurology, 1981, 23, 217-227.
Denckla, M. B. Childhood learning disabilities. In K. M. Heilman
and E. Valenstein (Eds.), Clinical Neuropsychology. New York:
Oxford University Press, 1979.
Fried, I., Tanguay, P. E., Boder. E., Doubleday, C. and Greensite,
M. Developmental dyslexia: Electrophysiological evidence of
clinical subgroups. Brain and Language, 1981, 12, 14-22.
Goodman, K. S. Analysis of oral reading miscues: Applied Psycho-
linguistics. Reading Research Quarterly, 1969, 5, 9-30.
Healy, J. M. The enigma of hyperlexia. Reading Research Quarterly,
1982, 17, 319-338.
Holmes, J. M. Dyslexia: A neurolinguistic study of traumatic and
developmental disorders of reading. Unpublished Ph. d. thesis,
University of Edinburgh, 1973.
Holmes, J. M. "Regression" and reading breakdown. In A. Caramazza
and E. B. Zurif (Eds.), Language Acquisition and Breakdown:
Parallels and Divergencies. Baltimore: Johns Hopkins Press, 1978.

Kean, M-L. Three perspectives for the anlayis of aphasic syndromes
    In M. A. Arbib, D. Caplan, and J. C. Marshall (Eds.), Neural
    Models of Language Processes. New York: Academic press, 1982.
Marcel, A. J. Surface dyslexia and beginning reading: A revised
    hypothesis of the pronunciation of print and its impairments.
    In M. Coltheart, K. E. Patterson and J. C. Marshall (Eds.),
    Deep Dylsexia. London: Routledge and Kegan Paul, 1980.
Marshall, J. C. and Newcombe, F. Patterns of paralexia: A psycho-
    linguistic approach. Journal of Psycholinguistic Research,
    1973, 2, 175-199.
Marshall, J. C., Newcombe, F. and Hiorns, R. W. Dyslexia: Patterns
    of disability and recovery. Scandinavian Journal of Rehabili-
    tation Medicine, 1975, 7, 37-43.
Marshall, J. C. Newcombe, F. and Holmes, J. M. (1975): Lexical
    memory: A linguistic approach. In A. Kennedy and A. Wilkes
    (Eds.), Studies in Long Term Memory. London; Wiley, 1975.
Massaro, D. W. and Klitzke, D. The role of lateral masking and
    orthographic structure in letter and word recognition. Acta
    Psychologica, 1979, 43, 413-426.
Mattis, S., French, J. H. and Rapin, I. Dyslexia in children and
    young adults: Three independent neuropsychological syndromes.
    Developmental Medicine and Child Neurology, 1975, 17, 150-163.
Morton, J. A model for continuous language behavior. Language and
    Speech, 1964, 7, 40-70.
Morton, J. Word recognition. In J. Morton and J. C. Marshall (Eds.),
    Psycholinguistic Series, Vol. 2. Cambridge, Mass.: M. I. T.
    Press, 1979.
Newcombe, F. and Marshall, J. C. Stages in recovery from dyslexia
    following a left cerebral abscess. Cortex, 1973, 9, 329-332.
Newcombe, F. and Marshall, J. C. On psycholinguistic classifications
    of the acquired dyslexias. Bulletin of the Orton Society, 1981,
    31, 29-46.
Nielsen, J. M. Agnosia, Apraxia, Aphasia: Their value in cerebral
    localization. New York: Hafner, 1946.
Patterson, K. E. The relation between reading and phonological co-
    ding: Further neuropsychological observations. In A. W. Ellis
    (Ed.), Normality and Pathology in Cognitive Functions. London:
    Academic Press, 1982.
Patterson, K. E. and Kay, J. Letter-by-letter reading: psycholo-
    gical descriptions of a neurological syndrome. Quarterly
    Journal of Experimental Psychology, 1982, 34A, 411-441.
Rutter, M. Prevalence and types of dyslexia. In A. L. Benton and
    D. Pearl (eds.), Dyslexia: An appraisal of current knowledge.
    New York: Oxford University Press, 1978.
Sartori, G. and Job, R. Phonological impairment in Italian acquired
    and developmental dyslexia. Paper presented to the NATO confe-
    rence on Acquisition of Symbolic Skills, Keele, England, 1982
Schwartz, M. F., Saffran, E. M. and Marin, O. S. M. Fractionating
    the reading process in dementia: Evidence for word-specific
    print-to-sound associations. In M. Coltheart, K. E. Patterson

and J. C. Marshall (Eds.), Deep Dyslexia. London: Routledge
and Kegan paul, 1980.

Shallice, T. Neurological impairment of cognitive processes. British Medical Bulletin, 1981, 37, 187-192.

Shallice, T. and Warrington, E. K. The possible role of selective attention in acquired dyslexia. Neuropsychologia, 1977, 15, 31-41.

Silberberg, N. and Silberberg, M. Hyperlexia: Specific word recognition skills in young children. Exceptional Children, 1967, 34, 41-42.

Temple, C. M. and Marshall, J. C. A case study of developmental phonological dyslexia. British Journal of psychology, In Press.

Venezky, R. L. The Structure of English Orthography. The Hague: Mouton, 1970.

Woodworth, R. S. Experimental Psychology. New York: Holt, 1938.

CLASSIFICATION ISSUES IN SUBTYPE RESEARCH:
AN APPLICATION OF SOME METHODS AND CONCEPTS

Robin Morris
Department of Psychology
Georgia State University
Atlanta, Georgia

Paul Satz
Neuropsychiatric Institute
University of California
Los Angeles, California

The search for subtypes of learning disabled children is of
recent origin. Most of this research has been confined to the past
decade as investigators have begun to recognize that traditional concepts of learning disabilities have been flawed by their presumpti-
on that these children constitute a homogeneous diagnostic class.
Such thinking, which ignored the heterogeneity of children subsumed
under these rather broad diagnostic labels, fostered rather simplistic explanatory models concerning causes, course and adaptation.
In the past decade, efforts have converged, using clinical and statistical approaches, to search for homogeneous subtypes of learning
disabled children. A critical review of this literature is presented in recent reports by Satz & Morris (1981).

Although a few definable subtypes have been identified across
various studies using clinical and/or statistical classification approaches, many other subtypes have been reported that could be criticized by the classification theory and methods used. More importantly, the conceptual framework underlying the use of various classification methods is not appreciated by many researchers. As a
result, the subtype literature, while committed to laudatory goals,
may be criticized in future years for its failure to understand and
document whether knowledge of subtypes helps in the diagnosis and
treatment of learning dislabled children.

The purpose of the present chapter is to present some of the
conceptual issues related to subtype classification and to use this
framework for discussing some of the recent findings from the Florida Longitudinal Project.

Classification

The literature on subtypes, although rarely identified as such, is concerned with the classification of learning disabled children. A basic assumption underlying subtyping is that there are children who show similarities and/or differences in their disabilities. By identifying these similarities and/or differences, or these "types" of children, it is thought that better understanding and research into their etiologies, prognosis, and treatments will be provided. Because these children have already been classified as learning disabled, the label "subtypes" represents a second order or "sub" classification. Since classification is a basic process in any science, the literature on the theoretical and practical issues involved in developing classifications will be discussed.

Kendell (1975), in an excellent book on the role of diagnosis, places the process of forming classifications into perspective:
Theories and therapeutic claims have no more chance of surviving than buildings if they are not built on secure foundations. Developing reliable diagnostic criteria and a valid classification may be tedious.....but provides the foundations on which all else will depend. (p. vii).

For those involved in the research on childhood disabilities, such a strong statement is somewhat unsettling because of the lack of interest historically in childhood classification systems. Achenbach and Edelbrock (1978) report that until the 1960s it was felt that a classification of childhood disorders was unnecessary. Even in the late 1960s there were only limited attempts to form child-oriented classification systems. It appears that most attempts at classifying children have been restricted to very specific subject areas such as learning disabilities, behavior disorders and mental retardation.

The term classification has been generally defined as the "ordering of concepts into groups (or sets) based on their relationship - their similarity" (Bailey, 1973). Sokal (1974) makes the important observation that "regardless of whether behavior is learned or instinctive, organisms must be able to perceive similarities in stimuli for survival" (p. 115). He further states that, "The paramount purpose of a classification is to describe the structure and relationship of the constituent objects to each other and to similar objects, and to simplify these relationships in such a way that general statements can be made about classes of objects" (p. 1116.).

Every noun we use constitutes an act of classification. Nomenclature, a system of names, is an alternative label for a classification system. Classification systems place their objects of study, in our case children, into groups so that in each group the children are more similar to each other than they are to children placed into another group. Classifications are used as a basis for communication, for information retrieval, as descriptive systems, to make predictions, and as a source of ideas (Blashfield & Draguns, 1976).

Although classification systems form the foundations of any of the major sciences, they possess both positive and negative attributes. This is because any classification system exerts a large influence on our approach to the child before us, the way we talk about the child to our colleagues, the ideas it provides about the causes and treatment of the child's disorder, and how we add to the theoretical models about the child's disorder. In these ways, such systems put limits on what and how we do our assessments and research. Noting such biases, Cattel and Coulter (1966) commented from a different perspective:

> Psychometrics has, in its main developments, ignored
> this granulation of its populations in favor of a sim-
> plified world of homogeneous normal distributions of
> characteristics and linear relations to them. Consi-
> derations of efficiency require that our models begin
> more explicitly to encompass types, and the nonlinear
> relations and pattern effects which go with them.
> (p. 238-239).

Another risk of classification systems is that by giving something a name, the illusion is conveyed that we clearly understand the object of study. A term such as dyslexia is an excellent example of this risk. It should be made clear that as Blashfield and Draguns (1976a, 1976b) point out, no classification label can "encompass all the relevant information about the individual". They also add that "a label generates expectations about a person's behavior. Once a person is diagnosed, predictions may be based on the diagnostic label and not the person's observed behavior".

The formation of a classification system is a complex process and there is an entire literature on the theoretical and practical issues involved in forming any classification system, regardless of subject content. Unfortunately, as Sokal (1974) points out, "in most classification research, theory has frequently followed methodology, and has generally only tried to formalize the work in the field. In a few instances, classification systems have been set up on a priori or philosophical grounds and the methodology made to fit into the principle" (p. 1116). Because there are empirical criteria which can be used to evaluate the adequacy of any classification system, the lack of an integration between classification theory and method should no longer be representative of this type of research (Skinner, 1981). Although psychologists have been testing the reliability and validity of the tests they have created for years, one has to question why they have not been using the same evaluative process with the classification systems they use. Classification systems should be developed as hypotheses which can be tested. Goodall (1966) has further suggested that the most practical null hypothesis in such research is that there are no sub-classes within the subject population being classified.

The ethical questions raised by the use of classification systems and diagnostic categories which may not be reliable or valid heighten these concerns. The unreliability of diagnostic labels is not limited to psychiatric or psychological systems (Koran, 1975). Those critics of diagnosis, those who think the labeling of children is more harmful than helpful, have cause to be alarmed with the current approach to classification research.

In general, classification research is looking for classification systems which are in accord with nature. Sokal (1974, p. 1116) states that, "It is the purpose of science to discover the true nature of things, and then form a correct classification to describe the object in such a way that their true relationships are displayed." Interestingly, logic is the science of relations among classes but cannot operate without clearly defined classes (Dreger, 1968).

To reach the goal of a "natural classification", Blashfield and Draguns (1976) have described four major criteria which need to be met in any adequate classification system. These are reliability, coverage, descriptive validity, and predictive validity.

Reliability is a term used to describe a group of criteria related to the consistency of a classificatory label. One type is inter-rater reliability. If a child is assessed by two different clinicians, will he/she be placed into the same subtype? Another aspect of reliability to be considered is intra-rater reliability: if the child is assessed by the same clinician over two occasions, will the child receive the same diagnosis?

Reliability is not equivalent to accuracy. Different assessors may agree but be wrong. A further important component of reliability is that it fixes the ceiling for validity. Validity can never be higher than the reliability.

In general, when a subtype is well-defined through operational specification of the specific attributes of each subtype, then the major job of the assessment is to correctly assess the attributes of the child. Those who develop computer classification systems have shown such systems to be totally consistent (Splitzer & Endicott, 1969). If the same data are put into such programs 100 times, they will place the child into the same group 100 times unless the computer fails. It should be made clear, though, that any classification is limited in its informational value by the variables on which it is based (Conger & Lipshitz, 1973). Also, no computer system can ever correct poor input data or programming.

Coverage refers to the 'applicability' of the classification to the children for which it is intended. If we have a group of 100 LD children, and our classification system can only place 30 of them into any subtype--the rest being undefined-- then such a classification system is not useful. Children have to be described as 'in' a subtype or not at any given time, although some have suggested that a degree of 'fitting' could be a useful concept. One of the major problems as described by Blashfield (1973) is that as coverage is increased, the reliability almost always decreases. In other words, by making the inclusion rules for a subtype somewhat looser, then we clearly make room for a broader use of the category and decrease the reliability. Canover (1972) has pointed out that intra-rater agreement increases with fewer number of and grosser criteria for the groups used in a classification system. Blashfield (1973) has suggested that this problem can be dealt with through the identification of homogeneous clusters of subjects within which there are distributions of attributes.

Descriptive validity refers to the homogeneity of the symptoms which are used to form a subtype. Homogeneity may have many different meanings. McQuitty (1967) has presented at least three definitions of a cluster in terms of its homogeneity:

1) A group in which every member of the group is more similar to at least one member of the same group than he or she is to any member of another group. 2) A group in which each member is more similar to all members of any other cluster. 3) A group in which each member has a greater average similarity to all members of the same cluster than with all members of any other group (Blashfield & Draguns, 1976b, p. 576).
Other alternatives have also been presented, although most research has not defined specific meanings for the concept of homogeneity. Each different definition of a homogeneous subtype could yield very different groupings.

Most researchers and clinicians have argued that predictive validity is the primary goal and purpose of any classification system. If the classification system being used does not help in predicting any future behavior, or the consequences of being placed in such a group, many feel it should be abandoned. Others, though, have argued that descriptive classification systems in psychology, psychiatry, and medicine are equally as important for the purpose of communication. If such systems help to describe and communicate better about the subjects in the clinic or in a research population, then it will be a major step forward from what is currently available.

A major problem with these two goals, prediction and

communication, is that they are in conflict. For good communication
purposes, a classification should be simple in structure; the diagnostic rules for identifying children into subtypes should be easy to
use; and the attributes on which the classification is based should
be the most frequently used in standard practice.

On the other hand, for predictive purposes, a classification needs to be highly complex; it should provide a basis for predicting
responses to many forms of treatment, for understanding of etiology,
and for making a prognosis. Because of this conflict, many have questioned whether there is need for two different classification systems, one for clinical practice and one for research.

With these criteria in mind, the development of a classification
system will be addressed. This development is highly dependent on
one's theoretical orientation and the purpose of the classification
system one is trying to form. Skinner (1981) suggests that, ideally,
one should be able to define each type and its attributes a priori.
An underlying issue involves the definition of "type". Cattell and
Coulter (1966) consider a type as "the most representative pattern
in a group of individuals located by a high relative frequency, a mode, in the distribution of persons in multidimensional space"(p. 240).
Typicality is based on how good an example it is of the class it is
attempting to describe.

Through this defining of "types" hypotheses are developed which
can be investigated. In this manner, such hypotheses can be refuted
as in most scientific endeavors. Unrefutable hypotheses are not useful in the development of a scientific theory.

There are three classification models which have been utilized
in a majority of the classification research. The first, hierarchical models, places children successively into specific nonoverlappi-
ng subsets which can be further subdivided into further subsets at
lower levels in the hierarchy. The second type, categorical models,
places children into discrete classes. The third type, dimensional
models, orders children along dimensional axes in a multidimensional
space. Of course, recently there have been hybrid combinations of
these different models. These new complex hybrids have not had a
great deal of study but hold promise since they attempt to alleviate
the limitations of the three basic models which have been used in
the past.

Kendell (1975) reports that the main strength of dimensional
models is that there is no loss of information, and maximal alternatives are possible along the dimensions. A problem with such models
is that any system with multiple dimensions has to be dealt with ge-
ometrically or algebraically. And, in a final analysis, most dimensional information is reduced to categories before clinicians will
use it. The main strength of a typology is the ease of description

it provides. A drawback is that a typology creates an expectation that all patients fit neatly into each category whether they actually do or not. Besides these considerations, Hempel (1961) has added a historical point which appears to relate to the developmental level of the scientific area of study. He notes that most sciences have started with dichotomous attributes but then replace them with dimensions, as more sophisticated and accurate attribute measurement becomes possible.

Related to the issue of selecting the model most appropriate to the question at hand is the entire debate about the nature of a "class". The term "class", at a theoretical level, is one which refers to a set whose boundaries are clear. That is, the classes are mutually exclusive and jointly exhaustive. Reality makes such "classes" less clear. In the abstract world all one needs to know are the attributes which define a class and the attributes of the child in order to place a child into a particular class. The problem comes in the real world where reality is oriented around inexact class definitions, inexact attribute measurement, and inexact class assignment. Bailey (1973) has discussed the implications of this distinction at some length. He described the differences in the following way.

A typology is monothetic if possession of a unique set of features is both necessary and sufficient for identifying a specimen as belonging to a particular cell in the typology. That is, each feature is necessary and the set is sufficient. In contrast, a polythetic typology is constructed by grouping together those individuals within a particular sample which have the greatest number of shared features. No single feature is either necessary or sufficient. The objects are grouped so as to maximize overall similarity within each group. Thus, polythetic types cannot be constructed prior to measurement. (p. 21).

An interesting issue is that monotheticism can be related to a simple order relationship in which there is only one way to get a certain score and therefore be assigned to a specific subtype. Polytheticism is related to a partial order relationship in which there are multiple ways to get a certain score and therefore be assigned to a specific subtype (Bailey, 1973).

An important consideration though is whether a 'class' approach is appropriate in developmental disabilities or childhood psychopathology. Kendell (1975) has reported that there has not been evidence of any natural boundary between any condition and others. For such classes to be considered 'real', then, one would expect to find multimodal distributions where there are points of rarity along the borders between the classes.

There has been some suggestion that there is such a bimodal

distribution in reading skills which represents the presence of dyslexic children (Yule, Rutter, Berger & Thompson, 1974). One has to
question whether the differences in the observed (3.5-6%) and expected (2.3%) frequency of deficient readers are based on a mirror artifact of a similar underlying bimodal distribution of intelligence.
The high correlations between the reading and IQ tests would lend support to this possibility. The research suggesting this distribution
is also based on a very limited assessment of reading abilities and
has not been replicated.

A major issue in the formation of any classification system is
the choice of attributes of which it is formed. For example, reading
deficits may be related to many complex and diverse factors. Also,
it may be neccessary to consider the course of the disorder and its
etiology in order to form an adequate classification system.

The use of etiology in research on learning disabilities does
not appear warranted at this time because most etiological attributes
are based on inferences. Such inferential etiological implications
have been at the root of many problems involving classification in
child psychiatry and psychology and are the result of theoretical
biases and extrapolations which cannot be operationally defined.

Some authors suggest that all classifications should be based
on attributes which exist at the time of assessment only. Others have suggested that time-linked changes in attributes should also be
considered which include past, present or future attributes. One
issue which appears clear throughout the present classification literature though, is that all attributes and their resulting classes require strict operational definitions.

From another perspective, if we look at the three attribute components of any child (a) those attributes that all children have
(lungs), (b) those attributes that only each individual child has
(3 moles on the inside of his left big toe in the shape of a triangle), and (c) those attributes which make an individual child more
similar to some children than to others (good in math), it is clear
that it is important to eliminate the first two components and focus
on the last.

Of course, the choice of attributes will be highly dependent on
one's theoretical orientation. A neuropsychologist may choose brain-
behavior relevant variables while a behaviorist may choose variables
related to specific environmental contingencies influencing specific
behaviors of the child. The number of attributes used in classification problems is a matter of some debate. On one hand, there are
those who feel that the lowest possible number of nonredundant variables should be used while others feel that as many possible variables from as many possible domains should be utilized. A related
issue surrounds syndromes, factor structures or the interrelation

among a group of variables. Many have mistakenly interpreted such factors within groups of children as being proof of clusters of children with such underlying attributes.

In the final analysis, however, the 'correctness' of one's choice of attributes will only be identified through an extensive validation and use of a classification system. It is, therefore, the validation phase of a classification project that represents the ultimate test of the many objective, subjective and theoretical decisions made in the forming of a classification system.

Once the decision about the basic attributes have been made, the next decision has to do with the actual methods used to create the classification system. These methods are just as diverse as other components of the process. Clinical experience and single-case paradigms have been the long-standing foundations of most psychiatric classification systems. More recently, multivariate statistical techniques (Blashfield, 1980; Garside & Roth, 1978; Kendall, 1975; Maxwell, 1971) have been utilized in conjunction with these clinically derived and oriented methods. It should be noted that clinical and statistical methods each have advantages and disadvantages and both are oriented toward the same goal from somewhat different approaches. Because of this, each can be used to validate classifications derived by the other and should be seen as mutually supportive process.

The validation phase in the development of any classification process includes both internal and external validation. Internal validation refers to evidence that a developed classification system meets the criteria of reliability, coverage, homogeneity, and replicability within a given sample. It should be noted that without adequate internal validity, the more important criterion of external validity probably cannot be achieved.

The external validity of a classification relates to the actual usefulness of a classification system. Questions of its value in predicting recovery, treatment type and results, descriptive validity, and generalizability to other populations are important considerations. The descriptive and predictive validity issues are probably the most important criteria related to the successfulness of any new classification. One approach to these issues is the use of alternative external, or independent attributes for discrimination purposes. Validity across these measures is important to support the distinctiveness or boundaries of the individual classes. The relationship of classes in predicting future behavior or relationships is the most important consideration.

The preceding section has attempted to provide a brief overview of some of the basic issues and approaches to classification that are seldom considered in the search for learning disability subtypes. The following section presents an application of some of the methods

and concepts involved in subtype classification using data from the
Florida Longitudinal Project.

Application

Previous reports on some of the Florida Longitudinal Project
subtype research can be found in Satz & Morris (1981) and Morris,
Blashfield & Satz (1981). A unique feature of this research was the
use of special clustering methods to identify the index cases (i.e.,
learning disabled subgroups) before searching for subtypes. This
was accomplished by first analyzing the WRAT achievement scores on a
large and generally unselected sample (n = 236) of white boys who[1] remained in Alachua County at the end of Grade 5 (six years later).
The sample (mean age = 11) included children at all levels of achievement. This approach used cluster analysis to define the target
subgroup and comparison subgroups prior to the search for subtypes.
This approach avoided the use of exclusionary criteria in the selection of learning disabled subjects, and provided a more objective
and statistical classification of index cases. Cluster analysis is
a procedure designed to facilitate the creation of classification
schemes (Morris, Blashfield & Satz, 1981). It has been defined as a
procedure which groups individuals into homogeneous clusters based
on each subject's performance on the clustering variables.

Phase I: Classification on Achievement Variables

The WRAT data were subjected to an average linkage hierarchical
agglomerative clustering method utilizing a square Euclidian distance similarity measure. The average linkage method combined with the
Euclidian distance measure was used because of its sensitivity to
elevation in a data set. This method was likely to permit clusters
to emerge which are different on their levels of achievement.

Nine clusters (subgroups) emerged, which were then subjected to
a K-means iterative partioning clustering method. This additional
method was used because of the fact that an individual, once placed
in a given cluster by a hierarchical agglomerative method, is not
able to be reassigned to a later forming cluster, even if its similarity to the later formed cluster is greater.[2] This method attempts to reduce within-cluster variance (increase homogeneity) while
increasing between-cluster variance (decrease overlap), thus attempting to clarify the cluster solution.

The nine subgroups, which included 230 of the 236 subjects, revealed a number of interesting patterns of reading, spelling and arithmetic skill.[3] These subjects are presented in Figure 1, where
the scores on each WRAT subtests are expressed on a scale with a population mean of zero and a standard deviation of one. This method
permits visualization of the subgroups in terms of both pattern and
elevation. Subgroups 1 and 2 both obtained superior scores in

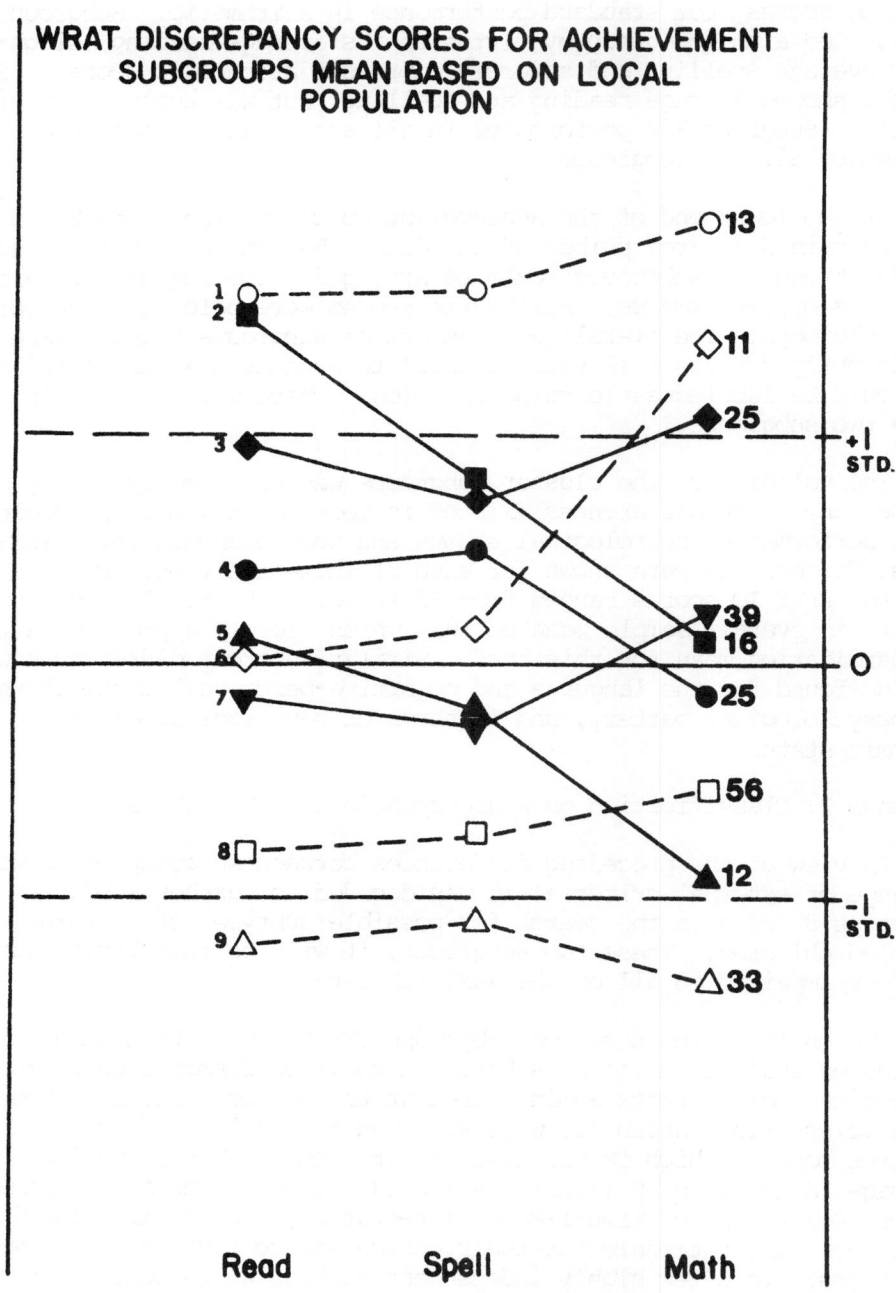

WRAT DISCREPANCY SCORES FOR ACHIEVEMENT
SUBGROUPS MEAN BASED ON LOCAL
POPULATION

FIGURE   1

reading, but subgroup 3 achieved high reading, spelling and arithmetic scores. Subgroup 4 emerged as a group with adequate reading and
spelling scores, but standard performance in arithmetic. Subgroup 5
constituted a unique group by virtue of its average reading, slightly
below average spelling and severely depressed arithmetic scores. Subgroup 6 showed average reading and spelling, but was superior in arithmetic. Subgroup 7's performance in all areas was the most nearly
average of all the subgroups.

At the lower end of the achievement spectrum, subgroups 8 and 9
each contained a large number of children. Reading and spelling scores for these two subgroups could be arranged according to increasing levels of performance. Arithmetic scores were below average for
both subgroups. The overall achievement of subgroups 8 and 9 were
sufficiently depressed (2 year deficit) to suggest that these children could be labeled as learning disabled. There were 89 boys in
these two subgroups.

The validity of the cluster subgroups was examined by asking
whether any group differences existed in terms of IQ, neuropsychological performance, neurological status and socioeconomic level (SES).
Robust differences were shown for each of these analyses. For example, the PPVT IQ scores ranged from 90 (subgroup 9) to 116 (subgroup
1) with an overall sample mean of 103, which closely approximates the
standardization mean for this test. Similar subgroup differences were also found for the language and cognitive-perceptual tests of the
neuropsychological battery, and in terms of neurological and socio-
economic status.

Phase 2: Classification on Neuropsychological Variables

In view of the preceding differences between subgroups on a wide range of external criteria, it was decided to further subdivide
subgroups 8 and 9 in the search for possible subtypes of learning
disabled children. These two subgroups, it will be remembered, were
severely impaired on all of the WRAT subtests.

The children in these two subgroups (N= 89) were then subjected
to cluster analytic techniques based on their performance on four
neuropsychological tests administered at the end of Grade 5. These
tests (clustering variables) were selected from a larger group of
measures based on high factor loadings (Fletcher & Satz, 1980) on a
language factor (WISC Similarities, Verbal Fluency) and a perceptual
factor (Beery Test of Visual-Motor Integration, Recognition Discrimination). The rationale for their choice was to restrict the number of tests to a few highly independent factors which would reduce
redundancy, random error variance, and increase subtype interpreta-
bility. Reliable variables yield a more reliable classification.
A number of clustering techniques were used to ensure that subtypes
were replicable across different clustering methods, a mandatory step

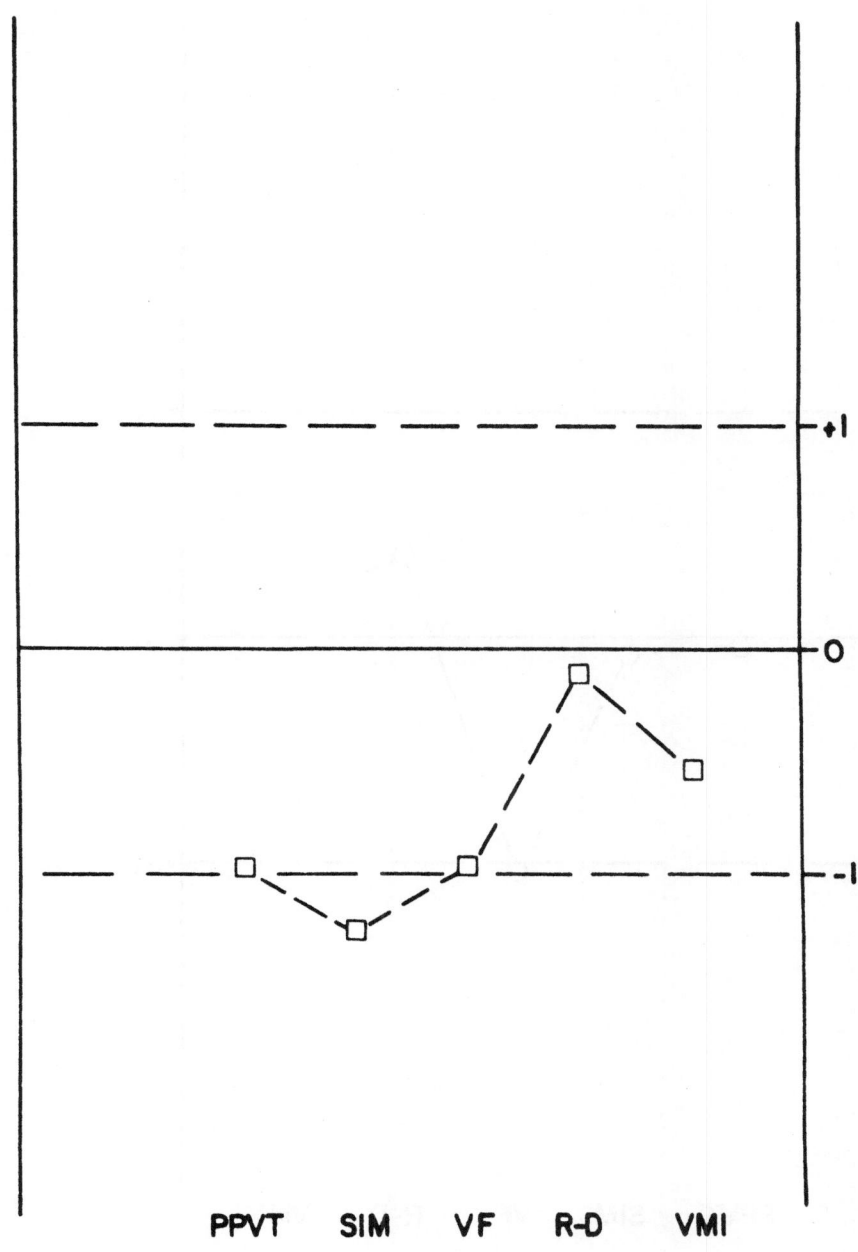

FIGURE 2. Ward's method with square Euclidian distance
6 cluster solution with relocate

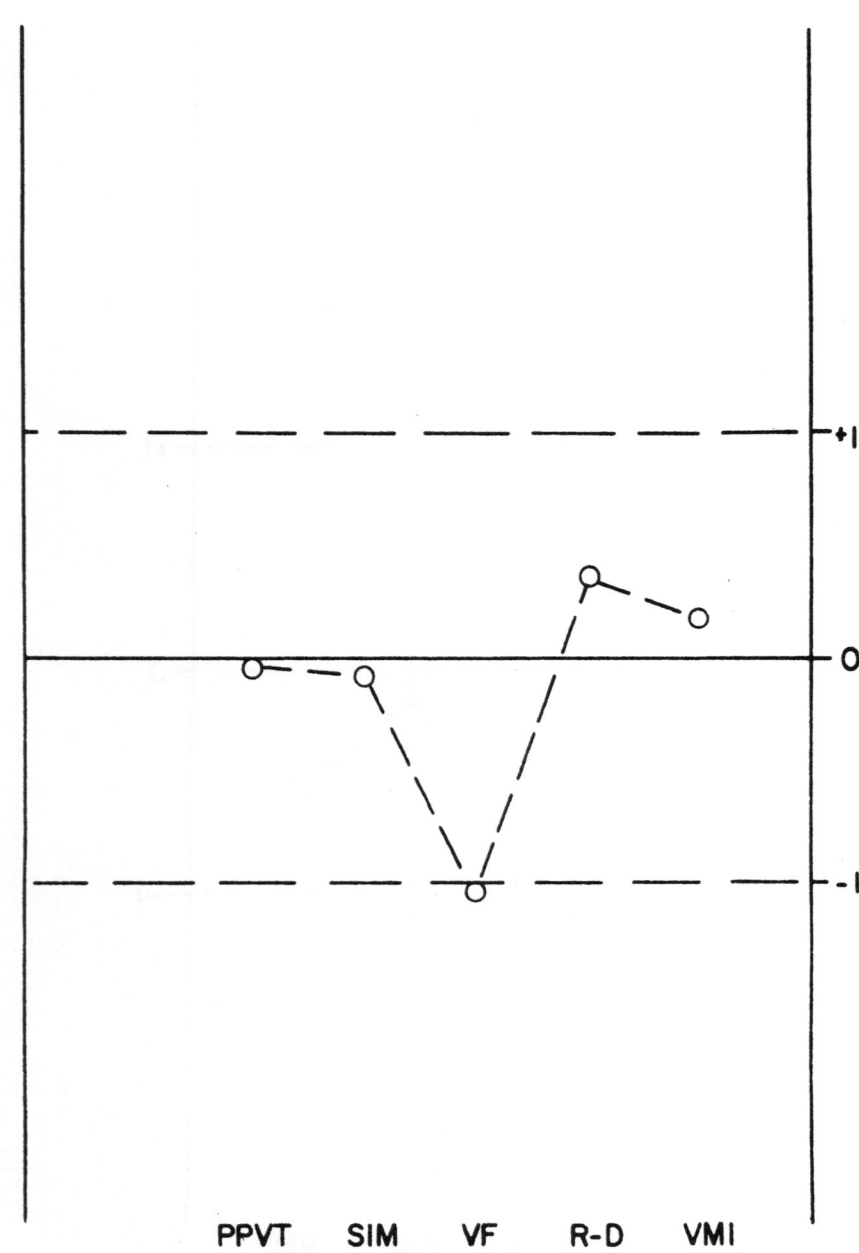

FIGURE 3. Ward's method with square Euclidian distance
          6 cluster solution with relocate

in view of the controversy surrounding the potential uses and misuses of cluster analysis (Everitt, 1980).

Four hierarchical agglomerative techniques utilizing two distance measures were employed. Following each cluster analysis, the individual solutions were subjected to a K-means iterative partioning method.

Five distinct clusters (subtypes) emerged from each of the cluster analytic methods. In fact, the subtypes were virtually identical in terms of profile elevation, pattern and sample sizes. The subtypes are presented separately in Figures 2-6. The subtypes are based on performance on the four neuropsychological tests which have been converted to standard scores with a population mean of zero and a standard deviation of one. Subtype 1 (Figure 2) were severely impaired on both of the language measures (Similarity and Verbal Fluency) and in terms of PPVT IQ (used as a marker variable). In contrast, performance on the non-language perceptual tests was within normal limits for this subtype ("normal" defined in terms of the scaled mean for the total sample, n = 236). This subtype (N = 27) was defined as a global language impairment type. Subtype 2 (Figure 3) was selectively impaired on only the verbal fluency test. Performance on the remaining neuropsychological tests was within normal limits. This subtype (N = 14) was defined as a specific language type.

Subtype 3 (Figure 4) was severely impaired on all of the neuropsychological tests (language and perceptual), including the PPVT IQ. This subtype (N = 10) was defined as a global language and perceptual impaired type (mixed). Subtype 4 (Figure 5) was selectively impaired on only the nonlanguage perceptual tests. In contrast, their performance on the language tests, including PPVT IQ, were within the normal range. This subtype (N = 27) was defined as a visual-perceptual-motor impaired type. Subtype 5 (Figure 6), in contrast to the preceding four subtypes, showed no impairment on any of the neuropsychological tests; in fact, their subtype profile was characterized by average to superior performance on each of the cognitive tests, including PPVT IQ. As such they were defined as an unexpected learning disabled subtype (N = 12).

Separate analyses were conducted comparing differences between subtypes on various external criteria including WRAT scores, SES level, neurological status and parental reading levels. A multivariate analysis of variance was first run on the WRAT scores to see whether the subtypes varied by achievement level. This analysis was prompted in part by the high neuropsychological performance of children in Subtype 5 (unexpected). No significant main effect was found, which supports the concept that these children are not different on achievement levels. Significant differences between subtypes were observed, however, in terms of neurological status, SES, and parental reading levels.

R. Morris and P. Satz

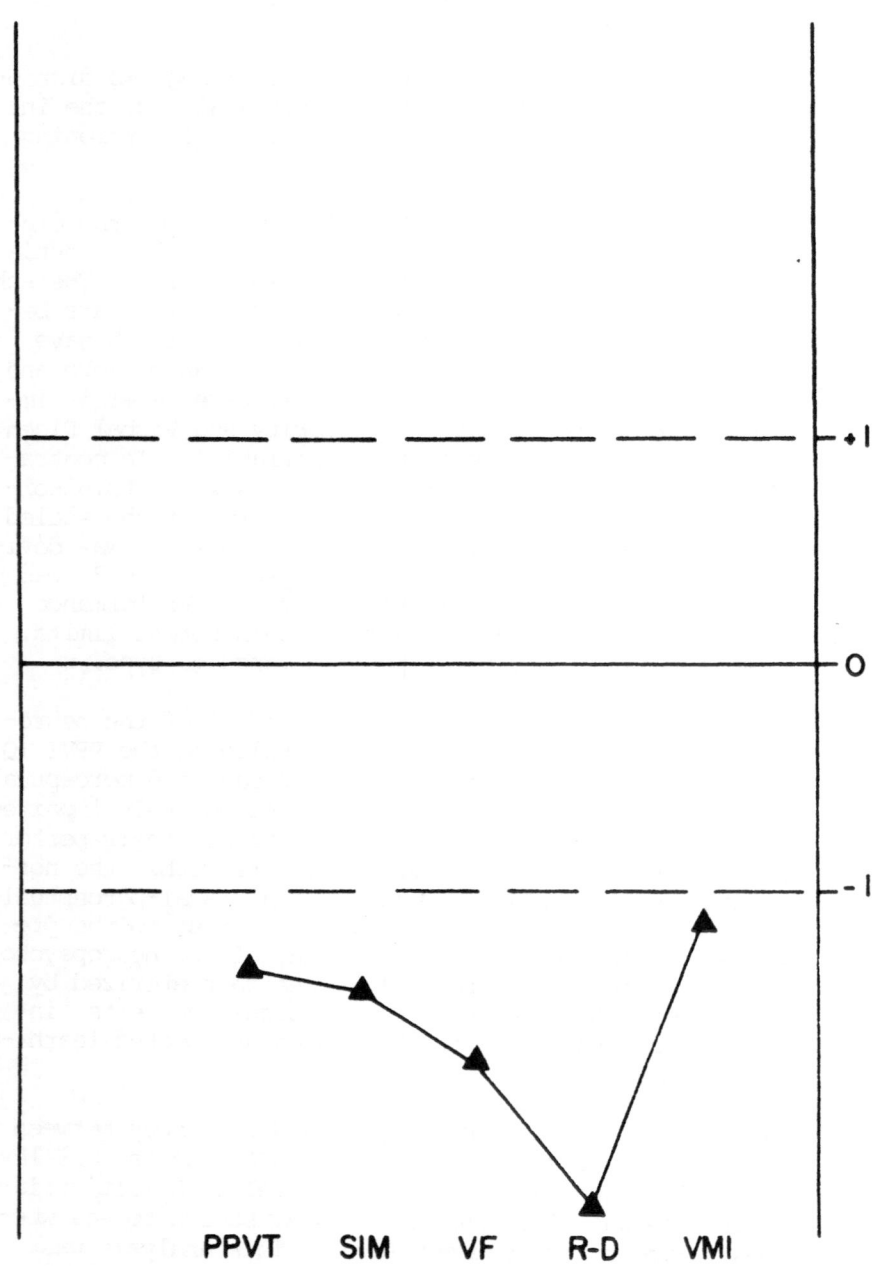

FIGURE 4. Ward's method with square Euclidian distance
6 cluster solution with relocate

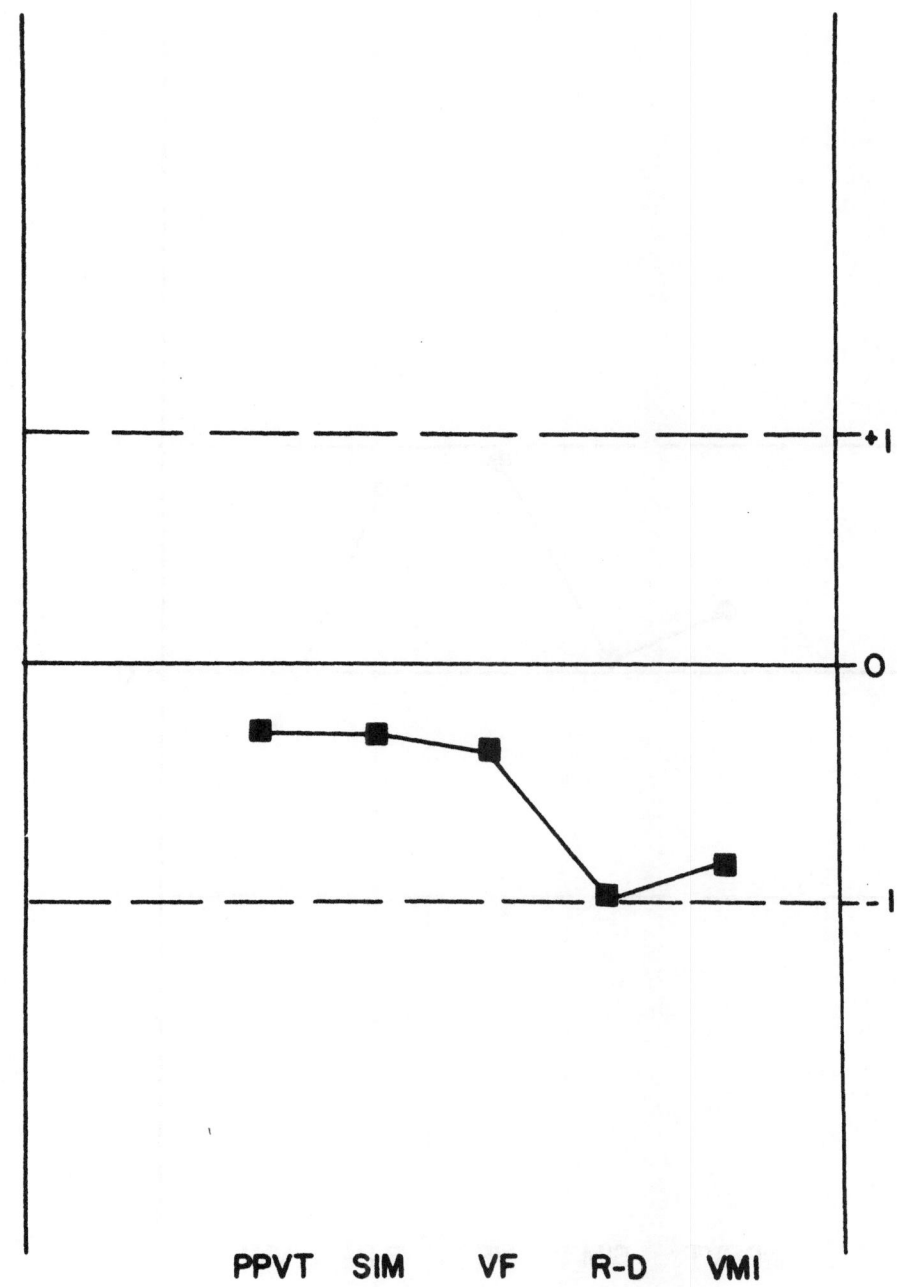

FIGURE 5. Ward's method with square Euclidian distance
           6 cluster solution with relocate

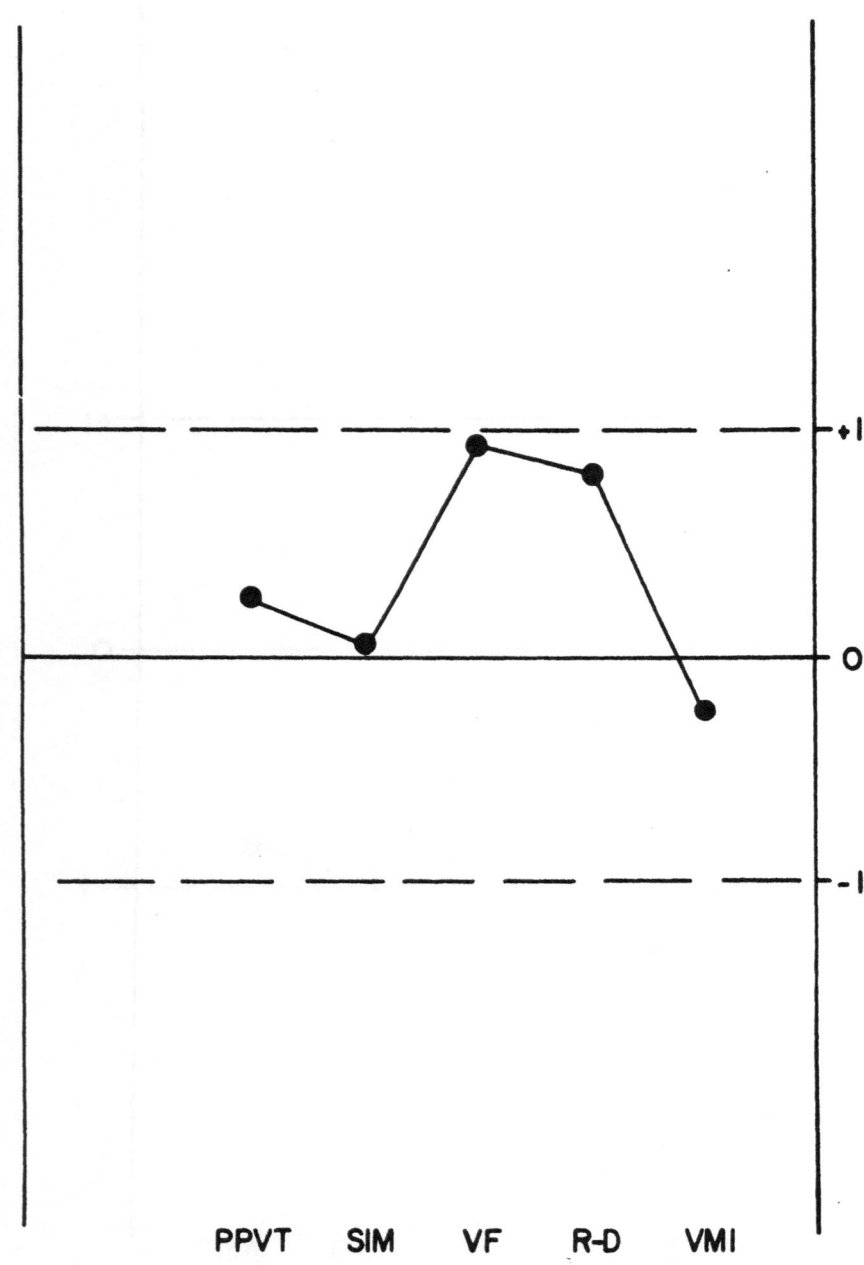

FIGURE 6.   Ward's method with square Euclidian distance
            6 cluster solution with relocate

In terms of neurological status, children in Subtypes 1 (global language), 3 (global language and perceptual) and 4 (visual-perceptual-motor) had a significantly higher proportion of positive findings (soft neurological signs). When parental reading levels were examined (WRAT) across subtypes, it was found that the blood parents of subtypes (2 & 5) achieved higher scores than those of the other subtypes; in fact, their WRAT scores, when adjusted for education and SES level, were shown to be higher than the total sample mean. This latter finding further underscores the need for subdividing learning disabled children into more homogeneous subtypes in the search for familial-genetic determinants (Taylor, Satz & Friel, 1979).

On the basis of the preceding analyses, one might conclude that the subtypes represent distinctive clusters of children who share a number of common attributes and remain relatively distinct when compared with various external criteria. However, the interpretation one assigns to these subtypes is another matter. At this level, caution should be exercised. Intuitively, the subtypes, at least types 1 - 4, are compatible with other studies (clinical and statistical) which typically report a language, perceptual and/or mixed subgroup of learning disabled children. Lacking additional clinical or neuro-radiologic information on these subtypes both cautions and restricts premature inferences concerning etiology. On the other hand, any advance in the etiology or causes of learning disabilities must first rest on a firm basis of classification and definition. The present results provide some beginning steps in this direction.

Despite the promise that this study holds, particularly for establishing an approach to classification, the results were viewed as preliminary. None of the subtype studies reviewed have been free of criticism. The present study is no exception. One should note the following concerns.

First, one must continue to question the use of achievement measures that sample such a restricted range of reading skills. The WRAT is notoriously limited in this respect. In fact, it provides no measure of reading comprehension that could have improved the search for subgroups and subtypes in this study.

Second, one could fault the use of such a small number of neuropsychological tests as clustering variables in the search for subtypes. One must still ask whether the same subtype clusters would have emerged with a larger number of neuropsychological variables. One might predict a similar subtype division if similar factor-loaded tests were clustered. However, this prediction remains to be confirmed empirically. More difficult to predict is the cluster typing that would emerge with other factor tests. The study also would have been strengthened by the use of more formal psycholinguistic measures that came into use after the Florida Longitudinal Project was launched (1970). The choice of attributes for classification was limited.

Third, one should note that the subtype analyses were conducted on only Subgroups 8 and 9, both of whom showed marked and uniform impairment on each of the WRAT subtests. However, Subgroup 5 showed a severe though selective impairment in arithmetic, which would have justified their inclusion in the learning disability subgroups.

Fourth, each of the subtypes was derived on a highly homogeneous group of children with respect to age (11 years), sex (male) and race (white). This factor significantly restricts any extrapolation to disabled learners in the general population.

Fifth, the validity of the subtypes would have been strengthened by the use of additional validation measures. For example, the relationship between subtypes and teacher observations, remedial programs, developmental histories and measures of personality functioning may have provided additional information which could have proved helpful.

Finally, the use of cluster analysis as a multivariate classification method has its own inherent limitations. Its limitations are somewhat different from those of Q-technique factor analysis, but are no less important to examine. Cluster analysis includes numerous methods, many of which have never been critically examined, nor clearly defined. This problem has only served to increase confusion and communication in the area. Different classification problems require different methods which can create problems not always apparent. There are also many different algorithms and computer software packages which may yield different results from the same procedures. In general, clustering methods are not built upon a firm statistical foundation and are basically only heuristic. In addition, only limited attempts have been made to validate cluster results. Thus, validation of cluster solutions is especially critical since most methods will 'find' solutions in random data (Morris, Blashfield & Satz, 1981).

Phase 3: Data Manipulation & Further Validation of Subtypes

As was pointed out earlier in this chapter, a useful classification schema must demonstrate adequate reliability, coverage and validity (descriptive and/or predictive). Despite the limited efforts made to address these issues, problems still remained as was noted in the last phase. Some of these problems were in the nature of the partioning method employed - in the present case, cluster analysis. Replication of the subtypes across different clustering techniques did provide some assurance of reliability and stability. Moreover, these techniques were felt to allow for the emergence of polythetic clusters, which if real, should yield better classification coverage. It was found that these techniques managed to classify 96 percent of the subjects into distinctive subtypes.

Still one might ask whether the various subtypes represent arti-
facts of the clustering methods rather than the true hidden structure of the data. Clustering techniques have been known to find clusters even in random data. As such, this could lead to premature mis-
conceptions by the unsuspecting investigator. With these reservations in mind, it was decided to subject the data to a further series
of statistical manipulations and validations.

First, a split-half design was employed which randomly assigned
the 89 children into two subsamples. It was expected that if the methods and subtypes are reliable, then the subsamples should yield
similar results, both between them and with the original subtypes.
Both subsamples yielded the same basic results, both of which replicated the original subtypes.

A Monte Carlo approach was utilized as a second validation schema. Since clustering methods find clusters even in random data, a
data set which mimics the known parameters of the original data, but
includes only randomly generated subject profiles, could be used to
test the null hypothesis that no actual clusters exist in one's data.

Such data sets were generated which had the same number of subjects, variables, means, and standard deviations, and the same correlation matrix between variables as the original data. 'Subjects' in
these data were generated by a multivariate random number generator,
thus the data contained no clusters. These data sets were clustered
using the original methods and the results compared to the original
subtypes. In general, the Monte Carlo technique yielded a different pattern of subtypes. Hence the null hypothesis was not supported. (A more detailed discussion of this hypothesis test is reported
in the paper by Morris et al., 1981).

It was next asked what would happen if additional variables were used for clustering the same subjects. The Peabody Picture Vocabulary Test (PPVT) and the Embedded Figures Test (EF) were added to
the original four clustering variables. This yielded a 6 variable
problem which was again clustered using the original procedure. The
subtype clusters and the cluster means did not change appreciably.

The addition of other subjects into the classification process
was also used to test subtype stability. In the first addition, the
12 children in Subgroup 5 (math disability) were added to the original 89 children and then subjected to the original clustering procedure. All five of the original subtypes maintained their original
profiles. The 12 children which were added clustered into two subtypes, with 4 (33%) going into Subtype 5 (unexpected subtype), and
6 (50%) going into Subtype 4 (visual-perceptual-motor subtype).
This supported the stability of the original cluster solution and

also provided new information about possible processes involved in math disabilities.

In a second addition, the 25 children from Subgroup 3 (above average achievement) were added to the original 89 children and clustered. For diagnostic and theoretical purposes it was expected that these average children would form a new cluster. This average subgroup did not fall into any deficit subtype but rather formed a new cluster of average or above average abilities.

The preceding results, in summary, present an application of some of the concepts, decisions, and methods involved in subtype classification described at the beginning of this chapter. Despite the promise that these methods of classification hold - as well as subtypes that emerged - the ultimate test will rest on whether this knowledge leads to improved diagnosis and treatment of learning disabled children. This test directly addresses the issues of subtype validation and utility. Unfortunately, the present results represent but a beginning step in the process of identifying valid subtypes of learning disabled children - but hopefully a step in the right direction.

The present chapter has attempted to show that the search for such subtypes is an enormously complex process that involves an appreciation of classification theory and methods regardless of whether statistical or clinical approaches are used. It is at least reassuring that other investigators are beginning to be concerned about issues in the classification process, and to replicate some of these subtypes using different statistical approaches and/or cultural samples. Through this process, they are expanding this knowledge to address the more important issues of etiology and treatment (Rourke, 1982; Lyon, in press; Van der Vlugt, in press).

FOOTNOTES

1. The sample comprised all learning disabled boys from the original standardized population who continued to reside in Alachua County, plus their matched and/or secondary controls. In this respect, only the learning disabled children were really unselected although they had been earlier defined on an a priori basis.

2. During each iterative partioning phase, each individual is statistically removed from its parent cluster and its similarity to all other clusters is computed. If its similarity to another cluster is greater, the individual is placed in that cluster.

3. Three small clusters, consisting of only 6 subjects resisted incorporation into the large clusters until a four cluster solution.

Following the recommendation of Everitt (1980), they were considered
'outliers' and were dropped from further analysis.

REFERENCES

Achenbach, T. M., & Edelbrock, C. S. The classification of child
    psychopathology: A review and analysis of empirical efforts.
    Psychological Bulletin, 1978, 85(6), 1275-1301.
Bailey, K. D. Monothetic and polythetic typologies and their rela-
    tion to conceptualization, measurement and scaling. American
    Sociological Review, 1973, 38, 18-33.
Blashfield, R. K. Evaluation of the DSM-III classification of schi-
    zophrenia as a nomenclature. Journal of Abnormal Psychology,
    1973, 82, 382-389.
Blashfield, R. K. Propositions regarding the use of cluster analy-
    sis in clinical research. Journal of Consulting and Clinical
    Psychology, 1980, 43(4), 456-459.
Blashfield, R. K., & Draguns, J. Evaluative criteria for psychia-
    tric classification. Journal of Abnormal Psychology, 1976,
    85, 140-150, a.
Blashfield, R. K., & Draguns, J. Toward a taxonomy of psychopatho-
    logy: The purpose of psychiatric classification. British Jour-
    nal of Psychiatry, 1976, 129, 574-583, b.
Canover, D. Psychiatric distinctions: New and old approaches.
    Journal of Health and Social Behavior, 1972, 13, 167-180.
Cattell, R. B., & Coulter, M. A. Principles of behavioral taxonomy
    and the mathematical basis of the taxonome computer program.
    British Journal of Mathematical and Statistical Psychology,
    1966, 19(2), 237-269.
Conger, A. J., & Lipshitz, R. Measures of reliability for profiles
    and test batteries. Psychometrika, 1973, 38, 411-427.
Dreger, R. M. Aristotle, Linnaaeus, and Lewin, or the place of
    classification in the evaluative-therapeutic process. The Jour-
    nal of General Psychology, 1968, 78, 41-59.
Everitt, H. Cluster analysis. London: Heineman Educational Books,
    1980.
Fletcher, J. M., & Satz, P. Developmental changes in the neuropsy-
    chological correlates of reading achievement: A six year longi-
    tudinal follow-up. Journal of Clinical Neuropsychology, 1980,
    2, 23-37.
Garside, R. F., & Roth, M. Multivariate statistical methods and
    problems of classification in psychiatry. British Journal of
    Psychiatry, 1978, 133, 53-67.
Goodall, D. W. Hypothesis-testing in classification. Nature, 1966,
    211, 329-330.
Hempel, C. G. Introduction to problems of taxonomy. In J. Zubin
    (Ed.,), Field studies in the mental disorders. New York: Grune

and Stratton, 1961.

Kendell, R. E. The role of diagnosis in psychiatry. London: Black-
    well Scientific Publications, 1975.

Koran, L. M. The reliability of clinical methods, data and judgemen-
    ts. (Parts 1 & 2). The New England Journal of Medicine, 1975,
    293(13), 642-626, 695-701.

Lyon, R. Subgroups of LD Readers: Clinical and Empirical Identifica-
    tion. In Myklebust, H. (Ed.), Progress in Learning Disabiliti-
    es, (Vol. V), Grune and Stratton, in press.

Maxwell, A. E. Multivariate statistical methods and classification
    problems. British Journal of Psychiatry, 1971, 119, 121-127.

McQuitty, L. L. A mutual development of some typological theories
    and pattern analytic methods. Educational and Psychological
    Measurement, 1967, 27, 21-46.

Morris, R., Blashfield, R., & Satz, P. Neuropsychology and cluster
    analysis: Potentials and problems. Journal of Clinical Neuro-
    psychology, 1981, 3, 79-99.

Rourke, B. P. Central processing deficiencies in children: Toward
    a developmental neuropsychological model. Journal of Clinical
    Neuropsychology, 1982, 4, 1-18.

Satz, P., & Morris, R. Learning disability subtypes: A review. In
    F. J. Pirozzolo & M. C. Wittrock (Eds.), Neuropsychological and
    cognitive processes in reading. New York: Academic Press, 1981.

Skinner, H. A. Toward the integration of classification theory and
    methods. Journal of Abnormal Psychology, 1981, 90(1), 68-87.

Sokal, R. R. Classification: Purposes, Principles, Progress, Pros-
    pects. Science, 1974, 185(4157), 1115-1123.

Spitzer, R. L., & Endicott, J, DIAGNO II. American Journal of
    Psychiatry, 1969, 125(7), 12-27.

Taylor, H. G., Satz, P., & Friel, J. Developmental dyslexia in
    relation to other childhood reading disorders: Significance
    and utility. Reading Research Quarterly, 1979, 15, 84-101.

Van der Vlugt, H. Reading disability subtypes: A cross-cultural
    validation. In Rourke, B. (Ed.), Learning disabilities in
    children: Advances in subtype analysis, Guilford Press, in press.

Yule, W., Rutter, M., Berger, M., & Thomson, J. Over and under-
    achievement in reading: Distribution in the general population.
    British Journal of Educational Psychology, 1974, 44, 1-12.

SPECIFIC SPELLING PROBLEMS

Uta Frith
MRC Cognitive Development Unit
London WClH OAH

INTRODUCTION

     Roderick was a 15 year old pupil at a London private school
with high academic standards when a teacher asked me to see if he was
dyslexic. He feared that Roderick might fail some of his pending O-
level examinations, even though he was sure that the boy was very
bright. Expecting a classic case of specific reading failure, I was
very surprised when on the first test I administered, the Schonell
Graded Word Reading Test, Roderick performed near ceiling level. In
other reading tests too he showed the competence of an adult fluent
reader. I quickly found out that he never had a reading problem,
had learned to read very early, and was in fact an avid and very fast
reader. When I queried him further it became clear that his only
problem was spelling but that it was a very serious handicap. Roderick was the first case of specific spelling failure that I had come
across and set me off on a long search to find out how it is possible
to be unable to spell the same words that one is easily able to recognize when reading. The existence of excellent readers who are
atrocious spellers challenges some implicitly held assumptions about
reading and writing. How can there be a dissociation of such closely
related skills as recognizing and reproducing a written word? Should
these two processes not be two sides of the same coin?

TWO MEANINGS OF SPELLING

     Spelling as Orthographic Structure

     First of all it seemed necessary to question what is meant by
"spelling'. The word "spelling" can be applied to both recognizing
and producing a written word, but there are two quite different

meanings involved: One (the spelling of a word) to do with the structure of the word on the page, the other (spelling a word) with the
production of the word from memory. Let us consider each meaning in
turn. The spelling of a word is the letter-by-letter sequence that
makes up a written word. The spelling of a word is not totally arbitrary but is governed by rules and precedents. In English these
rules have historically evolved into a highly complex system and it
is not surprising that a definitive description, a "grammar" of orthography, is not yet available. Chomsky and Halle (1968), Haas
(1969, 1970) Klima (1972), Scragg (1974), and Coulmas (1981) have all
provided stimulating and sometimes provocative accounts of orthography from the point of view of linguistics. An excellent discussion
from the point of view of cognitive psychology is provided by Henderson (1982).

Without going into detail a number of points on the nature of
English orthography, a few points need to be mentioned as they are
relevant to the present context. English orthography is notorious
if one just considers letter-sound correspondence. However, it is
an unwarranted limitation to evaluate English orthography only in
terms of how well it reflects spoken language. The notion of orthographic structure as a reflection of speech is extremely interesting,
but also problematic. For instance, spoken language changes markedly
over time and is continually changing while written language has the
potential of being laid down forever. Therefore, written spelling,
if it were intended to reflect speech faithfully would have to change
in line with spoken language, which loses some of its special advantages. Spelling reforms usually involve some compromise with the
conflicting demands of the two language systems. Languages with relatively recent spelling reforms e. g., Finnish, Turkish, Serbocroat,
often reflect current pronunciation satisfactorily and their orthography is said to be phonetic. However, this may change with time,
if and when pronunciation in these languages changes. In addition
to the problem of change, there is the problem of dialect representation. Also, the nature of the phonology of a particular language is
an extremely important factor in determining the complexity of spellin.
English has highly complex phonolgy and spelling is equally complex.

Apart from these aspects of English orthography that can be considered in terms of past or present phonology there are many other
factors which are not reflected in the pronunciation but are reflected in certain grapheme patterns. Examples are plural S (regardless
of its pronunciation as Z or S), semantically related words that so-
und different (muscle/musculature), and semantically unrelated words
that sound the same (muscle vs. mussel). The key to many of the seemingly idiosyncratic features of English orthography is the realization that English is a language created mainly from Germanic and
Romance elements but also several other languages and has a mix-
ture of orthographies (e. g., Ph = f in Greek words only). The
origin of many English words is preserved in their spelling, even if

the spoken form does not reflect this at all (psychology vs. sicology). The knowledge of word origin is not necessarily conscious in literate people, but subtle experiments (Baker, 1980; Smith, 1980a, b) have revealed that people are surprisingly sensitive to this aspect. Similarly, it is surprising that misspellings often retain etymologically based graphemic features.

Some neglected aspects of orthography are the rules of punctuation and the use of small or capital letters. There are also conventions about abbreviation, hyphenation and segmentation of written words. Intentional phonetic renderings of speech, e. g. eye dialect (Bowdre, 1982) are also subject to restrictions from standard spelling. All these aspects of written language are influenced by many different factors, including social and political ones (Venezky, 1980).

These brief considerations make clear that the mastery of spelling for word recognition is not a trivial accomplishment. Considering spelling for word production in the next section will perhaps elucidate some similarities and differences between the two meanings of spelling.

Spelling as Word Production

Spelling a word means letter-by-letter production and this is specific to alphabetic scripts. The concept of the alphabet is based on the principle that speech sound is represented visually. The process of phonographic translation (Haas, 1970) is highly complex. The main problem is that speech sound is continuous and written letters are discrete units. The discrete letter units are mapped onto discrete sound units that are not naturally given, but artificially created. This discovery was made by Liberman et al (1967) when they attempted to build a device that translated letters into sounds to assist the blind in reading. They found that it was not feasible to create an alphabet of sounds to match the alphabet of letters. Gleitman and Rozin (1977) showed that to become literate in an alphabetic script involves a major psychological effort: it is necessary to learn about the artificial speech-sound units (phonemes) and to relate them to letters (graphemes). This skill has often been described as segmentation.

Much of the early stages in learning to spell is taken up by learning to segment words into units that make sense as phonemes. Some phonemes are represented by one letter, others by 2 or more (-sh- for $\int$; -eau- for -O-). One particular problem is presented by certain consonant clusters (Marcel, 1980), such as in hint or lamp. These clusters are late in the acquisition of phonology in spoken language. In many cases children reduce the clusters and the same phenomenon can be seen in early spelling attempts (Read, 1971; Chomsky, 1971). Examples from Read (1978) are : bopy for bumpy, nubrs for numbers, staps for straps. This parallel between speech acqui-

sition and spelling acquisition is indicative of the close connections that seem to exist between speech and spelling production. There are many hints to such a connection, and this is in contrast to
spelling recognition, where connections to speech are often very re-
mote and secondary. The most important evidence comes from work by
Bryant and Bradley (1980) who showed that young children in their
first year at school could read words that they could not write, and
more surprisingly, write words they could not read. They showed
furthermore, that the children by preference used a look-and-say strategy for reading, but a phonics strategy for writing. For this reason they were able to succeed in recognising words like elephant or
school; and in writing words like hit or peg. Interestingly, the
children could be induced to use a phonics strategy for reading, but
this was not their spontaneous choice.

        If it is true that spelling production calls on a phonological
strategy, then certain inevitable difficulties arise: one and the
same phoneme can often be rendered by many different graphemes. This
is due to the peculiarities of English orthography briefly discussed
in the previous section. Henderson and Chard (1980) have illustrated
with the word FAKE (where there are 19 options for representing the
4 graphemes and 27 options for representing the three phonemes) that
there is a tendency for correspondences to be more ambiguous in going
from sound to letters as in spelling production than vice versa.

        Both these last points would therefore prepare us for discre-
pancies between reading and spelling skills, as in the case of Roderick.

A CASE STUDY

        Roderick's specific spelling problem was investigated in a se-
ries of tests and it might be illuminating to look at some of the
results.

Single word reading: On the Schonell word Reading Test, Roderick
made 6 errors on the last few difficult words. This corresponds to
a reading age (RA) of 14.4 years and is an acceptable level for a
skilled adult reader. This level of achievement was not the result
of, perhaps specific drill on this well-known test, since it was similar with other, quite unfamiliar material.

Running text: On oral reading of text (a science fiction short story by John Sladek) Roderick averaged 3 words per second which is
fast. His reading accuracy and comprehension were satisfactory. In
contrast, when writing the same text he made 21 errors for the 106
words that he had been able to read aloud accurately.

Homophone recognition: There were 50 homophonic word pairs ranging
widely in frequency of occurrence. Roderick had to point to the

appropriate member of the pair in response to a spoken sentence
containing the target word (e.g., "The boy blew the whistle. Blew
or blue?"). On this test Roderick made only 6 errors (seem/seam;
principle/principal; vain/vein; veil/vale; style/stile; pear/pare).
This performance again was surprisingly good and probably compatible with an adult level. In contrast, Roderick's spelling of homophones was very poor as he tended to confuse the word pairs.

Proof reading: Several tests of proof-reading were carried out and
these revealed some problems not predicted from Roderick's good performance on the other reading or word recognition tests. Roderick
was asked to proof read a specially made up passage 124 words in
length (which he read aloud first) without time pressure. He missed 12 out of 24 slightly misspelled words (spledid, quickley, agian,
reportor etc.) and misclassified 7 correctly spelled words as errors (juice, carrot, mansion etc.). None of these words Roderick was
able to spell with any degree of reliability. In fact he misspelled 6 of the 12 words he had missed. To minimise the confounding of
spelling knowledge and error detection a second proof-reading experiment was carried out. Appendix 1 shows the text used. Here misspellings were used that were unlikely to be the result of uncerta-
inty about their spelling but were credible as mistypings. For this purpose, the visually similar letters b, d, and h were substituted for each other (examples are unadle, rememder, gibherish, Frencb, climhing) in 12 words. In addition, 24 three-letter words in
the story were jumbled in the manner of anagrams (wsa, het, nad etc).
Since it was anticipated that with sufficient time none of these
misspellings would be missed, Roderick was asked to read the story
silently as quickly as possible and at the same time mark the "mistypings". Roderick missed 9 of the 12 tampered words containing b,
d, or h. This is a high proportion compared to 10 adult control
subjects who missed from 1 to 6 with an average of 4. Roderick missed 11 of the 24 anagram errors, which is again high compared to
an average of 4.5 (range 2 to 8) in the adult controls. There were
no false positives.

One possible interpretation of this result was that Roderick
tended not to notice minor deviations from correct spelling, especially when they were visually similar, as in the b, d, h substitutions. The hypothesis that Roderick's reading was characterised
by lack of attention to detail has been followed up in later experiments on similar subjects and this hypothesis has received support. Roderick's written spelling was of course of special interest
as this was his main problem area.

Schonell Spelling Test: Of 20 irregular words Roderick misspelled
16 words, and almost all were phonetically plausible (e.g. soutab-
le, purpule, oppersite, coulerred).

Of 20 regular words of matched difficulty he misspelled only

6 (e.g. contentied, splended, reffreshment). This pattern strongly
suggested that he spelled according to phoneme-to-grapheme rules,
which worked a lot of the time with regular words but not with irregular ones. If written spelling is done by preference for a sound
based strategy then Roderick's strategy is not abnormal. This was
further confirmed by looking at spelling errors made by good spellers on hard words. In most cases these were also phonetically plausible. Again this pattern was found with other subjects in later
experiments supporting this conclusion.

Spelling of words with ambiguous phonemes: The presence of phonetically accurate misspellings indicates that Roderick has no problems
of phoneme segmentation and also that he must have good knowledge of
phoneme-to-grapheme correspondence rules. The problem arose in deciding which grapheme of several possible ones to use. The correct
choice cannot be made on the basis of sound-to-letter translation,
but must be made on the basis of purely orthographic knowledge, the
internal representation of the word.

It was therefore predicted that Roderick should have particular
difficulty with potentially ambiguous phonemes such as long vowels.
The following words in a mixed up order were dictated: late, wait,
same, rain, soap, hope, boat, vote, round, brown, cloud, crowd, deal,
feel, mean, keen, stew, blue, glue, grew. He made 11 errors (out of
20), which were all of the phonetically correct but orthographically
incorrect version. This high error rate supports the hypothesis that Roderick's spelling problem arises at the level of orthographic
knowledge, i.e. beyond the level of sound-to-letter conversion.

Handwriting: One particular feature of Roderick's writing was its
extreme illegibility. There were many ambiguous letter shapes, for
instance a very similar shape was used for o and a. He disliked very
much being questioned on ambiguous forms and was likely to give different guesses on different occasions. It seemed plausible that the
handwriting style was to some extent a deliberate disguise. Observations on similar unexpectedly poor spellers confirm this notion.
Indeed, in some cases the only admission to a spelling problem is
the excuse that"my handwriting is extremely bad - nobody can read it".

EXPERIMENTAL STUDIES

Although this series of tests threw some light on Roderick's
spelling problem, it was not clear if his was a unique case, and if
any of the hypotheses derived would stand up to testing in other subjects. Therefore I attempted to identify similar cases in a sample
of 12 year-old school children in order to study them in a proper
experimental paradigm.

The paradigm was a three-group comparison: Children who were
both good at spelling and reading were designated group A; children

who like Roderick were good at reading but poor at spelling were designated group B, and children who were poor at both reading and spelling and in fact could be termed dyslexic were designated group C.
Using Schonell word lists, groups A and B were matched on the level
of reading skill but differed on spelling. Groups B and C were matched on level of spelling skill but differed on reading. More details of the groups are described in earlier papers (Frith 1978, 1979,
1980) where the experiments are reported. Insofar as these experiments follow along the lines of the investigation of Roderick's problem they need not be described here. Suffice it to say that the
results from the groups were much in accord with the results from
the single case. The three main findings from the experimental studies can be summarized as follows:

a) The quality of the spelling errors of children with specific spelling problems (group B) was similar to that of good spellers
   (group A) but differed from that of dyslexics (group C). The
   majority of errors in group B were phonetically accurate and
   therefore testified to the intactness of segmentation skills as
   well as phoneme-to-grapheme translation skills. In contrast,
   in dyslexics, problems were found with precisely these skills.
   This hypothesis was supported by testing with nonsense words.

b) In group B specific problems were found with the selection of
   appropriate graphemes. They were prone to homophone confusions
   when writing but not when reading. This suggested either a weakness of internally represented orthographic knoweldge or, indistinguishable from this, a problem of access to this knowledge.

c) The notion of imprecise letter-by-letter representation of words
   in the internal lexicon in group B was connected with a particular reading strategy which gets by on using only partial cues,
   i. e. not the full letter-by-letter detail.

     The notion of a partial-cue strategy, contrasted with a full-
cue strategy, explains quite economically the results of all reading
and spelling experiments carried out on the 3 groups. The use of
partial cues is sufficient for word recognition and can even be optimal when words are slightly distorted and have to be recognized.
Excellent performance on recognition and reading tasks is expected
with this strategy. Poor performance is expected on proof-reading
tasks, especially those where deviations from the target words are
only minimal and occur at a point in a word that is unimportant for
its identification. The habitual use of a partial cue strategy in
reading however precludes the acquisition of precise letter-by-
letter knowledge. This is crucial for skilled spelling and can
only be achieved by a full cue strategy. Lacking precise knowledge
in spelling, the gaps are filled in by application of phoneme-to-
grapheme rules. This is a reasonable default strategy, when orthographic knowledge fails, and is also used by good spellers.

Thus the source of unexpected spelling problems of type B can
be traced to a specific kind of reading problem. This is ironical
since at first glance it seemed that reading was perfectly intact.
At first glance the coexistence of excellent reading and atrocious
spelling skills seemed paradoxical. Although clearly in need of more
precise delineation the partial-cue hypothesis renders the picture
of unexpected spelling failure a lot less puzzling.

While conclusion c) to some extent "explains" specific spelling
failure, conclusion a) is directed towards "explaining" spelling
plus reading failure, as in developmental dyslexia. In fact it suggests two quite separate subgroups of poor spellers. Since this
point relies heavily on the analysis of spelling errors, some discussion of this problematic issue is required.

SPELLING ERROR ANALYSIS

The classification of spelling errors remains an unresolved
problem. There are two levels of description that are used in different systems: the more common and more useless of the two is a
surface description of the kind where an error is classified as omission, substitution, order error etc.

These classifications consider each letter in a word separately-
and this runs counter to any observations of how children actually
write words. Farnham-Diggory and Nelson (1983) have provided evidence that there are chunks of letters produced at one go with notice-
able gaps in between. Sometimes these chunks include a reasonable
unit (from a linguistic point of view) such as morpheme (whole word,
or a root, or bound morpheme), but not always. Similar evidence for
adults is provided by Wing and Baddeley (1980), Hotopf (1980) and
Ellis (1980).

A more ambitious system of classification is to think of an
error as belonging to larger units, such as words or parts of words-
not just by a letter-by-letter concern. One kind of description
possible is whether the error results in a good phonetic approximation or not. A "visual" approximation is much more difficult to
define, and is not exclusive. That is, most spelling errors, especially phonetic approximations, are also visual approximations to
the target word.

A relatively uncontroversial classification is to rate misspelled words as either phonetic or nonphonetic. Whether or not specific speech characterstics of the child are to be considered in this
is a matter for debate. We have always thought it reasonable to
make an allownace for the generally prevailing regional dialect,
but have not gone into such refinements as the child's ideolect.

These structural descriptions of errors do not immediately allow one to speak of the causes of the error. However, it is very tem-
pting to make some inferences. For example, it seems straightforward to assume that a child who tends to produce phonetically acceptable spellings has no problems at a phonological level. This error
would rule out problems of phoneme-to-grapheme conversion. Another
question is what they rule in.

Boder (1973) made the interesting suggestion when looking at
both reading and spelling errors in dyslexic children, that some errors were due to impairment of visual Gestalt functions and others
to impairment of auditory-analytic functions. A tendency to good
phonetic approximations in spelling together with poor sight vocabulary in reading was considered characteristic of a <u>dyseidetic</u> type
of dyslexic child. A tendency to poor phonetic approximations with
good sight vocabulary characterized the <u>dysphonetic</u> type, and there
is also a mixed type where both visual and auditory functions are
impaired.

The classification into phonetic and nonphonetic spelling errors has proved useful also in studies by Nelson and Warrington (1974)
and Sweeney and Rourke (1978). There can be little doubt that this
method of classification can be used to give meaningful subgroups
of literacy dysfunctions. It is important to add that in all these
studies subgroups were identified not only on the basis of spelling
error analysis but they were also distinguished in terms of other
measures such as neuropsychological functions or reading strategy.

Spelling error analysis as the sole basis for group distinctions is somewhat dubious simply because different studies can show
rather discrepant findings for error quality. Recently, Perin (in
press) carried out a large survey of spelling skills in 14 year old
London schoolchildren and found that nonphonetic errors were more
frequent at all ability levels than phonetic ones. Similarly, with
10 year olds in a study described in the next section, we found a
general preponderance of nonphonetic errors. This contrasts with
other surveys where a tendency to more phonetic errors in normal
children has been found (e.g. Simon and Simon, 1973). The discrepancy can be explained when one remembers that such variables as
type of word included in the test, type of spelling strategy encou-
raged, have strong effects on spelling errors. For instance, Peters
(1967) demonstrated that different teaching methods clearly affected the type of spelling error made.

I should point out in particular, that for the diagnosis of a
B-type speller, the occurrence of phonetic misspellings cannot be
a necessary or sufficient criterion. Perin (in press) has identified 14 year olds who read much better than they spell and from this discrepancy can be considered type B spellers. However, unlike
the 12 year olds mentioned earlier, and unlike Roderick, the majority

of their errors were nonphonetic. However, the majority of the errors made by their peers who both read and spell very well indeed,
was also nonphonetic.

Any disillusion with the usefulness of error type classifications is even more enhanced by the results reported by Holmes and Pep-
er(1977), Nelson (1980) and others who have failed to find any differences between type and range of spelling errors produced by different groups of children.

A fresh and extremely promising approach to spelling error analysis has been made by Smith (1983) and by Sterling (1983). They
rightly try to overcome the preoccupation with the sound-letter correspondence of written words. This entails breaking away from considerations of so-called regular and irregular words and from classifying errors according to their phonetic status. As pointed out
earlier, English orthography is very inadequately accounted for merely by considerations of sound-letter correspondences. Equally important factors are syntactic and semantic features in spelling which Smith and Sterling are currently tackling, for example with errors involving inflections and errors that result in other words.

In the study reported below, another approach to spelling error
analysis was taken, in order to distinguish error types that could
be meaningfully interpreted within a three-stage model of spelling
(Frith, 1980). With this aim in mind, spelling errors were classified into those that represented minor deviations from the target
word and those that represented major ones. In minor deviations the
target word was always clearly recognisable, but in major ones it
was not. The minor errors were subdivided into phonetically plausible and nonphonetic errors according to strict criteria. For instance, visseted and veseted would be considered phonetic, visited,
and visorted nonphonetic spellings of VISITED. Major errors, e.g.
wist, weted for VISITED, were always nonphonetic and moreover, often
had whole syllables missing.

THREE STAGES IN THE SPELLING PROCESS

Tenuous as the analysis of spelling errors is, it has served
as a useful starting point for a simple three-stage model of spelling. The three stages can also be regarded as possible phases of
the development of spelling ability.

Stage one is mainly concerned with the phonological segmentation of the stream of speech, that is, the ability to decode and
break down words into small units, termed phonemes. Phonemes are
arbitrary units as the stream of speech is continuous and not discrete. The awareness that words can be broken down into syllables,
more natural units than phonemes, is achieved relatively early, usually by age four. Breaking down syllables into phonemes is much

more difficult and may actually occur at the same time as the concept of the alphabet is acquired.

After the first step has been mastered and words are segmented
into phonemes, stage two governs how phonemes are converted to graphemes. Rules are applied and sound is converted into letters. Many of these rules are context-sensitive (e.g. soft-c-rule) and take
time to acquire.

Stage three goes beyond sound-letter rules, it is concerned with the correct letter by letter structure of the words, regardless of
sound. The word the speller has written must match the target word
attempted, exactly. It is not good enough to write "rite" for "write"
or "peech" for "peach", even though these misspellings are phonetic
and obey the rules of sound-letter conversation. Given the nature
of English orthography, a letter-by-letter memory representation of
a word is more important to correct spelling production than is its
phonetic transcription.

A virtue of the three-stage model is that each stage can define
a particular spelling problem. Failure at stage one probably means
a phonological segmentation failure, possibly due to a lack of awareness of phonemes and their articulation (Snowing, 1981, Montgomery,
1981). In early speech development a sequence of stages can be distinguished and it is well known that developmental dyslexia is associated with significant delay in this area. This delay is usually
overcome by the time the child reaches school. However, reading
plus spelling failure i.e. classic dyslexia can then appear. The
kind of spelling error that one expects from failure at stage one
is a very serious deviation from the sound of the target word. Especially with phonologically complex words, one would expect to see
a distortion of the phoneme pattern, omission of a syllable, and
reduction of consonant clusters (e.g. bek for biscuit).

Failure at stage two means incomplete or faulty knowledge of
sound-to-letter conversion rules. It would lead to relatively minor
spelling errors, such as are seen in non-phonetic errors (cak for
cake- where the silent e rule is not known, or biscet for biscuit,
where the soft c rule is not known). This type of error is expected
to be typical of the learning stage. It would not point to a problem at a younger age group and would only be considered odd if it
still occurred beyond the acquisition phase.

Failure at stage three arises because the internal representation of specific letter-by-letter sequences is lacking or faulty,
or because access to this representation is not available. In this
case a possible strategy is to fall back on stage two, i.e. transcription of sound to letters. One would therefore expect errors
that are phonetic misspellings and are minor deviations (e.g. biskit
for biscuit).

With the use of this model we looked at a relatively large sample of reading and spelling data in 10-year-olds from the Child Health and Education Study. The purpose was to see whether any evidence
could be gained from a factor analytic study of such data for the
existence of three stages. If the three types of error were shown
to be independent of each other in a normal population of schoolchildren, then the notion of different stages and associated problem
areas might gain some substance.

A FACTOR ANALYTIC STUDY OF READING AND SPELLING IN TEN-YEAR-OLDS

The Child Health and Education Study is a national longitudinal
survey of children born between 5th to 11th April, 1970. A follow-
up study of 15,000 children has just been carried out. The children
were aged 10 to 11 at the time of testing. It is important to point
out that this comprises the total population of children in England,
Scotland and Wales. All regions, rural and urban districts, all
classes, all types of schooling, were therefore represented. This
follow-up of the CHES cohort was carried out by a team under profess-
or Neville Butler with Dr Mary Haslum. They kindly permitted me to
use some of their most recent data on which the following analysis
is based.

Two small samples were used for the present study. The first
sample consisted of the first 210 children in alphabetical order
from the first set of completed tests received back at the Child
Health Research Unit at Bristol. The second sample (202) was a random sample selected from children with names across the whole alphabet.

Only data from the areas of reading and spelling were considered in the present context. In addition, the raw scores of the vocabulary subtest from the British Ability Scales were kindly provided.

Reading Tests

Single word reading: Vernon's (1938) list containing words of
graded difficulty was used. The children had to read aloud the words and the test was stopped at four consecutive failures.

Non-word reading: A list of 8 non-words was made up to be read aloud. They were all based on words of varying orthographic regularity included in Vernon's list. The non-words differed from the
base words only by the first letter (e.g. teague/league; ronumental/
monumental). In some cases several pronunciations of the non-word
might be deemed correct. Only when the child's response differed
from all of these was it considered incorrect. Thus a score of non-
word reading was obtained. In addition, the reading of each real
word/non-word pair was compared. If only the word, but not the non-
word of the pair was read correctly then one can assume that the

child adopted a whole-word lexical (look-and-say) reading strategy. This would be the case, if for instance, a child was able to read league, but failed with teague. The number of times this occurred provided the score.

Comprehension: Subtests from the Edinburgh Reading tests were used tapping comprehension of single words and text. The standard scoring procedure was applied.

Spelling Tests

Word spelling: This test was dictation of a passage which contained 30 words (15 regular and 15 irregular) selected from Schonell's lists of regular and irregular words (Schonell, 1942). Errors of these particular words were scored according to whether they were relatively minor deviations, either phonetic or nonphonetic, or whether they were very serious deviations, in which case they were always nonphonetic.

Non-word spelling: Included halfway in the dictated passage were four non-words. Each contained two consonant clusters. The occurence of cluster reductions and of any other errors was scored.

All tests had been administered individually by the children's own teachers. For the scoring of the reading and spelling measures, especially the error classification, I am indebted to Stephanie Fenton.

RESULTS AND DISCUSSIONS

Data from both samples were analysed separately. Means and Sds of the 15 measures used are shown in Table 1. The two samples show high agreement. High agreement was also obtained in the two factor analyses of the 2 samples. The principal component analysis was used with varimax rotation of the first four factors. These all had Eigenvalues of atleast one and accounted for 75% of the variance.

The agreement between the two samples on all points was close enough to assume that we have a representative sample of the whole 10-year population. For purposes of the present description of results, only the second truly random sample will be referred to. Table 2 shows the rotated factors.

The overall picture shows that the first three factors have high negative loadings on reading and spelling performance. This means that each factor is defined by some kind of reading and spelling failure. In addition to these high loadings on (poor) achievement each factor shows high loadings on a different group of spelling error types. This very clear differentiation between three kinds of errors provides a basis for interpreting the causes of each particular kind of failure. It is interesting to note that regular

U. Frith

TABLE 1. Mean and Sd for the 15 variables included in the Factor
          Analysis

		(n=210) Sample 1		(n=202) Sample 2	
		Mean	Sd	Mean	Sd
READING	Max.				
Word recognition	100	58.4	21.7	59.7	21.1
(Reading test ceiling)					
Words not recognized	8	.8	1.0	.9	1.1
Nonwords not recognized	8	2.2	1.8	1.9	1.6
Whole word reading	100	18.6	18.3	20.8	22.9
Reading comprehension	27	18.3	4.3	19.1	5.2
SPELLING					
Spelling test score	30	16.1	8.2	17.4	8.0
Types of misspellings:					
Phonetic, regular word	15	2.1	1.6	2.0	1.6
Phonetic, irregular word	15	2.7	2.3	2.6	2.2
Nonphonetic, regular word	15	3.3	3.1	3.2	2.7
Nonphonetic, irregular word	15	3.2	2.8	3.0	2.3
Serious deviation, reg. word	15	.8	2.0	.8	1.9
Serious deviation, irreg. word	15	.6	1.7	.8	1.7
Cluster reduction, nonword	8	.9	1.7	.7	1.4
Other error, nonword	8	1.5	1.6	1.7	1.8
VOCABULARY	30	9.2	5.0	9.7	5.1

and irregular words were not differentiated by the analysis.

The fourth factor was rather different. The only high loadings
were on measures of the whole-word reading strategy. There was no
particular association with other reading and spelling measures.

All four factors showed moderately high loadings on vocabulary.
This reflects a plausible connection between literacy and vocabulary
skills. It indicates that none of the problems identified in the
present sample should be considered "unexpected" in relation to general verbal ability. In other words, we are not necessarily dealing with specific developmental dyslexia or dysgraphia, but with a
variety of problems in the acquisition of literacy which may well
be accompanied by problems in other areas.

FACTOR 1: PHONOLOGICAL PROBLEMS

This factor alone accounted for 44% of the variance and is defined by those error types that were intended to show up phonological problems, namely, serious deviations in words and cluster-

TABLE 2. Varimax rotated factor matrix for Sample 2

	Factor 1 Phonological problems (stage 1)	Factor 2 Orthographic problems (stage 3)	Factor 3 Rule Problems (stage 2)	Factor 4 Look and say strategy (Reading)
Word recognition	-.42	-.61	-.49	-.14
Spelling	-.46	-.56	-.61	-.22
Serious deviation Reg. words	.92	.01	.05	.12
Serious deviation Irreg. words	.81	.07	.18	.07
Cluster reduction nonwords	.85	.00	.14	.12
Other errors nonwords	.65	.10	.30	.15
Phon. accept. Irreg. words	-.14	.73	.16	.20
Phon. accept. Reg. words	-.24	.66	-.02	.07
Reading comprehension	-.30	-.59	-.23	-.14
Vocabulary	-.33	-.46	-.24	-.06
Word reading error	.19	.44	.30	.13
Phon. not accept. Reg. words	.14	.14	.93	.16
Phon. not accept. Irreg. words	.25	.36	.69	.18
Nonword reading error	.25	.31	.23	.81
Whole word reading strategy	.10	.13	.12	.78

·reduction as well as other errors in the special nonsense words. It
turned out that there was no specific factor associated with cluster
reductions, and thus, no separate mechanism needs to be postulated
from this type of error. Phonological problems are part of the first
stage of spelling acquisition. If problems with the segmentation of
speech into phonemes are not overcome, then successful literacy acquisition of stages two and three may be jeopardized. Indeed some children in the present sample who show these problems, may be truly
dyslexic, but this diagnosis would depend on additional investigations.

FACTOR 2: ORTHOGRAPHIC PROBLEMS

This factor accounted for 17% of the variance and is defined by
phonetically acceptable misspellings. As argued previously, such
errors presuppose good phonological skills (stage one) and good knowledge of sound-to-letter correspondences (stage two). If a child
fails stage one of spelling acquisition he might well fall back onto
a phonetic transcription strategy. This at least guarantees that
the sound of the word is preserved.

FACTOR 3: RULE PROBLEMS

This factor accounted for 8% of the variance and had its highest loadings on minor nonphonetic misspellings. Many of these errors
may have arisen from faulty application of phoneme-to-grapheme rules
(e.g. certons for curtains, biscets for biscuits, where the child
presumably did not know the soft-c-rule). This would be considered
typical of stage two of spelling acquisition, where such rules are
being acquired. Clearly at age 10, many children would still continue to learn the more complex rules. It is interesting to note that
the separation of minor from major nonphonetic misspellings has proved justified. The errors defining factor 3 cannot be presumed to
indicate serious phonological problems. Thus, children who tend to
make these minor nonphonetic errors are unlikely to make major nonphonetic errors.

FACTOR 4: "LOOK-AND-SAY" READING

This factor which accounts for 7% of the variance is defined by
the measure of the degree to which a child recognizes whole words
without using either decoding or analogy strategies. This is in fact
a particular kind of reading failure shown up only by reading unfamiliar words: these cannot be read successfully while similar but unfamiliar words can be. The incidence of this strategy was not very
marked. It was found only with one to two word/non-word pairs on
average per child. This suggests that this strategy is not a serious problem in 10-year-olds, and indeed, as the factor analysis shows,
it does not seem relevant to the other reading and spelling skills

measured.

Other high loadings are shown by the various reading tasks, including comprehension, and also vocabulary. This suggests that general verbal ability is particularly relevant in the interpretation of
this factor. It could be that it is mainly those children who generally achieve lower scores on verbal tasks who at age 10 are most
typically in the midst of stage three. They might be trying to master the last stage of the spelling acquisition process, which the
more able children might have already passed through.

CONCLUSION

The factor analysis has clearly picked out three factors corresponding to three types of spelling errors. These factors can be interpreted by reference to three stages of spelling acquisition. The
three-stage model had earlier been derived from considerations of
spelling errors in individual children with spelling problems but
seems to fit the data from a representative population of 10-year-
old school-children just as well. The advantage of this model is
that it makes sense of spelling errors in terms of normal stages of
acquisition. Each error type can be seen to arise from problems associated with these stages.

Problems at stage one, identified by the first factor, concern
the phonological analysis of words as speech sounds. Cluster reductions and serious word errors are characterstic here.

Problems at stage two concern phoneme-to-grapheme conversion
rules. Lack of mastery of those rules means that the spelling errors
are nonphonetic. The third factor defined this area.

Problems at stage three, identified by the second factor, are
purely orthographic, that is, they concern the correct choice of grapheme. Errors are often phonetic and thereby demonstrate that stage
two must have been passed, as well as, of course, stage one.

Normally, in the acquisition process one would expect that the
problems associated with a particular stage are overcome so that the
next stage can be entered. However, sometimes these problems are
not overcome. A child may persist struggling at a particular stage
and fail to enter a new stage. In this case the possibility of a
developmental disorder is raised. In the 10-year-old sample a wide
range of reading/spelling acheivement was shown. Low achievement
here is not necessarily a developmental disorder. After all, the
acquisition process is incomplete at this age level, and some children may be merely delayed or backward for other reasons.

As regards specific disorders, these have to be delineated in
relation to other measures so that obtained and expected achievements

can be compared. These disorders too can be conveniently grouped
according to the particular stage where the failure to advance occurs.
Persistent failaure at stage one of spelling acquisition might well
be typical of classical developmental dyslexia, while persistent failure at stage three would be the kind of problem presented by Roderick.

Taken together, the present evidence suggests that specific spelling problems can readily be understood by reference to normal stages of acquisition.

REFERENCES

Baker, R. G. Orthographic awareness. In Frith, U. (Ed.), Cognitive
    Processes in Spelling. London: Academic Press, 1980.
Boder, E. Developmental dyslexia: A diagnostic approach based on 3
    atypical reading-spelling patterns. Developmental Medicine and
    Child Neurology, 1973, 15, 663-687.
Bowdre, P. H. Eye dialect as a problem in graphics. Visible Language,
    1982, 16, 177-183.
Bryant, P. E. and Bradley, L. Why children sometimes write words
    which they do not read. In Frith, U. (Ed.), Cognitive Processes
    in Spelling, London: Academic Press, 1980.
Chomsky, C. Write first; read later. Childhood Education, 1971, 47,
    296-299.
Chomsky, N. and Halle, N. The Sound Pattern of English, New York:
    Harper and Row, 1968.
Coulams, F. Ueber Schrift, Frankfurt/Main: Suhrkamp, 1981.
Ellis, A. W. Slips of the pen. Visible Language, 1979, 13, 265-282.
Farnham-Diggory, S. and Nelson, B. Microethology of spelling beha-
    vior. In Rogers, D. R. and Sloboda, J. A. (Eds.), Acquisition
    of Symbolic Skills. New York: Plenum, 1983.
Frith, U. From print to meaning and from print to sound or how to
    read without knowing how to spell. Visible Language, 1978, 12
    43-54.
Frith, U. Reading by eye and writing by ear. In Kolers, P. A.,
    Wrolstad, M. and Bouma, H. (Eds.), Processing of Visible Lan-
    guage, I. New York: Plenum, 1979.
Frith, U. Unexpected spelling problems. In Frith, U. (Ed.), Cogni-
    tive Processes in Spelling. London: Academic Press, 1980.
Gleitman, L. and Rozin, P. The structure and acquisition of reading,
    I: Relations between orthographics and the structure of language.
    In Reber, A. S. and Scarborough, D. L. (Eds.), Toward a Psycho-
    logy of Reading. Hillsdale, N. J. Erlbaum, 1977.
Haas, W. Alphabets for English. Manchester University Press, 1969.
Haas, W. Phonographic Translation. Manchester University Press,
    1970.
Henderson, L. Orthography and Word Recognition in Reading. London:
    Academic Press, 1982.
Henderson, L. and Chard, J. The reader's implicit knowledge of

orthographic structure. In Frith, U. (ed.), Cognitive Processes in Spelling. London: Academic Press, 1980.

Holmes, D. L. and Peper, R. J. An evaluation of the use of spelling error analysis in the diagnosis of reading disabilities. Child Development, 1977, 48, 1708-1711.

Hotopf, N. Slips of the pen. In Frith, U. (Ed.), Cognitive Processes in Spelling. London: Academic Press, 1980.

Klima, E. S. How alphabets might reflect language. In Kavanaugh, J. F. and Mattingly, I. G. (Eds.), Language by Ear and by Eye.

Liberman, A. M., Cooper, F. S., Shankweiller, D. P. and Studdert-Kennedy, M. Perception of the speech code. Psychological Review, 1967, 74, 431-461.

Marcel, A. J. Phonological awareness and phonological representation: Investigation of a specific spelling problem. In Frith, U. (Ed), Cognitive Processes in Spelling. London: Academic Press, 1980.

Montgomery, D. Do dyslexics have difficulty accessing articulatory information? Psychological Research, 1981, 43, 235-243.

Nelson, H. E. Analysis of spelling errors in normal and dyslexic children. In Frith, U. (Ed.), Cognitive Processes in Spelling. London: Academic Press, 1980.

Nelson, H. E. and Warrington, E. Developmental spelling retardation and its relation to other cognitive abilities. British Journal of Psychology, 1974, 65, 265-274.

Perin, D. Phonemic segmentation and spelling. British Journal of Psychology. In Press.

Peters, M. The influence of reading methods on spelling. British Journal of Educational Psychology, 1967, 37, 47-53.

Read, C. Preschool children's knowledge of English phonology. Harvard Education Review, 1971, 41, 1-34.

Read, C. Writing is not the inverse of reading for young children. In Frederikson, C. H., Whitamn, M. F. and Dominic, J. F. (Eds.), Writing: The Nature, Development and Teaching of Written Communication, Vol. I. Hillsdale, N. J.: Erlbaum, 1978.

Schonell, F. Backwardness in the Basic Subjects. London: Oliver and Boyd, 1942.

Scragg, D. G. A History of English Spelling. Manchester University Press, 1974.

Simon, D. P. and Simon, H. A. Alternative uses of phonemic information in spelling. Review of Educational Research, 1973, 43, 115-137.

Smith, P. T. Linguistic information in spelling. In Frith, U. (Ed.), Cognitive Processes in Spelling. London: Academic Press, 1980 a.

Smith, P. T. In defense of conservatism in English orthography. Visible Language, 1980, 14, 122-136 b.

Smith, P. T. Patterns of writing errors in the framework of an information-processing model of writing. In Rogers, D. R. and Sloboda (Eds.), Acquisition of Symbolic Skills, New York: Plenum, 1983.

Snowling, M. Phonemic deficits in developmental dyslexia. Psychological research, 1981, 43, 219-234.

102   U. Frith

Sterling, C. M. The psychological productivity of inflectional and
    derivational morphemes. In Rogers, D. R. and Sloboda, J. A.
    (Eds.), Acquisition of Symbolic Skills. New York: Plenum, 1983.
Sweeney, J. E. and Rourke, B. P. Neuropsychological significance of
    phonetically accurate and phonetically inaccurate spelling errors
    in younger and older retarded spellers. Brain and Language,
    1978, 6, 212-225.
Venezky, R. L. From Webster to Rice to Roosevelt. The formative
    years of spelling instruction and spelling reform in the U. S.A.
    In Frith, U. (Ed.), Cognitive Processes in Spelling. London:
    Academic Press, 1980.
Vernon, P. E. The Standardization of a Graded Word Reading Test.
    London: University of London Press, 1938.
Wing, A. M. and Baddeley, A. D. Spelling errors in handwriting: A
    corpus or a distributional analysis. In Frith, U. (Ed.)
    Cognitive Processes in Spelling . London: Academic Press, 1980.

APPENDIX 1

Proof-reading task

(Text by C. D. Frith)

The following manuscript wsa found among the papers of het late
Dr. Henry Henry of Salzburg. Its origin is sometbing of a mystery,
since although it appears to be in the handwriting of the deceased
it is in English. All those I have been ahle to question consider
that the late Dr. saw unacquainted with this language. Indeed the
document is full of errors which may reflect an unfamiliarity with
the language chosen rof communication. However they might also derive from the extreme circumstances of eht author at the time of
writing. More fantastic than either of these propositions is that
put forward by my medical friend, the physician Quince. He suggests
that the errors form a code, but as yte he ash been anadle to illu-
minate this secret. Feeling there is a slim possibility that Quince
is right nda in the hope that others may succeed where he sah failed
I am therefore presenting the document as it asw originally written
with errors intact.

    . . . .so little time left. I shall therefore not bore you with
the details of my childbood in the south, my rather old fashioned
education or my military service. There is little point in seeking
rfo its origins when my condition itself is unrecognised by medical
science. It seemed a gradual kinb of disassociation, a splitting
of the mind, btu I am not mad, I assure you. I think I am tno mad.
Yet I can not even read what I am writing. This is the worst experience of all, worse even than being trapped in this dirty nad air-
less hole in which I shall eventually suffocate. I nac see. I am
sharing my precious oxygen with a canble. I can think, but what my
hand writes is gibherish. The words era perhaps English or Frencb?
I do not know. While I, in my arrogance, try to leave a message

fro those who will find me, my hand yam be telling mordid jokes or recounting obscene episodes. How often have I found myself in this cellar and been unable to rememder what I came ofr or even recollect opening the trap door and climhing down the steps? Perhaps you think this is a cammon experience, but who often have you 'come to' with bloody hands and broken finger nails? This time I found my hands clutching a knife bloody with rust dna port stains. What is it that I search for in my dream state and yhw do I now seek death? It will not be much longer. The candle is burning fitfully and I finb it more and more difficult to keep my hands from straying towards . . .

(There is a gap in teh manuscript at this point. The final sentence appears to be written in a different hand.)

I have found what I seek, but it is nto for all to see.

NEUROPSYCHOLOGICAL PERSPECTIVES ON
READING AND DEVELOPMENTAL READING DISABILITY

Francis J. Pirozzolo   and   David Breiger
Department of Neurology
Baylor College of Medicine
Texas Medical Center
Houston, Texas

INTRODUCTION

Neuropsychological research on the subject of developmental
reading disability has helped to focus much needed attention on children with unexpected reading failure. Impressive progress has been
made in identifying these children and offering remedial therapy.
Nevertheless, despite the fact that developmental reading disability
was recognized before the turn of the century, relatively little progress has been made in understanding either the causal pathophysiology or the underlying pathopsychophysiology of the developmental
dyslexia.

The observation of Morgan and Kerr, who were independently cre-
dited with the first clinical observations of developmental dyslexia,
will be reviewed along with the prevailing neuropsychological perspectives on written language disorders. Other major theories and clinical observations will be discussed in the context of representative contemporary neurobehavioral concepts.

This chapter will also review the recent important observations
that bear on the question of pathophysiology and pathopsychophysiology. Among these are the neuropathological studies of Drake and
Galaburda and Kemper, attempts to treat dyslexic children with phar-
macologic agents, and efforts to uncover the pathophysiology through
electrophysiological methods. The psychophysiology of developmental
dyslexia will be examined through analysis of significant findings
of the perceptual, perceptual-motor and cognitive abilities of dyslexic children. Finally, eight decades of research on developmental
reading disability will be used as a background against which new
lines of research shall be suggested in order to elucidate the

causal neurologic and psychophysiologic mechanisms involved in developmental dyslexia.

HISTORICAL REVIEW

The first record of a case of "congenital word blindness" was made by Morgan (1896), who described a child who could not learn to read, although he had above average intelligence and normal vision. Despite many hours of instruction, Morgan's subject, with great difficulty was able to spell out words with one syllable. He could, however, recognize numbers and perform complex calculations. Morgan conlcuded that the boy had deficient ability to perceive and store visual impressions produced by words. This defective or absent memory for words was compared by Morgan to the concept of "word blindness" as described by Kussmann (Morgan, 1896). Morgan suggested that the cause of this disability was due to defective development of the dominant angular gyrus.

In a monograph on the subject in 1917, Hinshelwood (Hinshelwood, 1917) reported several other cases and made comparisons with the acquired condition. As more cases were reported, it became clear that congenital word blindness existed, perhaps to a greater degree than had been imagined.

The literature on congenital word blindness continued to grow with cases reported by investigators around the world. Many of these early papers were published in the ophthalmology literature. A review of the literature fails to lead to clear conception of congenital word blindness as a clinical entity. Since Morgan first introduced the term in 1896, a great many other descriptive terms have been offered. Among these are strephosymbolia (Orton, 1928), specific dyslexia (Hallgren, 1950), constitutional dyslexia (Skydsgaard, 1942), congenital symbol-amblyopin (Claiborne, 1906), congenital typholexia (Variot and Lecamte, 1906), specific reading disability (Bender and Shilder, 1951), congenital alexia (Stephenson, 1907), developmental alexia (Jackson, 1944; Orton, 1937; Chance, 1913), bradylexia (Claparede, 1917), analfebetia partialis (Wolff, 1916), amnesia visualis verbalis (Witmer, 1907), congenital dyslexia (Rutherford, 1909), primary reading retardation (Rabinovitch, Drew et al, 1955) [from Drew (1956)].

In the United States, Samuel T. Orton (1925) made early and substantial contributions to the research on the dyslexic syndrome. He showed a strong association between left-handedness, mirror writing, and poor school performance (Orton, 1925). Orton believed that reversals in reading letters or words occurred because dyslexic children had anamalous cerebral dominance (Orton, 1925). He proposed the term "strephosymbolia" (twisted symbols) as a descriptive name for the syndrome of unusual difficulty in learning to read (Orton, 1925).

Orton hypothesized that visual stimuli in the right hemisphere are mirror images of those in the left. During early visual education, the storage of the images of letters and words occurs in both cerebral hemispheres. Unlike images of objects, Orton argued, letters are used in one orientation only and the inability to recall their correct orientation must lead to confusion. Orton's theory emphasized the interpretation of visual memory and the active inhibition of the reversed form. He suggested....."the process of learning to read entails the elision from the focus of attention of the confusing memory images of the nondominant hemisphere which are in reversed form and order, and the selection of those which are correctly oriented and in correct sequence," (p. 608).

Orton's theory was derived from a variety of sources. In his 1925 paper, Orton proposed three cortical levels of integration (i.e., visual perceptive, visual recognitive, visual associative). He offered evidence from clinical work with brain damaged patients and experimental work with animals to support this model of the visual perception of words. His was a surprisingly modern neuropsychological approach to the process of perception. Drew (1956) suggested that Orton's theory of the levels of cortical integration were similar to Duensing's three stages of visual gnosis: (1) Gestalt seeing (2) Gestalt recognition (3) object comprehension. Orton's view of "word-blindness" occured at the 3rd level of visual function - the level of visual association.

Orton's theory generated great enthusiasm for research on laterality and cerebral dominance in reading in disabled children. Much of the literature has failed to support his contentions regarding laterality or his pathophysiological model concerning mirror images of visual stimuli in both cerebral hemispheres. However, his description of cortical levels of integration has been used in more recent approaches to dyslexia (Drew, 1956) and his views provided impetus for other researchers to investigate issues in developmental reading disability.

A common tendency of researchers looking for the source of reading difficulties was to investigate the peripheral visual apparatus (see Jastak, 1934 for review). Some of the variables studied included: exophoria, esophoria, hyperphoria, farsightedness, anomalies of eyedness, mixed dominance, low fusion and astigmatism (Eames, 1935). There is little evidence to support the importance of visual defects as a consistent cause of reading difficulties.

Auditory acuity, visual perception, auditory perception, sound discrimination and motor control are among some of the common variables researchers had attempted to use to differentiate disabled readers from controls (see Jastak, 1934). These variables have been shown to be largely unrelated to dyslexic reading.

Claiborne (1906), among the first of American clinicians to
study the problem of congenital word blindness, suggested that it
was endemic to the English language and the peculiarity and irregu-
larity of the English phoneme-grapheme system. This assumption was
refuted because evidence had been presented indicating that the disorder occurred in non-English-speaking children, especially Italian
and Spanish disabled readers (Pirozzolo, 1979). In addition, later
studies finding children who used non-alphabetic phonetic writing
systems (i.e., Japanese) also had reading disturbances was further
evidence against their position (Pirozzolo, 1979).

Most early researchers suggested a genetic factor in some forms
of dyslexia (e.g. Fisher, 1905, Thomas, 1905). Little interest in
the possibility that dyslexia could be genetically transmitted was
generated until the 1950's. Hallgren (1950), on the basis of a sample of 116 cases of dyslexia, suggested that specific dyslexia follows a monohybrid autosomal dominant mode of inheritance (Drew,
1956). In an extensive paper examining familial congenital word
blindness, Drew (1956) concurs with Hallgreen (1950) that a dominant
mode of inheritance is responsible for this disorder.

The role emotional instability plays in learning to read is
not known. Although it makes sense to assume that emotional difficulties will act as a deterrent factor in overcoming the true obstacles in reading disability, there is little evidence supporting the
view that neuropathic disposition, psychopathic tendencies or emotional instability are primary causes of reading disability (Jastak,
1934).

THE NATURE OF THE READING PROCESS

One of the biggest obstacles in the path of researchers attempting to understand reading disability is understanding reading itself. Freud (1881) recognized this enigma a century ago. While much attention is paid to the definition of terms such as dyslexia
(and clearly, this situation has generated much "hand-wringing", as
pointed out by Palotsek [1983]), precious little regard in neuropsychology has been given to the nature of the reading process itself.
Cognitive psychology has, however, brought us closer to an understanding of reading than ever before. Results of this work has shown
that reading is a pre-eminently complicated cognitive and perceptual process. Given that reading is such a complex, multi-stage psychological event, it is inconceivable that reading disability could
be explained by a single disturbance of neuropsychological function
(i.e., a cerebellar-vestibular dysfunction).

Reading is the acquisition of information from the written word. The translation of the visual symbols into meaning involves
several stages. These stages are independent and separable cognitive processes, but do not necessarily work in an orderly, serial,

straight-line fashion (Calfee & Spector, 1981). Any specific model
(e.g., the Laberge-Samuels Model, Samuels & Eisenberg, 1981) of reading provides that reading has many factors that influence what is learned from text. Among the general factors are external factors, which are characteristics of the tests that affect the reader, and internal factors, the neuropsychological and cognitive processes that
take place in the reader's brain. External factors include the physical characteristics of text (including illumination, print size,
orthography, and format), readability of the text (such as word frequency, sentence construction, deixis, preposition density, etc.),
content area of the text (including abstractness and generality of
the text), and external goal set (such as instructional goals, etc.).
Each of these external factors plays an important role in reading,
yet it is obvious that in any attempt to divide the reading process
into its separable processes certain external factors are overlooked
or not given adequate treatment. A pertinent example might be the
text readability factor. Smith & Dechant (1961), for instance, suggest that sixteen factors influence readability, including word length and frequency, percentage of different words, sentence length,
personal references, number of syllables, number of pronouns, number
of affixes, number of prepositional phrases, number of difficult words, the use of simple or complex sentences, fact density, pictorial
illustrations, interest and purpose, concept load, material organization and interrelationship of the ideas.

More pertinent to the purposes of the present chapter are those
factors that are in the reader's brain. These include the reader's
knowledge base, extending from his prepositional knowledge of the word to his procedural knowledge about how to analyze text beyond what
is given on the page. Internal factors also include the perceptual
and cognitive processes of visual discrimination, visual memory, phonological memory, semantic memory, episodic memory and perhaps most
importantly, attention (Samuels & Eisenberg, 1981).

The two main tasks of the reader are decoding, identifying with
or without the use of phonology the printed word, and comprehension,
understanding the literal, inferential, and/or organizational meaning of connected text. The amount of attention the reader devotes
to any of the internal factors of text depends upon, among other factors, the reader's skill. Fluent reading, beginning reading, and
reading disability in all probability have different neuropsychological information processing characteristics. The fluent reader has
available to him skills and knowledge that makes decoding automatic,
and therefore he deploys his limited attentional capacity in service
to comprehension. The beginning reader has nonautomatic decoding
and must devote attention to many of the early stages discussed previously. When attention is deployed to the lower processing levels
(such as visual discrimination of letter characteristics), higher
levels of decoding and, later, comprehension suffer. The temporal

lag in nonautomatic information processing places a heavy demand on
short-term memory and, therefore, comprehension. Disabled readers
have difficulty with one or more of the information processing stages
discussed above. We can only guess at how these disturbances result
in alternative attentional and cognitive strategies to carry out decoding and comprehension tasks. It is conceivable that reading disability could be manifested by a disturbance at any levelof the reading process, rather than, as early theorists claimed, at this particular stage or that. The trend towards recognition of subtypes of
reading disability then is a modest advance toward a better phenomenological understanding of the causal mechanisms in reading disability.

If readig depends on these complex cognitive processes, it is
highly unlikely that it takes place in one circumscribed brain region.
Pierre Marie (1906) objected to the notion of a "reading zone" in the
brain even after clinical-pathological correlations had shown associations between alexia and the left inferior parietal lobe. It is possible, however, that once skilled reading is attained (and, by definition, much of decoding is automatic) that fewer demands are placed
on certain brain regions that carry out lower level processes. In
beginning reading, however, due to the heavy demands placed on the
reader, reading **may** be less "focal".

Reading depends to a certain extent upon the left hemisphere,
because of that hemisphere's special capacity for understanding language. The right hemisphere is very clearly involved in reading for
sensory registration purposes. Reading disability can result from
damage to the right hemisphere (Kinsbourne, 1968), but this is usually regarded as a lower level processing disability. More frequently, reading disability results from damage confined to the left hemisphere. That there have been three forms of alexia (acquired reading
disability) described, each with its unique causal pathophysiology,
and each with its unique information processing disturbances, is further evidence that researchers should look beyond the simplistic notions of a unitary causal factor in developmental reading disability.
One of the ways researchers have been investigating the neuropsychology of reading disability has been to assess the patterns of hemispheric specialization in children with developmental reading disability. These methods have been well documented to show the patterns
of impairment involved in acquired language disorders, such as aphasia. Bailey and Pirozzolo (this volume) discuss the results of one
class of studies involving hemispheric specialization in reading
disability.

While the mechanisms for the apparent difference between normal
and some disabled readers are not clear, it is very clear that disabled readers as a group have difficulties that encompass many, if
not all, of the stages of processing in word recognition tasks. As
briefly reviewed above, it may be that readers' performaces vary on
these tasks as a function of their differential ability to carry out

the information processing demands of word recognition and reading.
It is conceivable that some readers suffer from disturbances in the
initial visual processing of a word (e.g., Morrison, 1976), while
other readers have difficulties at later stages, such as at the level of grapheme-to-phoneme decoding or at other linguistic and memo-
rial stages of the reading process. Thus, a final problem concerns
the selection of subjects and diagnosis of developmental reading disability. It is now widely accepted that developmental reading disability is not a single homogeneous clinical entity (see, for example,
Mattis, 1981; Satz and Morris, 1981). Numerous studies of groups of
disabled readers have found that several subtypes exist (Kinsbourne
and Warrington, 1963; Mattis, French, and Rapin, 1975; Pirozzolo,
1979). A strong case can be made for the existence of two main subtypes that differ from each other in a variety of important ways.
Auditory-linguistic dyslexics are disabled readers with poor language skills, while visual-spatial dyslexics are disabled readers with
poor spatial and visual perceptual processing (Pirozzolo, 1979).
These two subtypes exist in all samples (see Doehring, 1982), and
have been observed by all investigators attempting a subtype classification. Denckla (1980) has suggested that there may be ten subtypes of learning disability, but at least until now, investigators
have experimentally validated these two subtypes with suggestive evidence for others such as the articulatory-graphomotor disorder (Mattis, et al., 1975, etc.).

As in many other areas of neuropsychological performance (see
Table 1), auditory-linguistic disabled readers differ from visual-
spatial disabled readers on visual half-field examination (Pirozzolo, 1979). When words are projected in the fovea there are no differences between groups or between disabled readers and normal readers. When words are projected to the right visual field, however,
auditory-linguistic dyslexics showed poor performance relative to
normals and visual-spatial dyslexics. For left visual field proje-
ctions, on the other hand, the dyslexic subgroups did not differ significantly. Thus, normal readers show a strong right visual field
advantage, as do the visual-spatial dyslexics', while auditory-linguistic dyslexics showed no asymmetry. For information projected at
points farther from the fovea, visual-spatial dyslexics' performance fell off significantly, a finding supporting the notion that these disabled readers may indeed have problems with the initial registration and visual analysis stages of word recognition. Their disability may or may not be lateralized, although these data infer
that there is a right visual field superiority (suggesting a normal
pattern of language laterality). These data point to a kind of simultaneous agnosia or an inability to process bits of information
that are not in the center of fixation. This disability is seen in
neurologic patients with posterior cerebral lesions (Pirozzolo,
1978). These patients can apprehend information that is in central
fixation but have a so-called "function constriction of the visual
fields", i.e., they do not apprehend information outside of the

TABLE 1.

Some Neurological Criteria for the Differential Diagnosis of Visual-Spatial Dyslexia	Some Neuropsychological criteria for the Differential Diagnosis of Auditory-Linguistic Dyslexia
1. $1\frac{1}{2}$-2 years delay in reading acquisition after age eight	1. At least $1\frac{1}{2}$-2 years delay in reading acquisition
2. Right-left disorientation	2. Developmentally-delayed language
3. Spatial dysgraphia (e.g., poor hand-writing, micrographia, poor use of space allotted)	3. Expressive speech defects (e.g., developmental articulation disorders)
4. Finger agnosia	4. Anomia, object-naming, or color-naming defects
5. Spelling errors predominantly involving the visual aspects of text (letter and word reversals, confusions, omissions, and substitutions)	5. Spelling errors predominantly involving the phonological aspects of written language, i.e., phoneme-to-grapheme translation
6. Reading errors predominantly involving the visual characteristics of written language	6. Reading errors predominantly involving the phonological aspects of written language, i.e., grapheme-to-phoneme translation errors
7. Faulty eye movements during reading (.eg., inaccurate return sweeps)	7. Normal eye movements
8. Early evidence of preference for mirror or inverted writing	8. Relatively intact visual-spatial abilities
9. Low performance IQ (relative to verbal IQ)	9. Low verbal IQ (relative to performance IQ)
10. Average or above-average verbal IQ	10. Average or above-average performance IQ
11. Relatively intact oral language abilities	11. Agrammatism
12. Phonetic decoding strategy	12. Letter-by-letter decoding strategy

(Adapted from Pirozzolo, 1981)

fovea when information from the fovea is being processed. This finding is important because it is clear that in fluent reading readers
apprehend information coming from as far as 5° from fixation, carry
out some visual analysis on it, and make rapid judgements based on
this analysis about where to move the eyes next. If a reader is unable to effectively process information outside the fovea, severe
constraints would be placed on his ability to read. These constraints would be manifested in slow reading, an unusual pattern of eye
fixation and movement across a page of text, and most importantly
poor comprehension due to the non-automaticity of the decoding process.

These studies await replication using more advanced eye moveme-
nt/visual perception technology now available. In addition to suggesting some of the possible mechanisms in one form of reading disability, they also strongly suggest that the selection of subjects
for entry into the disabled reader group is an important factor that
influences group performance data.

Other Studies of Orton's Theory

Hier, LeMay, Rosenburger and Perlo (1978) have studied the CT
scans of normal and disabled readers. They found that good readers
have a larger left (than right) parieto-occipital region. Previous
work (e.g., Geschwind and Levitsky, 1968) had suggested the language
representation in the left hemisphere was correlated with larger left hemisphere language zones relative to their homologous regions in
the right hemisphere. Some disabled readers in the Hier, et al. study had evidence of a "reversal of cerebral dominance," i.e., a wider right parieto-occipital region.

Autopsy studies have produced somewhat similar findings. For
example, a recent study by Galaburda and Kemper (1979) of the brain
of a dyslexic young man showed that the left hemisphere was wider
than the right in virtually the whole cerebral hemisphere. However,
the right and left planum temporale (the region shown by Geschwind
and Levitsky to be larger on the left) were equivalent in size in
this dyslexic. This finding suggests that in reading disability,
the left hemisphere may not be specially endowed (as many have suggested it is in normals) to carry on language functions. Orton had
suggested that faulty lateralization was somehow the causal mechanism in reading disability, but his theory had little empirical foundation. As it turns out, however, many lines of evidence have
shown that faulty lateralization is quite likely to hold at least
for many dyslexics. A cause-and-effect relationship is far from
clear, however. It is only clear that some abnormal neuropsychological mechanisms are important factors in developmental reading disability. Neuropsychological studies have shown many factors throughout the stages of information processing in word recognition and

reading to be possible problems for disabled readers. These information processing stages may or may not be carried out in single (i.e., the left hemisphere). It is a virtual certainty that beginning reading, when readers do not have a high level of automatic information processing (decoding), depends upon both hemispheres. It is unlikely that all disabled readers have the same neuropsychological disturbance, although it remains a possibility that a left hemisphere dysfunction causes reading disability, since all of the problem stages could be interfered with by the left hemisphere abnormality. Results of the work of Duffy, et al. (1980a) suggest such a conclusion. What may be observed in these data, as well as many other studies of reading disability, may be the two or more subtypes of deficit. The existence of these subtypes could explain many of the apparent contradictions in the literature on dyslexic. The lines of research discussed in this chapter are likely to provide clues to the causal mechanisms in the not too distant future. Of greatest importance is the continued progress in measuring the visual information processing characteristics of normal and disabled readers while they are engaged in reading (cf. Rayner, 1983), better empirical verification and validation of subtypes of dyslexia, and careful neuroanatomical studies of the brains of normal and disabled readers.

REFERENCES

Boder, E. Development dyslexia: A diagnostic approach based on three atypical reading-spelling patterns. Developmental Medicine and Child Neurology, 1973, 15, 663-687.
Calfee, R. C. and Spector, J. E. Separable processes in reading. In F. J. Pirozzolo and M. C. Wittrock (Eds.), Neuropsychological and cognitive processes in reading. New York: Academic Press, 1981.
Claiborne, J. H. Types of congenital symbol amblyopia, Journal of the American Medical Association, 1906, 47, 1813-1816.
Denckla, M. B. Learning disability. In K. Heilman and E. Valeretein (Eds.), Clinical Neuropsychology. New York: Oxford, 1980.
Drew, A. A neurological appraisal of familial congenital word blindness. Brain, 1956, 79, 440-460.
Duffy, F. H., Denckla, M. B., Bartels, P. H. and Sandini, G. Dyslexia: Regional differences in brain electrical activity by topographic mapping. Annals of Neurology, 1980a, 7, 412-420.
Duffy, F. H., Denckla, M. B., Bartels, P. H., Sandini, G., and Kiessling, L. S. Dyslexia: Automated diagnosis of computerized classification of brain electrical activity. Annals of Neurology, 1980b, 7, 421-428.
Eames, T. H. The anatomical basis of lateral dominance anomalies. American Journal of Orthopsychiatry, 1934, 4, 524-528.

Eames, T. H. A frequency study of physical handicaps in reading disability and unselected groups. Journal of Educational Research, 1935, 29, 1-5.

Fisher, J. H. A case of congenital word blindness (inability to learn to read). Ophthalmological Review, 1905, 24, 315.

Galaburda, A. and Kemper, T. Cytoarchitectonic abnormalities in developmental dyslexia: A case study. Annals of Neurology, 1979, 6, 94-100.

Geschwind, N. and Levitsky, W. Human brain: Left-right asymmetries in temporal speech region. Science, 1968, 161, 186-188.

Hallgren, B. Specific dyslexia (congenital word blindness), a clinical genetic study. Acta Psychiatrica et Neurologica, 1950, 65, Supplementum.

Hier, D. B., LeMay, M., Rosenberger, P. and Perlo, V. P. Developmental dyslexia. Archives of Neurology, 1978, 35, 90-92.

Hinshelwood, J. Congenital word blindness. London: Lewis, 1917.

Jastak, J. Interferences in reading. Psychological Bulletin, 1934, 21, 244-272.

Kinsbourne, M. and Warrington, E. K. Developmental factors in reading and writing backwards. British Journal of Psychology, 1963, 54, 145-156.

Marie, P. Revision de laquestion de l'aphasie: Le 3^e circonvolution frontale gauche ne jove aucun rule speciale dans la fonction du language. Semaire Medicale, 1906, May 23, 241-247.

Marshall, W. and Ferguson, J. Hereditary word blindness as a defect of selective association. Journal of Nervous and Mental Disease, 1939, 89, 165-173.

Mattis, S. Dyslexia syndromes in children: Toward the development of syndrome-specific treatment programs. In F. J. Pirozzolo and M. C. Wittrock (Eds.), Neuropsychological and cognitive processes in reading. New York: Academic Press, 1981.

Mattis, S., French, J. and Rapin, E. Dyslexia in children and young adults: Three independent neuropsychological syndromes. Developmental Medicine and Child Neurology, 1975, 17, 150-163.

Morgan, W. P. A case of congenital word blindness. British Medical Journal, 1896, 2, 1378.

Orton, S. T. Word blindness in school children. Archives of Neurology and Psychiatry, 1925, 14, 581-615.

Orton, S. T. Reading, Writing and Speech Problems in Children. New York: Norton, 1937.

Pirozzolo, F. J. Disorders of perceptual processing. In E. Carterette and M. Friedman (Eds.), Handbook of Perception, Vol. IX. New York: Academic Press, 1978.

Pirozzolo, F. J. and Rayner, K. Hemispheric specialization in reading and word recognition. Brain and Language, 1977, 4, 248-261.

Pirozzolo, F. J. and Rayner, K. Cerebral organization and reading disability. Neuropsychologia, 1979, 17, 485-491.

Pirozzolo, F. J., Rayner, K. and Hynd, G. The measurement of cerebral hemispheric asymmetries in children with developmental

reading disability. In J. Hellige (Ed.), <u>Cerebral Hemisphere</u>
<u>Asymmetry: Method, Theory and Application.</u> New York: Praeger,
1982.

Pirozzolo, F. J. <u>The Neuropsychology of Developmental Reading Dis-</u>
<u>orders</u>. New York: Praeger, 1979.

Pirozzolo, F. J. Language and brain: Neuropsychological aspects of
developmental reading disability. <u>School Psychological Review</u>,
1981, <u>10</u>, 350-355.

Pollatsek, A. What can eye movements tell us about dyslexia? In
K. Rayner (Ed.), <u>Eye movements in reading: Perceptual and lan-</u>
<u>guage processes.</u> New York: Academic Press, 1983.

Rayner, K. (Ed.), <u>Eye Movements in Reading: Perceptual and Lingui-</u>
<u>stic Aspects.</u> New York: Academic Press, 1983.

Samuels, S. J. and Eisenberg, P. A framework for understanding the
reading process. In F. J. Pirozzolo and M. C. Wittrock (Eds.),
<u>Neuropsychological and cognitive processes in reading</u>. New York:
Academic Press, 1981.

Satz, P. and Morris, R. Learning disability subtypes. A review.
In F. J. Pirozzolo and M. C. Wittrock (Eds.), <u>Neuropsychologi-</u>
<u>cal and cognitive processes in reading</u>. New York: Academic
Press, 1981.

Smith, H. P. and Dechant, E. V. <u>Psychology in teaching reading</u>.
Englewood Cliffs, New Jersey: Prentice Hall, 1961.

Thomas, C. J. Congenital word blindness and its treatment. <u>Ophtha-</u>
<u>lmoscope</u>, 1905, <u>3</u>, 380-385.

Yeni-Komshian, G., Isenberg, D. and Goldberg, H. Cerebral dominance
and reading disability: Left visual field deficit in poor readers. <u>Neuropsychologia</u>, 1975, <u>13</u>, 83-94.

IN SEARCH OF THE CORE OF DYSLEXIA:
ANALYSIS OF THE READING PROCESS OF DYSLECTIC CHILDREN

H. Bouma   and   Ch. P. Legein
Institute for Perception Research, IPR,
P. O. Box 513,
5600 MB Eindhoven
The Netherlands

INTRODUCTION

One of the changes which has taken place in our society is that reading now plays an increasingly important part. Books, magazi-
nes, newspapers, circulars, checks and television subtitles are all
based on the assumption that nearly everyone can read. And yet there are many people who have difficulty in reading. These people thus have an obvious handicap, which may have a number of causes. These include, for example, poor eyesight or a general lack of mental
development. However, there are also cases of children who have difficulty in reading without there being any apparent cause. They have good eyes, a good intellect, there is nothing wrong socially or
emotionally, but still they cannot properly learn how to read. This
phenomenon is known by a number of names, such as word blindness or
developmental dyslexia.

The term word blindness incorrectly suggests that the person concerned cannot read any words at all. In fact, although they do have
trouble reading words, they are certainly able to read short, everyday words. We will stick here to the term dyslexia.

To find out what percentage of children is dyslectic, we shall
have to make definitions and agree which children we are going to call dyslectic. If we take children who are two years or more behind
at primary school as a guideline, then we get a rough estimate of about five per cent of boys and one per cent of girls. The discrepancy
between boys and girls indicates that a hereditary factor is involved
which is sex-linked. In this respect, the situation can be compared
to color blindness, which it might be better to call color defective-

ness. One difference between them, however, is that with good teaching the reading lag need not become greater as time goes by, whereas with color defectiveness, on the other hand, little can be done to improve the ability to perceive colors.

Researchers and therapists from many fields have been working
intensively on the problem of dyslexia. An almost endless series
of publications has resulted from this. But the concepts and hypotheses concerning the question of where the core of the reading difficulty is situated reveal a multiplicity which comes across as
confusing rather than enlightening. Anyone wishing to find this out
for himself should read the survey by Vernon: "Reading and its difficulties" (1971).

The hypotheses can be divided into a number of criteria. Some
are of a neuro-anatomical nature (in which part of the brain is the
defect located ?), some are of a functional nature (which functional
defect underlies the problem ?) and others are of a pedagogical nature (on what base can I build the most productive therapy ?). A
different classification could be made based on the degree of specificity of the hypotheses. Thus, there are rather extremely precise
hypotheses (there is a defect in the left parietal lobe; it is a
result of being left-handed) and rather broad hypotheses (there is
a minimal diffuse cerebral lesion, there is a slight general retardation in development).

The various hypotheses do not necessarily exclude one another,
but they do make it difficult to obtain a general picture of what
the trouble actually is. The cause of this confusion must be looked
for primarily in the complex background of the phenomenon. Until
we find out exactly how the normal reading process works, how this
is acquired, and which perceptual, motor and intellectual skills are
used in doing it, it is extremely unlikely that we shall be able to
explain precisely defects in that process.

Another reason for the difficulties is that it is not easy to
distinguish between cause and effect. If someone cannot read particularly well, differences in skills soon arise which are based directly or indirectly on this reading. Also, the children concerned
will generally be dealt with differently, because their reading problem is considered to be laziness or unwillingness if they are of
normal intellect, for example, or precisely because they are pampe-
red more. Then when these children are about ten or eleven, it is
extremely difficult to make out which phenomena should be regarded
more as the cause and which as the effect. Add to this the fact that any extra attention which those children are given seems to have
a positive effect on learning to read, and you can form some picture
of the multiplicity mentioned.

Before giving an overall description of research that we have

carried out at the Institute for Perception Research during the last
few years, we should first like to describe our position with regard
to the many possibilities mentioned. Our starting-point is: insight
already gained into normal reading processes, whereby we are primarily oriented towards visual processes, including visual recognition. In the experiments with dyslectic children, we thus concentrate
mainly on the extent to which the results deviate from those of children of the same age-group who read normallly. We are thus opting
for a functional approach.

A further aim is to find as specific a hypothesis as possible
for dyslexia. In doing so, we went on the fact that it has been fo-
und over the years that the defect itself has an extremely specific
character. All this means that we tend primarily towards handling
alphabetical material and we shall for the moment not consider the
often smaller effects which have been reported outside this field.

ANALYSIS OF NORMAL READING

The purpose of the approach which we are using here is to split
reading into sub-processes in such a way that we obtain a clear picture of the whole. In doing this, we hope to obtain insight into
the sub-processes and the way in which they fit together, which will
give us an overall picture. The skill lies in finding an arrangement such that the chosen sub-processes lend themselves to being dealt
with separately, so that they can be isolated for the purpose of experiments. It should also preferably be possible to give a straightforward description. The approach which we have used is therefore
certainly not the only one possible and its value must be assessed
according to the insights obtained.

However, this does not mean that this choice is an arbitrary
one. We have based our choice on the fact that when a stationary
text is being read the eye does not glide over the lines, but moves
in jumps. The jumps take only a few hundredths of a second and during each jump the retina image moves so rapidly that no useful visual information can be absorbed. The absorption of information takes place during the eye pauses, which vary in duration from about
150 to 500 milliseconds. Visual text information is thus absorbed
by the retina from stationary retina pictures which change several
times per second. These observations have led to a distinction being made between the following three visual reading processes.

a) The control of eye jumps during reading: These jumps can be
sub-divided into normal forward jumps, which we shall call reading
jumps; small backward jumps in a line (correction jumps), and large
backward jumps at the beginning of a new line (line jumps). Line
jumps are often followed immediately by a small correction jump.

A lot of research has been carried out in recent years into the

control of eye jumps, and our knowledge of this has thus increased
considerably. As a result, we have good reason to make a distinction between an independent basic rhythm, control from rough data such as word length, observed to the right of the visual focus, and
control from centres of memory and comprehension. A treatment of
this falls outside the scope of this article.

b) Word recognition during an eye pause: The processing of visual
information which is absorbed during one eye pause can only comprise
those letters and words which are situated relatively close to the
visual focus, i.e. the centre of the retinal fovea. This is because
the visual analysis capability decreases rapidly from the fovea out-
words. This is not only the result of a decreasing visual acuity,
as used to be assumed, but rather a result of increasing masking between adjacent contour elements. The subsidiary problem which we
come up against here is therefore the visual recognition of words in
and around the fovea. In this field, too, considerable progress has
been made during the last few years. We now have an adequate supported theory for visual word recognition, in which it is assumed that
the visual information and the context information contribute independently to the recognition. The visual information contribution
is part of this sub-theme, the context information contribution is
part of the interaction with other sub-processes.

Visual recognition can be examined with no context by just presenting a single word, or a combination of words which are not connected. Instead of using words, meaningless letter combinations can
also be presented, which may or may not be pronounceable. The view
which has come to the fore as a result of this type of experiment
is that visual word recognition is based on the recognition both of
some letters and of their position in the word. The moment of recognition occurs as soon as the accumulated visual information activates a certain word from the internal lexicon more than other words
which resemble it to some extent. The situation in the fovea and to
the left and right of the fovea differs to the extent that the contour masking increases rapidly as the distance from the fovea increases, and also increases less rapidly to the right of the visual focus than to the left. Fig. 1 shows the percentages of correctly recognised words as a function of the distance from the visual focus.
It can also be seen from the figure that the percentage of incorrectly recognised words may rise considerably before the answer "un-
readable" is given. It is clear that the choice between alternatives is not made very selectively.

By carrying out experiments of this sort, it is possible to
estimate the width of the field of vision from which useful visual
information can be absorbed during an eye pause. This area is known as the reading field of vision.

By means of ingenious techniques, measurements have now been

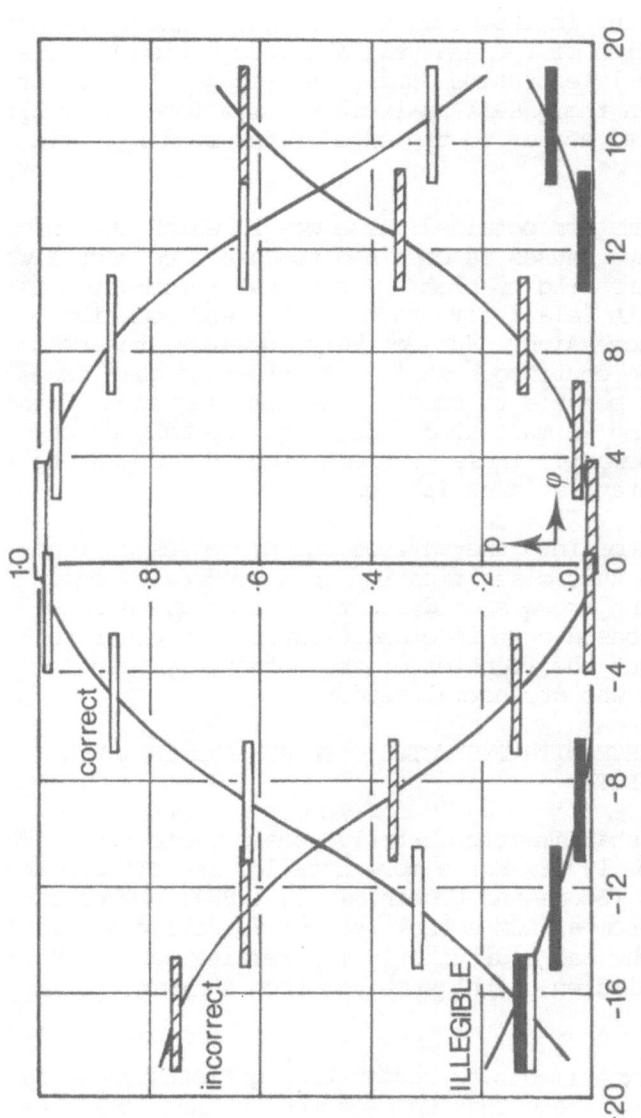

DISTANCE FROM VISUAL FOCUS (NUMBER OF LETTERS)

FIGURE 1.   Recognition scores of Dutch words (length 3 to 6 letters) for various distances from the visual focus. Presentation time 100 msec. Mean scores of a group of 11 adult test persons with good reading ability.

taken of the reading field of vision during the reading process.
For the right-hand visual field, the measurements for disconnected
words and for connected text correspond very well, whereas hardly
any information appears to be absorbed in the left-hand field of vision during the reading of connected text, although visually this
ought in fact to be possible. Our understanding in this area is certainly not yet complete.

A factor still lacking in the present recognition theory is an
explanation of the duration of the analysis and recognition processes. We do know that the latency time during the recognition of words increases rapidly when the visual analysis becomes more difficult,
as when words are situated nearer to the edge of the reading field
of vision.

c) Integration of Information obtained: The way in which the information from successive eye pauses is combined to make a connected whole is an extremely interesting problem. The visual information is
received intermittently in relatively random units, and sometimes
even several times in succession. Subjectively, however, the reading process occurs as one continuous whole. In order to gain access
to this problem, we must be able to specify the time sequence of the
recognition processes, and we must also understand the make-up of
the short-term working memory. These problems, too, now appear to
be accessible for quantitative investigation.

The insights obtainted into the various sub-processes of reading lead us to hope that this classification is a productive one.
With regard to the reading process of dyslectic children, we shall
now discuss experiments based on this classification, in order to
develop a hypothesis about the location of the defect, by means of
comparison with children who are normal readers.

RESULTS OF READING RESEARCH WITH DYSLECTIC CHILDREN AND CHILDREN
WITH AVERAGE READING ABILITY

In this section we shall mention briefly some experiments which
we have carried out since 1974. For a more detailed report, see several other publications (Bouma and Legein, 1977, 1980). We compared groups of children from an LOM school (school for children with
educational problems), who had a distinctly low reading age and normal intelligence, and children of the same age from a normal primary
school.

We restricted the experiments to recognition of letters, words
and figures, because it was here that we expected the most characteristic discrepancies. The recognition experiments were carried out
tachistoscopically with a fixed presentation time of 100 milliseconds, with the same word generally being presented once in the same
experiment. The stimuli were usually presented both in the visual

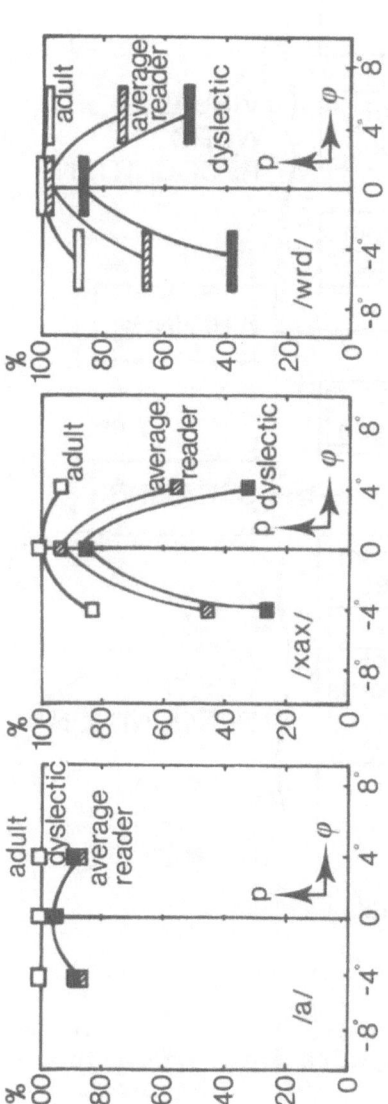

DISTANCE FROM VISUAL FOCUS (NUMBER OF LETTERS)

FIGURE 2.   Recognition scores of disconnected letters (a), embedded letters (xax) and words of 3-5 letters (wrd) for three places in the field of vision.   Groups of approx. 10 children.   The results of a group of adults with good reading ability are also given for purposes of comparison.

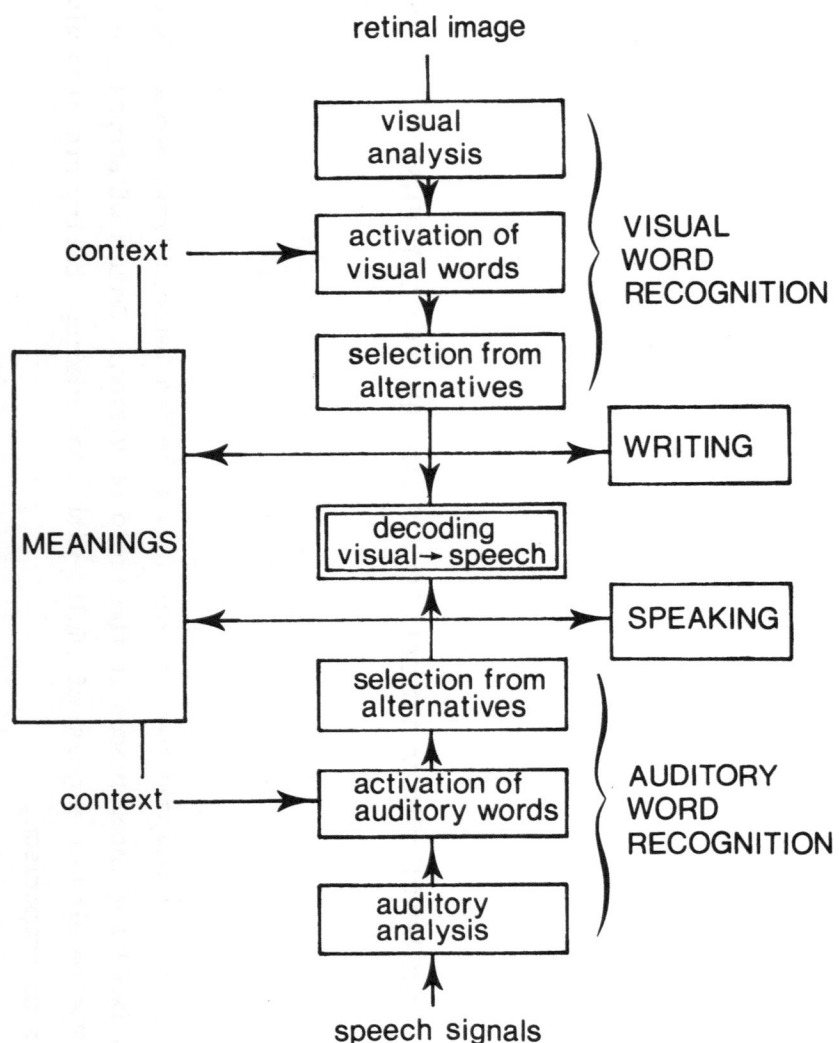

FIGURE 3. Table of some processes which are a factor in word
            recognition.

focus (foveal), as well as approximately four letters to the left and right of the visual focus (parafoveal). We were particularly interested in the parafoveal results, because we thought it possible that the reading field of vision would not be as wide in the case of dyslectic children.

A few characteristic results of the experiments were:
a) Recognition of disconnected letters: Both dyslectic children and children with average reading ability obtained high scores: in the visual focus about 95%, and outside the visual focus almost 90% correct.

In any case the conclusion is that dyslectics, too, are fully aware of the shapes of letters. We found scarcely any indications of the "mirror transpositions", for example between b, p, d and q, which have received quite a lot of attention in literature. In this age group these difficulties are obviously a thing of the past, even with dyslectics.

b) Recognition of embedded letters: Since we knew that significant contour maskings occur with good adult readers, we also carried out an experiment in which the letter to be recognised had an x on either side of it, with normal typewriter spacing. In this experiment there did turn out to be discrepancies between dyslectic children and children with average reading ability: in the visual focus approximately 85% compared to 95%, and outside the visual focus, too, a discrepancy of around 30% compared to 50%. The first conclusion is that the effect of contour masking is considerable for both groups of children, but that the dyslectics have considerably more difficulty in this case than the average readers.

It is also interesting to note that for stimuli just outside the visual focus, - and this is also true of adult readers - recognition in the right-hand field of vision turns out to be somewhat better than to the left of the visual focus, both for dyslectics and for average readers.

c) Recognition of disconnected words: For this we whose normal Dutch words, (nouns) of four to six letters in length; as was expected, the correct scores of the dyslectic children were lower than those of the children with average reading ability. Nevertheless, the dyslectic children still got 85% correct in the visual focus(children with average reading ability 95) and about 45% outside the visual focus (children with average reading ability 70%). The dyslectic children can thus recognise words, but not so well as the children with average reading abiltiy. An analysis of the words given incorrectly revealed nothing special, to the extent that the mistakes made by the children with average reading ability and by the dyslectic children had the same character. The word-recognition process clearly does not work quite so well, but does not differ very greatly in quality. It is also interesting that word recognition by both groups of children is better to the right of the visual focus than to the left of the visual focus. Since this discrepancy is presumably linked to training in reading direction from left to right, we can say that in this respect dyslectic children display a normal development.

d) Recognition of long words: When listening to dyslectic children aloud, it is immediately obvious that it is the long words in particular which give a lot of difficulty. We were able to confirm this in a recognition experiment in which words of various lengths were presented once in the centre of the field of vision. Whereas children with average reading ability made virtually no mistakes up to a length of ten letters, in the case of dyslectic children the score fell as the word-length increased, to about 30% at ten letters.

e) Latency times: In general it can be said that the latency time of correct recognitions increases as the degree of difficulty increases (i.e. as the recognition score decreases). This is the case both for dyslectic children and for children with average reading ability. Thus, recognition outside the fovea generally gives longer latency times than in the fovea and recognition of embedded letters gives a longer latency time than with disconnected letters. It was found, however, that with dyslectic children there was an additional delay, which was dependent solely on the type of recognition, i.e. letters or words, and not on the degree of difficulty of the recognition. This came as a surprise to us and gave rise to the hypothesis which we shall discuss in the next section.

f) In the case of long words, we checked whether recognition improved when the words were split into two parts. For this we used words whose parts themselves also form words, such as headlamp. If the contour masking is relatively great for dyslectic children, one would expect that the insertion of a space in between might improve recognition. However, this did not on the whole prove to be the case. We also presented the component words in quick succession with regard to time. This did bring about a significant improvement in the recognition score. This, too, is an indication that something peculiar is going on, particularly in the time sequence of the recognition processes.

GENERAL TABLE OF READING PROCESSES

In order to relate the phenomena discovered to one another, we have drawn up a table. This table is based on current ideas about recognition and on what we consider to be characteristic results published in literature (Morton 1969 and others).

The table is a general one because at the moment we are not yet in a position to supplement it quantitatively for dyslexia. This would be more easily possible for average readers. This table now looks as follows (fig. 3):

TABLE 1. Latency times (msec) for visual recognition of letters and words, foveal and parafoveal (roughly four letter positions from the centre). Mean figures from a group of nine dyslectics and nine average readers. The figures in brackets are the standard deviations of the distribution of individual means.

This data is from a different experiment to the data in Fig. 2.

	Dyslectics	Average readers	Discrepancy
Disconnected letters a) foveal	910 (260)	770 (120)	140
Disconnected letters b) Parafoveal	840 (140)	740 (110)	100
Embedded letters (xax), foveal	940 (240)	830 (170)	110
Embedded letters (xax), parafoveal	1040 (120)	920 (130)	120
Disconnected words (wrd), foveal	900 (190)	680 (100)	220
Disconnected words (wrd), parafoveal	940 (150)	730 (90)	210

TABLE 2. Recognition scores (%) for words of 8 letters, made up of two words of 4 letters, (e.g. headlamp). Foveal, single presentation. Each group consisted of 12 children. Spatial splitting does not help recognition, temporal splitting does. Only answers which were completely right were counted.

	Dyslectics	Average readers
Typed normally (1 = 8)	21%	85%
Split in space (1= 4//4)	18%	79%
Split in time (1= 4, Δt, 1 = 4)	36%	88%

After the retina image on which the printed text is shown, there next comes a stage of visual analysis, followed by an activation

of units of recognition, for example words, by which is meant strictly a visual image, with no meanings yet being involved. Next, from a number of more or less strongly activated units of recognition,
one is selected which thus becomes internally available as a mental
unit. To get from this unit to the meaning, there are two routes:
one is by direct access, the other goes by means of translation into
a corresponding speech code. The internal speech then has further
access to the meanings store. In the case of a child learning to
read alphabetical script, the direct-access route from visual code
to meaning has not yet been formed. In this case the visual image
first has to be translated into speech. As reading skill improves,
this route has to be used less and less.

THE POSSIBLE NATURE OF DYSLEXIA

    The hypothesis which at the moment seems to correspond best wi-
th the available information is that the entire visual process is
fundamentally normal in the case of dyslectics, as is the speaking
and understanding process. However, what does not proceed normally
in dyslectics is the translation from the visual code to the speech
code. To be more specific, we can only assume that this process is
delayed. We should now like to find out how a number of findings
fit into this schematic picture.

Non-alphabetical material: Clear indications that the visual system
in itself functions normally in dyslectics have been uncovered by
Vellutino and colleagues. He got children to copy down all kinds
of figures which resembled letters but which were not actually letters. Average readers and dyslectics performed equally well. It thus appears that the difficulties for dyslectics only arise when letters and words are involved, i.e. when some kind of recoding into
speech enters into it. But not all recoding causes difficulties for
dyslectic children. If they perceive a tree or a football, they have no difficulty in finding the correct word for it. The difference
between images which can be named immediately and images for which
this is difficult is to be found in the symbolic character of the
alphabetic system, in which the shape and meaning of letters and words is based on general conventions. In this connection it is interesting to report that there seems to be virtually no dyslexia in
Japanese children. In the writing system known as Kanji, each visual symbol has a particular meaning, as in Chinese. Learning to recognise visually these complicated ideograms appears to proceed without any particular difficulties. The second Japanese writing system, the Kana, is a syllabic writing system in which each symbol
corresponds directly to a pronounced syllable. In this system, too,
the difficulties do not seem to arise which occur in the Western
languages, in which there is a more complicated relationship between
spelling and pronunciation.

    In view of the fact that dyslectic children in everyday life speak normally and understand speech, it is also reasonable to assume that the speech system in itself also functions normally. This then evokes the image of a visual system functioning normally and a speech system functioning normally, in which the connections between the visual system and the speech system are inadequately developed.

Certainly during the learning-to-read phase, these connections are indispensable for forming the link between visual image and meaning, so that this causes in dyslectic children the development of an inadequate connection between the visual word image and the meaning.

Alphabetic material: If we now look closely at the table it will be possible to discover a difference in analysis difficulty in the score and latency time of recognition. For letters and words outside the visual focus we would expect a more difficult analysis than in the visual focus, and for embedded letters, owing to the contour masking, a more difficult analysis than for disconnected letters. However, since dyslectic children's difficulty is not situated in visual analysis, the extra time required for the more complicated analysis should be the same for dyslectics and average readers, and this was found to be the case.

The fact that the recognition scores for both groups of children become lower as the visual analysis becomes more difficult may be due to two factors: firstly, the spatial analysis itself may be inadequate, and secondly the analysis may take longer than the information can be retained. We still do not know enough about how visual information is stored in the short-term, but it seems certain that language information in the form of speech can be retained for longer.

The simple fact that it takes dyslectics longer to code visual information into speech form means that the score will also be lower. Also, delayed answers will more often be wrong than rapid answers, a fact that has been shown to be the case both for average readers and for dyslectic children.

That dyslectic children experience difficulties with long words in particular follows directly from this observation. They have so much difficulty in translating long words into speech code that they have forgotten the word, as it were, before it has been properly converted into speech. If they convert a small part of it first, they have to try to retain this first piece as speech (rehearsal) and then in the meantime "translate" the second part of the word. Average readers are not troubled by this memory load. The improved recognition of long words when we present the parts in succession is then explained primarily by the fact that we are eliminating problems of temporary storage of information.

We still need to know whether the purely visual word images are
formed normally in the case of dyslectics, but do not make any contact with the meanings, in the way we have outlined, or whether it
is precisely the lack of connection with the meaning which causes
the purely visual word images to be inadequately formed.

As well as having difficulties in reading, dyslectic children
also have great difficulty in spelling. This indicates that the reverse translating process, i.e. from a speech code into a visual code, also functions inadequately.

Of course, reading is more than visual word recognition. But
visual word recognition is such an integral component of the reading
process that a deficiency in this makes normal reading extremely difficult. It is easily possible for average readers to check this
for themselves, for example if they try to read a foreign language
which they have only a partial command of. Decoding the words then
gives them so much trouble that the meaning of large sections is easily lost. At the end of a sentence you can't remember what was said at the beginning. The comparison is certainly not completely valid, partly because the reader cannot usually speak the foreign language well, either. But it is quite obvious that the difficulty in
visual word recognition alone is sufficient to seriously impede the
entire reading process. It goes without saying that the eye-moveme-
nt pattern of dyslectics and of average readers will also differ,
but that the cause of the reading difficulties need not be looked
for there. Notions which look for the main cause of dyslexia in inadequate development of a right/left body layout, or in a motor weakness, also fit badly into the hypothesis which is proposed here.
On the other hand, there are also many theories which in themselves
are quite compatible with our hypothesis, such as a neuro-anatomic
theory, since the translation from visual image to speech image must
take place somewhere in the brain.

On the therapeutic side, we would not like to draw many conclusions from our experimental and theoretical observations. We do think that some possibility of help is afforded by supplying the speech image while the word image is being looked at, but without experimental foundations this is rather speculative. Luckily, any serious help and attention which dyslectic children are given contribu-
tes to improving reading performances, so that the reading lag is
not increased further. This fortunate circumstance, however, makes
it difficult to test ideas which underlie the therapy, since an improvement in reading performances cannot in itself be taken as evidence that the ideas underlying the therapy are thereby well-founded.

On the other hand, there is also no reason to stop using a reasonably effective therapy as long as a better one has not been developed. Nevertheless, all these pitfalls need not prevent us from
continuing to look for as straightforward a cause as possible or

from building in due course a therapeutic structure upon the foundations of basic research.

REFERENCES

Bouma, H. and Legein, Ch. P. - Foveal and parafoveal recognition
    of letters and words by dyslexics and by average readers.
    Neuropsychologia, 1977, 15, 69-80.
Bouma, H. and Legein, Ch. P. - Dyslexia: a specific recoding de-
    fiency. An analysis of response latencies for letters and wor-
    ds in dyslectics and in average readers. Neuropsychologia, 1980.
Morton, J. - Interaction of information in word recognition.
    Psyhcological Review, 1969, 76, 165-178.
Vellutino, F. R., Smith, H., Steger, J. A. and Kaman, M. -
    Reading disability: age differences and the perceptual deficit
    hypothesis. Child Development, 1975, 46, 487-493.
Vernon, M. D. - Reading and its difficulties. Cambridge Univer-
    sity Press, London, 1971.

DEVELOPMENTAL SURFACE DYSLEXIA IN ITALIAN

Remo Job   Giuseppe Sartori   Jacqueline Masterson Max Coltheart

University   U. S. L. - Tre-   Department of Psychology
di Padova   viso, Italy   University of London
Padova,   London, U. K.
Italy

INTRODUCTION

Surface dyslexia is a reading disorder characterized by a disproportionate difficulty in reading irregular words, i.e. words for
which the application of parsing procedures and phoneme assignment
rules such as those proposed by Wijk (1966) and Venezky (1970) would
yield incorrect phonological representations (cf. blood versus sham-
poo, pint versus pine). The errors produced by surface dyslexics
when they try to read irregular words are often "regularization errors" (Marshall and Newcombe, 1973; Coltheart, Masterson, Byng, Prior,
and Riddoch, in press), i.e. reading gauge as "gorge" and are as
"air". Stress placement errors on polysyllabic words are also observed, so that omit may be stressed on the first syllable (Marshall
and Newcombe, 1973) and recent may be read as "resent" (Holmes, 19-
78). Another type of error made by surface dyslexics concerns non-
homographic homophones. Patients may in fact correctly read aloud
a given homophone, but may be unable to assign it the correct meaning. For example, Newcombe and Marshall (1981) report that the patient JC correctly read the noun bee, but glossed is as "To be or
not to be, that is the question".

This syndrome has recently received a great deal of attention,
and detailed analyses of a number of patients' reading performance
are now available (see Coltheart, 1982, for a review). Most of the
data have been collected from adult patients who became dyslexic
after brain damage. However, surface dyslexia is one of the acquired reading disorders for which a developmental analog has been reported. For example, Holmes (1973, 1978) showed that the four dyslexic children she studied exhibited a pattern of reading errors similar to that observed in two acquired dyslexics. Similarly,

Coltheart et al. (in press), comparing a developmental and an acquired dyslexic, found a very close similarity in their reading and spelling performance. As the authors point out, the errors made by the
two subjects to a given stimulus were sometimes the same.

From a theoretical point of view, surface dyslexia may be explained in the framework of what has been classically called the dual-
route model of reading (see Marshall, this volume, for a detailed discussion of the model). Very briefly, two routes are postulated in
the model for accessing the mental lexicon: A visual route and a phonological route. The first route allows the reader to access the meaning of a word directly from the printed stimulus; the second requires a conversion of the graphemes comprising a word into the corresponding phonemes. Only after this operation has been performed is
it possible to access the lexical entry. Logical arguments, as well
as empirical evidence have been offered (cf. Coltheart, 1981) to support the view that in normal readers both routes are operating, though, depending on several factors such as task requirements, age of
the readers, and material employed, one or the other may be favored.
On the assumption of modularity of the cognitive processes (see Shallice, 1981), it can be postulated that damage to the reading system
may impair either one of the two routes, or both. In the former case,
a person may still be able to read through the spared route; however
the flexibility of the system arising from the interplay of both surface dyslexia is interpreted to arise because of a selective breakdown, from mild to complete, of the visual route. Therefore, only
the phonological route can be used by the patients, and words have
to be read via grapheme-to-phoneme conversion rules. When the word
to be read is regular, these rules may productively be applied, and
the word may be successfully read; however, irregular words are, by
definition, correctly read only through the visual route, since the
general parsing procedures and rules for converting the parsed elements into phonemes cannot be applied to them. Therefore, reading
irregular words via the phonological route will be inadequate, and
regularization errors will arise.

From the pattern of reading performance observed in surface dyslexics, and from the given theoretical interpretation, it should follow that this reading disorder should manifest itself only in readers of languages in which either irregular words or non-homographic
homophones, or both, exist. Therefore, for readers of languages with a regular and one-to-one grapheme-to-phoneme and phoneme-to-grapheme correspondence system, surface dyslexia should pass undetected.
In these languages, in fact, all words can be correctly read using
the phonological route. There are, however, two symptoms of surface
dyslexia which are not "tied" to irregular words and homophones:
The first, which we already mentioned, is given by stress errors;
the second by orthographic errors (cf. Coltheart et al., in press).
The latter consists of letter substitution, addition, omissions, and
transposition, or a combination of them. This symptom is quite non-

specific, since orthographic errors can be observed in most dyslexic syndromes. The former errors, instead, are specific to surface dyslexia, and even if not very frequent, they can be considered critical for diagnosing this reading disorder. The interesting fact about these errors is that they can, of course, occur also in languages with a regular grapheme-to-phoneme correspondence system, provided that they do not have a regular stress placement system.

Italian is one of such languages. Its grapheme-to-phoneme and phoneme-to-grapheme correspondence rules are in fact highly regular, while stress assignment is not very consistent. Given the first of these two characteristics, no irregular word exist in Italian. Also, no homophones which are not also homographs exist in this language, with only a few exceptions. The exceptions are due to three inflected forms of the verb avere (to have). The first letter of these inflected forms is h, which is never pronounced in Italian. Thus, the following word pairs are homophones:

ha (he/she/it has)	a (to)
hai (you have)	ai (to the)
hanno (they have)	anno (year).

As far as stress assignment is concerned, Italian is a "free stress" language (Lepschy and Lepschy, 1981). This means that some polysyllabic words are stressed on the first syllable [e.g. orfano/'orfæno/ (orphan)], some on the last syllable [e.g. liberta'/ɪˈbɛrtæ/ (freedom)], and some on one of the intermediate syllables [e.g. cavallo /kæˈvælːo/ (horse)]. However, most Italian polysyllabic words are stressed on the penultimate syllable, and this is almost always the case when the penultimate syllable ends with a consonant [e.g. ca-val-lo (horse)]. If, as discussed above, the visual route is impaired in surface dyslexia, then word-specific information such as stress should not always be available to the subject; hence we would expect that he/she should sometimes give the wrong stress to a word, particularly to a word which is not stressed on the penultimate syllable.

Case Study

Luigi is an 11.5-year-old right-handed male. He was referred to the Neurology Department of Treviso Hospital for reading problems by the school psychologist in June 1982 but is reported as having had difficulty with reading throughout his school career. Physical development and onset of speech were both normal and he has no known history of neurological abnormality. No other member of his family suffers from reading disability and all of them are right-handed. Standard neurological examination and EEG (carried out in June 1982) were normal. Neuropsychological testing revealed that his general IQ is 96 (verbal IQ = 100, Performance IQ = 93). The range of standard scores of the sub-tests in the verbal section was

8-12 and the worst performance was with the Arithmetic sub-test. With regard to Performance sub-tests the range was 8-12 and the worst performance was on the Coding sub-test where he scored 4. He has no short-term memory problem since he scored in the normal range on the Digit Span test. His score on the Progressive Matrices is 28/36 (which is in the 25th percentile). His score on the Oseresky Motor Development test was within the normal range as was his score on the Complex Figure Coping test. His comprehension of sentences was assessed with the TROG test (Bishop, personal communication) and he scored in the normal range for auditory and visual presentation (70/80 for both). His performance on the sub-tests of a standardised Italian reading test (Faglioni, Gatti, Paganoni, and Robutti, 1967) was as follows: 1) word comprehension (visual presentation) 26/50 correct; 2) non-word matching (visual presentation) 35/50; 3) writing to dictation - 34 errors. His overall score on the test is below the first percentile.

Results of reading tests

Luigi's reading ability has been tested on a number of occasions within a time span of six months. A description of the reading tests administered together with the results obtained follows. The analysis takes into account initial responses only.

Forty-Word List

This test consisted of 40 nouns all five letters in length, with orthogonal rotation of the factors of frequency and concreteness (so that ten nouns were concrete and of high frequency, ten were abstract and of high frequency, ten were concrete and of low frequency and ten were abstract and of low frequency). The items in the test were randomized and were presented typed in upper-case in a list. Luigi read 83% of the words in the test correctly. Both factors of concreteness and frequency were found to have an effect on Luigi's reading (with 100% of concrete but 65% of abstract nouns read correctly; and 95% of high frequency and 75% of low frequency nouns read correctly).

Eighty-Word and Eighty-Non-Word List

This test consisted of 80 nouns with orthogonal rotation of the factors of length (4,5, 7 or 8 letters), frequently and concreteness (so that five nouns were four letters long, frequent and concrete, five were four letters long, frequent and abstract, and so on). Eighty non-words were derived from the nouns by changing one letter in each item. The order of the nouns and the non-words was randomized and they were presented in a mixed list, typed in upper-case. Considering the results for the words first, in this test concreteness had a reverse effect on Luigi's reading performance with more abstract than concrete words read aloud correctly (78%

vs. 65% respectively). However more words of high frequency were read aloud correctly, replicating the result of the first test with regard to the effect of frequency. Word length had a variable effect on Luigi's reading performance since only 55% of four-letter words were read aloud correctly whereas 70% of five-letter words, 85% of seven-letter words, and 75% of eight-letter words were read aloud correctly.

To consider next the results for the non-words, a comparison of word and non-word reading reveals that whereas 71% of the nouns were read aloud correctly, only 44% of the non-words were. This result was not due to a tendency to give words (rather than neologisms) as responses, since analysis of Luigi's errors to words and non-words in this test reveals that 12/23 errors to words were lexicalisations, whereas only 14/45 errors to non-words were. Length did not have a pronounced effect on the reading of non-words since 50% of four-letter non-words, 45% of five-letter non-words, 45% of seven-letter non-words, and 35% of eight-letter non-words were read aloud correctly.

Error Analysis

Luigi's reading aloud performance was found to be sensitive to frequency in both the forty-word list and the eighty-word list, with words of high frequency being read aloud with more accuracy than words of low frequency. Concreteness had an inconsistent effect with concrete words being read aloud with greater accuracy than abstract words in the forty-word list but not in the eighty-word list. Word length had a variable effect with seven-letter words read aloud with the greatest accuracy, followed by eight-letter words, and five-letter words. Four-letter words produced the least accurate performance. Words were read aloud with more accuracy than non-words and there was a slight length effect with the latter, since increasing length led to a decrease in accuracy.

The errors made in reading aloud words were of two types: orthographic errors and stress placement errors. The first type consisted of the substitution, insertion or deletion of one or more letters or of a combination of these. This type of error was also made in reading aloud non-words. Table 1 gives examples of such errors taken from Luigi's corpus.

Since many of the orthographic errors involved visually similar letters investigations were made of Luigi's visual feature analysis abilities. He was required to name the 21 letters of the Italian alphabet which were typed individually in upper-case on cards. He made only one error (g -> c), although on 4 occassions he provided the sounds of the letters and not their names (for the letters v, p, d, s). Second, he was asked to name a given letter embedded in a sequence. The letter to be named was underlined while the others were not (e.g. azfelm). Again, he scored 95.24% correct. Finally,

TABLE 1. Examples of orthographic errors in reading aloud

RESPONSE

		WORD	NON-WORD
	ADD	case -> casse	-
WORD	DEL	dazio -> dio	pace -> ace
	SUB	sale -> sole	lampo -> lampa
STIMULUS			
	ADD	scipo -> scippo	cona -> conna
NON-WORD	DEL	-	alimerto -> alimer
	SUB	cabe -> cade	nadre -> nodre

he was given a cross-case matching task. Two letters, one in upper
case and one in lower case, were presented on a single card. There
were 58 cards, half requiring a same response (e.g. A a) and half a
different response (e.g. b A). On this task Luigi was correct 90.00%
of the time.

From these tests it is clear that Luigi's reading impairment
is not due to difficulties at the letter identification level.

The second type of error Luigi made when reading words concerns
stress assignment. These arose because he sometimes shifted the stress of polysyllabic words from the correct syllable to the penultimate one. Since the words used in the reading task were not matched
for locus of stress, a new list was constructed. It consisted of
60 words matched for length and grammatical class: Half of them had
stress on the penultimate syllable, the other half on syllables other than the last but one. Luigi gave erroneous responses to 12 words. Of these errors, 3 were stress placement errors and in all cases they regarded words with stress on syllables other than the last
but one.

Thus, Luigi presents both of the symptoms of surface dyslexia
that do not depend on grapheme-to-phoneme conversion rules: The
non-specific orthographic errors and the specific stress assignment
errors. However stronger evidence for a diagnosis of surface dyslexia was provided in the next test. For this, we constructed a test
for homophonic confusion, since both Newcombe and Marshall (1981)
and Coltheart et al. (in press) showed this to be a critical symptom
of surface dyslexia. As pointed out above, non-homographic homophones are practically absent in Italian. However, some sequences of
the type "article + apostrophe + noun" sound exactly the same as some words in this language. For example, the sequence l'ago (the
needle) and the word lago (lake) are pronounced in the same way.

TABLE 2. Examples of the material used in the homophones task

L'AGO e' fatto di   ACQUA   LEGNO   TERRA   FERRO
LAGO e' fatto di   ACQUA   LEGNO   TERRA   FERRO

(THE NEEDLE is made of WATER   WOOD   GROUND   METAL)

(LAKE   is made of WATER   WOOD   GROUND   METAL)

L'IRA   vuol dire PUZZA   RABBIA   SOLDI   AEREO
LIRA   vuol dire PUZZA   RABBIA   SOLDI   AEREO

(THE ANGER means SMELL   FURY   MONEY   AEROPLANE)

(LIRA   means SMELL   FURY   MONEY   AEROPLANE)

Therefore, we have pairs of letter strings (that we will call words for short) which sound the same but differ at the orthohraphic level in the presence or absence of the apostrophe.

A list of 16 pairs of such words were selected. For each word of a pair both a synonym, or a closely related word, and an unrelated word of the same grammatical class were selected. Luigi was presented with the 32 words in random order and the corresponding 4 alternatives, and was asked to mark the word that meant the same thing as, or was related to, the target word (examples of the material are presented in Table 2).

Luigi chose an unrelated word only once. For the remaining 31 words he was at chance level in choosing between the two synonyms. That is to say, he chose the correct synonym 16 times and the wrong one 15 times. This result strongly suggests that in reading Luigi is not using orthographic knowledge to retrieve the meaning of some words; rather, he relies on the phonological representation of the word to access the lexicon. In order to further investigage this point we used a writing to dictation task. Fifteen of the word pairs used in the preceding task and three new ones were utilized. Each word pair was used in a single sentence of the type:

La mamma seduta in riva al lago cuce i pantaloni con l'ago.
(the mother seated by the lake sewed the trousers with the needle).

First, the whole sentence was read aloud to Luigi who was instructed to listen carefully; then, the sentence was re-read to him, a few words at a time, and he wrote them down. After he completed a sentence, the next one was presented, and so on.

Only the results for the homophonic pairs will be presented here, even if Luigi made a number of other errors. In this task

too the child was at chance level with this type of stimuli: He correctly wrote 18/36 words, the remaining 18 being homophonic errors.

A comparison of the performance on those 15 word pairs common
to both tasks shows that to the 15 words he correctly comprehended
in the first task he made 5 errors in writing, while he correctly wrote 4 of the fourteen words he was wrong with in the first task.

Concluding Remarks

The pattern of reading performance, and the types of errors made
by the subject presented here suggest that he is unable to productively use the visual route for accessing the lexicon. We know in fact
from experimental evidence (Sartori and Masutto, 1982) that both this
route and the phonological route are available to Italian readers,
even if the orthographic structure of this language means that it is
possible to read virtually all words by using the latter route. However, when presented with material that could only be correctly read
with reference to its graphemic configuration, Luigi was unable to
use this information. We may conclude that Luigi cannot adequately
use the visual route, and that his reading disorder may properly be
classified as developmental surface dyslexia. Thus, although at the
beginning of this chapter it was suggested that surface dyslexia could pass undetected in readers of Italian because of the nature of
the relationship between spelling and sound in that language we have
seen that it is possible to demonstrate the disorder in readers of
Italian. It seems likely that further cross-language research on
dyslexia will give us insights in the relationship between scripts
and reading.

REFERENCES

Coltheart, M. Disorders of reading and their implications for models
    of normal reading. Visible Language, 1981, 15, 245-286.
Coltheart, M. The psycholinguistic analysis of acquired dyslexias:
    some illustrations. Philosophical Transactions Of The Royal
    Society Of London, 1982, B 298, 151-164.
Coltheart, M., Masterson, J., Byng, S., Prior, M., and Riddoch, J.
    Surface Dyslexia. Quarterly Journal of Experimental Psychology,
    In press.
Faglioni, P., Gatti, B., Paganoni, A. M., and Robutti, A. La valu-
    tazione psychometrica della dislessia. Infanzia Anormale,
    1967, 81, 628-644.
Holmes, J. M. Dyslexia: A neurolinguistic study of traumatic and
    developmental disorders of reading. Unpublished Ph. D. thesis,
    University of Edinburgh, 1973.
Holmes, J. M. Regression and reading breakdown. In A. Caramazza
    and E. Zurif (Eds.) The acquisition and breakdown of language:

Parallels and divergencies. Baltimore: Johns Hopkins University Press, 1978.

Lepschy, A. L. and Lepschy, G. La lingua italiana. Milano: Bompiani, 1981.

Marshall, J. C. and Newcombe, F. Patterns of paralexia. *Journal of Psycholinguistic Research*, 1973, 2, 175-199.

Newcombe, F. and Marshall, J. C. On psycholinguistic classifications of the acquired dyslexias. *Bulletin of the Orton Society*, 1981, 31, 29-46.

Sartori, G. and Masutto, S. Visual access and phonological recoding in reading Italian. *Psychological Research*, 1982, 44, 243-256.

Shallice, T. Neurological impairment of cognitive processes. *British Medical Bulletin*, 1981, 37, 187-192.

Venezky, R. L. *The structure of English orthography.* The Hague: Mouton, 1970.

Wijk, A. *Rules of pronunciation for the English language.* London: Oxford University Press, 1966.

DEVELOPMENTAL ANALOGUES TO ACQUIRED PHONOLOGICAL DYSLEXIA[1]

Christine M. Temple
Neuropsychology Unit
Radcliffe Infirmary
Oxford OX2 6HE

This chapter will present details of two cases of developmental dyslexia. It is my contention that these two cases represent the first developmental analogues to acquired phonological alexia and henceforth children of this type should be called developmental phonological dyslexics.

The general theoretical issues concerned in drawing comparisons between acquired and developmental dyslexia, within an information processing model, have been addressed elsewhere (Marshall, this volume), and therefore, not be dealt with here. In 1973, Holmes pointed out in her doctoral dissertation that some developmental dyslexics exhibit reading patterns very similar to those shown by acquired surface dyslexics. This work has been confirmed and greatly expanded by Coltheart and his colleagues (1982, Coltheart, Masterson, Byng, Prior and Riddoch, 1983). Aram, Rose, and Horwitz (this volume) have discussed the syndrome of hyperlexia in children which may parallel the acquired disorder of direct dyslexia (Schwartz, Saffran and Marin, 1980). I will consider parallels to another acquired reading disorder, phonological dyslexia.

Phonological dyslexia was first reported in France by Beauvois and Dérouesne (1979). The syndrome has been discussed fairly extensively elsewhere (Coltheart, this volume) but since, for

---

1. I wish to thank Dr. Nigel Hyman, consultant neurologist at the Radcliffe infirmary, Oxford, for referring H. M. Thanks also to John Marshall for comments on an earlier version of this manuscript and to Perdy Dobson for secretarial assistance. This work was supported by an MRC studentship.

comparative purposes, it is important to be clear what the characteristics of acquired phonological dyslexia are and just how much
variation there is within the features exhibited, I shall reiterate
them.

CHARACTERISTICS OF PHONOLOGICAL DYSLEXIA

Phonological dyslexics have difficulty reading non-words in
comparison to their ability to read words. This difficulty is not
as severe as that found in deep dyslexia (Marshall and Newcombe,
1966), where there is often complete failure to read any non-words.
Although the phonological dyslexic of Funnell (1983) reads virtually
no non-words, it is more common for some non-word reading skills to
be present. Indeed, the patient A. M. of Patterson (1982) reads
23% of non-words and B. T. T. (Shallice and Warrington, 1980) reads
50% of non-words. When non-words were read erroneously they are frequently lexicalised. That is, they are read as words which bear some
orthographic resemblance to the stimulus item. Regardless of the level of non-word reading, the level of word reading is always higher.

For some phonological dyslexics word reading performance is so
good that their error corpus is small. However, even amongst these
cases a characteristic error pattern has emerged. Words that are
morphologically complex with derivational and inflectional affixes
are frequently misread; the usual term for these errors is 'derivational'. In addition to the derivational errors, 'visual' errors
are made. Originally, these errors were misleadingly labelled and
are probably better considered as invalid errors. They were called
visual errors (Marshall and Newcombe, 1973) as the responses bear
a visual resemblance to the stimulus items. They also, however,
bear a phonological resemblance by virtue of the structure of an
alphabetic orthography. The term does not imply that the errors
result from any peripheral difficulties with the visuo-sensory
system. Examples of visual errors are:

                    goat -> get
                    place ->palace
                    grow -> grop   /gɾɒp/

In phonological dyslexia we are concerned with visual errors like
the first two above, i. e. with visual paralexias. Visual errors
in phonological dyslexics do not generally result in neologistic
responses. In fact, very few, if any, of the responses of a phonological dyslexic are neologistic. When errors are made by phonological dyslexics they are visual or derivational in nature, although
the incidence of one or other type may be small. Thus A. M. (Patterson, 1982) makes very few visual errors and W. B. (Funnell, 1983)
makes few derivational errors.

Visual and derivational errors are also characteristic of deep dyslexics. However, the most salient feature in the syndrome of deep dyslexia is the presence of semantic errors. Semantic errors have only ever been reported in one phonological dyslexic patient (Funnell, 1983) and in this case their incidence was extremely rare. With the exception of the three or four errors in this case, one may say that semantic errors are absent in phonological dyslexia. Nonetheless, in a number of cases of phonological alexia the occasional error has been reported which bears both a visual and a semantic relation to the stimulus item (Funnell, 1983; Job and Sartori, 1982; Patterson, 1982; Kremin, this volume) e. g., satirical -> "sarcastic".

Just as the semantic error of the deep dyslexic is absent in phonological dyslexia, so the regularisation error characterstic of the surface dyslexic is also absent. Thus, one does not find errors of the sort sweat -> "sweet".

A number of phonological dyslexics have been reported to have difficulty reading function words in isolation (e. g. Beauvois and Dérouesné, 1979; Patterson, 1982), whilst other phonological dyslexics have been reported to have no such difficulty (Shallice and Warrington, 1980; Dérouesné and Beauvois, 1982). Since this feature is variable it cannot be considered as a crucial or defin- ing characteristic of phonological dyslexia. However, it is begi- nning to emerge that even those phonological dyslexics who do not have difficulty with reading function words in isolation have extreme difficulty reading function words within text (Kremin, this volume; Shallice, personal communication). Normal adult readers make some errors reading function words in text but the difficulties observed in the cases of phonological dyslexia is much more severe. It remains to be seen whether the difficulty in text will prove to be true for all phonological dyslexics.

Reading through the cases of phonological dyslexia reported in the literature one is struck by the number of left handers. About half of the reported cases are left-handed individuals. Clearly this is much higher than the proportion of left handers in the population as a whole. There is also at least one case of a right hander becoming a phonological dyslexic after a right hemi- sphere lesion (Beauvois, personal communication). The question arises as to whether phonological dyslexics are prone to lie with- in an unusual neurological subpopulation. This concludes the discussion of the characterstics of phonological dyslexia. A summary in presented in Table 1.

THEORETICAL EXPLANATION

The syndrome of acquired phonological dyslexia has been expla- ined as resulting from damage to the grapheme-phoneme conversion

Table 1. The characterstics of acquired phonological dyslexia

---

1. Non word reading poor in comparison to word reading

2. Presence of derivational paralexias, e. g.
            children -> "child"

3. Presence of visual paralexias, e. g.
            goat   ->   "get"

4. Virtual absence of semantic errors

5. Virtual absence of regularisations

6. Function word difficulties in isolation or in text
    (to be confirmed)

7. Unusual neurological subpopulation (?)

Fig. 1. A simplified reading model showing the G. P. C. route,
         the semantic route and the direct route

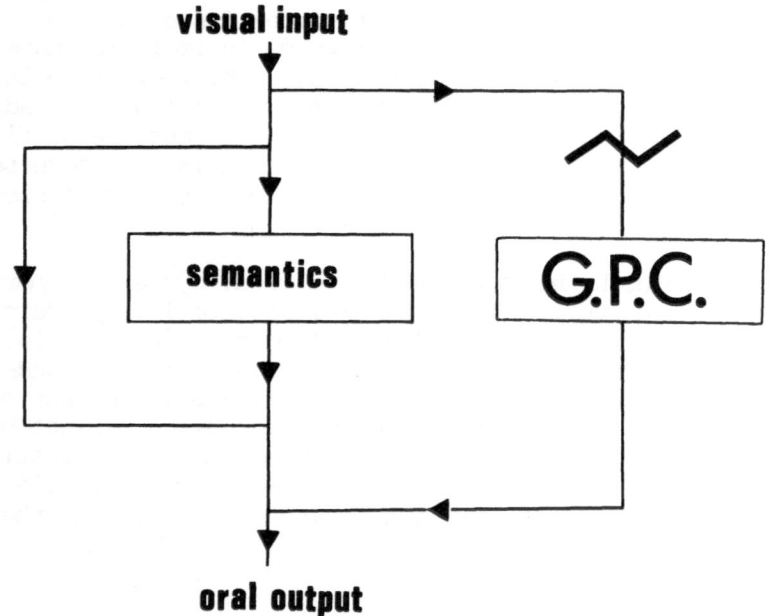

system, one of three hypothesized reading routes. A simplified
version of the reading models presented in other chapters in this
volume is given in Figure 1.

The three reading routes are all marked. The "G. P. C. route"
contains the grapheme-phoneme conversion system. The "semantic
route" passes through semantic representations. The "direct route"
bypasses semantics. The lightning bolt represents the hypothesized
functional disconnection of the G. P. C. route. Non-words, which
require the grapheme-phoneme conversion system to be read are thus
difficult, whereas words can be read relatively efficiently by use
of the direct route or the semantic route. In terms of a triple
route model this is similar to the theoretical interpretation that
has been proferred for deep dyslexia. The differences between the
two may be explained in at least two ways on this model. In phonological dyslexia we may be seeing the true normal functioning of
the semantic route. The direct route may or may not be intact.
In deep dyslexia there may be additional lesions to both the direct
route and also to the semantics box resulting in the production of
semantic errors. In other words, by this explanation of phonological dyslexia the semantic route is intact and possibly also the
direct route but the G. P. C. route is functionally disconnected,
the direct route is functionally disconnected and the semantic
system is impaired. An alternative explanation suggests that in
deep dyslexia we may be seeing the true normal functioning of the
direct route which is intrinsically unstable, resulting in semantic
errors. In phonological dyslexia these errors may be prevented by
the minimal phonology that remains intact in the G. P. C. system.
This explanation would implicate the same sites of disconnection
for phonological dyslexia as the first explanation but for deep
dyslexia it would posit only two impairments, not three. That
is, in deep dyslexia both the G. P. C. route and the direct route
would be functionally disconnected but the semantic route would be
intact.

Just as there are two explanations for the differences between
deep and phonological dyslexia on this model, so there are at least
two explanations for the presence of derivational errors. One explanation, however, would require considerable restructuring of
our notions of how the G.P. C. system works. If one wishes to
argue that phonological dyslexia is caused by a single functional
lesion, then one may suggest that affix stripping (Taft, 1981;
Morton, 1981) occurs early in processing with base lexical item
travelling down the direct route. It is processed via semantics
which is unimpaired. The affix, however, is processed via the
grapheme-phoneme conversion system. We know that in phonological
dyslexia this system is disrupted. The current formulation of the
G. P. C. system would permit that when the system was malfunctioning affixes or indeed any letter groups could be dropped. It would
not permit that affixes could be added or substituted. Shallice,

Warrington and McCarthy (1983) have suggested that an expansion of
our notions of the phonological system may be necessary. The system
may not merely operate at the level of the grapheme but "can operate
on a number of different types of orthographic units, namely, graphemes, consonant clusters, sub-syllabic units, syllables and morphemes." If this notion was extended to suggest that one unit which
could be operated on was the affix, then a deficit in the phonological route could produce errors of omission, substitution and addition of affixes to stimulus words. Although this explanation would
require an expansion of the phonological route and a clearer formulation of exactly what constraints govern it and how they may be
disrupted, it would permit the full syndrome of phonological dyslexia to be explained from one "lesion." It would also be consistent with the observation that in all reported cases to date of
patients who have difficulty reading nonsense words, derivational
reading errors are also made.

The alternative explanation for the presence of derivational
errors may be made using the model as it stands, but the explanation
requires a second "lesion" to the model. In this explanation both
base lexical item and affix may be processed via the semantic route.
A deficit at some point in the system results in the production of
a word orthographically (visually) and semantically related to the
stimulus item. This type of error could occur at one of several
sites within the semantic route.

THE CASES

   1. H. M.

   H. M. is a seventeen year old girl with developmental dyslexia.
She is left-handed. There is no family history of reading or spelling disability. She has never received remedial treatment, and
survived within the normal school system until concern arose after
failure in state examinations. She was referred for assessment of
reading and spelling difficulties.

   The standardized test results that H. M. attained are presented
in Table II. It can be seen that H. M. is of at least average
intelligence. The decline in WISC scores over five years does not
reflect intellectual deterioration. The pattern is characteristic
of dyslexic children. The test is scored from age norms. Each year
the special handicap of these children causes them to fall further
and further behind their peers. Thus, although absolute scores
increase, age scaled scores are lower and IQ's appear to drop.

   It is interesting to note that H. M.'s digit span is average
for age. Digit span is a test of auditory sequential short term
memory. In Baddeley's terms (Baddeley, 1981), it would be a test of
working memory. It has been claimed that dyslexic children have

TABLE II. Standardized test results of H. M.

H. M.   Age 17

Wechsler Intelligence Scale for children

1976 Verbal IQ 114   Performance IQ 115
1981 Verbal IQ 105   Performance IQ   86

Raven's Progressive Matrices

IQ 107-111

Peabody Picture Vocabulary Test

IQ 113

Digit span

6 forward   4 backward

Schonell Single Word Reading

10 years 11 months

Neale Text Reading

9 years 7 months

Schonell Single Word Spelling

10 years 7 months

Arithmetic - very poor

---

reduced digit spans and if one looks at group data or indeed at
most individual cases this is true. The reading pattern to be
described occurs with normal auditory sequential short term memory.

       H. M.'s reading level is 10 years and 11 months. This clearly
shows reading retardation but does not reflect a gross impairment.
It is considered that many adult readers may not have a reading age
above 12 years 6 months on this test. Certainly H. M.'s reading
level lies within that spanned by adult phonological dyslexics.
H. M.'s text reading score is lower than her single word reading
score. One often sees the reverse pattern because of the facilitating effects of context. The pattern here results from a function
word deficit in text which will be discussed later. Table II indicates that spelling is also well below expectation.

2. J. E.

J. E. is a sixteen and a half year old girl. She is right handed. Her father is a research engineer but is reported to have had reading and spelling difficulties. Her elder sister has a good university degree and excellent academic record but complains of spelling difficulties and mild difficulties reading aloud. Detailed examination revealed a mild but not handicapping disability. Both sisters have right-left confusions. J. E.'s results on standardized test are shown in Table III. She is of high average intelligence.

TABLE III. Standardized test results of J. E.

J. E. Age 16½

Wechsler Intelligence Scale for Children

1982 Verbal IQ 115   Performance IQ 112

Raven's Progressive Matrices

IQ 97

Digit span

4 forward   3 backward

Schonell Single Word Reading

12 years 4 months

Neale Text Reading

9 years 2 months

Schonell Single Word Spelling

10 years 7 months

Arithmetic - very poor

Digit span in this case is reduced. J. E.'s single word reading level is higher than H. M.'s, but once again the difficulty in text reading is manifest: the cause again a function word difficulty. Spelling and arithmetic are also poor. In addition, J. E. has visuo-spatial and sequencing problems which H. M. does not have.

J. E. still makes many b-d reversals.

Before even turning to the character of the reading performance
it is apparent that one of the tentative characterstics in Table I
has a parallel. It was suggested that acquired phonological dyslexia might occur in an unusual neurological subpopulation. The two
developmental cases here are females and one is left-handed. The
sex differnce in the number of boys and girls who are affected by
dyslexia is well documented. Estimates vary from a ratio of 4:1
to that of 6:1, boys always being more affected than girls. My own
experience with referrals is that the sex ratio is about 10:1.
Social factors may be involved here as there may still be more
concern produced by a boy failing academically than a girl who may
be permitted to concentrate instead on less intellectually demanding activities. Whatever the cause, having seen very few dyslexic
girls, I found the presence of the disorder to be described very
striking. I will rashly predict that developmental phonological
dyslexia will be more common amongst girls and amongst left-handers
than overall population estimates would predict.

READING OF NON-WORDS

It will be recalled that the crucial characterstic of phonological dyslexia is the discrepancy between word reading and non-
word reading. Table IV presents examples of the reading errors
which J. E. and H. M. make to non-words.

TABLE IV. Examples of reading errors to non-words

H. M.

vissil	->	vessel	
glud	->	blood	
grele	->	grill	
rond	->	rod	
etum	->	etrum	/ɛtrʌm/
fide	->	frid	/frɪd/

J. E.

goom	->	gloom	
falad	->	floor	
grele	->	grill	
duss	->	dusk	
pume	->	perume	/pɛrum/
hice	->	hins	/hɪns/

They are impaired at non-word reading and many of their erroneous responses are lexicalisations. Some neologistic responses
are made. The response item bears at least some similarity to the
stimulus item. The performance on non-word reading is significantly
worse than the performance on word reading. This is a consistent
effect true for both the subjects. One example will be given here.
H. M. was presented with a random list of 25 words and 25 non-words
to read aloud. Each non-word differed from one of the words by one
letter. The stimuli were taken from an unpublished list constructed
by Coltheart (1981). A full list of these stimuli and the responses
to them is presented in Table V. H. M. read all 25 of the words

TABLE V. H. M.'s reading responses to a balanced word/non-word list

NON WORD		WORD	
floon	"flown"	floor	✔
gouse	"goose"	house	✔
fime	"firm"	fine	✔
noor	"nor"	door	✔
doney	"donkey"	money	✔
foom	"foam"	room	✔
chold	"cold"	child	✔
foop	"flop"	food	✔
garl	"gall"	girl	✔
moman	"mormon"	woman	✔
boak	"book"	book	✔
streed	"stress"	street	✔
cimy	"clammy"	city	✔
ede	"Ed"	eye	✔
fape	"fap" /fæp/	face	✔
charch	"chark" /tʃɑrk/	church	✔
pand	✔	hand	✔
doy	✔	boy	✔
cag	✔	car	✔
schoom	✔	school	✔
mun	✔	man	✔
heam	✔	head	✔
poad	✔	road	✔
nater	✔	water	✔
toble	✔	table	✔

correctly but only read 9/25 of the non-words correctly. This was despite a lenient scoring criterion for non-words in which any reasonable interpretation was accepted. Of the sixteen errors to non-words,
fourteen were lexicalisations and two were neologisms.

ERRORS ON WORD READING ALOUD

Derivational errors are made by both the subjects. Examples
of these are given in Table VI. About a quarter of H. M.'s errors
are derivational in nature and about half of J. E.'s errors are
derivational. The number of derivational errors elicited varies
slightly from list to list. Amongst the other reading errors a

TABLE VI. Derivational errors

H. M. eg:

weigh	->	weight
instance	->	instant
appeared	->	appearance ⌒ 25% of errors
imagine	->	image
smoulder	->	smouldering

J. E. eg:

amusement	->	amused
refuse	->	refusal
political	->	politician ⌒ 50% of errors
cautious	->	caution
children	->	child

---

large proportion are "visual". J. E. makes the errors:

politics	->	"polite"
archer	->	"anchors"
bouquet	->	"boutique"
persuade	->	"pursued"

and H. M. makes the errors:

secret	->	"scarlet"
press	->	"pass"
strength	->	"strange"
harsh	->	"haste"

Regularisation errors are not present, nor are semantic errors.
However, one or two other interesting errors occur which are "pseudoderivational" or visuo-semantic. H. M. reads conscience as "con-
scient" /kɒnsəɪənt/ . The response is neologistic but it would
seem that a similar mechanism may be involved in its production as
in the production of derivational errors. Another example of this
sort is the error unjust ->"injust", although admittedly this could
merely be a visual error. J. E. makes the error conscience ->"con/

science"/kɒnllsəɪəns/. Once again, this error may be related to a
derivational error. J. E. has particular difficulty with affixes.
It was noted that 50% of her errors are derivational. She also often
reads a word omitting the suffix; sufficient time will elapse for me
to write down the stimulus and mark it wrong and I will be about to
present a subsequent stimulus when suddenly she says the suffix:
instantly ->"instant. . . . . . ."ly". This occurs with some consistency. It may be of interest to note that a deep dyslexic patient,
Y. N., that Marshall and I have recently had the opportunity to study
also makes "pseudoderivational" errors. She, of course, as a deep
dyslexic makes many derivational errors. Examples of Y. N.'s "pseudoderivational" errors include:

> lush   -> "lushed"
> corner -> "corn"
> design -> "sign"
> round -> "rounders"

It was noted in the introduction that acquired phonological
dyslexics sometimes make errors which are both visually and semantically related to the stimulus item. H. M. made five errors of this
sort: thinness ->"thickness", gaoled -> "gallowed", politics ->
"policies", arrangement ->"agreement" and simile ->similar. J. E.
made the identical error gaoled -> "gallowed" and also made the
errors insufficient ->"insignificant", naive ->"native", naughty ->
"caught". Observing these latter errors I became interested in what
meaning the subjects were deriving from print. The question of the
meaning that is derived by the reader has arisen recently with respect to surface dyslexia. In the original patients of Marshall and
Newcombe (1973) meaning was attributed to the response. For example,
patient J. C. made the error begin->"beggin" and glossed the meaning
as " collected money". He thus interpreted his own response not the
stimulus. However, Kremin (1983) has recently reported a patient
who, despite making regularisation errors, attributes meaning correctly to the original stimulus item.

H. M. and J. E. do not make regularisation errors. However, they
do make visual errors. I asked J. E. the meaning of a few words immediately after she had made visual errors to them. For some words
meaning was attributed to the response: pneumonia-> "pandemonia". .
"everything going wrong." However, for a number of others the meaning
of the original stimulus was given despite an erroneous vacalisation:

> soloist   -> "solicit" . . . "sings alone"
> slovenly -> "solvently" . . "sort of lounges about"
>   . . . "I don't really know."
> preliminary->"peliminary" /pɛlɪmɪndrel/ . "basic"

There were also instances when the meaning of both the stimulus
and response appeared to be conveyed. The following conversation

illustrates this:
J. E. was presented with the word <u>colonel</u>:

        J. E.:   "Cologne"
        C. T.:   "Can you tell me what it means?"
        J. E.:   "Is it perfume or is it a colonel?"
        C. T.:   "If you had to pick one which would you pick?"
        J. E.:   "I don't know. It's either perfume or it's a
                   sergeant."
        C. T.:   "Would you like to try and read it again?"
        J. E.:   "Cologne."

It is of particular interest that J. E. articulates the correct word
when describing the meaning of the word, yet still does not seem to
realize that this was the original stimulus item.

This pattern of performance is characterstic of words of intermediate difficulty. Easy words are read correctly. Harder words are
treated like nonsense words. The neologistic responses arise to
these, e. g., <u>scintillate</u> -> signitate   /Saɪnɪteɪt/
When asked the meaning of this she had no idea.

One relevant aspect of the reading of the two subjects had not
yet been mentioned. Both subjects are very good at reading function
words presented in isolation. However, when the function words occur
in text problems are created. A substantial proportion of the errors
in text reading are on function words and this disability accounts in
large part for the low Neale text reading age of each subject in comparison to her Schonell single word reading age. Many children and
even adults reading aloud make errors on function words, but the severity of the problem in the cases of these two subjects is striking.

Combined together all these reading errors produce impaired reading of text. An example for each subject is given below. The sentences are taken from the Neale Analysis of Reading Test. H. M. was
presented with the sentences:

        Among animals the fox has no rival for cunning. Sus-
        picious of man, who is its only natural enemy, it will,
        when pursued, perform extraordinary feats, even alighting
        on the backs of sheep to divert its scent trail.

She read it as follows:

        "Am<u>ongst</u> animals the fox has no rival<u>s</u> for cunning.
        <u>Surprisingly</u> of man, who <u>is</u> its only natural enemy <u>at</u>
        will, <u>with</u> pursued perform<u>ance</u> extraordinary feat<u>_</u>,
        even alighting on the backs of sheep to divert its
        scent <u>trial</u>."

J. E. was presented with the following sentence:

> Each April, at the reappearance of the cuckoo in its
> familiar haunts, bird-watchers must marvel at the
> accurate flights with which birds span the distances
> between their seasonal abodes.

She read it:

> "Each April, at the reappearance of the cuckoo in the
> familiar haunts, the bird-watchers must marvel at the
> accent flights, which the birds span the distance_
> between the_ seasonal abdoze."

It is readily apparent that both subjects' reading is paragrammatic
(Kleist, 1934). To the listener the sentences also became less comprehensible. Given that J. E. often comprehends correctly words
that she had read incorrectly, it is not clear whether to her the
passage remains fully comprehensible.

THE QUESTION OF THE PARALLEL

At the beginning of this chapter the characterstics of acquired
phonological dyslexia were discussed, and then summarized in Table I.
The current contention is that these two developmental cases form
analogues to acquired phonological dyslexia. Having presented the
data it is worthwhile now referring back to Table I and checking
which of the adult characterstics have also been observed in the
developmental cases. It has been shown that the non-word reading
of H. M. and J. E. is poor in comparison to word reading. Amongst
the error data of both subjects there are derivational paralexias
and visual paralexias. There are no semantic errors or regularisation errors. Function word difficulties occur in text reading.
Both subjects are females, which in view of the sex ratio in developmental dyslexia, may suggest an unusual subpopulation is involved.

All the characterstics of acquired phonological dyslexia have
been found in the two developmental cases described here. It would
seem we may now refer to developmental phonological dyslexia.

QUESTIONS FOR THE FUTURE

The existence of developmental phonological dyslexia raises a
number of interesting questions. Firstly, how are we to conceptua-
lize the development of reading in the normal child, when acquisition of reading, to the level of competency described here, is possible in the presence of only minimal phonics. It has been considered that the phonological route is needed to learn to read. Is
H. M. atypical or do our theories require revision? Secondly, given

that developmental parallels have now been found to acquired surface dyslexia (Coltheart, 1982; Coltheart et al., 1983) and to acquired phonological dyslexia, how many of the other acquired reading disorders also have parallels amongst the developmental dyslexias. Is there, for example, a parallel to acquired deep dyslexia? Do children exist who make semantic errors to single words presented in isolation and who also have very poor phonics? Suppose, for the moment, that parallels to <u>all</u> the acquired reading disorders were found in developmental cases. That is, whenever reading broke down in a literate adult the pattern of dissolution was very similar to one of the patterns of difficulty seen in the acquisition of reading. Would it be necessary to assume that much more of the reading system is prewired then one might have thought? What then would be the role of learning? Even if parallels are not found to all the acquired reading disorders an explanation is required for those parallels that do exist. Finally, moving from theoretical to practical considerations, do these subtypes of developmental dyslexia, respond differently to different remedial strategies? This question can also be addressed with respect to the acquired subtypes. Can we learn anything about the most fruitful way to remediate the adult from the study of the child parallels or vice versa? Are the recovery paths of acquired and developmental parallels the same qualitatively or quantitatively?

These are some of the questions raised by the existence of developmental phonological dyslexia. No doubt, there are many more. It is to be hoped that in the years to come at least some of them will be answered.

REFERENCES

Aram, D. M., Rose, D. F. and Horowitz, S. J. Hyperlexia: Developmental reading without meaning. (This volume)
Baddely, A. The concept of working memory: A view of its current state and probable future developments. <u>Cognition</u>, 1981, <u>10</u>, 17-23.
Beauvois, M. F. and Dérouesné, J. Phonological processes in reading: data from alexia. <u>Journal of Neurology, Neurosurgery, and Psychiatry</u>, 1979, <u>42</u>, 1125-1132.
Coltheart, M. Analyzing acquired disorders of reading. Unpublished manuscript, Birkbeck college, 1981.
Coltheart, M. Surface dyslexia and its implications for models of normal reading. In D. E. Broadbent and L. Weiskrantz (Eds.) <u>The Neuropsychology of Cognitive Function</u>. London: The Royal Society, 1982.
Coltheart, M., Masterson, J., Byng, S., Prior, M. and Riddoch, J. Surface dyslexia. <u>Quarterly Journal of Experimental Psychology</u>, (In Press).

Dérouesné, J. and Beauvois, M. F. Phonological alexia. Paper pre-
    sented at the V European Conference of the I. N. S., Deauville,
    France, June 15-18, 1982.
Funnell, E.   Phonological processes in reading: New evidence from
    acquired dyslexia. British Journal of Psychology, (In Press).
Goldblum, M. C. and Kremin, H. Semantic processing of words in sur-
    face dyslexia. In J. C. Marshall, K. E. Patterson and M. Colt-
    heart (Eds.), Surface Dyslexia, London: Routledge and Kegan
    Paul, 1983.
Holmes, J. M. Dyslexia: A neurolinguistic study of traumatic and
    developmental disorders of reading. Ph. D. Thesis, University
    of Edinburgh, 1973.
Job, R. and Sartori, G. Prelexical decomposition. University of
    Padua Institute of Psychology, Report 62, 1982.
Kleist, K. Gehirnpathologie. Barth: Leipzig, 1934.
Marshall, J. C. and Newcombe, F. Syntactic and semantic errors in
    paralexia. Neuropsychologia, 1966, 4, 169-176.
Marshall, J. C. and Newcombe, F. Patterns of paralexia: A psycho-
    linguistic approach. Journal of Psycholinguistic Research,
    1973, 2, 175-199.
Morton, J. The status of information processing models of language.
    Philosophical Transactions of the Royal Society, London, B295,
    1981, 387-396.
Patterson, K. E. The relation between reading and phonological co-
    ding: Further neuropsychological observations. In A. W.
    Ellis (Ed.), Normality and Pathology in Cognitive Functions,
    London: Academic Press, 1982.
Schwartz, M. F., Saffran, E. M. and Marin, O. S. M. Fractionating
    the reading process in dementia: Evidence for word-specific
    print-to-sound associations. In M. Coltheart, K. Patterson
    and J. C. Marshall (Eds.), Deep Dyslexia, London: Routledge and
    Kegan Paul, 1980.
Shallice, T. and Warrington, E. K. Single and multiple component
    central dyslexic syndromes. In M. Coltheart, K. Patterson and
    J. C. Marshall (Eds.), Deep Dyslexia, London: Routledge and
    Kegan Paul, 1980.
Shallice, T., Warrington, E. K. and McCarthy, R. Reading without
    semantics. Quarterly Journal of Experimental Psychology, (In
    press).
Taft, M. Prefix stripping revisited. Journal of Verbal Learning
    and Verbal Behavior, 1981, 20, 289-297.

LETTER NAMING AS A SPELLING STRATEGY[1]

Philip A Luelsdorff
Institut Fur Anglistic
Univesität Regensburg
Regesnburg, 1 West Germany

INTRODUCTION

Poor performance in spelling has frequently been cited as a characteristic of dyslexics (Critchley, 1975; Naidoo, 1972; Orton, 1966; Rutter, 1978), although little attention has been devoted to its study (Cook, 1981) and remediation (Bradley, 1981) in dyslexic monolinguals and even less in dyslexic bilinguals (Luelsdorff, 1981; Luelsdorff and Marshall, 1982).

The purpose of this paper is to discuss the use of letter naming as a spelling strategy based on an analysis of the vowel errors attributable to letter naming in a corpus of sentences containing 6,162 words with 2,138 errors dictated to a 12-year-old incipient English/ German bilingual over a 14month period (cf. Luelsdorff 1981 for methodological details) and to propose extended letter naming as a technique for the prevention and remediation of spelling errors.

PRECONVENTIONAL SPELLING

Studies of preschool children's prephonic, preliterate, "invented" spelling (Read, 1971) indicate that such children spell on the basis of their phonetic analysis of the spoken word and their knowledge of the written alphabet and letter names, a spelling strategy which was pointed out by Cook (1981) to be also frequently observable in the misspellings of older dyslexic children. That knowledge of letter names plays the key role in preconventional spelling becomes

1. The major portion of the research for this paper was made possible by a grant from the Fritz Thyssen Stiftung.

apparent on the inspection of the list of preconventional error types, reproduced here from Cook (1981) as Table 1.

TABLE 1

I.   Consonant Phonetic Spellings (Preconventional)

      A. Nasal omitted before a final stop consonant, as WET/went;
          DOT/don't.

      B. Use of letter whose name contains the phoneme, as Y for
          /w/ and H for /ch/:YOH/watch; YEL/will.

      C. Spelling initial /dr/ as JR (JRS/dress) and initial /tr/
          as CHR (CHRAN/train).

      D. Representation of surface phonetic detail, such as the re-
          duction of medial /t/, as in LIDL/little.

II.   Vowel Phonetic Spellings (Preconventional)

      A. Letter name for long vowel sound, as in MAK/make; FEL/feel;
          SNO/snow.

      B. Short vowel sound spelled with letter name articulated in
          same place, such as BAD/bed; KIT/cut; SET/sit; JRO/draw.

      C. Representaion of elongation, rounding, or glide on vowels,
          such as BOE/boy; GOW/go; MEE/me.

III. Syllabic Phonetic Spellings (Preconventional)

      A. Letter name used for syllable or part of syllable, as RGU/
          argue; XPRS/express.

      B. Final syllables (vowel-consonant segments) as in ENTR/ent-
          er; MITN/mitten; LIDL/little.

LITERAL USE AND MENTION

       To Carnap we owe the expression "autonymous" in reference to
the use of words as the names of the same words, as in "The word
'man' is spelled with three letters" or "The word 'man' is a mono-
syllable." To this expression we would like to add "visual autonymous use" and "audio autonymous use" in order to distinguish between
the two essentially different autonymous uses of names exemplified
by "The word 'man' begins with the letter m," in which 'man' is used
to refer to the sequence of letters which constitute its legitimate
spelling, and by "The word 'man' initiates in a voiced bilabial nasal," in which 'man' is used to refer to its pronunciation. Both these autonymous uses of the word 'man', in which 'man' appears as the
proper name of its spelling, on the one hand, and as the proper name
of its pronunciation, on the other, sharply contrast with the deno-
tative use of 'man', in which 'man' is used to refer to a featherless,
plantigrade, biped animal. Cast in terms of Quine's distinction

between the mention of a word and its use, we may mention a word to refer to either its spoken or written shape, or use it to denote.

The distinction between visual and audio autonymous use pertains to the names of letters as well as to the names of words, as in "The word 'salmon' is spelled with an <u>l</u>" and "<u>L</u> is a consonant whose name begins with a vowel". Thus letters, like words, can be either signifiers or signifieds. The sounds which the letter is used to represent are its signifieds and the letter itself their signifier; the name of the letter is the signifier and the letter itself the signified. When the sound of the name of the letter and the sound the letter is used to represent fully coincide, as in the free alternate pronunciation of the "primary vowels" <u>a</u>, <u>e</u>, <u>i</u>, <u>o</u>, and <u>u</u> in English (cf. Venezky 1970), that is, <u>when the mention of a letter is identical with its</u> use, we speak of <u>complete echoicity</u> and propose ranking the alphabets of the world according to the extent to which their letters are echoic

LETTER NAMING

Letter naming, i.e., pronouncing the names of the letters of the alphabet, e.g., English <u>a</u> = [e ɪ], <u>e</u> = [ɪ], <u>i</u> = [a ɪ], <u>o</u> = [o y], <u>u</u> = [j o y], or German <u>a</u> = [d:], <u>e</u> = [e:], <u>i</u> = [i:], <u>o</u> = [o:], <u>u</u> = [u:] has been described as one of the devices characteristic of the invented spelling of young children (Read, 1971; Schreiber and Read, 1980; Cook, 1981) where letter symbols are generated on the basis of preliterate children's knowledge of the written alphabet and letter names.

We place three conditions on a theory of letter-naming used as a strategy for spelling: 1) that the informant know the names of the letters; 2) that the names of the letters be either identical with, closely approximate, or contain the sounds of the words they are used to represent; and 3) that the letters not correspond to those used in the standard spelling. (If the letters do correspond to those used in the standard spelling, it is clearly impossible to distinguish between letter-naming used as a spelling strategy, on the one hand, and letter-sounding used as a spelling strategy, on the other). Under these three conditions we find ample evidence of both English and German letter-naming used as a spelling strategy in the attempts of our incipient English/German bilingual to spell English words. We view this phenomenon as an overgeneralization of those instances where the names of the letters partially resemble the sounds the letters are used to legitimately represent, hence the abilities to 1) letter name and 2) use letter naming as a spelling strategy as constituent components of the spelling competence of the normal, fluent writer. Since this relationship is one of similarity between the sound of the letter name and the sound of the words the letter - name or the sequence of letter names is used to represent, it is echoic. Were this relationship completely regular,

whereby the names of the letters were identical with the constituent sounds of the words, or the sounds of the words predictably derivable from the names of the letters, such as appears to be
the case, or nearly the case, in Japanese kana, the orthography
would be optimally echoic.

As mentioned above, Cook (1981) has shown that letter-naming,
which is employed as a spelling strategy by preliterate, monolingual
children using "invented" spelling, is also characteristic of monolingual, developmentally dyslexic children, decreasingly in direct proportion to age, for children diagnosed as dyslexic on independent
grounds. We now have evidence to suggest that both native and target
language letter-naming interference in spelling be used as one of the
symptoms characteristic of the foreign-language dyslexia syndrome, the
additional attributes of which are yet to be ascertained.

Clear examples of English letter-naming in the Bernhard corpus
include the Vowels a, e, i, and u:

TABLE 2.   English Letter-Naming

Vowel	Target	Attempt	Page
a	paints	pans	A 2(2)
e	here	her	A 6, A 9(2)
	jeans	jens	A 75
i	likes	liks	A 5
	nine	nin	A 9
u	juice	just	A 20

Unambiguous examples of German letter-naming include the letters a, e, i, and u:

TABLE 3.   German Letter-Naming

Vowel	Target	Attempt	Page
a	John	Jam	A 14
	on	an	A 75(2)
e	cornflakes	cornfleks	A 2
	eighth	egth	A 11
i	evening	ivening	A 1
	sleeps	shlips	A 5
u	to	tu	A 9
	soup	sup	A 49

Apparently interpretable as examples of either English or German letter-naming are English or German o, which were pronounced virtually the same by the person administering the dictation:

o	toast	tost	A 6
	bones	bons	A 49

MAJOR PATTERN FOR PRIMARY VOWELS:

Venezky (1970) shows that the vowel spellings a, e, i/y, o, and u, which he terms "primary vowel spellings", carry the major burden of vowel representaion in English, and that each of the primary vowel units corresponds regularly to two different "morphophonemes", a free one and a checked one, according to the morpheme structure of the word in which it occurs and the consonant and vowel units which follow it.   These correspondences are given in Table IV, reproduced from Venezky (1970):

TABLE 4. Major Pattern for Primary Vowels

Spelling	Free Alternate	Checked Alternate
a	{e} sane mate ration	{æ} sanity mat rattle
e	{i} athlete mete penal	{ɛ} athletic met pennant
i	{ai} rise malign site	{ɪ} risen malignant sit
o	{o} cone robe posy	{a} conic rob possible
u	{ju} induce rude lucre	{ə} induction rudder luxury

In order to avoid repetition, a statement of the environmental determinants of the pronunciation of the primary vowel spellings will be defrayed until immediately below. Be it noted, however, that the names of the primary vowel letters are identical to the free alternat realizations listed in Table 4.

SPELLING: A TEACHING STRATEGY

It has been established that a major factor in the spelling strategy of both preschool, preconventional spellers and older dyslexic children is letter-naming. This strategy is maximally effective to the extent that there exists a one-to-one correspondence between the grapheme name and phoneme, which, in English, is notoriously not the case. Given the stated predisposition of preliterate, normal children and older dyslexic children to use letter-naming as a spelling strategy, we suggest naming each letter with an additional name such that the additional name is identical with the other predictable phoneme correspondence of the grapheme in question. This having been done, the task of the speller then amounts to correctly identifying the sound to be spelled with the sounds of the names of the grapheme and spelling accordingly. In the case of the primary vowel units a, e, i, o, u, this entails supplementing the established names of the letters [eɪ, Ik, ar, oʊ, joʊ], the free alternates, with the new letter names [æ, ɛ, I, a, ʌ   ], the checked alternates, respectively, with the instruction that the marker e be appended to words containing free alternates in their final syllables.

As a strategy for oral reading, the primary vowel letters are to be pronounced with their free alternates when they are followed by 1) a functionally simple consonant unit which in turn is followed by another vowel unit (including final e) or 2) a functionally simple consonant unit, followed by l or r, and then another vowel unit (including final e). Continuing to recapitulate Venezky (1970), they correspond to their checked alternates in the remaining cases, i.e., when followed by 1) a functionally compound consonant unit, e.g., x, dg, 2) a cluster of consonant units, e.g., nn, lth or, 3) a word-final consonant unit or units. Venezky's examples are shown in Table 5.

TABLE 5. Examples of Primary Vowel Correspondences for Selected Environments

Spelling	Free Alternate		Checked Alternate		
	1	2	1	2	3
a	canine	ladle	badge	saddle	sat
e	median	zebra	exit	antenna	ebb
i	pilot	microbe	chicken	epistle	hitch
o	vogue	noble	pocket	cognate	sod
u	dubious	lucre	luxury	supper	rug

In the case of slower monolingual and bilingual learners we suggest augmenting the bimodal, audio-visual approach of extended letter-naming proposed above with the trimodal audio-visual-tactile method partially developed and demonstrated to be effective by Bradley (1981). This method consists of the following series of ordered steps:

1) The student proposes the word he wants to learn. Clearly, in the case of the primary vowel units, the words proposed must be restricted to those containing either the free or the checked alternate.

2) The word is written correctly for him (or made with plastic script letters).

3) The student names the word.

4) He then writes the word himself, saying the alphabetic name of each letter of the word as it is written. Here the teacher should control to see that the letter names which are used are the English letter names and not the letter names in the native language.

5) He names the word again. He checks to see that the word has been written correctly so as to avoid inaccurate copying. Repeat steps 2 to 5 twice more, covering or disregarding the stimulus word as soon as the student feels he can manage without it.

6) The student practices the word in this way for six consecutive days.

Bradley reports that 80% of the words learned with this method were still spelled correctly four weeks later. It is hoped that the method of augmented letter naming proposed herein will yet improve this already impressive statistic.

REFERENCES

Bradley, L. The organization of motor patterns for spelling: An effective remedial strategy for backward readers. Developmental Medicine and Child Neurology, 1981, 23, 83-91.
Cook, L. Misspelling analysis in dyslexia: Observation of developmental strategy shifts. Bulletin of the Orton Society, 1981, 31, 123-134.
Critchley, M. Specific developmental dyslexia. In E. H. Lenneberg and E. Lenneberg (Eds.), Foundations of Language Development:

A multidisciplinary approach. Vol. II. New York: Academic
    Press, 1975.
Luelsdorff, P. A. Foreign language dyslexia: A research report,
    Linguistic Agency University of Trier, series B, Paper No. 71A,
    1981.
Luelsdorff, P. A. and Marshall, J. C. On putative 'transpositions'
    in spelling. Unpublished manuscript.
Naidoo, S. Specific Dyslexia, New York: Wiley & Sons, 1972.
Orton, J. L. The Orton-Gillingham approach. In J. Money (Ed.),
    The Disabled Reader. Baltimore: The Johns Hopkins Press, 1966.
Read, C. Preschool children's knowledge of English phonology.
    Harvard Educational Review, 1971, 41, 1-34.
Rutter, M. Prevalence and types of dyslexia. In A. Benton and
    D. Pearl (Eds.), Dyslexia: An appraisal of current knowledge,
    New York: Oxford University Press, 1978.
Schreiber, P. and Read, C. Children's use of phonetic cues in
    spelling, parsing, and ---- may be ------- reading. Bulletin
    of the Orton Society, 1980, 30, 209-224.
Venezky, R. L. The structure of English orthography. Janua Lingua-
    rum, Series Minor, No. 82. The Hague: Mouton, 1970.

TEMPORAL ORDER PERCEPTION
AND
LATERALIZATION IN DYSLEXIC CHILDREN

Paul Eling [1]
Max-Planck-Institut fur
Psycholinguistik
Berg en Dalseweg 79
6522 BC Nijmegen
The Netherlands

INTRODUCTION

In the literature on developmental dyslexia a large number of suggestions have been offered for explaining the 'unexpected inability to learn to read' in a certain proportion of the children. Reference is often made to theoretical notions that have been introduced in other, usually more basic areas of research in order to explain this disability to learn to read. One example is the concept of temporal order perception (Bakker, 1972) or sequential analysis. Comparing visual and auditory modes of processing, it is often observed that auditory information, for instance speech, has to be perceived by integration over time: the whole stimulus is not present on a single moment in time and in order to perceive the stimulus successive 'snapshots' have to be integrated. Several authors have suggested that dyslexic children have specific problems with this process of sequential analysis. However if one carefully reads what is meant by this process by the different authors, or more particularly how it is measured, it appears that the notion of sequential analysis has been used for many different functions (for an overview, see Bakker, 1972). The present study is not designed to test the hypothesis that dyslexic children have specific problems with temporal order perception, because it appears from the literature that this 'fact' seems to be agreed upon generally.

Rather the aim is to demonstrate that under certain conditions dyslexic don't show these problems. Although it is obvious that one should not try to establish the null hypothesis (note 1) we assume that in this way we can point to the shortcomings of the indiscrimi-

1. The author gratefully acknowledges the assistance of Magriet Gal in collecting the data.

nate use of the concept of sequential analysis in the literature.

This study takes as a starting point the work of Orton (1937) and of Bakker (1972). In my opinion both authors predict on different grounds that dyslexic children make more errors in the recall of acoustically presented reversable words. By reversable words, a term used by Orton, I mean words in which the order of 'phonemes' can be reversed so that they produce a new meaningful word, e.g., 'straat' vs. 'staart' (= street vs. tail) or 'naam' vs. 'maan' (=name vs. mone). Orton and Bakker do not only predict problems in temporal order perception in dyslexic children but they also argue that these children are not lateralized like normal reading children. Both aspects, temporal order perception and laterality, are claimed to be interrelated, although in a different manner for Orton than for Bakker. First, I will briefly describe Orton's position, followed by Bakker's T. O. P. - theory.

The first assumption Orton made was that stimuli, visual as well as acoustical, are recorded in the brain in 'engrams'. In each hemisphere an engram will be laid down, the 'correct' one in the dominant left hemisphere and a 'mirror image' one in the right hemisphere. If the child fails to inhibit the functioning of the nondominant hemisphere, mirror image engrams may be activated when an attempt is made to recall particular words. Orton explicitly states that, although in the speech of reading disordered children only rarely complete reversals of words or parts of words occur, nevertheless sounds towards the end are distorted in order frequently when words previously heard are recalled.

Bakker's position is somewhat different. He is perfectly aware of the fact that temporal order perception has been studied in normal and reading retarded children in many different ways. In his review he mentions studies in which children are asked to reproduce rhythamic patterns that have been tapped out to them; in other studies series of digits are presented and the child has to recall the series or give the position of a particular item in the whole series of digits. According to Bakker there is a relation between temporal order perception and reading: children poor in temporal order perception tend to have low scores on reading tests. Furthermore, he clams that this relation is a causal one. The argument for this conclusion is one that can be found at many places in the literature on hemisphere specialization, in particular in those studies, that try to give an answer to the question what is the basic principle underlying the functions for which the left hemisphere is specialized. The argument runs as follows. Temporal order perception is a function of the left hemisphere or rather the left hemisphere is specialized in temporal analysis and therefore specialized in language processes like speech and reading. If the left hemisphere does not function properly temporal order perception will be disturbed and therefore problems will arise in acquiring reading.

The main difference between the explanations of Orton and Bakker is the following: for Orton problems will arise due to an active nondominant hemisphere. According to Bakker the disturbance in the development of the dominant hemisphere is the fact on causing problems in the functioning of language processes. On the other hand, both Orton and Bakker predict (1) that reading disordered children will make more errors in recalling audiotorily presented words and (2) that they will show a pattern of laterality different from that of normal children.

EXPERIMENT

To study these hypotheses the following experiment was done. As stimuli, 48 orthographically regular, monosyllabic Dutch words were used, all of which children of 7 years are supposed to know very well (Kohnstamm and De Vries, 1969). Half of the words were reversable words and the other half were not reversable. A word is called reversable if by changing the order of some 'phonemes', usually two, a new meaningful word is formed. The words were recorded from a female speaker. Using a PDP 11/45 computer they were digitized and stored on disk. A dichotic tape of 16 trials was produced with these tokens. Each trial consisted of three pairs of words; all words were either reversable or non-reversable words. The reversed version of a particular word was not presented in the same trial as the word from which it was formed: that is, words like 'maan' and 'naam' were not presented on the same trial. All stimuli were presented once to the right ear and once to the left ear. They were presented at a rate of 1 pair per second, with a recall period of 15 seconds. The headphone position was reversed for half of the subjects.

The experimental group consisted of 13 dyslexic children with a mean chronological age of 9 years. The control group consisted of 13 normal children of the same age. In addition to the dichotic task, laterality was measured in both groups of children using the Annett questionnaire and Annett's peg board (Annett, 1970a; 1970b).

We will first describe the results of the laterality measures. On the basis of the questionnaire children can be divided into three groups: consistent left-handers, consistent right-handers and a mixed group. For the normal children the number of children in each of these categories is 7, 2 and 4 respectively. Of the dyslexic children 7 are right handed and 6 are mixed. There does not appear to be a significant difference between the two groups of children in this respect.

The results of the peg board task are as follows: for both groups the right hand was significantly faster than the left hand. For the dyslexics the difference between the hands is 0.52 sec. (t = 1.96, p <0. 5). For the normals this difference is 1.16 sec.

($\underline{t}$ = 2.49, $\underline{p}$ < .05). However, if we compare the between-hand differences of the dyslexic children with those of the normal children
there does not appear to be a statistically significant effect ($\underline{t}$ =
1.17, $\underline{p}$ > .10).

I will now turn to the results of the dichotic task. All answers were recorded during recall. First an analysis of variance was
performed on the number of correctly recalled words. A significant
right ear advantage was found (F ($\underline{df}$ 24, 1) + 6.94, p < .05) of approximately 10% (see also Fig. 1). The ear advantage was similar for
both groups of children. Furthermore, it appears that reversable words are recalled more often correctly than non-reversable words (F
($\underline{df}$ 24, 1) = 8.36, $\underline{p}$ < .05).

We also looked at the number of children that show a right ear
advantage, a left ear advantage or no difference between ear scores.
The results are as follows: of the normal children 10 had a REA and
3 a LEA; of the dyslexic children 8 show a REA, 4 a LEA and 1 had no
difference between ear scores. No significant difference between
the two groups of children arises from the three measures of laterality we have used. This is not surprising considering the many negative results that have been published in the literature (for overvi-
ews, see Benton, 1975 and Satz, 1976).

The more interesting question, namely the perception and recall
of reversable words, was studied by looking at the errors produced
during recall. The total amount of reversal errors produced by the
dyslexic children is 13 (=2%): 8 errors to stimuli presented to the
right ear and 5 to left sided stimuli. For the normals these data
are: 16 reversal errors (=2.5%) of which 10 are to right ear stimuli
and 6 are to left ear stimuli. The great majority of errors for both groups of children consists of omissions. From these results, we
can conclude that in our study dyslexic children did not make more
errors than normal controls in the recalling of words and did not demonstrate specific problems in the perception of temporal order of
auditorily presented words.

DISCUSSION

A number of remarks can be made with respect to our study. The
number of trials in the dichotic task is rather low: only 16 trials
of three pairs of words. Nevertheless, a significant right ear advantage is demonstrated. Furthermore, the number of reversal errors
is also low. Perhaps it can be argued that what is observed here is
a floor effect and no meaningful comparison between dyslexic and normal children can be made. However, it must be noted that the childr-
en were far from being perfect in recalling the words. It appears
that they tend to omit the words they cannot recall correctly.

What is more important than discussing the strengths and

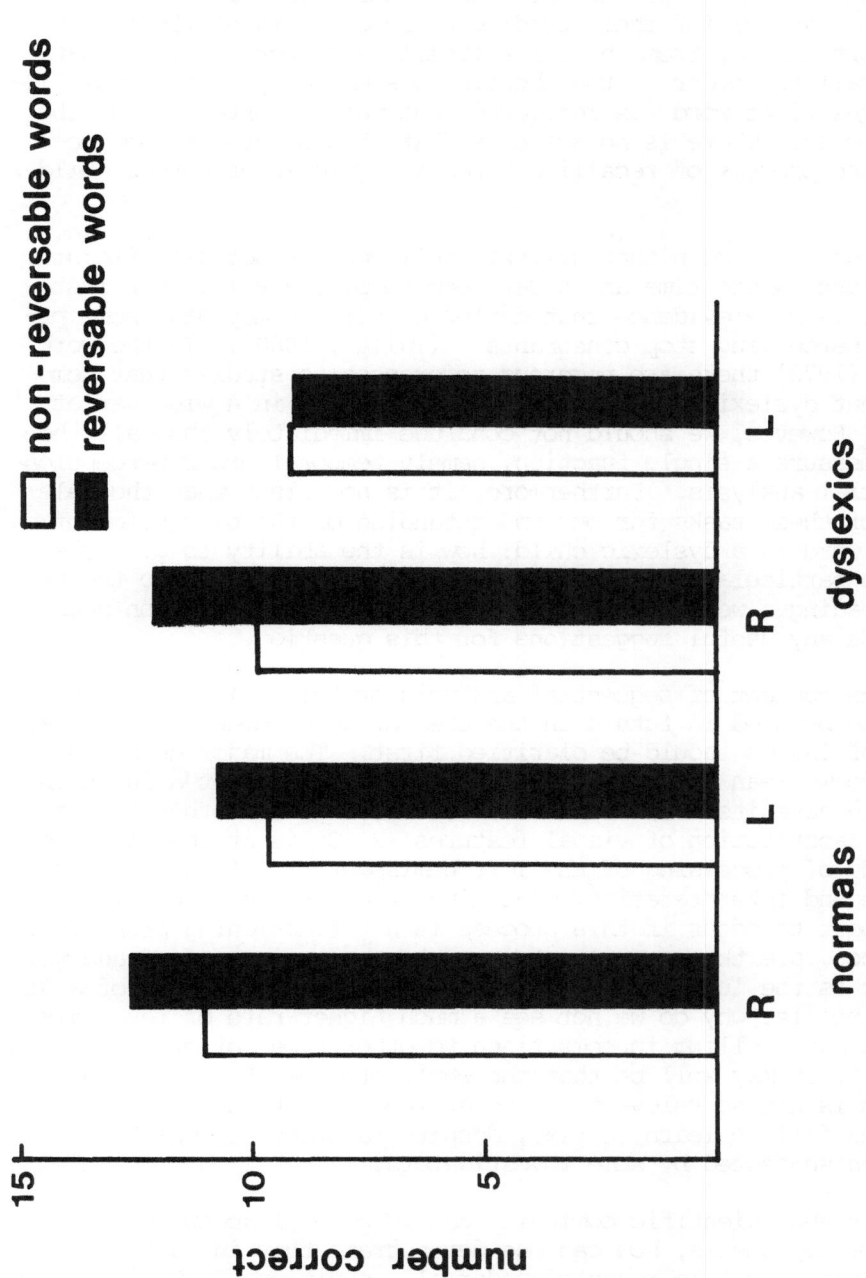

FIGURE 1.   Mean number of correct reversable and non-reversable words for normal and dyslexic children

weaknesses of this experiment, is the conclusion that dyslexic children can recall words previously heard quite well without distorting the order of phonemes. To my knowledge there is no reliable evidence that dyslexic children have specific problems in auditorily perceiving words. In reading aloud or in writing they may produce a word that is comparable to the target word except for the fact that some of the 'phonemes' are in the wrong order. This is certainly not an error typical for their reading behavior (Wissel 1963; Bakker, 1965). Furthermore, from the error itself we cannot conclude that during recall the order of the phonemes was mixed up. This would imply that the right word was retrieved, but was distorted during the output process. There is no evidence that this occurs at some occasions in the process of recalling words in dyslexic or normal children.

This does not mean that dyslexic children are not significantly worse in tasks where time and order seem to play a role. For instance, there is some evidence that dyslexic children may have some problems in perceiving stop consonants   (Tallal, 1980). In the work of Bakker (1972) there are numerous references to studies that demonstrate that dyslexics perform worse than normals in a wide variety of tasks. However, we should not conclude immediately that all these tasks measure a single function, namely temporal order perception or sequential analysis. Furthermore, it is not clear what the relevance is of these tasks for our understanding of the perception of a printed word in a dyslexic child: how is the ability to give the place of a particular digit in a series of digits related to the ability to reading a word ? The literature on speech perception does not provide any useful suggestions for this question.

If the concept of sequential analysis or temporal order perception is to be used in future in the area of developmental dyslexia, a number of issues should be clarified first. The major question is: what do we mean by temporal order perception. Is it a function that should have its 'box' in a model of reading like other functions, e.g., 'abstraction of visual features' ? Or is it the characteristic mode of processing of the left hemisphere ? If one chooses for the second interpretation, what kind of errors in temporal order can we expect to occur if this process is not functioning properly ? For instance, are the errors restricted to errors in reading and writing; what is the 'unit' that can be displaced ? A question of a different level is: why do we not see a much higher rate of reversals in reading and spelling in comparison to other types of errors in dyslexics ? It may well be that the whole problem of temporal order perception is not so relevant to the explanation of the fact that some children fail to learn to read, despite favorable circumstances as has been suggested by some investigators.

NOTE 1. If the scientific community has in general accepted the alternative hypothesis, how can one demonstrate that in fact the null hypothesis cannot be rejected under all conditions ? One solution would be to redefine the null hypothesis as the hypotheses that is held by the majority of the researchers in a particular area.

REFERENCES

Annett, M. A classification of hand preference by association ana-lysis. British Journal of Psychology, 1970, 61, 303-312, a
Annett, M. The growth of manual preference and speed. British Journal of Psychology, 1970, 61, 545-558, b
Bakker, D. J. Leerstoornissen: een fouten-analyse Nederlands Tijd-schrift voor de Psychologie, 1965, 20, 173-183.
Bakker, D. J. Temporal order in disturbed reading. Rotterdam: University Press 1972.
Benton, A. L. Developmental Dyslexia: Neurological aspects. In: W. J. Friedlander (Ed), Advances in Neurology. New York: Raven Press, 1975.
Kohnstamm, G. A., & De Vries, A. K. Streeflijst woordenschat by de overgang van kleuteronderwijs naar basis onderwijs. IJmuiden: Vermande en Zonen, 1969.
Orton, S. Reading, writing and speech-problems in children. London: Norton & Co., 1937.
Satz, P. Cerebral dominance and reading disability. In: R. Knights & D. J. Bakker, The neuropsychology of learning disorders. Baltimore: University park Press, 1976.
Tallal, P. Auditory temporal perception, phonics, and reading dis-abilities in children. Brain and Language, 1980, 9, 182-198.
Wissel, A. van de Spellings moeilijkheden, minus-variant of dysor-thografie. Nederlands Tijdschrift voor de Psychologie, 1963, 18, 13-42.

EYE MOVEMENTS IN DEVELOPMENTAL DYSLEXIA

Kay P. Dunn
Department of Psychology
University of Houston
Houston, Texas

Francis J. Pirozzolo
Department of Neurology
Baylor College of Medicine
Houston, Texas

It has been suggested that faulty eye movements secondary to cerebellar-vestibular dysfunction are the primary cause of developmental dyslexia. Since this notion appears to be attracting a good amount of attention, it seems worthwhile to tackle the issue of eye movements and their relationship to developmental dyslexia in light of recent research findings. In order to do this, we will discuss eye movements in normal reading, disorders of the saccadic eye movement system, and recent eye movement research in our laboratory pertaining specifically to developmental dyslexia.

Eye movements during normal reading have at least three major components. Saccades are a series of very rapid movements that attempt to bring visual information to the fovea, the area of highest visual acuity. These movements last approximately 20-40 ms and cover an area of about eight character spaces. The second component is the period during which the eye is relatively still -- the fixation. It is during this fixation period (with an average duration of 200-250 ms) that information is processed to higher centres in the brain. Lastly, there are right-to-left movements called regressions, which account for approximately 10-15% of a normal reader's saccades. The eye, then, is fixated for about 90% of the time during reading, and moving 10% of the time.

With respect to these components, there are important factors to note pertaining to normal information processing and individual variability. First, the saccade is a ballistic movement, and once programmed cannot be redirected. Information from the text is not picked up during this movement due to partial visual suppression which prevents the reader from perceiving the blur that would otherwise result from the great speed (100@-740@/sec) with which the eye

moves. Since this saccadic suppression begins some 30 ms prior to
launching the saccade and persists for a short time after the eye
comes to rest, it also serves to minimize the effects of masking.
It is also important to note that there is a great deal of variability within and between Ss, in latency for a saccade (116 ms to over
280 ms): length of a saccade (2 to 18 character spaces) and duration
of fixation (100 to over 500 ms). As such, although saccadic latency, saccadic length and fixation duration are usually cited as fairly
stable indices of EM's during reading, they are actually susceptible
to variability both as a result of individual differences such as cognitive factors (e.g., senile dementia patients have greatly increased saccadic latencies) and, more importantly for our purposes -- task demands.

     Developmental studies indicate that in the normal course of rea-
ding acquisition, saccade lengths increase while mean fixation duration and number of regressions decrease; at any given age level, th-
en, poor readers generally make shorter saccades, have longer fixation durations and make more regressions than their more skilled peers.
Interestingly, if task difficulty is manipulated (e.g., reading a
story versus technical material versus a foreign language), the EM's
of skilled readers become more like those of poor readers as difficulty increases. The point here is that if many different factors,
such as task demands and individual differences, can result in eli-
citation of entirely different EM's from normal, competent readers,
then caution must be exercised when using EM's as a criterion for
distinguishing between normal and disabled readers.

     Since good readers are highly variable in their EM behavior,
and regressions have been shown to aid comprehension rather than hin-
dering it, the once popular belief that the difference between good
and poor readers is that good readers make smooth, rhythmic EM's over the text and poor readers do not, simply cannot be supported. This belief became popular largely because researchers could not specify the mechanism that guided the ballistic saccade and concluded that the movement was so brief that precise programming was impossible.
Recently, however, Rayner (1978) and Rayner and McConkie (1976) have
demonstrated in a series of experiments that cognitive processing
does influence saccadic length as well as fixation duration and number of regressions; information from parafoveal vision involves gross feature discrimination such as word length, and is probably used
by the reader to aid integration of information from one fixation to
the next as well as providing a rough guide for the length of the
next saccade. Results also indicate that this "perceptual span" is
asymmetric and varies according to culturally-determined attentional
mechanisms, with more information being obtained from the right as
opposed to the left of fixation for English readers, while the converse is true for Hebrew readers. A final important note with respect to normal EM's is that the latency for rightward saccades is
shorter than that for leftward saccades, and this difference appears

to be due to a structural factor rather than a learning effect (Pirozzolo and Rayner, 1980), since it occurs for both left and right handers.

Since some researchers (e.g, Levinson and Pavlides) support the
notion that faulty eye movements as a result of possible cerebellar-
vestibular dysfunction are the primary cause of developmental dyslexia, it would seem appropriate to discuss reading characteristics
in individuals who have oculomotor disorders.

It is not surprising that clinicians note that problems in reading are among the first complaints of many patients afflicted with
oculomotor problems.

In the case of paralytic or slow saccades (resulting from lesions involving the basal ganglia, brainstem and cerebral cortex) patients make saccades as slowly as 30@-40@/sec, as compared with a
normal speed of up to 740@/sec. As a compensatory strategy, these
patients make head movements and smooth following movements
of the eyes; in this fashion they are able to read.

Acquired and congenital apraxias involving the left and right
parietal lobes can impair initiation of saccades, but evidence suggests that the strategy of head movements is again used successfully
as a compensatory mechanism in the majority of these patients.

However, quite contrary to the foregoing, Prechtl and Stemmer
(1959) noted reading problems in all of a group of 50 children with
"hyperactive syndrome" whose eye muscles were affected by the disorder, indicating that reading acquisition was retarded in these children as a result of their involuntary eye movements.

Likewise, cerebellar disorders resulting in the incorrect programming of saccades and other coordinated neuromuscular activities,
can have a profound effect on reading ability. Pirozzolo and Rayner
(1978) noted that comprehension was impaired in one such patient with Freidreich's ataxia, a hereditary spinocerebellar degeneration,
and concluded that saccadic dysmetria and slow saccades severely affected this patient's performance, and that visual disorientation and
the greater time the eye was in movement resulted in an ability to
read on a level remotely compatible with the S's intellectual ability. This patient's eye movements were characterized not only by the
large increase in time that the eye was in flight (170 ms versus 35
ms normal), but also by overshoots at the end of a line and hypome-
tric return sweeps. This patient's last saccade would overshoot the
end of the line (as opposed to the normal pattern of 4-5 characters
before the end), and would be followed by a series of right to left
saccades until his gaze rested at the beginning of the next line.

It would seem, then, that although it is possible to read in the absence of eye movements (e.g., Moebius syndrome) and compensate by head turning in the case of some acquired disorders, evidence strongly suggests that disorders of oculomotor control are responsible for reading disturbances observed in patients with basal ganglia and cerebellar disorders.

Turning now to the issue of faulty eye movements and their relationship to developmental dyslexia; it seems logical to propose that since EM's are an essential element of the reading process, and since disorders of EM's can cause acquired reading problems, then, congenital eye movement problems could be the underlying cause of developmental dyslexia. Levinson and colleagues propose that cerebellar-vestibular dysfunction and subsequent eye movement problems were the cause of reading disability in 97% of 250 cases that they studied. Eye movement studies have demonstrated faulty eye movements in many dyslexics. So why not conclude, then, that EM problems are the cause of developmental dyslexia?

Firstly, all studies of developmental dyslexia (DD) are, of necessity, strictly correlational, and as such the direction of cause and effect is called into serious question; that is to say: Do faulty EM's cause DD, or does DD result in faulty EM's? Secondly, as mentioned earlier in this presentation, EM data varies widely as a function of both individual differences and task demands. Lastly, developmental dyslexics are a heterogeneous - not homogeneous - group; as such the search for etiology is confounded before it is begun and it is realistically impossible for any one factor to be cited as the cause since there are probably as many, if not more, causes than identified subtypes of DD.

With respect to EM's during reading, Pirozzolo, in association with Rayner and others, identified EM patterns consistent with the hypothesis that at least two subtypes of DD exist. One group whose neuropsychological profile is characterized by low performance scores on standard IQ tests, finger agnosia, directional disorientation, dysgraphia, dyscalculia, difficulty with spatial and constructional tasks and letter reversals during reading, has abnormal EM patterns characterized by a high percentage of right to left saccades. The EM's of a patient studied by Pirozzolo and Rayner (1978) are depicted in Figure 1 and demonstrate this phenomenon.

Also, after dropping her eyes to a new line of text, this patient would often begin a series of right to left saccades. After three or four of these saccades, she would correct herself, move to the left margin and start a series of left to right EM's. Errors in oral reading primarily involved her ending one line and then reading the last words on the next. Interestingly, upon rotating the test 180@, her EM's showed a normal, "staircase pattern", and her comprehension improved from the sixth to the tenth grade level.

Figure 1.

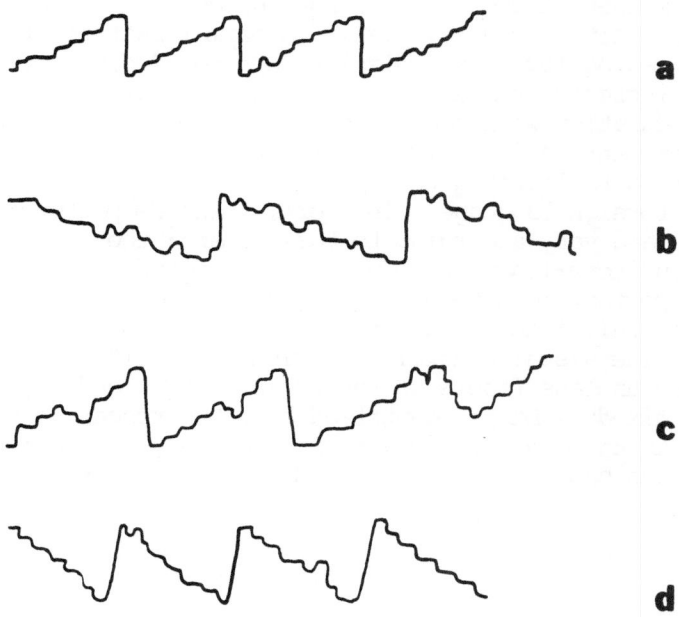

The second subgroup apparent from EM research is the auditory-linguistic subtype. Neuropsychological performance is characterized by adequate or superior visuospatial abilities, low verbal scores on standard IQ tests, and low auditory-vocal and high visual-motor channel scores on the ITPA psycholinguistic profile, and reading errors involving faulty grapheme to phoneme translocations. The patient studied by Pirozzolo, Rayner and Whitaker, (1977), had EM's that were not significantly different from normal when for reading text at his comprehension level, but when reading difficult passages, he made a larger number of fixations, and short regressions within words(see Figure 2).

When he encountered an unfamiliar word he would search for contextual cues in the words preceding or following, and would then adopt an almost letter-by-letter strategy which is characteristic of children learning to read. There was <u>no</u> evidence of an increased number of right to left saccades, or a tendency to overshoot or undershoot the first word of the next line of print.

Evidence from EM studies in DD from Pirozzolo and colleagues, then, suggest that v-s dyslexics do have abnormal EM's characterised by return sweep inaccuracies and frequent instances of right to left scanning. They also have shorter saccadic latencies to the left parafovea as opposed to the right (see Figure 3).

Given the neuropsychological profiles of these patients, it would appear that these faulty EM patterns are secondary to a dysfunction spatial mechanism that, among other things, guides EM's. Auditory-linguistic dyslexics, alternatively, display a normal pattern of EM's for text at their reading level, and display "apparent" oculomotor "deficits" such as increased number of fixations and regressions and increased fixation duration when reading difficult text. Note, however, that these forementioned "deficits" are the very same characteristics of normal readers learning to read, reading technical material or reading in a foreign language. In short, these EM patterns are essentially normal, and vary according to task demand; the apparent EM dysfunction in auditory-linguistic dyslexia is <u>secondary</u> to the dyslexic. It is important to note here that the greatest number of DD's seen in our lab fall into the auditory-linguistic subtype - approximately 50-60%. The visual-spatial dyslexics number 10-12%. The remaining 28-40% are unclassifiable on the basis of EM's and may correspond with the "mixed" subtype identified by other researchers. The most important thing to note, however, is that only one patient of 212 seen in our lab had DD <u>secondary</u> to EM dysfunction as a result

FIGURE 2

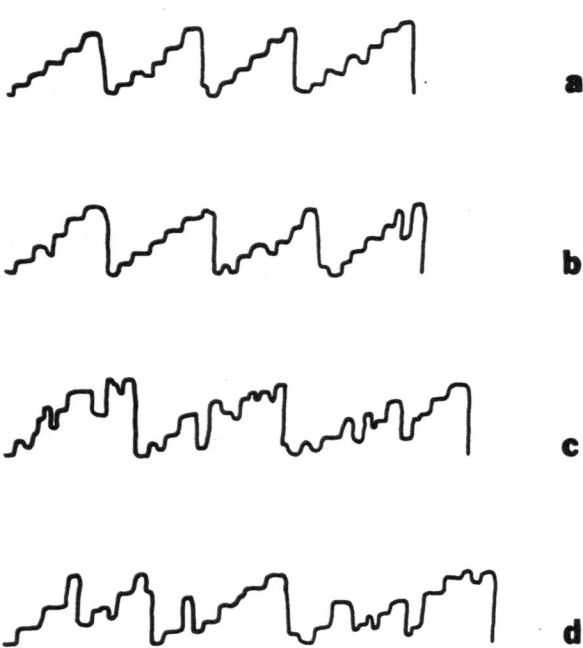

FIGURE 3

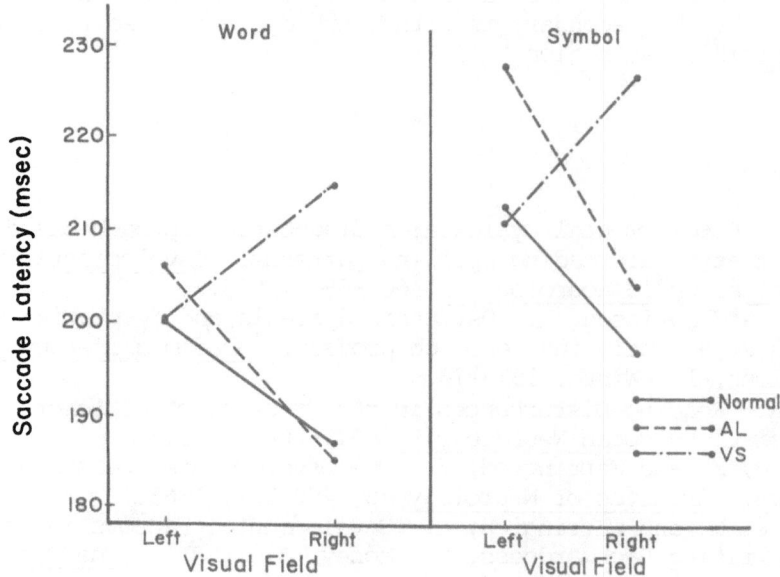

of cerebellar-vestibular dysfunction!   So what of work by Levinson
and colleagues, and Pavlides? Levinson's claim that 97% of dyslexics have c-v dysfunction is not supported.   Pavlides' claim that the
faulty EM's of dyslexics can be remediated by having subjects follow
a series of lights, and thus encourage regular EM's, has not been
supported in a recent replication by Gordon Stanley in England, and
does not succeed on theoretical grounds since in almost all developmental dyslexics the EM patterns are not the cause of the dyslexia,
but rather are secondary to either the dyslexia or a visuospatial
dysfunction.

    In addition, patients with acquired dyslexia caused by faulty
EM's as a result of spinocerebellar degeneration, for example, have
qualitatively different EM's from both EM derived subtypes of DD.
Whereas auditory-linguistic dyslexics have EM's similar to those of
normal readers learning to read, and visual-spatial dyslexics have
EM problems characterized by right to left saccades, shorter latencies for leftward saccades and return sweep inaccuracies that sometimes land them on the wrong line of print, neither group displays
evidence of slow saccades, or the phenomenon of dysmetria where the
last saccade consistently overshoots the line of print by several
degrees and the return sweep consistently undershoots the next line
by several more degrees.

Finally, if the qualitative differences in the EM patterns are not evidence enough, the fact that EM's are not necessary for reading and EM dysfunction can be compensated for in a great number of cases by head movement indicates that atypical EM's are not the cause of DD, but are secondary to either the dyslexia itself, or to visual-spatial dysfunction.

REFERENCES

Boder, E. Developmental Dyslexia: A diagnostic approach based on three atypical reading-spelling patterns. Developmental Medicine and Child Neurology, 15, 663-687, 1973.

Frank, J. and Levinson, H. Dsymetric dyslexia and dyspraxia: Synopsis of a continuing research project. Academic Therapy publications, 11, Winter 1975-76.

Hartje, W. Reading Disturbances in the Presence of Oculomotor Disorders. European Neurology, 7, 249-264, 1972.

Kinsbourne, M. and Warrington, E. The Developmental Gerstmann Syndrome. Archives of Neurology, 8, 490-501, 1963.

Kinsbourne, M. and Warrington, E. Developmental Factors in Reading and Writing Backwardness. In Money, J. (Ed.). The Disabled Reader, Baltimore, MD: Johns Hopkins University Press, 1965.

Levinson, F. Dyslexia: A Solution to the Riddle, New York: Springer-Verlag, 1981.

Pavlides, G. Do eye movements hold the key to dyslexia? Neuropsychologia, 19, 57-64, 1981.

Pirozzolo, F. J. The Neuropsychology of Developmental Reading Disorders, New York: Praeger, 1979.

Pirozzolo, F. J. Eye Movements and Reading Disability, in Rayner, K. (Ed.). Eye Movements in Reading: Perceptual and Language Processes, New York: Academic Press, 1982.

Pirozzolo, F. J. and Rayner, K. Hemispheric Specialization in Reading and Word Recognition. Brain and Language, 4, 248-261, 1977.

Pirozzolo, F. J. and Rayner, K. Disorders of Oculomotor Scanning and Graphic Orientation in Developmental Gerstmann Syndrome. Brain and Language, 5, 119-126, 1978.

Pirozzolo, F. J. and Rayner, K. The Neural Control of Eye Movements in Acquired and Developmental Reading Disorders. In Whitaker, H. and Whitaker, H. A. (Eds.). Studies in Neurolinguistics, Vol. 4, New York: Academic Press, 1979.

Rayner, K. Saccadic Latencies for Parafoveally Presented Words. Bulletin of the Psychonomic Society, 11, 13-16, 1978.

Rayner, K. and McConkie, G. What guides a reader's eye movements? Vision Research, 16, 829-837, 1976.

Rubino, C. A. and Minden, H. A. An analysis of eye-movements in children with a reading disability. Cortex, 9, 217-220, 1973.

Tinker, M. A. Recent Studies of Eye Movements in Reading. Psychological Bulletin, 55, 215-231, 1958.

VISUAL HALF-FIELD STUDIES OF DEVELOPMENTAL
READING DISABILITY

Cynthia A. Bailey
Department of Psychology
University of Houston,
Houston, Texas

Francis J. Pirozzolo
Department of Neurology
Baylor College of Medicine
Houston, Texas

INTRODUCTION

Reading disabilities were first proposed to be related to deficiencies in hemispheric specialization by Orton in 1937. He utilized hand and eye preference to determine the degree of cerebral lateralization because of the prevailing belief that this preference indicated hemispheric dominance, and that a large proportion of the
reading disabled are left handed or ambidextrous. Benton and Kemble
(1980) suggested that handedness is an unreliable indicant of cerebral dominance, which has been confirmed by numerous empirical studies. Therefore, it is necessary to find a valid measure of differential hemispheric processing.

Visual half field studies may provide such a measure. This method is based on the anatomical fact that each lateral visual half
field projects to the contralateral occipital lobe. Stimuli which
are presented tachistoscopically to the right visual field (RVF) will be conveyed directly to the left hemisphere and vice versa.

It has been demonstrated that normal readers show a RVF advantage and LVF advantage for faces (Pirozzolo, 1977; 1979). Stimulus
parameters can be manipulated and presentations may be made unilaterally or bilaterally. The duration of exposure varies from study to
study but ideally should be less than the time required to initiate
and execute a saccadic eye movement (150-200 msec). The stimuli used in the studies reviewed here have been words, letters, numbers
or faces. Size, complexity, contrast and position can be changed.

HEMISPHERIC ROLES IN READING

Reading is often presumed to be exclusively a left hemisphere activity because of its linguistic nature. However, the right hemisphere may be extremely important in reading. Psycholinguistic theories state that perceptual analysis of the printed material (i.e., shape, orientation) is more prominent in early unskilled readers. As the perceptual analysis became automatized, linguistic analysis predominates (Fries, 1963; Smith, 1971).

The right hemisphere is specialized in discriminating difficult visuospatial relationships. Bryden & Allard (1976) demonstrated that the right hemisphere is predominant when unusual, novel or complex print types are presented. As Bakker (1979) points out, all printed material is unusual novel and complex to the novice reader. Gibson (1968) theorizes that unskilled readers attend to the graphic orthographic and phonological aspects of words. This would indicate a large involvement of the right hemisphere in beginning readers.

The left hemisphere begins to gain an advantage when visuospatial perceptual analysis becomes automated. Linguistic processing, including grapheme to phoneme translation and semantic analysis, takes precedence in the skilled reader. Fluent readers of all ages show a left hemisphere (RVF) superiority in word recognition.

EARLY VISUAL HALF FIELD STUDIES

Mishkin & Forgays (1952) found that English speaking fluent readers had a RVF advantage, while bilinguals showed a LVF advantage. They attributed these results to the overlearned scanning mechanisms used in each language (left to right in English, right to left in Hebrew). Kimura (1961) postulated that the differential field asymmetries are due to the functional specialization of the two hemispheres. Barton et al., (1965) demonstrated that the RVF advantage is independent of scanning mechanisms by presenting vertically arranged words. Kinsbourne (1970) and Dimond (1972) hypothesized that the RVF superiority is due to attentional bias caused by the selective "priming" of the left hemisphere by the linguistic nature of the task, and concurrent suppression of the right hemisphere. Hines (1975) and Pirozzolo & Rayner (1977) have shown that subjects presented with words in the right visual field -- faces in the left visual field can process both simultaneously, which argues against the attentional hypothesis.

Once it was established that fluent speakers showed these assymmetries, investigations of poor readers were inevitable. Marcel, Katz & Smith (1974) found that the poor readers in their study had a decreased RVF advantage in comparison to normals, but the superiority still existed. They interpreted this as a result of greater differential lateralization in good readers. Yeni-Komshian et al.,

(1975) found increased right visual field superiority. This was attributed to a right hemisphere or a callosal transfer defect because the poor readers performed much worse than normals when stimuli were presented to the LVF and about the same when presented in the RVF. However, the controls did not exhibit a RVF superiority, which indicates the task they used may not have been measuring differential lateralization. McKeever & Huling (1970) found a RVF superiority in poor readers which was similar to controls. Other visual half field studies comparing poor and good readers have found the similar results: increased RVF advantage, no RVF advantage, or normal RVF superiority. These studies are presumably investigating the same population with presumably the same method with strikingly discrepant results.

METHODOLOGICAL PROBLEMS

Young & Ellis (1981) and Young (1982) thoroughly discuss many of the methodological problems that plague these studies. Fixation on a central point must be monitored, eye movements controlled, and the stimulus located such that it does not fall into the central visual field. The duration time of the stimulus must be long enough to ensure perception. Gross et al (1978) observed that some disabled readers have longer thresholds for identifying words. The dependent variable chosen (accuracy vs. response time) can greatly affect the results. Young suggested that response time may be a better measure because it is more sensitive and direct. Reliability of visual half field studies is an important issue that has not been adequately studied.

Selection of subjects is of paramount importance in these studies as in any other experimental procedure. Young (1982) states that only right-handed subjects should be used to ensure left cerebral dominance for language. Sex and age are important subject variables that need to be controlled. The ratio of male dyslexics to female dyslexics has been reported to be 7:1, and in order to increase generalizability of the results, the sample should reflect this. In addition, some researchers (Witelson, 1976; Grant, 1981) have found different patterns or asymmetry in boys and girls. In view of these possible differences, results should be analyzed separately for male and female subjects. Witelson also found differences in young (less than ten years old) and older (greater than ten years old) dyslexics. These differences may account for some of the conflicting results found, especially when the mean age of the sample is 10 years old. Severity of reading disability has also been shown to affect results. Kirsner (1977) found the RVF advantage was inversely related to degree of reading disability. Garren (1980) showed that only those readers who were 18 months or more below their grade level differed significantly from controls.

Another problem in the selection of subjects is that of classi-

fication. It has been suggested that there are at least two subtypes
of dyslexia; auditory-linguistic and visuo-spatial. Differing proportions of these subtypes in a sample would lead to varying results.
Keefe & Swinney (1979) found that even though their dyslexic subjects
showed cerebral asymmetry similar to controls, a closer look showed
that the dyslexic sample was bimodally distributed about the mean,
whereas the controls were normally distributed. Some of the dyslexics exhibited greater lateralization and some less lateralization.
They interpreted these results to be consistent with a Right Hemisphere (visuospatial) deficit and Left Hemisphere (auditory-linguistic)
deficit paradigm. The visuo-spatial dyslexics showed a right visual
field advantage similar to controls. The auditory linguistic dyslexics demonstrated a decreased right visual field superiority. Pirozzolo (1979) found the same results. Another problem in interpreting
the results of these studies is the lack of a consistent laterality
index. Such an index is necessary in order to control for accurate
vs. inaccurate results as well as number of trails successfully completed in order to compare subjects. Unfortunately, different expe-
rimenters have utilized different indices, and it is difficult, if
not impossible, to compare results across experiments. None of the
indices that have been used are satisfactory.

INFORMATION PROCESSING AND DYSLEXIA

    An information processing model of reading can be used to expla-
in many of these conflicting results. The first step in reading is
to analyze the physical characteristics of the stimuli presented.
It is generally agreed that most dyslexics are able to do this adequately. The percept must then be stored in the visual iconic store
or sensory store. There is evidence that this is a stumbling block
for some dyslexics. Lovegrove et al., (1980) tested the VIS deviation at different spatial frequencies in reading disabled and normal
children. They found that in low spatial frequencies (1, 2, 4 cycles per second) the VIS deviation was longer for reading disabled children. At medium frequencies (8 cps) there were no significant differences and at high frequencies (12 cps) the VIS deviation of reading disabled children was shorter than controls. The implications
of these results for reading are as follows. Low spatial frequency
receptors are more dominant in the periphery. In normal readers these are active in guidance and peripheral processing. They save the
function or noting length of the word, punctuation markers and other
general guidance. The short duration of the VIS aids in this rapid
processing of data. The longer VIS duration in reading disabled children would tend to trip up this guidance system since information
would not clear fast enough to allow for incoming data. High frequency receptors are found predominantly in the fovea. In normal readers the increased VIS duration allows more time for processing of
internal details. Dyslexics, with their shorter VIS durations, would not be able to process details as complete. In fact, Gross et
al., (1976) demonstrated that dyslexics do process visual information

more slowly. It is at this point that visuo-spatial dyslexics may
encounter difficulties.

Information must be transferred into visual short-term memory
from the VIS. This may be defective as well in visuo-spatial dyslexics (Pirozzolo & Pirozzolo, 1978). Gildemeister & Friedman (1980)
found that their reading disabled subjects were worse on visual memory and visual analytical tasks. They also demonstrated that the reading disabled group was more field dependent.

The information must be recoded into speech patterns from visual
short-term memory. This requires interhemispheric processing and may
be the site of the critical defect in auditory linguistic duslexics.
Bouma & Leguen (1980) found that reading disabled subjects exhibited
a longer latency in recognizing letters and words. They attributed
this latency to defects in visual to speech recoding process. Pirozzolo and Pirozzolo (1978) found that grapheme to phoneme transfer
was faulty. Words must be semantically processed once recoding. Dyslexics may have difficulties here as well, but this has not been
extensively researched.

SUMMARY AND CONCLUSION

Visual half field studies have been fraught with methodological
and interpretive problems. The methodological issues include control
and consistency of experimental parameters, choice of dependent variable, choice of subjects and methods or analysis.

Interpretation of the results might best be done by considering
classification of subtypes and an information processing scheme of
reading. It is important to determine whether or not the disabled
reader is able to process information in the same way as the skilled
reader, and if or where the breakdowns occur.

REFERENCES

Bakker, D. J. Cerebral Lateralization and Reading Proficiency.
    Paper presented at the international symposium on "Cerebral La-
    teralization of Language Functions and Its Role in Language
    Development and Language Disorders in Children"; Lavacherie,
    Belgium, October, 1979.
Barton, M., Goodglass, H., and Shai, A. Differential recognition of
    tachistoscopically presented English and Hebrew words in right
    and left visual fields. Perceptual and Motor Skills, 1965,
    21, 431-437.
Benton, A. L. and Kemble, V. D. Right-left orientation and reading
    disabilities. Psych. Neurol., 1960, 139, 49-60.

188 C. Bailey and F. Pirozzolo

Bouma, H. and Leguin, C. P. Dyslexia: A specific recoding deficit?
An analysis of response latencies for letters and words in dyslexics and in average readers. Neuropsychologia, 1980, 18,
285-298.

Bryden, M. P. and Allard, F. Visual hemifield differences depend on
typeface. Brain and Language, 1976, 3, 463-469.

Dimond, S. J. The Double Brain. Baltimore: Williams and Wilkins,
1972.

Fries, C. C. Linguistics and Reading. New York: Holt, Rinehart,
and Winston, 1963.

Garrén, R. B. Hemispheric laterality differences among four levels
of reading achievement. Perceptual and Motor Skills, 1980, 50,
119-123.

Gibson, E. Learning to read. In N. S. Endler, L. R. Boulter and
H. Osser (Eds.), Contemporary Issues in Developmental Psychology.
New York: Holt, Rinehart and Winston, 1968.

Gildemeister, V. E. and Friedman, P. Differences in visual analysis
and sequence memory of skilled and poor readers. Perceptual
and Motor Skills, 1980, 51, 582.

Grant, D. W. Sex, reading disability, and visual half-field test-
retest reliability. Perceptual and Motor Skills, 1982, 54,
49-50.

Gross, K., Rothenberg, S., and Schottenfield, S. Duration thresholds
for letter identification in left and right visual fields for
normal and reading-disabled children. Neuropsychologia, 1978,
16, 709-715.

Hines, D. Independent functioning of the two cerebral hemispheres
for recognizing bilaterally presented tachistoscopic visual
half-field stimuli. Cortex, 1975, 11, 132-143.

Keffe, B. and Swinney, D. On the relationship of hemispheric specialization and developmental dyslexia. Cortex, 1979, 15,
471-481.

Kershner, J. R. Cerebral dominance in disabled readers, good readers and gifted children: Search for a valid model. Child Development, 1977, 45, 61-67.

Kimura, D. Cerebral dominance and the perception of verbal stimuli.
Canadian Journal of Psychology, 1961, 15, 166-171.

Kinsbourne, M. The cerebral basis of lateral asymmetries in attention. Acta Psychologica, 1970, 33, 193-201.

Lovegrove, W. J., Heddle, M. and Slaghuis, W. Reading disability:
Spatial frequency deficits in visual information store. Neuropsychologia, 1980, 18, 111-115.

McKeever, W. and Huling, M. Lateral dominance in tachistoscopic
word recognition of children at two levels of ability. Quarterly Journal of Experimental Psychology, 1970, 22, 600-604.

Marcel, T., Katz, L. and Smith, M. Laterality and reading proficiency. Neuropsychologia, 1974, 12, 131-139.

Mishkin, M. and Forgays, D. G. Word recognition as a function of
retinal locus. Journal of Experimental Psychology, 1952, 43,
43-48.

Pirozzolo, F. J.   Lateral asymmetry in visual perception: A review of tachistoscopic visual half-field studies. Perceptual and Motor Skills, 1977, 45, 695-701.

Pirozzolo, F. J.   The Neuropsychology of Developmental Reading Disorders. New York: Praeger, 1979.

Pirozzolo, F. J. and Pirozzolo, P. H.   A model of brain function in dyslexia. SISTM Quarterly, 1978, 2, 20-21.

Pirozzolo, F. J. and Rayner, K.   Hemispheric specialization in reading and word recognition. Brain and Language, 1977, 4, 248-261.

Pirozzolo, F. J., Rayner, K. and Hynd, G. W.   The measurement of hemispheric asymmetries in children with developmental reading disabilities in J. B. Hellige (Ed.). Cerebral Hemisphere Asymmetry: Method, Theory and Application. New York: Praeger, 1982.

Smith, F.   Understanding Reading. New York: Holt, Rinehart and Winston, 1971.

Witelson, S. F.   Abnormal right hemisphere specialization in developmental dyslexia.   In R. M. Knights, D. J. Bakker (Eds.), The Neurospychology of Learning Disabilities. Baltimore: University Park Press, 1976.

Yeni-Komshian, G. H., Isenberg, D. and Goldberg, H.   Cerebral dominance and reading disability: Left visual field deficit in poor readers. Neurospychologia, 1975, 13, 83-94.

Young, A. W. and Ellis, A. W.   Asymmetry of cerebral hemispheric function in normal and poor readers. Psychological Bulletin, 1981, 89, 183-190.

Young, A. W.   Methodological and theoretical bases of visual hemifield studies.   In J. G. Beaumont (Ed.), Divided Visual Field Studies of Cerebral Organization, London: Academic Press, 1982.

ALEXIA IN RELATION TO APHASIA AND AGNOSIA

Yvan Lebrun
Vrije Universiteit
Brussels

Françoise Devreux
Foundation Universitaire
Luxembourgeoise

For many years acquired reading disorders were classified with
reference to the other verbal deficits which accompanied the reading
impairment. Alexia without concomitant impairment of spoken language
was distinguised from alexia associated with aphasia. Following Dejerine's lead (1892), the former was usually subdivided into pure
alexia and alexia with agraphia. As regards alexia with aphasia, a
distinction was made according to whether the accompanying speech
disorder was sensory or motor. Alexia occurring in the context of
motor aphasia was termed third alexia by Benson (1977), who contrasted
it with pure alexia on the one hand and with alexia accompanied by
agraphia but without disturbance of spoken language, on the other hand.
Goldstein (1948, p. 120-125), as for one, regarded pure alexia and
alexia with agraphia as primary alexias, and alexia with aphasia as
a secondary alexia.

In the last decade, however, a new taxonomy of acquired reading
disorders was introduced which is based on the types of reading errors
and on the kinds of words most affected by them, rather than on the
verbal deficits concomitant with the reading impairment. To be sure,
traditional classification did not completely ignore error types.
Pure alexia was often subdivided into literal, verbal, and global
alexia according to whether letters were more difficult to read than
words, or words were more difficult than letters, or letters and
words were equally difficult. Sometimes (e. g.Dubois-Charlier, 1971)
a fourth subdivision was made: sentence alexia.

In recent years, however, attention was shifted from the syntagmatic to the paradigmatic axis and stress laid on the classes of
words which patients found the most difficult to read as well as on
the kinds of paralexias they made. This approach has generally

resulted in a classification of acquired reading impairments into
visual, surface, and deep dyslexia. The new typology has the advantage of highlighting features of the patients' reading behavior which
the traditional classification tended to ignore. On the other hand,
it runs the risk of lumping together cases which are but superfici-
ally similar and thus of obscuring the distinctive pathophysiology
of the reading disorders under consideration. Let us try to validate
this caveat. In a recent paper, Marshall and Newcome (1980) mention
Beringer and Stein's case (1930) and Goldstein's case no. 23 (1948,
p. 310-316) as instances of deep dyslexia. At first sight, the two
cases resemble one another: either patient made semantic paralexias
and found function words more difficult to read aloud than content
words. These features are generally considered essential characteristics of deep dyslexia. Indeed, Coltheart (1980) holds semantic
paralexias to be pathognomonic of the disorder. He calls the semantic reading error the linchpin of deep dyslexia, for the occurrence
of semantic paralexias guarantees that the other components of the
syndrome will also be present. However, while Beringer and Stein's
patient and Goldstein's patient both made semantic errors when reading aloud, the mechanism underlying these misreadings does not seem
to have been the same in the two cases. Comments spontaneously offered by the patient clearly indicate that the word which she was to
read aloud, often evoked some semantic field, to which it actually
belonged, but it could not be more specifically identified. For instance, the patient misread <u>Indien</u> (India) as <u>Elephant</u> (elephant)
and commented: "It is a foreign word. I could immediately see that
it was something which is far away, in the tropics, it is hot, and I
came to think of elephants. I have always liked elephants." When
she misread <u>Reichstag</u> (which was the name of the German parliament)
as <u>Berlin</u>, she said: "I had the impression of somewhere I had been,
where there was so much to see and to look at, one just sits down on
a park bench and then looks at it all, the whole picture." Nothing
in the patient's comments or in Beringer and Stein's description
suggests that the patient could correctly identify the word to be
read but was unable to sound it out or could not help uttering a semantically related word. Instead, the visual word form appears to
have been apprehended globally and to have conjured up a vague sce-
nary (a hot tropical, far away country or a large city worth visit-
ing), which in turn evoked a concept (elephant, capital town) which
the patient then named effortless. When she was requested to take
a second look at the word to be read, sometimes it then evoked the
appropriate concept. For instance, having misread <u>Reichstag</u> as
<u>Berlin</u>, she was asked to try again and she said: "Oh no, it's some-
thing in Berlin, that's it, Reichstag." Having to read the name
<u>Goethe</u>, she said: "It's a man, a poet, I know, but I can't name him,
Uhland, no, not Uhland, he belongs to the Biedermeier period." She
then proceeded to spell the beginning of the word and suddenly ex-
claimed: "The name is Goethe!". Such comments clearly indicate that
the difficulty was on the input, not on the output side. Once the
patient had succeded in recognizing a written word, she had no trouble

at all sounding it out. She could say whatever she wanted. She was
not aphasic, as Beringer and Stein point out. Her problem was the
identification of written words: often this identification remained
partial and thus entailed a semantic paralexia. This view is confirmed by the fact that when she was given a semantic clue her reading
improved considerably. For instance, one day she was shown a list
of 12 words but she could not recognize any of them. She was then
told that these words all denoted tools. Thanks to this semantic
indication she was able to read 11 of the 12 words.

The situation appears to have been completely different in the
case described by Goldstein, who says that "from the beginning the
patient seemed to 'recognize' a number of [written] words even if he
could not read them aloud" (p. 312). Often the patient indicated
that he understood the word but could not speak it, or else he said
a word which was semantically related to the target word. Sometimes,
when he could not speak the word, he would start to copy it, and the
graphomotor activity more often than not enabled him to suddenly recognize the desired item. Goldstein concluded therefore that his
patient "seemed to recognize a number of words and understand them
without being able to read them [aloud] correctly." This description
strongly suggests that in this case the difficulty was, at least in
part, on the output side: the patient, who by the way had a severe
motor aphasia, could not always pronounce the words he had identified.
It appears then that while Beringer and Stein's patient and Goldstein's patient both made semantic reading errors, the pathogenesis of
these mistakes was not the same in the two cases. This conclusion
holds also true in respect of the difficulty in reading function words aloud. As was mentioned above, the two patients found function
words more difficult to read aloud than the content words. However,
Beringer and Stein's patient could and did use functors adequately
in spoken language, while Goldstein explicitly states that his patient could neither employ function words spontaneously nor repeat them,
even though he could repeat other parts of speech. In all likelihood, Beringer and Stein's patient was unable to identify function
words because, in contradistinction to content words, they failed
to evoke any semantic field; they could not conjure up an image or
scenery, however vague. Goldstein's patient, on the contrary, could
identify function words far better than he could sound them out.
How is this output difficulty to be explained? Goldstein observes
that his patient could read aloud the figure <u>four</u> but not the preposition <u>for</u> (p. 313), although the two words sound alike. A similar dissoiciation was noted in a case reported by Andreewsky and Seron
(1975) and considered by Coltheart (1980) to be an instance of deep
dyslexia. When requested to read aloud the French sentence <u>Le car</u>
<u>ralentit car le moteur chauffe</u> (the bus slows down because the bus
overheats), Andrewsky and Seron's patient said <u>car ralentit moteur</u>
<u>chauffe</u>. Thus he read aloud the second but not the fourth word al-
though they are homophones. However, the former is a content while

the latter is a function word. When requested to read aloud the anomalous sentence <u>Le train ralentit mer le moteur chauffe</u> (the train
slows down ocean the engine overheats), the patient said <u>train ralentit moteur chauffe</u>. Thus he skipped the substantive <u>mer</u> (ocean),
although he could read it aloud when it was presented isolated or
when it was not used anomalously as a conjunction. Again, when asked
to read aloud a list of seven French conjunctions, he sounded only
two of them out, <u>or</u> and <u>car</u>, which happen to be homophones with sub-
stantives, and he misread <u>mais</u> as the substantive <u>maïs</u>, which is
written nearly the same. This behavior indicates that the patient
identified function words for what they were and possibly understood
them, but was prevented from pronouncing them. He therefore resembles a patient who was described by Morton and Patterson (1980b)
and who had also great difficulty in reading aloud function words.
However, he could correctly discriminate functors from non-words in
a lexical decision task, and specially devised tests showed that he
could extract "quite a lot of information from written function
words." In conclusion, all three patients evidenced the same feature:
they were far better at identifying function words than at reading
them aloud. The fact that these patients were all agrammatic may
explain the observed dissociation. It has been argued (Lebrun et
al., 1971) that the basic difficulty in agrammatism is competition
along the syntagmatic as well as along the paradigmatic axis. More
specifically, when an agrammatic patient has to utter one particular
word, semantically related words tend to be activated at the same
time and to render the emission of the desired item difficult. An
agrammatic patient of Luria's (1966, p. 363) used to complain that
when he wanted to say a word, related words crossed his mind making
it hard for him to pick out and utter the desired item. Could it
not be that this spreading activation, i. e. the troublesome arousal
of related verbal engrams, is more frequent and more paralyzing when
the word to be pronounced belongs to the group of functors, i. e.
to a limited class of items that very much resemble one another from
a distributional, connotative and affective point of view? If this
is the case, then it may be predicted that if a patient with that
kind of problem makes a paralexia when attempting to read aloud a
function word, the paralexia is likely to be a member of the same
syntactical class. Now, this is precisely what has been observed
in a number of patients, as Coltheart himself points out (1980):
many deep dyslexics tend to make function word substitutions. In
the case reported by Morton and Patterson (1980b), when function
words were misread, the paralexias were function words in more than
two thirds of the cases. This percentage would even be higher, if,
in contradistinction to Morton and Patterson, one considers such
misreadings as <u>downstairs</u> for <u>beneath</u> and <u>two</u> for <u>both</u> to be functor
substitutions.

The comparison of Beringer and Stein's case with the cases
reported by Goldstein, by Andreewsky and Seron, and by Morton and
Patterson shows that semantic paralexias may have different origins

in different patients and that function words may be difficult to
read for various reasons. The comparison indicates further that the
pathophysiology of the individual cases can hardly be understood if
one does not take into account the other verbal deficits which may
accompany the alexia. As a matter of fact, when alexia is concomitant with aphasia there is often a close relationship between the
two disorders. This was recently recognized and documented by
Nolan and Caramazza (1982) who in a case of deep dyslexia identified
by Marin, Saffran and Schwartz (1976) and considered as such by
Coltheart (1980), found that "reading performance is but one expression of a more general deficit which affects the patient's ability
to deal with language in all input and response modalities." Accordingly, they concluded that "any model proposed to account for deep
dyslexic reading must be able to account for similar impairments in
other modalities of input and response."

As a matter of fact, Nolan and Caramazza's patient was classified as Broca's aphasic on the basis of the Boston Diagnostic Aphasia Examination. This battery does not distinguish between Broca's
aphasia and agrammatism. Indeed, it holds the latter to be a frequent feature of the former. In Nolan and Caramazza's paper there
is a suggestion that the patient did have agrammatic speech. Moreover, as is the rule in true agrammatism (Lebrun et al., 1971) the
patient found infinitive verb forms and uninflected noun forms easier
to repeat than inflected verb and noun forms; and he found nonwords
harder to repeat than words. It may be assumed, therefore, that he
actually had agrammatism like the patients described by Goldstein,
by Andrewsky and Seron, and by Morton and Patterson and discussed
above.

Typically, in Nolan and Caramazza's case there was as much as
83% functor substitutions in oral reading. Moreover, the patient's
identification of written words was far better than his reading
aloud of them. And his behavior when asked to rate his confidence
in each of his responses "supports the view that semantic reading
errors occur when the correct word has been accessed but is not....
available for output." Such feature could also be observed in the
three cases previously discussed.

Last but not least, in order to account for functor substitutions in their case, Nolan and Caramazza found it necessary to assume that function words "constitute a close-knit associative network
by virtue of their shared form class, and presentation of one functor will cause a great deal of spreading activation to other functors." This is exactly what has been suggested above.

It has been shown (Dubois et al., 1967) that patients with severe agrammatism find nonsense words noticeably harder to repeat
than real words. Indeed, they may be completely unable to reproduce non-words. Accordingly, deep dyslexics who are agrammatic and

find the repetition of nonsense words impossible, may be unable to
read aloud non-words not because they cannot turn graphemes into
phonemes but because due to their agrammatism they cannot utter non-
existing words.

On the other hand, Nolan and Caramazza insist that, while agrammatism is frequent in deep dyslexics, yet the two disorders need
not necessarily co-occur. Beringer and Stein's case discussed above
verifies the last part of this statement.

It follows from all this that deep dyslexia is not a unitary
syndrome but rather, as Shallice and Warrington (1980) contend,
"a class of multi-component dyslexic syndromes". In trying to account
for these various forms of dyslexia it is often necessary to take
into consideration the other verbal deficits which accompany to
reading impairment. Failure to do so may lead one completely astray
as to the pathophysiology of the observed reading difficulties. In
other words, it seems desirable to reconcile the new and the traditional typology of acquired reading disorders and to inquire e.g.
whether deep dyslexia occurs as pure alexia, (as in Beringer and
Stein's case), or is concomitant with agraphia but without accompanying disorder of spoken language, or is associated with aphasia.
If it is, then a possible relationship between the alexic and the
aphasic deficit should be looked for, as it may be difficult to
account for the former if one ignores the latter.

Alexia may be accompanied not only by aphasia but also by agnosia, especially visual agnosia. On the whole, classical authors
seem to have considered such an association to be anything but rare.
Indeed, Head (1926, I, P. 108-110) expressed the view that visual
agnosia always entails reading problems. In a number of modern publications, however, the existence of an agnosic component in cases of
alexia, especially of pure alexia, has been doubted. Geschwind (1965)
in particular has insisted that most instances of so-called visual
agnosia are in fact examples of a visuo-verbal disconnection syndrome.
In other words, the patient does recognize the objects he perceives
visually but he is unable to name them properly as long as they are
perceived by sight only.

Is the view really correct that most cases of visual agnosia
are in reality cases of optic aphasia? Does each wrong response of
such patients in the naming-on-confrontation test allow of an interpretation in terms of aphasia? In connection with alexia the question
can even be more specific. In 1976, Stachowiak and Poeck contended
that there was a continuum from pure alexia without any other verbal
deficit to the complete syndrome of optic aphasia. Does the continuum
never extend so as to include visual agnosia? The following clinical
case may help us answer this question:

The patient, Jeanne F., was a French-speaking, right-handed,
68-year-old female with a known heart disease. In 1980 she suffered

a first CVA which resulted in right hemiparesis and right homonymous hemianopia. The EEG evidenced left fronto-temporal anomalies. In May 1981 she had a second CVA. In addition to the previous symptoms she now had a global rightsided hypoesthesia with ataxic hand movements. Reflexes were brisk but plantar responses were flexor.

The patient was given an extensive neurolinguistic examination which was spread over several sessions.

LANGUAGE

Comprehension of speech

Simple verbal messages could be understood without difficulty. Longer utterances had sometimes to be repeated before their meaning could be grasped. The patient herself would occasionally repeat an instruction aloud before following it. The first two parts of Pierre Marie's three-paper-test were carried out correctly; as for the third part, the patient could not remember what it was.

Locative prepositions and temporal conjunctions similar to those used in the last part of the Token Test were understood correctly. The Token Test itself could not be administered because of the patient's color aphasia.

Oral expression

Jeanne's spontaneous speech was fluent, copious and adequate. From time to time she made a semantic paraphasia (e.g. lunch instead of dinner, words instead of letters). She made no verbal perseverations but the same themes (e.g. her illness) tended to recur in her conversation. There was no dysarthria.

The patient could easily give the feminine or the plural form of words mentioned by the examiner; she could find words beginning with a given syllable and she correctly completed 33 of 41 idiomatic expressions whose beginning had been enunciated by the examiner. Two of the erroneous answers indicated that she telescoped two different idioms. Twice her answer was incomplete. In the remaining cases, she happened not to know the proposed idiom. The patient could form sentences containing 1 or 2 words given by the examiner, but her answers were occasionally anomalous or not well-formed sentences.

Her score on Rey's 15-word-test (evocation 4, 5, 5, 3, 4 = 21; recognition: 6) revealed a severe impairment of short term verbal memory. The patient could hardly re-tell a 15-line story which had been read out to her.

Naming on confrontation was hesitant and often incorrect. In one naming test 29 different common objects were shown (two of them, the tooth brush and the scissors, being shown twice). Fourteen were named adequately; in 7 cases, the use of the object was described appropriately, though the object itself could not be named. In 2 cases, she spontaneously corrected her error: scissors -> hair brush, no, scissors; keys -> pincers, no, keys. Of the remaining 8 cases 2 can be regarded as semantic paraphasias: stork -> swan, toothbrush -> nail brush, and 4 were perseverations, e.g. razor -> fountain pen, ball point; tooth brush -> fountain pen, something to write with; fork -> to write with ?; scissors -> fountain pen.

On another occasion, 18 common objects were shown. Six could be named correctly and of another 5 the use was described adequately. One error was self-corrected. Five objects were misnamed (e.g. clothes-peg -> cork, corkscrew, I keep one in the drawer to use on bottles) and one could not be recognized at all. One of the 5 misnaming was perseverative in nature: scissors -> scissors; knife -> these are also scissors.

Naming of images, i.e. of depicted objects, was even more impaired. On one occasion only 2 out of 10 pictures were correctly named: a sheep and a snail. One picture could not be named at all. The remaining seven were misnamed. Two of the errors were perseverations. On another occasion, Jeanne correctly named 13 out of 26 pictures. Some of her correct answers were given in a hesitant tone of voice. Others were arrived at after much groping, e.g. Gruyere cheese -> it looks like meat: pork or lamb, I'd say...... it is not a cauliflower, Brussels sprouts...... I think there are small holes, it must be Gruyere cheese. One depicted object could not be named but its use could be adequately described. For 3 objects she could tell the conceptual category they belonged to, e.g. parrots -> animals; cherries -> fruit. There were 9 misnamings (e.g. ironing board -> to make coffee), some of which were perseverative in nature, e.g. endives -> bananas, endives; pile of plates -> endives, salad, chrysanthemums. In a few cases, the object named somewhat resembled the object depicted, e.g. burning candle -> rose.

One day the patient was asked to name 10 depicted professions or crafts. She named 4 of them correctly. As in the preceding tests, she sometimes arrived at the correct answer after having elimi-nated alternatives. For instance, being shown the picture of a police-man she said: "He is not a soldier, he is not Buffalo Bill (a few minutes earlier she had misread Clancy as Buffalo Bill). A kind of policeman". Curiously enough, in 4 cases, although she could not name the depicted profession she spontaneously named a detail repre-sented in the picture, e.g. a small tortoise near the fisherman's foot, a dog biting in the postman's trousers, or a little mouse on the wedding cake carried by the baker.

On the other hand, being shown a square whose sides were made
of small triangles and a triangle whose sides were made of small
squares, the patient immediately named the large geometrical forms.
Indeed, while she had more difficulty naming pictures than objects,
she could readily name geometrical forms.

Pointing to images of objects named by the examiner was considerably better than naming the images herself: 8/11 and 25/27.

Naming colors on confrontation was often erroneous, especially
after the patient had named a few of them correctly. Pointing to
colors mentioned by the examiner was slightly impaired. On the other
hand, the patient always answered correctly such questions as What
is the color of snow? of blood? of grass?

Matching of colors was faultless. And so was the coloring of
outlines of common objects, provided the patient had correctly identified the depicted subjects. But she sometimes made mistakes when
she had to point to the color corresponding to an object named by the
examiner. It should be noted that the patient tended to name the
color before pointing to it; generally the color was named appropriately, but she failed to point to the corresponding color patch, e.g.,
when the examiner said "tree leaf"' Jeanne said "green" but pointed
successively to the orange, brown, blue, red, and yellow patches.
She also erred or was very hesitant when she had to color a non-figu-
rative pattern according to a model, especially if several colors
had to be used.

Reading

Naming of isolated letters was impaired. For instance, on one
occasion the patient named correctly 10 letters out of 25, and on
another occasion 16 out of 25. She provided an answer for each of
the 50 letters. Errors were not systematic. They were neither predominantly morphological (confusing letters which look alike) nor
predominantly phonemic (confusing letters corresponding to phonemes
which sound alike). But R was often proposed as an answer. The
patient was never confident as to the correctness of her reading,
and she tended to make more errors at the end than at the beginning
of the test.

On the other hand, Jeanne succeeded in naming a series of 25
capital letters using Wildbrand's manoeuvre. Kinesthetic reading
then was undisturbed. So-called dynamic reading was also preserved,
as the patient could identify each of 25 capital letters which were
drawn in front of her by the examiner.

Sorting capital letters was possible and pointing to letters
named by the examiner (in an array of 5 letters) was often correct
(7/10). Jeanne could discriminate between alphabetical and non-

alphabetical symbols, and she could tell when a letter was presented upside down.

Reading aloud of isolated monosyllabic words was arduous,
often incorrect and perseverative. Words of more than one syllable
could almost never be read aloud correctly. Her misreadings included semantic paralexias [e.g. port(=harbor) -> moule(=mossel),
morue(=cod); escargot(=snail) -> crabe(crab); Venise(=Venice) ->
Salzbourg(=Salzburg)], morphological paralexias(visual errors)
[e.g. carrotte(=carrot) -> cacao], and unrelated errors[e.g. prune
(=plum) ->institut(=institute)]. More than once the answer consisted in a negative statement, e.g. vache(=cow) -> ce n'est pas du
vin(it's not wine). On the other hand, dynamic reading of short
words written in script was usually correct; however, dynamic reading of short words written in block letters was hardly better than
static readig. On the other hand, function words were not more
difficult to read aloud than content words.

The patient was more successful in selecting from among three
written words the item corresponding to a picture than in reading
aloud isolated words, provided she had correctly identified the
picture. Indeed, it happened a few times that she unhesitatingly
and correctly matched the word with the picture although she could
neither pronounce the word nor say what the picture represented, or
else she produced a totally different word. For instance, she
correctly matched the word cigarettes with the picture of a box of
cigarettes, but she said "Fish, fishing".

Jeanne could usually select from among three written words the
one that corresponded to a word pronounced by the examiner (9/10,
8/12, 3/6, 6/6, 18/24). In a series of three spoken words she
could generally indicate which item corresponded to a given written
word (8/10). In a series of three written words, she could often
pinpoint the one that did not belong to a semantic category mentioned
by the examiner; however, she was but rarely in a position to read
this odd word aloud correctly. Similarly, she usually was able to
choose from among three written words the one that belonged to a
semantic category specified by the examiner or that corresponded
to the definition the examiner had given; however, Jeanne was not
always able to read aloud the words she had selected.

Reading aloud of single figures was impaired(5/8) and reading
aloud of numbers was almost impossible (1/9, 0/5); however, using
Wildbrand's manoeuvre, numbers comprising up to three figures
could be read aloud.

Writing

Spelling common short words from memory was generally correct
(7/8, 4/5) and identification of short words spelled aloud by the

examiner was easy (5/5, 11/11).

Because of her rightsided paresis, the patient had to write with her left hand. Nonetheless, her handwriting was legible. Of 22 common words dictated by the examiner, 17 were written correctly. Four of the 5 errors consisted in the omission of one letter. When writing sentences (in total 40 words) under dictation, Jeanne made several grammatical mistakes, most of which concerned the agreement of past participles. She also left out a few letters.

Computation

As regards simple mental calculation, there were considerable fluctuations in the patient's performance from session to session. Sometimes she would produce the correct answer quickly; at other times she was off the mark and unable to correct herself. Written calculation was impossible.

Drawing

With her left hand the patient was able to produce acceptable drawings of common objects. She could not draw a cube, however, even if she was given a model.

Identification of individual fingers on the basis of tactile and proprioceptive sensations was correct. In other words, there was no finger agnosia. There was no finger aphasia either, the patient being able to name her fingers and to wiggle fingers named by the examiner.

The patient found it difficult to identify pictures of well-known politicians. On the other hand, she could recognize the faces of her relatives, friends, and doctors.

Her score on the Money Standardized Test of Direction Sense (1976) was dull-normal (23/32).

This case then very much resembles the one described by Stachowiak and Poeck (1976). Both patients had pure alexia, which was more pronounced for words than for letters. Identification of written words mentioned by the examiner was better than reading aloud. Recognition of words spelled by the examiner was correct. Spoken language and writing were noticeably less disturbed than reading. Spelling words from memory was normal or nearly so. On the other hand, both patients had color aphasia. They often erred when they had to name colors shown or to point to colors named. But, as is common in color aphasia, they could sort colors well and could tell the typical color of objects mentioned by the examiner. Finally, Stachowiak and Poeck's patient had a slight, and our patient a more pronounced, visual naming deficit. Was this deficit entirely

aphasic ? In other words, did the patients, and especially Jeanne,
evidence optic aphasia exclusively, or was there some degree of visual
agnosia as well ? Was there solely a difficulty in naming visually
presented stimuli, or was there in addition some visual recognition
problem ? That Jeanne had optic aphasia cannot be doubted: more than
once in the naming-on-confrontation test she indicated the use of an
object which she could not name. It is not quite clear, however,
whether in such a case she could not retrieve the name of the object
or could not say it. When she had to match written words with pictures or to choose from among three written words the one that belonged
to a semantic category specified by the examiner, she would often
perform the task adequately but could not always utter the words she
had identified. Or else she would produce a paralexia. May be a
similar output difficulty was present in the naming of objects on
confrontation. If this was actually the case, then it may be concluded that optic aphasia is more akin to Broca's aphasia than to amnestic aphasia. This in turn would account for the verbal perseverations and contaminations which mark some of Jeanne's answers. For
instance, on one occasion she was shown a picture of a piano, which
she named correctly. Then a picture of a score was presented, and
she said: "It's not a guitar, it's not a piano", but she could not
say what it was, and the examiner had to tell her: "It's a score,
a sheet of paper with staffs and music written on them". Next the
patient was shown a picture representing a pair of gloves of which
only four fingers were visible. She said: "It's music, a verse....
words, no not words, piano, guitar, a sheet which one follows, a
verse..... there should be 5 of them, but one can only see 4". The
last part of her response indicates that she had identified the
gloves, although she could not name them. What precedes the last
sentence seems to be vain attempts at saying the right word: instead
of producing the correct item she repeated words which she had just
been using (perseverations) or which the examiner had just been
using (contaminations).

    In some of her responses, Jeanne eliminated a few possibilities
before giving the object or the picture its correct name. The rejected possibilities often referred to objects or pictures that had
just been named and may therefore be perseverations which the patient
sought to repress. For instance, after she had misread Clancy as
Buffalo Bill she was shown the picture of a policeman. Her response
was: "He is not a soldier, he is not Buffalo Bill. A kind of police-
man".

    It is noteworthy that verbal perseverations were not observed
outside the naming-on-confrontation test. In particular, Jeanne
never perseverated in spontaneous speech. This dissociation was
also noted by Caplan and Hedley-Whyte (1974) in a case of alexia
without agraphia: the patient, though her spontaneous speech was
normal, yet made perseverations in visual naming.

In a similar case, Lhermitte and Beauvois (1973) made the interesting observation that the number of perseverations did not decrease in the naming-on-confrontation test when the patient engaged in a one-minute chat between the successive presentations of visual stimuli. This suggests that the visuo-verbal connections used in visual naming are relatively independent of the neurolinguistic mechanisms underlying conversation.

However, not all perseverations that were noted in the naming-on-confrontation tasks performed by Jeanne appear to be aphasic. At times, the patient seemed to really mean the word she was using. On one occasion, she was shown a picture of a razor, which she called "A fountain pen, a ball point". Next a picture of a tooth brush was presented, and she said: "Fountain pen, something to write with". Does the second part of the answer "something to write with" not indicate that Jeanne really meant a fountain pen or atleast something you use to write ? To be sure, it might be argued that we have here a double verbal perseveration, that the patient in fact wanted to say "Tooth brush, something to brush your teeth with" but that the word fountain pen and its semantic field could not be inhibited and therefore perseverated. But what about the following instance ? The patient was shown a picture representing a pair of scissors. She named it correctly. Then a picture of a knife was presented, and she said "These are also scissors". Similar examples can be found in Lhermitte and Beauvois' paper (1973). After having correctly named a picture of a kite balloon, their patient was shown a picture of a parachute, which he called "another kind of kite balloon". When a picture of a wrist watch and that of a pair of scissors were presented successively, he named the first correctly and identified the second as "a wrist watch again". The words also, another, and again which appear in these answers strongly suggest that the two patients did mean the name they applied to the second picture in each case. In other words: the perseveration here does not seem to be verbal in nature. It appears instead to pertain to the mechanisms of visual perception. It is as if the first percept has an exaggerated remanence and blocks out, or pervades, the new incoming percept.

Perseveration of visual sensations following posterior cerebral damage is a well-documented phenomenon. Particularly relevant in the present context is the obliteration or modification of a new incoming percept by a preceding one. For instance, a prosopagnosic patient of Lhermitte et al.'s (1972) explained that when he glanced at his wife's face after having looked at somebody else's face, he had the impression that she had taken on some of the facial features of the person he had just been looking at. And at a Christmas Party, a patient of Meadows and Munro (1977) "noticed that a replica of the white beard of the attendant Santa Claus was superimposed upon the face of everyone she spoke to".

Perceptual perseverations may also occur when looking at

written words. At the onset of his alexia, a patient of Alajouanine's
(1968, p.128) had the impression that every article in his newspaper
began with the same sentence, which presumably was the one he had
deciphered when starting to read. A patient of ours (M. S.) who,
following removal of a left parieto-occipital tumor had alexia with
agraphia and right homonymous hemianopia, had frequently the impression that the words she was to read were longer than they actually
were. When she looked at a word she would see additional letters to
the right of it which actually were not there. This patient had verbal alexia: she could read letters and would often try to recognize
a word by identifying its letters one by one. But she was often led
astray by the additional letters she saw. After she had experienced
this deception for a few days, she took the precaution, before attempting to read a word, to look at it as a black spot on a white page
and to put her finger to the right of it. Then she proceeded to
identify the letters of the word one by one. The presence of her
finger marking the end of the word precluded the sensory illusion,
which was clearly perseverative in nature, as the additional letters
the patient saw corresponded to letters perceived earlier in the word.

It appears then that identification of objects, of pictures,
and of written material on confrontation may be rendered difficult
by perceptual perseveration. Obviously, misnamings which result from
perceptual perseveration are not aphasic in nature. But they cannot
be said to be agnosic either, since agnosia by definition precludes
perceptual disturbances. As was argued above, Jeanne most probably
experienced visual perseveration in naming-on-confrontation tests.
Did she, in addition, have any agnosic deficit ? Some of her answers
suggest that she did. For instance, on one occasion she was shown
a clothes-peg and said: "A cork, a corkscrew. I keep one in the
drawer to use on bottles". The last part of this answer seems to
indicate that the patient really mistook the clothes-peg for a corkscrew. On another occasion she was shown a fork, and she said: "A
tin-opener, when one wants to eat tinned sardines". In this case
too, the second part of the answer suggests that the patient did
mean tin-opener, that is to say that the patient made a paragnosia.
One day she was shown a picture of a piece of Gruyere cheese and
said: "It looks like meat: pork or lamb, I'd say..... it's not a
cauliflower, Brussels sprouts..... I think there are small holes;
it must be Gruyere cheese". It looks as if the patient at first did
not recognize the cheese; it was not until she noticed the holes that
she realized it must be Gruyere. Such responses strongly suggest
that in addition to optic aphasia Jeanne had some degree of visual
agnosia. That this was visual agnosia and not dementia is demonstrated by the fact that after she had mistaken the clothes-peg for a
corkscrew, she was allowed to handle the object, and she immediately
identified it correctly. Just the same happened with the fork, which
she had first mistaken for a tin-opener. Her agnosia then was restricted to the visual modality and no sign of mental confusion could
be observed.

As was noted above, Jeanne's capability to understand written words was less disturbed than her ability to read these words aloud. Indeed, it happened repeatedly in the tests that the patient identified a word but could not say it or said another word, as when she appropriately matched the written word cigarettes with the picture of a cigarette box but called it "Fish, fishing'.

Correct identification with false naming was also observed in Caplan and Hedley-Whyte's case (1974) when the patient had to tell some ten letters alphabetically: she aligned the letters properly despite frequent misnaming of them. She would generally complete letters adequately in words or appropriately cover extra letters with her hand, although she read the words aloud erroneously. For instance, being shown the anomalous word CATAT, she covered the last two letters but said "Boy". She changed RACF into RACE but said "Dog".

A similar discrepancy between silent and oral reading was also noted in the case reported by Albert et al. (1973). The patient was shown a single written word and was asked to select from among 3 pictures the one that corresponded to the word. He selected the correct alternative in 8 of 10 items of this kind. However, he could read aloud correctly only 3 of the 8 words he had appropriately matched with the picture. One of his failures concerned the word shoe: he pointed to the correct picture but said: "I can't name it. I can't name it. I can't read it. I know what it is. I can't read". He then tried to identify the individual letters which the word comprised, but he failed: "g-m-o-a, t-o-m-o". On another occasion, he was shown a picture of a lion and was requested to point to the correct word from among the written alternatives cat, lion, and bear. He correctly designated the word lion, but read it aloud as "Black. No. Horse, I imagine. Yeah, black". In this response black was a perseverative segment from the immediately preceding answer. The four agrammatic patients mentioned in the first part of this paper could also understand written words far better than they could read them aloud.

Oral reading then may be more severely impaired than silent reading. Written words which are correctly understood may be replaced by perseverations or paralexias when sounded out. In fact, in oral reading two mechanisms - one decoding and the other encoding- come into play, and they may be affected differently by cerebral damage. In Beringer and Stein's case, which was discussed above, only the decoding mechanism appears to have been disturbed. But the reverse may obtain: comprehension of written language may be preserved- at least to a larger extent- while the sounding out of what has been decoded is markedly impaired. Interestingly enough, when the output mechanism is disordered, having to use it may have a negative influence on the otherwise relatively intact input mechanism. Dennis (1980) has reported the case of a nine-year-old girl with acquired aphasia who could understand written words well and written sentences fairly well as long as she could read silently. Understanding was

considerably more impaired when she had to read aloud.   "Oral output was in fact disruptive of reading" Dennis writes.

   These various observations show how important it is to carefully
indicate in the description of alexic patients' verbal behavior whether one is referring to silent reading or, on the contrary, to oral
reading.   Indeed, errors made in reading aloud may not be reading
errors at all, but may result from a disruption in the mechanisms
used to verbalize what one has understood through reading.   In other
words, some paralexias are speech errors, not reading errors.

   The difference between reading for meaning and reading aloud
is further underscored by the existence of patients who can read
aloud but fail to understand what they read.   This dissociation may
occasionally be observed in the context of sensory aphasia.   One of
our patients with paraphasic speech and impaired comprehension of
spoken language could still read aloud correctly but he was unable
to read for meaning.   Nurses used to amuse themselves by having the
patient read aloud sentences which were derogatory to him, such as
I am a cuckold.   The patient would read such sentences most seriously
and be surprised by the ensuing laughter.

   Returning to the case of Jeanne, we may say that the optic
aphasia which affected naming of objects and pictures on confrontation also disturbed reading aloud of letters and words.   However,
as was shown above, not all of her misnamings can be considered to
be aphasic.   Visual perseveration and visual agnosia are responsible
for some of her errors.   Indeed, visual agnosia may be said to have
disturbed not only her identification of objects and pictures
but also her identification of written material.   Though silent reading was superior to oral reading, it was not normal.   The patient
had difficulty in understanding written commands and she performed
at chance level in written lexical decision tasks.   When she had to
match written words with pictures or to designate written words named
by the examiner she responded often, but not always, adequately.
In other words, Jeanne appears to have had an intrinsic reading disorder, which was complicated by optic aphasia and visual perseveration.
This symptomatology seemed to be three-staged.

   1. Visual percepts were sometimes altered by visual persevera-
       tion;

   2. Unaltered visual percepts could not always be correctly
       identified;

   3. Correctly identified visual percepts could not always be
       named appropriately.

   The first stage is perceptual, the second gnosic, and the third
verbal in nature.   They form a crescendo as more errors appear to

have resulted from stage 2 than from stage 1, and from stage 3 than from stage 2. Silent reading could be perturbed by any of the first two stages, while oral reading could be perturbed by any of the three stages.

Moreover, the naming problem in stage 3 appears more akin to Broca's aphasia than to amnestic aphasia, as the patient seemed to have difficulty not only in evoking the appropriate names but also in saying them. Interpreting these findings in terms of a logogen model such as the one proposed by Morton and Patterson (1980a), one might say that in Jeanne's case disturbances could occur at any of the four levels from visual analysis to visual input logogen to semantics to output logogens.

As was mentioned earlier in this paper, Stachowiak and Poeck (1976) have argued that there is an upward gradient from pure alexia to pure alexia with right hemianopia to pure alexia with hemianopia and color aphasia to the full syndrome of optic aphasia. Jeanne's deficits show that this gamut may extend so as to include visual agnosia and perseverative visual perception.

Finally, it should be recalled that Jeanne made semantic para-lexias. However, her condition was not identical with that of Berin-ger and Stein's patient, since Jeanne had optic aphasia while in Beringer and Stein's case there was no aphasia. Because she had aphasia and her difficulty in reading words aloud often resulted from her language impairment, Jeanne resembles the patients described by Goldstein, by Andrewsky and Seron, by Morton and Patterson, and by Nolan and Caramazza. Yet, her aphasia was different from theirs: she had optic aphasia while they all had agrammatism. This is proba-bly the reason why they found functors more difficult to read aloud than content words, while she did not. It appears then that the pathophysiology of acquired reading disorders may be complex and variegated. Different patients make (semantic) paralexias for diffe-rent reasons. In trying to explain their reading errors, one often has to take into account the deficits which may accompany the alexia, particularly aphasia and agnosia. In a way the classics had anti-cipated this, as they classified acquired disorders of reading with reference to the accompanying verbal impairments and called pure alexia agnostic or optic alexia (Alajouanine, 1968, p. 125). By highlighting the types of errors made by alexic patients and the types of words they find most difficult to read aloud, modern research has undoubtedly opened new vistas. However, the knowledge gained in this way does not supersede that of the classics but supplements it. The most profitable way to look at acquired reading disorders appears to be to integrate traditional teachings and modern discove-ries into a harmonious whole. In other words, there need be no rupture between the past and the present of alexia.

REFERENCES

Alajouanine, T. L'aphasie et le langage pathologique. Paris: Bai-
    llière, 1968.
Albert, M., Yamadori, A., Gardner, H. and Howes, D. Comprehension
    in alexia. Brain, 1973, 96, 317-328.
Andreewsky, E. and Seron, X. Implicit processing of grammatical
    rules in a case of agrammatism. Cortex, 1975, 11, 379-390.
Benson, F. The third alexia. Archives of Neurology, 1977, 34,
    327-331.
Beringer, K. and Stein, J. Analyse eines Falles von "reiner" Alexie.
    Zeitschrift für Neurologie, 1930, 123, 472-478.
Caplan, L. and Hedley-Whyte, T. Cuing and memory dysfunction in ale-
    xia without agraphia. Brain, 1974, 97, 251-262
Coltheart, M. Deep dyslexia: A review of the syndrome. In Coltheart,
    M., Patterson, K. and Marshall, J. (Eds.), Deep dyslexia. London:
    Routledge and Kegan Paul, 1980.
Dejerine, J. Contribution à l'étude anatomo-pathologique et clinique
    des différentes variétés de cécité verbale. Mémoires de la
    société de Biologie, 1892, 4, 61-90.
Dennis, M. Strokes in childhood I: Communicative intent, expression,
    and comprehension after left hemisphere arteriopathy in a right-
    handed nine-year-old. In Rieber, R. (Ed.), Language development
    and aphasia in children. New York: Academic Press, 1980.
Dubois-charlier, F. Approche neurolinguistique du problème de
    l'alexie pure. Journal de Psychologie Normale et Pathologique,
    1971, 39-68.
Dubois, J., Marcie, P.and Hecaen H. Description et classification
    des aphasies. Languages, 1967, 5, 18-36.
Geschwind, N. Disconnexion syndromes in animals and men. Brain, 1965,
    88, 237-294, 585-644.
Goldstein, K. Language and language disturbances. New York: Grune
    and Stratton, 1948.
Head, H. Aphasia and kindred disorders of speech. Cambridge:
    Cambridge University Press, 1926.
Lebrun, Y., Brihaye, J. and Lebrun, N. On expressive agrammatism.
    Journal of Communicative Disorders, 1971, 4, 126-133.
Lhermitte, F. and Beauvois, M. A visual-speech disconnexion syndrome.
    Brain, 1973, 96, 695-714.
Lhermitte, F., Chain, F., Escourolle, R., Ducarne, B. and Pillon, B.
    Etude anatomo-clinique d'un cas de prosopagnosie. Revue Neuro-
    logique, 1972, 126, 329-346.
Luria, A. Human brain and psychological processes. New York: Harper
    and Row, 1966.
Marin, O., Saffran. E., and Schwartz, M. Dissociations of language
    in aphasia: Implications for normal function. Annals of the
    New York Academy of Sciences, 1976, 280, 868-884.
Marshall, J. and Newcombe, F. The conceptual status of deep dysle-
    xia: An historical perspective. In Coltheart, M., Patterson, K.
    and Marshall, J. (Eds.), Deep dyslexia. London: Routledge and

Kegan Paul, 1980.

Meadows, J. and Munro, S. Palinopsia. Journal of Neurology, Neurosurgery, and Psychiatry, 1977, 40, 5-8.

Morton, J. and Patterson, K. A new attempt at an interpretation, or
an attempt at a new interpretation. In Coltheart, M., Patterson, K. and Marshall, J. (Eds.), Deep dyslexia. London: Routledge and Kegan Paul, 1980 (a).

Morton, J. and Patterson, K. 'Little words -No!' In Coltheart, M.,
Patterson, K. and Marshall, J. (Eds.), Deep dyslexia. London:
Routledge and Kegan Paul, 1980 (b).

Nolan, K. and Caramazza, A. Modality-independent impairments in word
processing in a deep dyslexic patient. Brain and Language,
1982, 16, 237-264.

Shallice, T. and Warrington, E. Single and multiple component central
dyslexic syndromes. In Coltheart, M., Patterson, K. and Marshall, J. (Eds.), Deep dyslexia. London: Routledge and Kegan
Pual, 1980.

Stachowiak, F. and Poeck, K. Functional disconnection in pure alexia
color naming deficit demonstrated by facilitating methods.
Brain and Language, 1976, 3, 135-143.

TOWARD A RATIONAL TAXONOMY OF THE ACQUIRED DYSLEXIAS

John C. Marshall
Neuropsychology Unit
The Radcliffe Infirmary
Oxford

The study of acquired disorders of written language has a history that extends for almost two millenia; in 30 C. E., Valerius
Maximus reported that an Athenian scholar lost the 'memory of letters'
after closed head injury whilst apparently retaining intact all his
other knowledge and skill (Kempf, 1888). Subsequently, scholars described such impairments in greater detail. For example: Schmidt
(1676) studied a man, N. C., who, after an attack of apoplexy, could
neither read words nor name individual letters, yet when words were
dictated to him he wrote them faultlessly. Schmidt was especially
surprised to discover that N. C. could not read back material that
the patient had himself written shortly beforehand; a century later,
Gesner (1770) described a case of neologistic jargon aphasia in which
both reading and writing were severly impaired. Gesner noted that,
when writing, the patient's output contained 'neographisms' that were
phonologically related to the neologisms that he produced in speaking.
At the end of the nineteenth century, Pitres (1894) discussed a case
of acquired dyslexia in which semantic errors and circumlocations
were made when reading aloud both individual words and text (see
Obler, This Volume). The varied nature of these previously literate
patients who, consequent upon brain-injury, have lost (in part) the
ability to read and write (despite adequate sight and motor control)
has continued to intrigue clinicians and theoreticians alike.

    A first step toward understanding the forms that acquired dysle-
xias (and dysgraphias) can take might be to group the patients on
the basis of their particularly outstanding characterstics. But in
any complex domain there will always be a wide variety of more or
less independent features that could, in principle, support classification; hence the distinct taxonomic classes that result from grouping according to one set of criteria could be largely orthogonal

212   J. Marshall

to the classes that emerge when other criteria are employed. It is
therefore mandatory that the striking characterstics on which a taxonomy is based are not only reliable but also pertinent. 'Pertinence',
however, is a two-place predicate and thus raises the question 'pertinent to what?' I shall accordingly outline some previous taxonomies of the acquired dyslexias with particular reference to the underlying grounds that motivate the taxonomy.

CLASSIFICATION BY ASSOCIATED SIGNS AND SYMPTOMS

     As Sherlock Holmes (almost) pointed out, one of the most outsta-
nding signs that can be associated with an acquired dyslexia is no
signs. That is, the patient who manifests a severe incapacity to
read (either aloud or silently with comprehension) despite (reasonably) intact writing, spelling and oral language will stand out in
even the most cursory clinical examination. If the patient's visual
system is sufficiently intact to support accurate (albeit slow and
laborious)copying of written words, as in the cases reported by Ajax
(1967), by Sroka, Solsi, and Bornstein (1973), and by Greenblatt
(1973), the 'purity' of the syndrome (dyslexia without dysgraphia)
becomes even more striking. Once such (relatively) pure cases of
dyslexia had been described (Broadbent, 1872; Charcot, 1889; Kussmaul, 1885) it seemed natural to classify other cases of acquired
reading disorder by the signs and symptoms that they displayed in
addition to their dyslexia.

     Thus most patients with dyslexia also show impairments of writ-
ing (both spontaneously and to dictation) and of oral spelling. Although many patients with dyslexia and dysgraphia also display 'sensory' (Wernicke's) aphasia (Starr, 1889), there are reports of severe reading and writing disorder in the context of minimal aphasia.
For example: the case of Dejerine (1891) showed an almost total abolition of reading and very limited writing in the presence of a mild
anomia. Similarly, the patient of Mohr (1976) had relatively well-
preserved oral language despite severe impairment of reading and
writing. Oral spelling, both expressive and receptive, was shared
in Mohr's case, although this positive feature is untypical of the
syndrome. Finally, in classification by association, it is customary
to distinguish aphasic dyslexia. That is, disorders of written language may co-occur with disorders of oral language which are of
(approximately) equal severity. The aphasic dyslexias will often
be further subdivided according to the type of aphasia with which
they co-exist. As mentioned previously, dyslexia and dysgraphia are
frequently found in conjunction with'fluent' aphasias. Thus Albert,
Goodglass, Helm, Rubens and Alexander (1981) report that most patients with Wernicke's aphasia have comparable reading and writing impairment whereby reading aloud is as paralexic and writing is as
paragraphic as their spoken language is paraphasic. Dyslexia can
also be seen in conjuction with a 'non-fluent' (Broca's or transcortical motor) aphasia. In some of these cases the dyslexia may be

restricted to reading aloud with relative preservation of comprehension (Nielsen, 1938); in other cases, however, comprehension of the closed-class vocabulary ('functors') may also be impaired and give rise to 'agrammatic' understanding of text (Benson, 1977).

Although the tripartite taxonomy of 'pure' dyslexia, dyslexia with dysgraphia, and aphasic dyslexia is still in widespread use it has, on the whole, not supported research programs that have cast much light on the functional decomposition of written language skills. Indeed it would seem that the notion of classifying by associated characteristics has directed attention away from the necessity of describing the fine detail of reading and writing impairments per se. Why then does taxonomy continue to exert such a powerful influence in some circles? When first outlined in the second half of the nineteenth century, the taxonomy showed promise of mapping onto a fairly well defined set of lesion-sites. That is, autopsy reports showed that in patients with 'pure' dyslexia there was brain-damage that disconnected primary visual cortex bilaterally from the left angular gyrus and the posterior part of the left superior temporal gyrus; that in dyslexia with dysgraphia there was often damage to the left angular gyrus itself; that in aphasic dyslexia there was damage either to the left superior temporal gyrus and the second temporal gyrus (dyslexia and dysgraphia with Wernicke's aphasia) or to the third left frontal gyrus (dyslexia and dysgraphia with Broca's aphasia). To a first approximation, these localizations have stood the test of time (although counterexamples are perhaps not as rare as one might wish). For the nineteenth century physician, lacking modern methods of in vivo brain visualization, the taxonomy was justified by its apparent success in predicting the likely locus of the patient's lesion before it could be seen by histology at autopsy. And the taxonomy has continued to support interesting research into the anatomy of the acquired dyslexias (Geschwind, 1962; Greenblatt, 1977). Neurological investigations of 'pure' dyslexia (see, for example, Ajax, Schenkenberg, and Kosteljanetz, 1977; Cohen, Salanga, Hully, Steinberg, and Hardy, 1976: Greenblatt, 1976; Kirshner, Staller, Webb, and Sachs, 1982) have been particularly productive in uncovering a large range of pathological conditions that can provoke the syndrome. In many papers, however, the detail and sophistication of anatomical description serves to conceal a paucity of information about the behavioral characterstics of the patient. It is worth reminding ourselves that intelligible structure-function correlations presuppose an adequate analysis of impaired and preserved functions.

CLASSIFICATION BY ORTHOGRAPHIC 'LEVELS'

In languages that are written alphabetically or syllabically it seems very reasonable to distinguish between the basic characters of the script, the words that are formed by concatenation of characters, and the sentences that are formed by concatenation of words. It accordingly occurred to a number of nineteenth century scholars (Hinshelwood, 1900; Elder, 1900) that one could attempt to classify

the acquired dyslexias in terms of the 'levels' of orthographic representaion (letters, words, or sentences) that the patient had greater difficulty in copying with. Being of a mathematical turn of
mind, Elder (1900) noted that from three features one can derive seven taxonomic classes. "It is possible", he writes, "for a person
to be letter-blind, word-blind, or sentence-blind; to be all three;
to be leter- and word- but not sentence-blind; to be word- and sen-
tence- but not letter-blind; to be letter- and sentence- but not word-
blind." Although all seven varieties of acquired dyslexia are logi-
cally possible, Elder is of the opinion that the empirical probability of encountering each and every subtype is not great: " . . . it
requires only a very cursory examination to see that some of these
varieties are not likely to occur, as, for instance, that in which a
person would be sentence- and letter- but not word-blind; or the opposite condition, where a person would be word-blind but not letter-
or sentence-blind." But in fact even these forms are not as odd as
Elder implies. It is not difficult to conceive that a patient could
be unable to name letters, could read individual words with fair comprehension, and yet fail to understand written sentences by virtue
of an incapacity to assign the correct grammatical relationships to
the constituents of the sentence. And indeed this variety sounds
quite similar to Benson's description of dyslexia in the context of
Broca's aphasia (Benson, 1977). Likewise one can at least imagine
conditions in which individual letter-naming is intact, individual
word-reading is impaired due, say, to lateral inhibition between letters, but sentence-reading is improved by virtue of contextual constraints facilitating word recognition. Be that as it may, the
three primary varieties of the Elder-Hinshelwood taxonomy continue
to be observed in more recent studies. Thus Hécaen and Kremin (1976)
have described cases of so-called 'verbal alexia' in which letter-
identification and naming is intact with gross impairment of word
reading (Elder's word-blindness); cases of 'literal alexia' in which
letter-naming is more impaired than the reading aloud of words (Elder's letter-blindness); and cases of 'sentence alexia' where isolated letters and words are read with fair accuracy (albeit with some
paralexic errors on suffixes) but comprehension of sentences and
text is very severely impaired.

Taxonomies based upon orthographic levels were usually justified
by an appeal to different methods for the teaching of reading and to
differential (qualitative) experience of reading. Thus Bramwell
(1887) argues that ". . . individual letters, which are generally
considered to be the most elementary parts (least highly specialised)
of written speech, as they are undoubtedly the first to be acquired,
are the last to be lost and destroyed." He notes, however, that
"after the preliminary difficulties of learning to read have been
overcome, and the act of reading has become facile, and has been
frequently repeated, the individual letters are, by some persons at
all events, ignored, and it is the combinations of letters, syllables, and individual words to which attention is chiefly directed."

Accordingly, Bramwell speculated that letter-without word-blindness would be "more frequent in well-educated and intelligent people, to whom the act of reading has, as it were, become automatic, than in uneducated persons, and those who before their illness, could only read with difficulty, and by spelling out (by the help of individual letters) the separate syllables and words." Elder (1900) continues this line of argument by observing that in "very modern" methods of education reading is taught by whole-word recognition. "The pupil is taught", he writes, "not by letters, but by words and sentences, so that he may be able to read quite well, and not know the individual letters of which the word is made up." A person who learned to read by this word-sentence method would, Elder claims, "probably show considerable variation in symptoms from the usual, if a pathological lesion affected the left angular gyrus, because, in such an individual, words and not letters are the elementary units." For Elder, then, the effects of this teaching method can mimic the manner in which "in some individuals, after much practice in reading, the words become practically the elementary units, the component letters scarcely at all being observed."

The taxonomy could also be justified by its success in mapping onto the results of contemporary studies of normal reading. For example: Erdmann and Dodge (1898) had shown, with normal subjects, that words could be correctly recognized at distances at which their letters, if presented individually, could not be identified. Could this demonstration that letter recognition is not an obligatory stage of analysis prior to word perception be an analogue of letter- without word-blindness? Later, Korte (1923) showed that in the recognition of non-word letter-strings, interior letters are masked by flanking letters. Interior letters could not be identified as eccentricities at which, if presented singly, recognition was invariably correct. Could the same mechanisms of lateral inhibition be implicated in some forms of word- without letter-blindness?

Although the primary criteria on which 'classification by association' and 'classification by level' are based are obviously disjoint, it could be the case that the two taxonomies pick out the same subgroups of patients. And, to some extent, this is indeed so. Thus patients with 'pure' dyslexia are frequently more impaired in word reading than in letter-naming; the converse pattern (letter-naming worse than word reading) is often seen in patients with dyslexia and dysgraphia and in cases of non-fluent dysphasic dyslexia (Benson, Brown, and Tomlinson, 1971). Likewise the ability to name letters and read words may be better preserved in Wernicke's aphasia than the ability to read (with understanding) sentences and continuous text.

CLASSIFICATION BY ERROR-TYPE

It is rare (although not unattested) for a dyslexic patient to be totally unable to respond when confronted with material for reading

aloud. Far more frequently, the patient will read some words correctly, will respond "Don't know" to others, and to yet other words
will make errors that bear some relationship to the stimulus items
presented. Likewise, a comparable range of phenomena will usually
be observed when the patient writes to dictation. Furthermore, the
qualitative nature of the errors made by one patient will often differ strikingly from the errors made by another. It is possible,
then, that a revealing taxonomy could be constructed from an analysis of error-types, a suggestion due originally to Newcombe and Marshall (1972).

Examples of the range of observed error-types in reading and
writing follow:

Patient A. G. (Marshall and Newcombe, 1977) had bilateral damage to the parieto-temporal region consequent upon a butterfly tumor
of the splenium of the corpus callosum. When reading single words
all his errors could be described as visual misidentifications and
omissions. Examples of his visual (or orthographic) errors include:

cat	->	"car"
sparrow	->	"narrow"
greet	->	"street"
intense	->	"incense"
village	->	"mileage"
pew	->	"few"

Patient J. C. (Newcombe and Marshall, 1972) sustained a large
left temporo-parietal injury when he was hit by a grenade fragment
in 1944. When reading individual words, a substantial proportion
of his errors are neologisms that bear both an orthographic and a
phonologic relationship to the stimulus. Examples of these errors
include:

bike	->	"bik"
devour	->	"dayver"
polite	->	"pollit"
hoof	->	"hoff"
broad	->	"brode"
aisle	->	"assell"

Patient H. A. (Marshall and Newcombe, 1977) was admitted to
hospital with a diagnosis of myocardial infarction. Despite anti-
coagulant treatment he later sustained a left-hemisphere stroke. A
substantial proportion of his errors on single word reading bore a
derivational relationship to the stimulus item. Examples of his
predicate to nominal and nominal to predicate misreadings include:

```
persuade  -> "persuasion"
defend    -> "defendant"
high      -> "height"
furniture ->"furnish"
truth     -> "true"
happiness -> "happy"
```

Patient Y. N. (Temple and Marshall, in preparation) suffered a left-hemisphere cerebro-vascular accident. She has chronic obstructive airways disease and had congestive cardiac failure at the time of her stroke. When first observed four months post-onset she made frank semantic errors when reading individual, unrelated words. Examples of her semantic paralexias include:

```
tree      -> "brook"
train     -> "aeroplane"
thirsty   -> "drink"
turquoise-> "mauve"
India     -> "Egypt"
weigh     -> "anchor"
```

Errors of these four types can also be seen when the task is writing to dictation.

Patient M. B. (Newcombe and Marshall, 1973) was admitted to surgery with angiographic evidence of a left occipital lobe mass. An osteoplastic occipital craniotomy was performed with needle aspiration of an intracranial abscess which was later evacuated. Her severe reading, writing, and spelling impairments gradually improved over the following two years,although residual deficits still remain. When writing to dictation a substantial number of her errors have a strong visuo-spatial relationship to the stimulus items. Examples of her errors follow:

```
"pig"  ->  big
"cat"  ->  cad
"den"  ->  dem
"rob"  ->  rub
"get"  ->  det
"mow"  ->  mon
```

Patient M. S. (Newcombe and Marshall, in preparation) sustained a severe closed head injury in a road traffic accident. CT scan (two years post-accident) showed slight generalized atrophy of the whole left hemisphere, most pronounced in the left temporo-parietal region, and of the right temporal region. His errors when writing to dictation were typically neologisms that bore a close orthographic and/or phonologic relationship to the stimulus. These 'neographisms' included:

"Chaos"	->	kos
"shoe"	->	shu
"guess"	->	ges
"honest"	->	onist
"click"	->	klik
"liquid"	->	likwid

Patient P. R. (Shallice, 1981a) had extensive internal carotid artery thrombosis that originated at the bifurcation on the left side. He sustained cerebral infarction that involved mainly the territory of the left middle cerebral artery. On writing to dictation, a notable proportion of his errors were derivationally related to the stimulus item. Examples include:

"defect"	->	defection
"injure"	->	injury
"coherent"	->	incoherent
"truth"	->	true
"hatred"	->	hateful
"loveliness"	->	lovely

Patient G. R. (Marshall and Newcombe, 1966) sustained a severe through-and-through penetrating missile injury to the left temporo-parietal region. A CT scan some thirty-five years post-injury showed a lesion that involved the left frontal, temporal and parietal lobe. There was sparing of the occipital lobe and part of the posterior temporal lobe on the left. The right hemisphere was well-preserved. When writing lists of unrelated words to dictation G. R. made numerous frank semantic errors. Examples include:

"star"	->	moon
"page"	->	read
"cake"	->	bun
"boat"	->	ship
"glove"	->	lace
"nephew"	->	uncle

The primary motivation for classifying patients on the basis of such differences in error-type is simply that the differences exist! An account of the acquired dyslexias and dysgraphias that

ignored the most striking characteristic of the data-base could
hardly lay claim even to observational adequacy (Chomsky, 1965).
Moreover, one might reasonably suppose that the nature of the errors
should give some insight into the mechanisms (impaired and preserved)
that give rise to them. Patients who display radically distinct
forms of paralexic and paragraphic error have been sporadically reported throughout the modern history of aphasiology (see, for example, Poppelreuter, 1917; Franz, 1930; and Luria, 1960), but it is
only recently that systematic attention has been paid to them (Marshall and Newcombe, 1973).

However, once one begins to regard the varieties of error as
more than interesting curiosities, it rapidly becomes obvious that
there is no intrinsic value in error-analysis per se. To base a
taxonomy upon the existence (or perhaps predominance) of qualitatively distinct errors in different patients is of limited interest
in itself. Error-analysis is valuable only in so far as it sheds
light upon the underlying structure of the reading and writing systems. And, one might stress, the same point holds with respect
to the criteria that are employed to construct any other taxonomy.
In short, the focus of attention must be shifted to the functional
architecture of normal visual language processing; the breakdown
of reading and writing skills must be explicitly related to the
pre-morbid structure of the relevant information-processing systems.

CLASSIFICATION OVER A FUNCTIONAL ARCHITECTURE

The moral of the preceding paragraph is far from novel
(although it is frequently forgotten). The chief insight of the
diagram-makers, from Wernicke (1874) to Bastian (1898), was precisely that the symptom-complexes of aphasia must be defined over
a model of normal functioning. And in 1885, Lichtheim produced
just such a model for the interpretation of the acquired dyslexias
and dysgraphias.

In the diagram (adapted from Lichtheim's Figure 4), A is the
center for auditory (language) engrams, M for motor (language) engrams, and B the 'concept' center. O is the center for visual (optic)
language engrams, and E the writing center (graphic engrams). The
representations assigned by these latter centers, specialized for
visual language, then map onto the spoken language system in the
fashion indicated by the arrows. By 'lesioning' the centers and
connections of the theoretical model Lichtheim attempts to predict
all the single and multi-symptom disorders of written language.
Thus, for example, he hypothesizes that copying may be intact (route
O -> E) in the context of impaired or abolished reading (lesion of
the connection between O and A); similarly, he predicts that reading
for meaning (route A -> B) may be abolished while reading aloud is

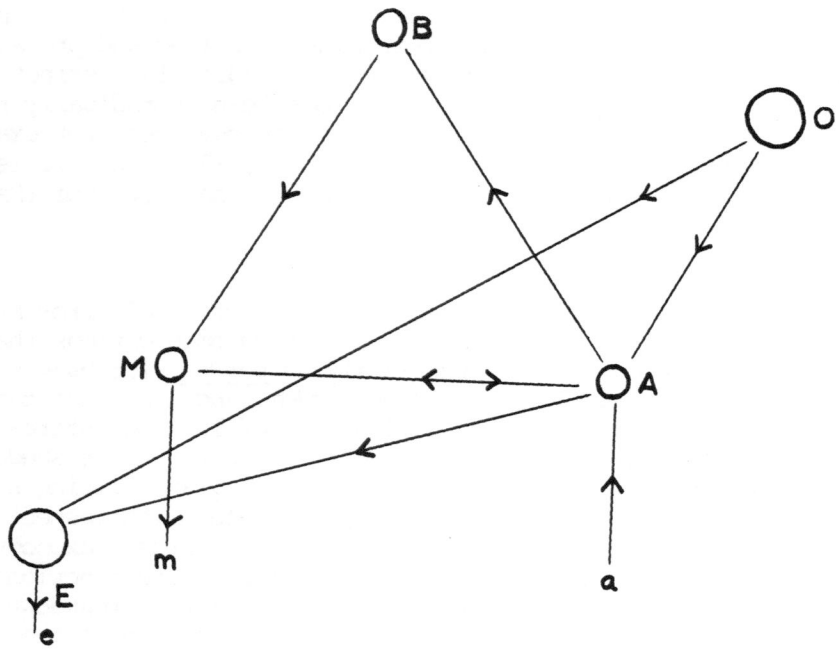

intact (route O -> A -> M). Confirmation(non-discrimination) of the
model would be obtained if all and only the clinically observed symptom-complexes of dyslexia and dysgraphia were those predicted by the
model. On the whole, the model is intuitively sensible (which is not
to say correct), although the route that seems to be demanded for spontaneous writing (B -> M -> A -> E ->e) is somewhat bizarre. For current purposes, however, the most interesting feature of Lichtheim's
schema is that it demands that, in reading, the sole mode of access
to meaning takes place via a phonologic ('auditory') re-coding of written material.

     Given the constraints on Lichtheim's manner of theorizing (i.e.
that syndromes should be defined over a normal functional architecture), it follows that it should be possible to obtain relevant evidence
(pro or con the hypothesis of obligatory phonological coding) from the
study of normal subjects. Lichtheim's extremely powerful conjecture
was (independently) revived by large numbers of scholars in the late
60s and early 70s of the suceeding century. It became popular to argue that ". . . written material must (my emphasis) be coded onto phonological form to be comprehended" (Laberge, 1972). At the time, it
seemed that one of the strongest lines of evidence in support of the
position came from experiments that used the technique of 'lexical
decision.' In this task, subjects are presented with a character

string and must judge whether or not the string is a word of their
language. Reaction times are taken and errors (false positives and
false negatives) are analysed. In a particularly ingeneous series of
experiments on normal subjects, Rubenstein, Lewis and Rubenstein (1971)
showed that reaction times for rejecting (as non-words) letter sequences which are homophonous with real words (e.g. rume -> room) are
longer than rejection times for orthographically legal non-homophonous
nonsense syllables (e.g. pake). It was also claimed that acceptance
times for homophonous words (e.g. maid -> made) are longer than for
those words that do not have homophones (e.g. lamp). These results,
are, of course, consistent with a model in which phonological recoding
precedes lexico-semantic access. That is, the processing stages in
the assignment of linguistic structure to written language are ordered
as: Stimulus -> Visual Form -> Phonologic Form -> Lexicon
But these processes must be supplemented by other mechanisms if observational adequacy is to be attained. Thus although rume takes longer
to reject it is indeed classified as a non-word; similarly, we can tell
the difference between pail and pale even if reaction times for acceptance of such stimuli are longer than for non-homophonous items. Rubenstein, Lewis and Rubenstein (1971) are accordingly forced to postulate that a post-lexical access 'spelling check' takes place before
stimuli are finally accepted or rejected. Although Rubenstein and his
colleagues do not themselves produce a diagram of their model it is
fairly clear what one would look like.

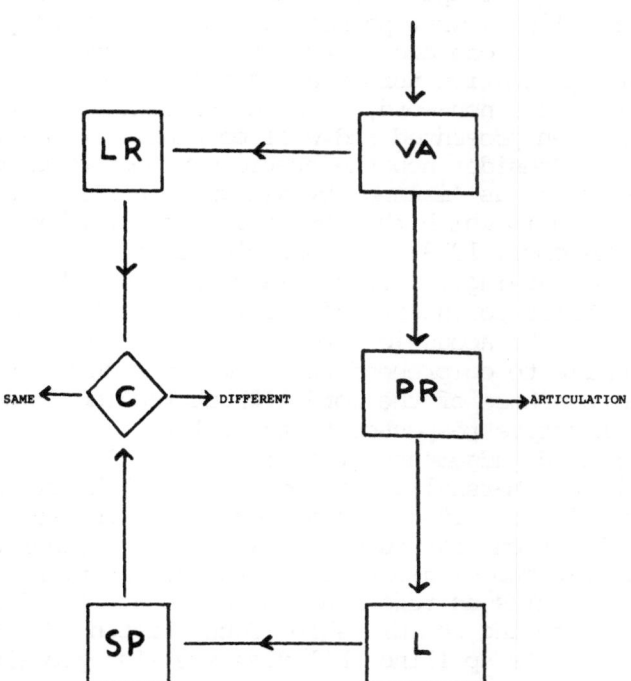

The labels on this 'reconstruction' of Rubenstein's theory are as follows: VA = Visual Analysis; LR = Letter Representations; PR = Phonological Representations; L = Lexicon; SP = Spelling Patterns; and C =
Comparator. The model would operate in the following fashion. Presented with a pronounceable letter-string, the phonologic form constructed in PR would be transmitted to L. If no corresponding entry
can be found (as for pake) rejection would follow immediately. If a
single entry was found (as for rume), then the spelling of the lexical address would be computed (room) and compared (in C) with the explicit letter-string derived from visual analysis of the stimulus presented. When these two forms failed to match, rejection would follow.
If two lexical entries were found, as when /peil/ addresses both 'bu-
cket' and 'light in color', then the spelling of one entry (e.g. pail)
would be compared against the letter-string presented; if it failed
to match, the spelling of the second lexical entry (pale) would be
compared against the original letter-string. Acceptance would follow
a successful match. It can readily be seen that the model accounts
well for the reaction-time data obtained in Rubenstein et al's experiment.

    The form of sight-to-sound conversion in the model is indiscri-
minate over the word/non-word status of the stimulus; it follows then
that phonologic recoding must take place over sub-word units. Following Venezky (1970) and Wijk (1966), let us assume that the mechanism
responsible operates with regular 'grapheme-to-phoneme correspondence
rules' of the form, for example, ai -> /ei/, s -> /s/ or /z/. or ch
-> /tʃ/. If, consequent upon brain damage, these rules are 'misapp-
lied' (or 'overapplied') what phenomena would the model predict in dyslexic subjects ? One can deduce from the structure of the model that if such a misapplication turned a visually-presented word into the
phonological form of a non-word, then the patient will not recognize
that a word has been presented and will be unable to assign a meaning
to the stimulus. Consider now the previously mentioned patient J. C.
This man reads island as "izland" by assigning a standard pronunciation of s to a word in which the letter is, non-standardly, silent
(Marshall and Newcombe, 1973); he then glosses his response by noting
"It doesn't mean anything......there is no such word". It is not the
case that J. C. fails to understand the (distal) stimulus because he
is 'lured away' by the acoustic form of his overt reading aloud; J. C.
is similarly unable to comprehend the stimulus when he is required
only to give a paraphase of the word without reading it aloud. And
he gives false negative responses to the relevant stimuli when just
making word/non-word judgements, that is, in the lexical decision paradigm (Newcombe and Marshall, 1981; see also Coltheart, Masterson,
Byng, Prior and Riddoch, 1983). Analogous phenomena are observed wh-
en rule mis-application transforms one word into another word. J. C.
assigns the regular phonologic value to the silent t in listen, and
interprets the stimulus as referring to the one-time holder of the
world heavyweight boxing championship, Sonny Liston (Marshall and Newcombe, 1973). J. C.'s spelling abilities are also grossly impaired.

It therefore follows from the Rubenstein model that J. C. will have peculiar problems with homophones even when he can <u>correctly</u> read them aloud (Coltheart, 1981). Thus <u>bee</u> is read correctly but interpreted as <u>be</u>; <u>billed</u> is read correctly and intrepreted as <u>build</u>; <u>sighs</u> is read correctly but interpreted as <u>size</u>; <u>pair</u> is read correctly and glossed "It's either two of a kind or it's the one for eating. I don't know which" (Newcombe and Marshall, 1981). Patients of this type (see Coltheart <u>et al</u>, 1983, for further examples) seem then to provide good evidence for the correctness of the Lichtheim-Rubenstein model. These patients do indeed access the lexicon via a phonological recoding of the written stimulus. It does not however follow that this is the <u>sole</u> route whereby the normal brain assigns meaning to the written word.

Morton (1969; 1979) has developed a model of word recognition in which abstract units (termed 'logogens') are postulated to underlie the perception and production of lexical formatives. The units of the 'internal dictionary' (or logogen system) have firing thresholds that are inversely correlated with the frequency of occurence of their respective words in the language. Sensory stimulation summates with the resting potential of all units that are 'physically' similar to the stimulus until one logogen reaches threshold. At this point, the word qua visual or auditory form is 'recognized', and, in parallel, made available for response and transmitted to the 'cognitive system' for the assignment of lexico-semantic features. A simplified diagram of one early version of this model follows.

In the drawing, VA = Visual Analysis; LS = Logogen System; RB = Response Buffer; and CS = Cognitive System. The model has been expressed mathematically (Morton, 1969) and gives a good quantitative account of the word-frequency effect in tachistoscopic perception and of the interaction between stimulus information and contextual evidence when words recognized in sentential frames.

For current purposes, however, the crucial characteristics of Morton's model is that, when single words are visually presented, word recognition takes place on the basis of purely visual cues, and cognitive interpretation is addressed by an abstract (non-modality specific) code; there is no recoding into phonological form <u>prior</u> to logogen activation and semantic access in the conceptual system. Phonologic coding is post-lexical in the sense that the <u>output</u> of the logogen system to the response buffer is a phonologic specification that can (eventually) trigger articulation of the word. The model in the early version I have described here is obviously incomplete. It provides no mechanism whereby (normal) subjects can read aloud pronounceable nonsense syllables written in an alphabetic or syllabic script; with respect to the lexical decision task, the model could account for 'Yes' responses to words, but no mechanism is provided whereby 'No' responses could be made to either legal or illegal non-word letter-strings (but see Coltheart, Davelaar, Jonasson and Besner, 1977).

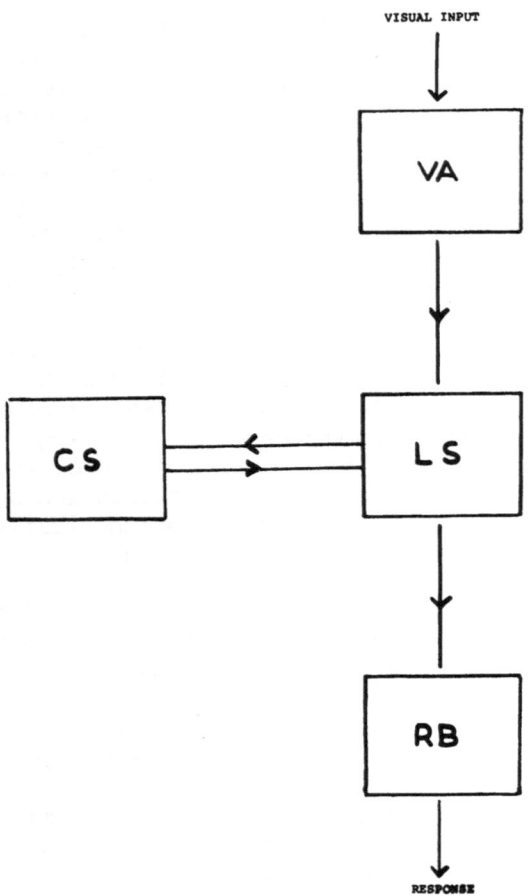

Nonetheless, we could speculate that some dyslexic subjects might read by the processes outlined in Morton's model and we can predict some phenomenological characteristics of impaired reading that
would follow from damage to particular components of the system.

In the first place, the patient would be totally unable to read
orthographically legal nonsense syllables aloud. If the patient responded at all to such stimuli, the best that might be expected is that the stimulus energy of the letter-string might exceed the threshold of a word that was visually highly similar to the nonsense syllable; this word would then be given in response. Second, recall that
the logogen system has two outputs, a phonologic code that is transmitted to the response buffer and an abstract code that addresses

lexico-semantic information. In effect, this is to claim that units of the logogen system have two thresholds. Let us conjecture (with Morton, 1968) that brain damage could raise one of these thresholds (the 'phonologic threshold') for certain words without altering the other (the 'cognitive system threshold'). If this was so, a stimulus, say, sick could activate the correct node within the logogen system, but fail to trigger the phonology of sick. Within the conceptual system sick would be associated with a range of semantically-related words, including, say, the synonym ill. If a code pertaining to this word was transmitted back to the logogen system, its phonologic realization might be readily available. The patient presented with sick would accordingly 'read' the word "ill".

Marshall and Newcombe (1966) reported a patient, G. R., whose pattern of reading impairment meets precisely the above characterization. As far as we know, G. R. has never, since sustaining brain injury, read correctly a single nonsense syllable, even of the simplest CVC form (e.g. nop). His typical response when presented with such stimuli is to say "Don't know", although he will on occasion produce a visually similar real word in response (e.g. zul -> "zulu"; wep -> "wet"). When reading words aloud his most characteristic error is to produce semantically related words. These range from quite close synonyms (e.g. ill -> "sick"; film -> "picture"; ancient -> "historic"; city -> "town") to more tangentially or distantly associated responses (e.g. envelope -> "letter"; fit -> "exercises"; glory -> "hero"; kitchen -> "oven"). It is clear that this pattern of performance has a very natural interpretation within the overall schema of Morton's model.

By contrast, the character of J. C.'s reading has no interpretation within the confines of (early versions of) Morton's theory, and G. R.'s reading has no interpretation within the Lichtheim/Rubenstein theory. An obvious (first) solution to this problem is to conjoin the two models, a step taken by Marshall and Newcombe (1973). Their very simple schema was diagramed as follows.

In this model, VR = Visual Representation; VA = Visual Addresses; PA = Phonological Addresses; SA = Semantic Addresses; T= Threshold; and AA = Articulatory Addresses. It will be seen that the model predicts the existence of 16, 383 distinct varieties of pure (single component) and mixed (multi-component) acquired dyslexia ($2^n - 1$, where n is the number of components, boxes plus arrows, represented in the diagram). From this multitude, three types were singled out for special attention: Visual Dyslexia, Surface Dyslexia, and Deep Dyslexia.

In the pure form of visual dyslexia the deficit is located in the box labelled VA, the 'store' of attested word forms. This component is closely analogous to Morton's 'Visual Input Logogens' (Morton, 1979). Noise within VA will result in misidentifications in

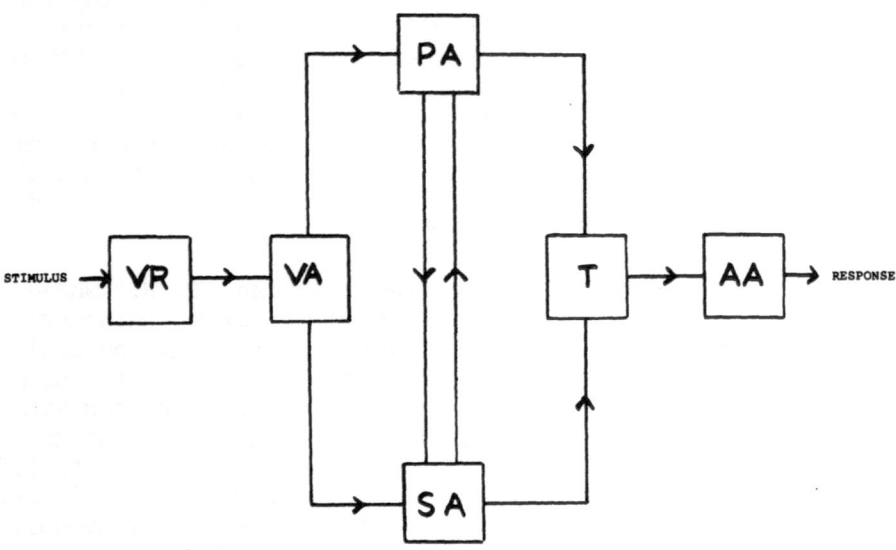

which there is a close visuo-spatial similarity between stimulus and
false response. All errors should be words of the language. To the
extent that this is not so and visually-related neologisms are produced, the errors must arise in the preceding component, VR; the neologistic letter-string will then be read via a connection (not given
in our original model) between VR and PA. On the assumption that word frequency effects arise within VA, and that the level of noise is
not so great as to totally over-ride or skew pre-morbid thresholds,
patients should be more accurate at reading high frequency words than
low frequency words, and false responses should, on average, be of
higher frequency than their respective stimuli. Performance should
not vary as a function of any linguistic or conceptual aspect of the
input words (e.g. part-of-speech, orthographic regularity, or 'concreteness'). To the extent that such variables do influence performance their effect must be attributed to later components. (A possible, although thus far unexplored, alternative would postulate that
pre-morbid thresholds within VA are set by linguistic variables in
addition to word-frequency).

        In the pure form of surface dyslexia, the deficit involves a
functional disconnection of VA from SA. On the assumption that the
alternative route (from VA to PA) operates by a system (not shown in
our original diagram) of regular grapheme-to-phoneme correspondence

rules, patients should be able to read aloud all regularly spelt words (and non-words). Irregularly spelt stimuli ('exception' words)
will fail to be read correctly, and errors will consist of 'regulari-
zations'. For example, pint will be read with the short i of pin;
the vowel digraph of broad will be realized as /ou/, its normal pronunciation in oak, boat, load etc. For regular words that can be read aloud accurately, semantic interpretation will be correct; the phonological code form PA will access the appropriate meaning via the
connection PA -> SA. Homophones may be exceptions to this claim;
thus pain could be read correctly and yet the patient be unable to
distinguish whether the stimulus was (semantically) pain or pane.
In these cases, one might expect that interpretation will be biased
by such factors as part-of-speech, 'concreteness', and word frequency. If a regularization error is made that results in another word
(e.g. bread -> /brɪːd/), then the meaning of breed will be assigned.
It can be seen that the diagram predicts a variant form of surface
dyslexia in which SA is functionally disconnected from T. In this
variety, reading aloud will be indistinguishable from the classical
form of surface dyslexia, but there will be good comprehension of words that are erroneously read aloud if the interpretive route VA ->
SA takes precedence over the route VA -> PA -> SA. Patients who me-
et this description have recently been discovered (Goldblum and Kremin, in preparation; Kay and Patterson, in preparation).

In deep dyslexia, the primary deficit involves the functional
disconnection of VA from PA. The patient is therefore unable to read pronounceable nonsense syllables, although word/non-word judgements may be made with remarkable accuracy. The recognition of rhyme
and homophony is seriously impaired when visually-presented stimuli
are orthographically distinct, e.g. soap and hope, wait and weight
(Patterson and Marcel, 1977; Saffran and Marin, 1977); words cannot
be accessed from pseudohomophones (e.g. kote, or lait). There are
no orthographic regularity effects in either reading aloud or comprehension. Semantic errors arise on the route VA -> SA -> T in reading
aloud and, sometimes, in comprehension (Newcombe and Marshall, 1980a).
There is at present no consensus concerning precisely where these semantic paralexias arise, and it seems likely that different mechanisms are responsible in different patients. In some patients, output
blocking at T may be involved, but this explanation appears not to
hold for G. R. (Newcombe and Marshall, 1980a). Friedman and Perlman
(1982) provide a good discussion of the issues at stake. It is usually argued that some pathological deficit (in lexical access, concept arousal, semantic knowledge, or output blocking) must be involved, although Newcombe and Marshall (1980b) have speculated that the
semantic route may be intrinsically unstable in the normal case and
requires input from phonologic coding if a unique entry is to be located. A number of other effects and deficits are also reliably fo-
und in deep dyslexia; patients show a strong part-of-speech effect,
whereby accuracy of reading is best for concrete nouns; adjectives,
verbs, and abstract nouns are of intermediate difficulty, and functors

are read worst (Marshall and Newcombe, 1966).   It is widely believed
that this part-of-speech hierarchy results from differences in the
subjective 'image-arousing' quality of the stimuli.   In addition to
semantic paralexias, patients with deep dyslexia make many visual and
derivational errors (see Patterson, 1980).   Current models provide no
truly convincing explanation for these latter phenomena.

CONCLUSION

     Over the last decade information-processing models have been
widely adopted as an appropriate framework within which to study disorders of cognition.   With specific respect to reading, the discovery
of such new syndromes as attentional dyslexia (Shallice and Warrington, 1977), direct dyslexia (Schwartz, Saffran and Marin, 1980) and
phonological dyslexia(Beauvois and Dérouesné, 1979) have necessitated
quite extensive modification and elaboration of the simple schema proposed by Marshall and Newcombe (1973); other changes and extensions
have been required to interpret more of the fine structure of the current range of syndromes and to incorporate phenomena such as letter-
by-letter reading, originally described in the nineteenth century but
only recently investigated in detail (Warrington and Shallice, 1980;
Patterson and Kay, 1982).   I have not covered this work here - many
of the relevant findings and theoretical extensions are outlined by
Coltheart (This Volume) - but rather concentrated on attempting to
show why modern studies have returned to the paradigm originally ex-
pounded so lucidly by Lichtheim (1885) and his fellow diagram-makers.

     A number of models of the reading system are now available with-
in the general framework discussed here (Morton and Patterson, 1980;
Marcel, 1980; Newcombe and Marshall, 1980b, 1981; Shallice, 1981b).
Although differing in exact execution, the schema all postulate a highly modular organization of the normal reading system in which multiple routes work in parallel to assign form, meaning, and sound with speed and accuracy.   To the extent that classification per se is
a rational enterprise, taxonomies of the acquired dyslexias must be
defined over an independently plausible functional architecture.

REFERENCES

Ajax. E. T. Dyslexia without agraphia: Prognostic considerations.
     Archives of Neurology, 1967, 17, 645-652.
Ajax, E. T., Schenkenberg, T. and Kosteljanetz, M. Alexia without
     agraphia and the inferior splenium. Neurology, 1977, 27, 685-688.
Albert M. L., Goodglass, H., Helm, N. A., Rubens, A. B. and Alexan-
     der, M. P. Clinical Aspects of Dysphasia. Vienna: Springer-
     Verlag, 1971.
Bastian, H. C. A treatise on aphasia and other speech deficits.
     London: H. K. Lewis, 1898.

Beauvois, M. F. and Dérouesné, J. Phonological alexia: Three disso-
    ciations. Journal of Neurology, Neurosurgery and Psychiatry,
    1979, 42, 1115-1124.
Benson, D. F. The third alexia. Archives of Neurology, 1977, 34,
    327-331.
Benson, D. F., Brown, J. and Tomlinson, E. B. Varieties of alexia:
    Word and letter blindness. Neurology, 1971, 21, 951-957.
Bramwell, B. Quoted in Elder (1900), 1887.
Broadbent, W. H. Cerebral mechanisms of speech and thought. Medi-
    cal and Chirurgical Transactions, 1872, 55, 145-194.
Charcot, J. M. On a case of word-blindness. Clinical lectures on
    diseases of the nervous system, Vol. 3, pp. 130-140. London:
    The New Sydenham Society. 1889.
Chomsky, N. Aspects of the Theory of Syntax. Cambridge, Mass.:
    MIT Press, 1965.
Cohen, D. N., Salanga, V. D., Hully, W., Steinberg, M. C. and Hardy,
    R. W. Alexia without agraphia. Neurology, 1976, 26,455-459.
Coltheart, M. Disorders of reading and their implications for models
    of normal reading. Visible Language, 1981, 15, 245-286.
Coltheart, M., Davelaar, E., Jonasson, J. T. and Besner, D. Access
    to the internal lexicon. In S. Dornic (ed.), Attention and per-
    formance, VI, Hillsdale: Erlbaum, 1977.
Coltheart, M., Masterson, J., Byng, S., Prior, M. and Riddoch, J.
    Surface dyslexia. Quarterly Journal of Experimental Psychology
    (In Press).
Déjerine, J. Sur un cas de cécité verbale avec agraphie, suivi
    d'autopsie. Mém. Soc. Biol. 1891, 3, 197-201.
Elder, W. The clinical varieties of visual aphasia. Edinburgh Me-
    dical Journal, 1900, 49, 433-454.
Erdmann, B. and Dodge, R. Psychologische Untersuchungen über das
    Lesen auf Experimenteller Grundlage. Halle: Neimeyer. 1898.
Franz, S. I. The relations of aphasia. Journal of General Psycho-
    logy, 1930, 3, 401-411.
Friedman, R. B. and Perlman, M. B. On the underlying causes of
    semantic paralexias in a patient with deep dyslexia. Neuropsy-
    chologia, 1982, 20, 559-568.
Geschwind, N. The anatomy of acquired disorders of reading. In
    J. Money (ed.), Reading Disorders. Baltimore: Johns Hopkins
    University Press, 1962.
Gesner, J. A. P. Die Sprachamnesie. Nordlingen: Beck, 1770.
Greenblatt, S. H. Alexia without agraphia or hemianopsia: Anatomi-
    cal analysis of an autopsied case. Brain, 1973, 96, 307-316.
Greenblatt, S. H. Subangular alexia without agraphia or hemianopsia.
    Brain and Language, 1976, 3, 229-245.
Greenblatt, S. H. Neurosurgery and the anatomy of reading: A practi-
    cal review. Neurosurgery, 1977, 1, 6-15.
Hecaen, H. and Kremin, H. Neurolinguistic research on reading dis-
    orders resulting from left hemisphere lesions: aphasic and
    "pure" alexias. In H. and H. A. Whitaker(eds.), Studies in
    Neurolinguistics, Vol. 2. New York: Academic Press, 1976.

Hinshelwood, J. Letter-, Word- and Mind-Blindness. London: H. K. Lewis. 1900.

Kempf, K. Valerii maximi factorum et dictorum memorabilium libri novem. Leipzig: Teubner. 1888.

Kirshner, H. S., Staller, J., Webb, W. and Sachs, P. Transtentorial herniation with posterior cerebral territory infarction: A new mechanism of the syndrome of alexia without agraphia. Stroke, 1982, 13, 243-246.

Korte, W. Studien über das Lesen. Zeitschrift für Psychologie,1923, 93, 17=82.

Kussmaul, A. Die Störungen der Sprache. Leipzig: Vogel, 1885.

LaBerge, D. Beyond auditory coding. In J. F. Kavanagh and I. G. Mattingly (eds.), Language by Ear and Eye. Cambridge, Mass; MIT Press, 1972.

Lichtheim, L. On aphasia. Brain, 1885, 7, 433-484.

Luria, A. R. Differences between disturbances of speech and writing in Russian and in French. International Journal of Slavic Linguistics and Poetics, 1960, 3, 13-22.

Marcel, A. J. Surface dyslexia and beginning reading: A revised hypothesis of the Pronunciation of print and its impairments. In M. Coltheart, K. Patterson, and J. C. Marshall (eds.), Deep Dyslexia. London: Routledge and Kegan Paul, 1980.

Marshall, J. C. and Newcombe, F. Syntactic and semantic errors in paralexia. Neuropsychologia, 1966, 4, 169-176.

Marshall, J. C. and Newcombe, F. Patterns of paralexia: A psycholinguistic approach. Journal of Psycholinguistic Research, 1973, 2, 175-199.

Marshall, J. C. and Newcombe, F. Variability and constraint in acquired dyslexia. In H. and H. A. Whitaker (eds.), Studies in Neurolinguistics, Vol.3. New York: Academic Press, 1977.

Mohr, J. P. An unusual case of dyslexia with dysgraphia. Brain and Language, 1976, 3, 324-334.

Morton, J. Grammar and Computation in language behavior. Progress Report No. 6, Center for Research in Language and Language Behavior, University of Michigan, 1968.

Morton, J. Interaction of information in word recognition. Psychological Review, 1969, 76, 165-178.

Morton, J. Word recognition. In J. Morton and J. C. Marshall(eds.), Psycholinguistics Series, Vol. 2. Cambridge, Mass.: MIT Press, 1979.

Morton, J. and Patterson, K. E. A new attempt at an interpretation, or, an attempt at a new interpretation. In M. Coltheart, K. Patterson and J. C. Marshall (eds.), Deep Dyslexia. London: Routledge and Kegan Paul, 1980.

Newcombe, F. and Marshall, J. C. Word retrieval in aphasia: Some recent findings. International Journal of Mental Health, 1972, 3, 38-45.

Newcombe, F. and Marshall, J. C. Stages in recovery from dyslexia following a left cerebral abscess. Cortex, 1973, 9, 329-332.

Newcombe, F. and Marshall, J. C. Response monitoring and response

blocking in deep dyslexia. In M. Coltheart, K. Patterson and
J. C. Marshall (eds.), Deep Dyslexia. London: Routledge and
Kegan Paul, 1980a.

Newcombe, F. and Marshall, J. C. Transcoding and lexical stabiliza-
tion in deep dyslexia. In M. Coltheart, K. Patterson and
J. C. Marshall (eds.), Deep Dyslexia. London: Routledge and
Kegan Paul, 1980b.

Newcombe, F. and Marshall, J. C. On psycholinguistic classifications
of the acquired dyslexias. Bulletin of the Orton Society, 1981,
31, 29-46.

Nielsen, J. M. The unsolved problems in aphasia. Part 1: Alexia in
motor aphasia. Bulletin of the Los Angeles Neurological Societies, 1938, 4, 114-122.

Patterson, K. E. Derivational errors. In M. Coltheart, K. patterson
and J. C. Marshall (eds.), Deep Dyslexia, London: Routledge and
Kegan Paul, 1980.

Patterson, K. E. The relation between reading and phonological coding: Further neuropsychological observations. In A. W. Ellis
(ed.), Normality and Pathology in Cognitive Functions. London:
Academic Press, 1982.

Patterson, K. E. and Kay, J. Letter-by-letter reading: Psyhcologi-
cal descriptions of a neurological syndrome. Quarterly Journal
of Experimental Psychology, 1982, 34A, 411- 441.

Patterson, K. E. and Marcel, A. J. Some Observations on aphasia and
dyslexia: Impairment in the phonological representation of
written words. Quarterly Journal of Experimental Psychology,
1977, 29, 307-318.

Poppelreuter, W. Die psychischen Schadigungen durch Kopfschuss im
Kriege 1914-1916. Leipzig: Voss, 1917.

Rubenstein, H., Lewis, S. S. and Rubenstein, M. Evidence for phonemic recoding in visual word recognition. Journal of Verbal
Learning and Verbal Behavior, 1971, 10, 645-657.

Saffran, E. M. and Marin, O. S. M. Reading without phonology: Evidence from aphasia. Quarterly Journal of Experimental Psychology, 1977, 29, 515-525.

Schmidt, J. De oblivione lectionis ex apoplexia slava scriptione.
Miscellanea curiosa medico-physica Academiae naturae curiosorum,
1676, 4, 195-197.

Schwartz, M. F., Saffran, E. M. and Marin, O. S. M. Fractionating
the reading process in dementia: Evidence for word-specific
print-to-sound associations. In M. Coltheart, K. Patterson and
J. C. Marshall (eds.), Deep Dyslexia. London: Routledge and
Kegan Paul, 1980.

Sroka, H., Solsi, P. and Bornstein, B. Alexia without agraphia with
complete recovery: Functional disconnection syndrome. Confinia
Neurologia, 1973, 35, 167-176.

Starr, A. The pathology of sensory aphasia. Brain, 1889, 12, 82-99.

Pitres, A. Rapport sur la question des aphasies. Bordeaux: Gounou-
ilhou, 1894.

Shallice, T. Phonological agraphia and the lexical route in writing.

Brain, 1981, 104, 413-429. a.

Shallice, T. Neurological impairment of cognitive processes. British Medical Bulletin, 1981, 37, 187-192. b.

Shallice, T. and Warrington, E. K. The possible role of selective attention in acquired dyslexia. Neuropsychologia, 1977, 15, 31-41.

Venezky, R. L. The Structure of English Orthography, The Hague: Mouton, 1970.

Warrington, E. K. and Shallice, T. Word-form dyslexia. Brain, 1980, 103, 99-112.

Wernicke, C. Der aphasische Symptomencomplex. Breslau: Cohn and Weigert, 1874.

Wijk, A. Rules of Pronunciation for the English Language. London: Oxford University Press, 1966.

WORD-RECOGNITION AND WORD-PRODUCTION:
DATA FROM PATHOLOGY

Helgard Kremin
Chargée de recherche au C. N. R. S.
Unité 111 de l' I. N. S. E. R. M.
2ter rue d'Alesia
75014 Paris - France

Brain injury may impair the components of language in a highly selective fashion. In many instances these dissociations are not transparent to our "common sense", and often they even resist smooth integration into existing linguistic and/or psychological models. This paper will furnish no answers. But we hope that it will help to ask more precise questions with regard to the processes involved in word recognition and in word production.

What might be surprising at first sight for the non-profession-al is an almost daily experience for neurologists, linguists, and therapists who work with brain damaged people: a patient who has ju-st uttered a given word in his spontaneous speech is unable to pro-duce the same word in a naming task, for example, or cannot repeat the item and/or read the word aloud and so on. In fact, modality-specific disturbances have been of crucial importance for the formu-lation of neuropsychological syndromes - usually by demonstrating that the disturbance was "pure", for example limited to reading (pu-re alexia), to writing (pure agraphia), to auditory analysis (pure word deafness), to naming (pure amnestic aphasia), to the recogniti-on of objects by sight (pure visual agnosia), by touch (pure tactile agnosia) or by sound (pure auditory agnosia), etc. These "pure" sy-ndromes, which are related to the channel or modality of the sensory input, were and remain of important theoretical concern for the des-cription of syndromes. But other forms of clinically observed diss-ociations are also to be taken into account : those related to the channel of motor output and those related to linguistic properties of the target. Indeed, brain damage may leave the sensory input in-tact but nonetheless prevent the production of the adequate verbal form. Thus a patient may "know" what he has seen, felt, or heard, but he cannot reproduce the target correctly at all or unless it is

experienced through another sensory channel. Moreover, the parallels
and divergencies of a patient's verbal behavior - compared over different modalities - can result in a pattern of such quantitative and
qualitative differences that it might be difficult to explain the patient's linguistic performances by just one causing disturbance. The
purpose of this paper is to review some data from pathology concerning word-recognition and word-production with regard to the tested modalities and the linguistic properties of the stimuli.

RECOGNITION VS PRODUCTION

     Formal testing of recognition vs production performances of sub-
jects suffering from aphasia has not often been systematically carried out. [One of the reasons might well be that aphasic disturbances
have been considered to be only disturbances of performance with the
underlying linguistic competence being spared (Weigl and Bierwisch,
1970) - although this view did not go without contradiction (see, for
example, Zurif, Caramazza and Myerson, 1972)].

     As we mentioned recognition and production performances of brain
damaged subjects have not often been comparatively investigated. Hecaen and Kremin (1976), however, carried out an analysis (based on
standardized principal components) of the relationship between the
(clustered) variables of recognition/comprehension and reading aloud.
(The data refer to the performances of 38 subjects with left-sided
lesions and oral language impairment on a battery of reading tests).
The first principal plan (83% of the variance) is shown in Figure 1.

     There is a clear dichotomy between recognition and reading aloud.
(Furthermore, a dichotomy between meaningful and non-meaningful material is very apparent - although the distinction between meaningful
and non-meaningful material is less marked in the case of reading
and tends instead to give way to a trichotomy between the reading of
meaningful material, the reading of nonsense syllables, and the reading
of isolated letters). It should be emphasized that this analysis does
not refer to the degree or the severity of the impairment; rather, it
shows the relative independence of both variables.

     In fact, patients might be able to recognize and understand
the graphic items without succeding in their oral production (see Figs.
2 and 3.)

     This pattern is typically found in cases with severe Broca's ap-
hasia where oral output might be almost impossible in spite of relatively preserved reading comprehension, at least at the level of isolated words. (Syntactic disorders, typical for anterior aphasics,
may, however, interfere with more complex tasks such as the reading and
comprehension of sentences - see Berndt and Caramazza, 1980). More
often, though, the relation of recognition and production is not a clear dissociation but rather a difference of degree. This might be

FIGURE 1. The relationship of the variables "recognition/comprehen-
sion" and "oral reading" (from Hecaen and Kremin, 1976,
Fig. 2, p. 303).

(1) Recognition of letters; (2) Recognition of words;
(3) Recognition of nonsense syllables; (4) Recognition/ comprehension of sentences; (5) Oral reading of letters; (6) Oral
reading of words; (7) Oral reading of sentences; (8) Oral
reading of nonsense syllables

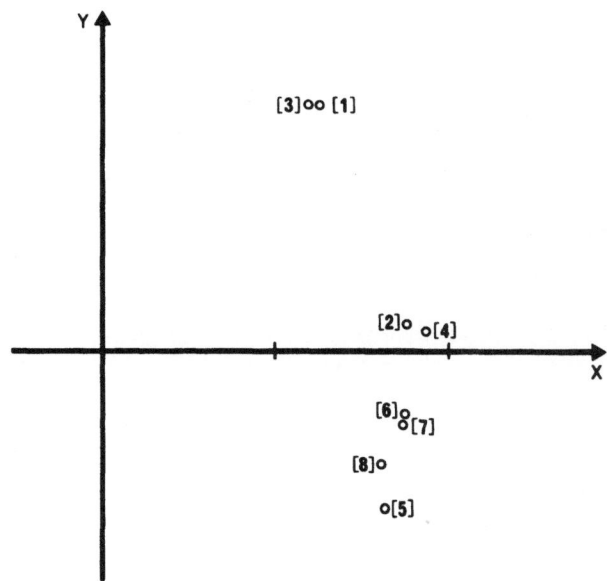

FIGURES 2 through 5: Reading and recognition performance (% error)
of 4 patients with left sided lesions. TEST DESCRIPTION

(1) Oral reading of isolated letters.

(2) Recognition of one letter in a group of ten letters (upper
or lower case, printed or handwritten).

(3) Recognition of Latin letters in a nonomeaningful context
(foreign characters)

(4) Recognition of a letter within a word - capital or lower
case, handwritten or printed (letters chosen on the basis
of thier similarity in terms of shape and position within
the word).

(5) Distinction between digits and letters from a set of letters and digits combined.

(6) Oral reading of words.

FIGURE 2.   Patient BRE

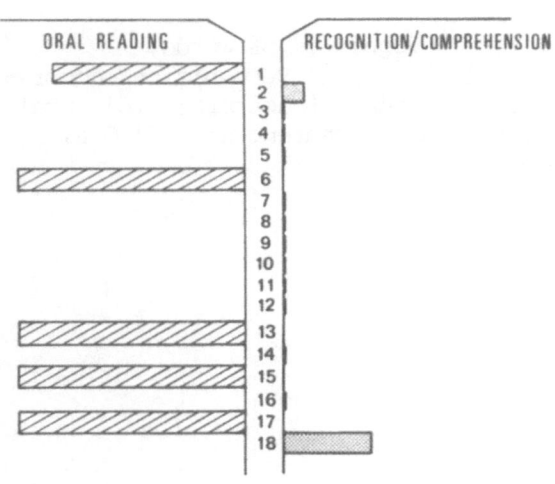

FIGURE 3. Patient FIG

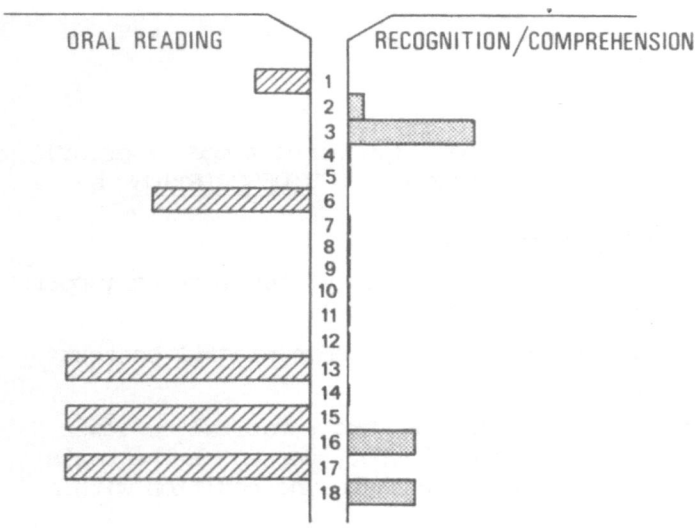

FIGURE 4. Patient PRA

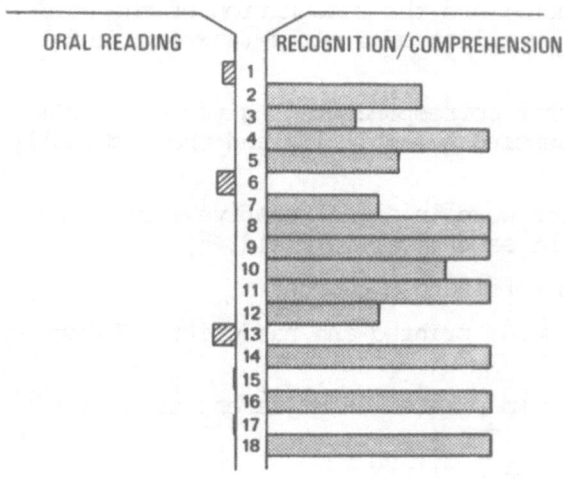

FIGURE 5. Patient CUS

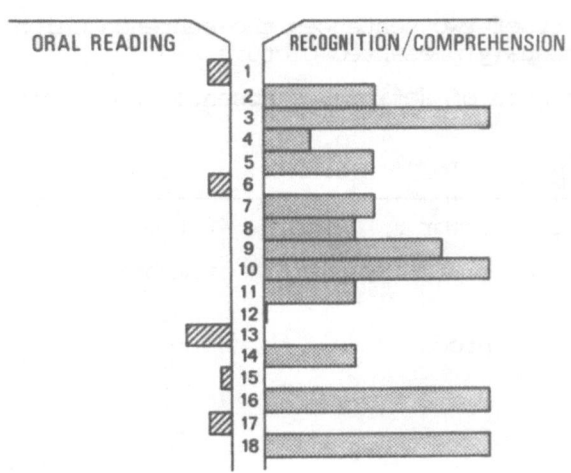

Figures 2-5 (contd.)

(7)   Recognition of the French word in a list of 5 words (4
      Hungarian and 1 French); and the recognition of the word
      which is not French in a list of 5 words (4 French and 1
      Hungarian).

(8)   Choose the picture that corresponds to a given word from
      four pictures representing semantically and phonologically
      similar words.

(9)   Recognition of the odd word in a list of five words four
      of which belong to the same semantic field.

(10) Lexical decisions on words and nonwords.

(11) Recognition of same word, printed and handwritten in an
      array of five.

(12) Recognition of same word printed in different size in an
      array of five.

(13) Oral reading of nonsense syllables.

(14) Recognition of one nonsense syllable in a set of five
      nonsense syllables.

(15) Oral reading of simple, semicomplex and complex commands.

(16) Execution of simple, semicomplex and complex commands.

(17) Oral reading of sentences.

(18) Recognition from a set of two sentences the sentence which
      describes a simultaneously presented picture.

ASSOCIATED DEFICITS   +=presence of deficit, o=absence of deficit

Patient	BRE	FIG	PRA	CUS
Etiology	vascular	tumor	tumor	tumor
Localization	?	?	parietal	temporal
Sensory aphasia	+		+	+
Motor aphasia	o	Broca	o	o
Agraphia	+	+	+	+
Apraxia: ideomotor	+	o	+	o
Ideatory	o	o	o	o
Visual Field Defect	o	o	o	o

Figure 2-5, Associated Deficits (Contd.)

Patient		BRE	FIG	PRA	CUS
Naming		100%	80%	20%	90%
Repetition	(errors)	100%	100%	20%	44%
Oral comprehension		52%	28%	44%	76%

illustrated by the reading comprehension profiles of some patients with deep dyslexia (taken from Patterson, 1981) and with surface dyslexia (taken from Kremin, 1983, in press) which are represented in Table 1. But the reverse pattern, relatively spared oral reading without comprehension, can also be found, although these occassions seem to be rare. (See Figures 4 and 5).

TABLE 1. Oral reading versus comprehension of written words.

	Reading	Comprehension	
	(error percentage)		
Deep Dyslexics			
B. B.	55	18.5	(word-picture matching)
D. E.	60	28	(word-picture matching)
P. W.	60	15	(word-picture matching)
LEC.	31	6	(word association)
Surface Dyslexics:			
FRA.	51	7	(word association)
HAM.	20	0	(word association)

Heilman, Tucker and Valenstein (1976) also mention a patient (with mixed transcortical aphasia) who "was able to read aloud but showed no comprehension of what he read" (p.423). Moreover, Schwartz, Marin and Saffran (1979) presented a case (of progressive dementia) in which the subject retained the ability to read words aloud in spite of a severe loss of semantic knowledge and the inability to access phonology for the purpose of naming or making reference. This patient could read words correctly, even words with similar spellings but dissimilar pronunciations (e.g. home /come; cost / post;

floor / flood), at a time where the patient's lexical loss is characterized by a severe loss of semantic features. (The picture of a
cat, for example, is associated with the word dog; the picture spoon
with fork, brush with comb, etc.).

In this respect (production better than recognition) a recently
described patient with surface dyslexia should also be mentioned (Deloche, Andreewsky and Desi, 1982) : A. D. incorrectly matched written
words to pictures and in a lexical decision task he committed 36%
errors on words and 12% errors on non-sense syllables. These performances in recognition contrast with his oral production : in fact,
reanalysis of the data shows that A. D. produced only 13% errors on
words and 7,6% errors on nonsense syllables while reading aloud (percentages are taken from last responses to the targets, that is autocorrections are included).

It should be underlined, however, that the mentioned dissociations of recognition and reading are characteristic only for patients
with aphasic disturbances. In cases of "pure" (verbal) alexia (without agraphia) there is generally a parallelism between recognition/
comprehension and oral reading.

Kremin (1981) furnished normative data for such a patient. Patient A was perfect in the visual matching of graphic stimuli, but
reading and comprehension of isolated words was equally impaired in
all tasks :
          - oral reading of words 50%
          - oral reading of nonsense syllables 48%
          - recognition of words (lexical decisions) 50%
          - comprehension of written words (multiple choice of
            written words) 50%
          - comprehension of written words (multiple choice of
            pictures) 50%

Only four exceptions to this general pattern have been reported
so far (Caplan and Hedley-White, 1974; Stachowiak and Poeck, 1976;
Warrington and Shallice, 1979; Landis, Regard and Serrat, 1980).

Caplan and Hedley-White (1974) presented a patient with pure
alexia - spontaneous language, writing, spelling, and repitition were intact - who showed problems in (visually) naming colors (74% errors) and objects (50% errors). The patient suffered from a global
reading impairment compromising letters and words. But when the recognition of graphic material was tested, the authors stated a dissociation between impaired reading and some spared comprehension.
Indeed, the patient was able to recognise the "gestalt" of words
which were embedded in parasite letters (e.g. Xedog) and he was able
to correct orthographic misspellings. Moreover, the patient was often able to indicate the category (colors, flowers, persons) of stimulus items. For example, when shown a list of words (red, hot,

brown, warm, pink, yellow) the patient could not read any of them
aloud. But when asked whether there were any colors, she responded
to the color words exclusively : pink -> tan, brown -> tan, yellow
-> brown. Furthermore, the patient correctly designated 2/3 of the
words spoken by the examinator (in a written multiple choice situation). Post mortem examination revealed a combined lesion of the
left occipital lobe (with involvement of the hippocampal region) and
the splenium. This case thus confirms and illustrates the reading
behavior of patients whose lesions correspond to Geschwind's disconnection syndrome.

Stachowiak and Poeck (1976) discussed their patient within the
same theoretical framework. Again, the patient showed a certain anomia for colors and objects. (It should be stressed, however, that
his spontaneous language revealed some semantic paraphasias). Oral
reading of letters induced 30% errors, oral reading of words was totally impossible. When the authors tried "deblocking" it turned out
that the patient recognised 3/4 of the written words when given a
tactile cue (touching of objects) or an acoustic cue (designation of
written words spelled out by the examinator). Visual cues (matching
of words with pictures) was less effective but still resulted in 42%
correct recognitions of the written words.

Landis, Regard and Serrat (1980) studied a case of pure verbal
alexia (with normal speech, spelling and naming of objects and colors). The patient correctly named isolated letters but he attempted
to read words by spelling aloud, correcting himself until the word
made sense. He read short words better than long ones, but when presented with nonsense syllables, he frequently gave up. After removal of a tumor (situated predominantly subcortically in the left occipital lobe but extending around the occipital horn to the trigone
and infiltrating medially to the splenium) the clinical picture remained unchanged. (It should be noted that in the early postoperati-
ve period tactile letter recognition was preserved with the left hand
but impaired with the right hand. One month after the surgical intervention the impairment of the right tactile letter recognition had
disappeared). Landis, Regard and Serrat tested the patient for tachistoscopic recognition of colors, objects, letters, and words one
week after the surgical intervention. At this time the patient showed the following "naming" performances with stimuli presented into
his left visual field : at an exposure of 50 msec he could read all
letters, at 200 msec he named all drawings of objects and all colors
correctly. However only at an exposure time of 1000 msec he correctly read one of ten words. The authors then presented, at an exposure
of only 30 msec, written names of familiar objects. (Objects, including those corresponding to the target words were placed in front of
the patient). Landis, Regard and Serrat observed that the patient
"instantly read the first eight names at this very short exposure,
but could not read aloud the remaining seven names and denied even

recognizing a single letter. He said : I do not see anything, it's just a flash of light; he was asked to point "intuitively" to the objects whose name he had not been able to see or read aloud. In five out of the remaining seven instances he pointed to the correct object, to his own astonishment" (p. 49).

When the same experiment was repeated 24 days later, the patient's tachistoscopic reading was improved: he named all letters at 10 msec; at 20 msec he correctly named 9/10 drawings and all colors; at the 20 msec exposure he read 4 out of 10 words aloud, and named some individual letters in the remaining words. "When asked to point to objects whose written names were exposed at 20 msec, he read only 2 out of 8 aloud and pointed incorrectly (based upon single recognized letters) in 5 instances" out of six (p. 49). Landis, Regard and Serrat think that only (!) in experiment I the patient performed a pure visual word-object association without knowledge of the associated spoken name. "We conjecture that in the case of our patient the written object names were not mediated through language areas, as suggested by the fact that he denied having seen more than a flash of light. It is likely that within the unimpaired right hemisphere the written name was associated with the object image and that this iconic reading strategy enabled him to point correctly to the correspondent object" (p. 51). The authors conclude that "two types of strategies exist for reading concrete nouns: visual-verbal reading, where a written word is associated with a spoken name, and iconic reading where a written word is associated with its image. The use of iconic reading appears impossible when visuo-verbal reading is available. Furthermore, it even appears compromised when visuo-verbal reading is sufficient to allow for letter reading. Only with the total absence of visuo-verbal reading ability or with complete disconnection does iconic reading seem to be available" (p. 52).

Warrignton and Shallice (1979) finally presented a case study of a patient who had preserved a certain capacity for categorizing words he was not able to read. Patient A. R. who presented this syndrome of "semantic access" dyslexia was classified by the authors as "dyslexia without dysgraphia". Some reserves may be made with regard to this classification since A. R. wrote only 66/100 words correctly to dictation (his oral spelling being somewhat better with 32/40 correct). Moreover, the data concerning his reading performance were collected during four years in which time "dysgraphia and dyslexia neither improved nor worsened" (p. 45). "His spoken speech was somewhat halting but for the most part accurate with regard to word choice and syntax" (p. 45). The most prominent feature was a marked anomia for objects and colors (optic aphasia).

A. R. had problems not only in reading isolated letters aloud, but, also, in their discrimination and categorization. Oral reading of isolated words varied between 22% and 49% correct for different lists. He succeeded in reading approximately 25% of (three letter)

nonsense syllables. (But the correct responses depended on sounding
out correctly all three letters of the nonsense syllable). Error
analysis of word reading permitted the classification of the patient
with regard to criteria for deep dyslexia : reading errors were mainly visual (57%) but A. R. produced 5% real semantic errors (e.g. month -> week). In lexical decisions and judgements about the visual
identity of words (e.g. along/ alone) A. R.'s performance was just
above chance. Clinical observation of A. R.'s failure to recognize
words and meanings suggested, however, that the patient was able to
derive partial meaning from written words: for example, for cereal
he said "it is something to eat"; for beaver he commented "could be
an animal, I have no idea which one"; confronted with drum, A. R.
carried out the appropriate miming and commented "I seem to imagine
I ought to be doing this but I don't know what it is". Then he said
"drum". Warrington and Shallice therefore formally tested the patient's ability to categorize words (which were presented tachistoscopically). A. R.'s categorization scores were significantly above
chance for concrete words and for non-concrete words. (Tested categories were surnames/forenames, boys/girls, authors/politicians, su-
bjects/measurements). For illustration we cite an example of performance with concrete words: at an exposure duration of 100 msec A. R.
read 5/20 words correctly and he was able to categorize 8/15 of the
not read words into one of the five given categories. It should be noted that A. R.'s performances did not depend - in contrast to Landis
et al.'s case (1980) - on exposure time: with unlimited presentation
time he scored 8/40 for correct reading and 22/32 for correct categorization. In contrast with the case presented by Landis et al.
(1980), A. R.'s reading of words improved much more with a spoken
prompt than with a visual prompt (20 vs 7 trials correct respectively). Although we do not agree with Warrington and Shallice's interpretation that the semantic priming effect provides evidence for
the relative independence of "semantic systems subserving object recognition and word comprehension" (p. 59), we think that the existence of a selective written word comprehension deficit is indeed evidence for an access specific to the written word to the semantic
system.

A related case has been described by Albert, Yamadori, Gardner and Howes (1973). The patient was aphasic with fluent speech
(with verbal paraphasia), agraphic and showed a certain degree on
anomia (likewise contaminated by verbal paraphasia). The patient
was unable to read letters, words or sentences aloud, or to carry
out written commands. He was, however, able to distinguish quite
easily between letters (correct identification of individual letters
presented verbally in a set of letters or as part of a word) and the
written forms of words (correct identification of words presented
in multiple choice). Furthermore, he was able to select a written
word on the basis of its relevant semantic category. Striking in
this case is, again, the dissociation of recognition/comprehension
and reading aloud. For example, when shown the picture of a lion

and required to chose the correct written word among cat, lion, bear, the patient succeeded. But when required to read aloud the same item, the patient produced : "black, No. Horse, I imagine. Yeah black". His reading errors included both comments and semantic paralexias, e.g. ant -> it's a small animal, jacket -> coat.

But, at least, with the last case we are definitely back to the first group of patients, these "non pure alexics" for whom a dissociation between oral reading and written comprehension is standard.

Most often, indeed, the recognition performances of aphasic subjects are superior to their oral productions. This holds not only for reading but for other tasks as well. Kremin and Koskas (1982), studying 50 subjects with lesions of the temporal lobe of the dominant hemipshere, found that, on average, patients committed 41% errors in oral naming as opposed to 7,5% recognition errors when the same targets had to be identified in a (written) multiple choice paradigm. Friederici, Schoenle and Goodglass (1981) studied the distribution of naming errors (oral and written) and recognition errors with regard to the two main aphasic groups, Broca's and Wernicke's.

They found that the difference between production (oral and written naming) and residual underlying knowledge (recognition) was highly significant for the Broca's aphasics but not significant for Wernicke's aphasics. In this connection one might also mention an investigation by Whitehouse, Caramazza and Zurif (1978). These authors studied the effects of forms and function of objects on name recognition. Subjects were shown line drawing of various food containers with varied perceptual dimensions such as height and width. The subjects were required to select a name for the object from a multiple choice list (cup, bowl, or glass). (Prototypical as well as nonprototypical objects were shown). The results show that Broca's aphasics exhibit relatively normal naming profiles; specifically, these patients seem to name the prototypes consistently. The anomic patients, in contrast, were unable to integrate perceptual and functional information with name recognition. The authors concluded that the posterior patients may suffer from an impairment in the underlying conceptual organization of the lexicon rather than from difficulties of word retrieval.

The common clinical picture of recognition being superior to production is accounted for by production models where word retrieval may be interfered with at different stages. In the most common view, step one entails recognition of the stimulus and arousal of its semantic representation. This stage is followed by retrieval of the phonological representation of the intended word and then by the realization of the phonological form into a motor articulary sequence. Thus the following error types can occur in different tasks (R = Reading, N = Naming, RPT = Repetition) requiring the production of an (isolated) word (examples are taken from the cited

literature) :
1)   Omission
2)   Circumlocution
     R : beaver -> could be an animal, I have no idea which one
     N : accordeon -> c'est un instrument de musique
     RPT : pheasant -> some kind of large bird

3)   Semantic association
     R : bush -> tree
     N : chair -> stool
     RPT : chausson -> pantoufle

4)   Semantic and phonological or visual association
     R   : paper -> page; flocon -> glaçon
     N   : broom -> brush
     RPT : auto -> moto

5)   Phonological and/or visual association
     R   : tired -> timed
     N   : wistle -> wisper
     RPT : front -> tronc

6)   Totally neologistic
     R   : hippopotamus -> apelafon
     N   : trellis -> tokel
     RPT : pipe -> nesava

     There seems to be no systematic investigation of the quantita-
tive distribution of error types with reference to the aphasic syndromes. Goodglass (1980), however, pointed to characteristic naming
errors with regard to the type of aphasia. Thus the stimulus picture of a chair may be misnamed by a patient with Broca's aphasia as
"tssair" (delayed access, articulatory disturbance), by a patient
with Wernicke's aphasia as "stool" (semantic paraphasia) or "chossl"
(neologistic jargon preserving minimal phonological similarity), by
an anomic patient as "I know what it is ......I have a lot of them"
(empty circumlocution), and by a patient with conduction aphasia as
"flair....no, swair.....tair...." (literal paraphasia, with repeated
attempts to reach the correct word).

     Furthermore, Cappa, Cavalotti and Vignolo (1981), examining 116
fluent aphasics, found - but only for some of these patients - a double dissociation. In fact, 10 patients showed an almost pure phonemic defect (that is phonemic paraphasias, "conduites d'approche",
neologisms, and phonemic jargon) and 11 patients represented an almost pure lexical defect (anomia, circumlocutions, verbal paraphasias, verbal jargon). Comparison of CT scan findings showed that phonemic disorders were associated with lesions nearer to the Sylvian fissure (comprising the inferior parietal lobule and the posterior part
of the superior temporal gyrus), whereas lexical disorders were

associated with lesions posterior to those of the phonemic group farther from the sylvian fissure (involving the temporo-parieto-occipi-
tal junction; encroaching on the superior temporal gyrus).   It should be noted that the experimental groups did not show any significant difference with regard to auditory comprehension on the Token
Test.

The relative distribution of phonological, semantic, and visual
errors in reading was checked by Gardner and Zurif (1975).   They analysed the occurence of these error types (in terms of identification errors on a multiple choice paradigm of written words) with reference to four different aphasic groups, Wernicke, global, anterior
and alexic (with agraphia).

Finally, Marshall and Newcombe (1973) distinguished three different types of reading disorders with respect to the relative occurence of different types of paralexias: visual dyslexia with mainly
visual errors, deep dyslexia with semantic paralexias and surface
dyslexia with phonological errors.   (We will come back to this later).

Several techniques have been applied to precisely determine
the extent of partial knowledge that aphasics may preserve when they
fail to produce a target word.   Goodglass, Kaplan, Weintraub and Ackerman (1976) studied the "tip-of-the-tongue" phenomenon in object
naming.   If a patient failed to respond (or responded inappropriate-
ly) to a given stimulus the patient was asked:

1) whether he had an idea if the correct word and knew what it
sounded like,
2) for syllable length of the target, and
3) for first-letter identification.
The results of this experiment are reproduced in Table 2.

TABLE 2:   Partial knowledge of words which are not named on picture
           presentation

% correct	Broca	Wernicke	Conduction	Anomic
"idea of word--Yes"	52.8	53.5	66.3	26.3
Number of syllables	20.1	13.8	34.3	9.8
Initial letter	20.6	13.8	34.1	5.5
(Naming failures:	16.71	23.50	20.85	16.00)

The main findings are that conduction aphasics identified both
first-letter and syllable length in 1/3 of the words which they could not name.   This pattern contrasts with the poor performances of
Wernicke and anomic aphasics.   (Broca aphasics could not be diffe-

rentiated from either the conduction group or the Wernicke/anomic
group). Goodglass et al. conclude that word finding is an "all or
none process for Wernicke and anomic patients in the sense that they
either recover a name well enough to produce it or they can give little evidence of partial knowledge. Words which are failed then seem
to be totally unavailable, as far as recall processes are concerned"
(p. 152). "In the case of the conduction aphasics the evidence of
tacit partial knowledge of many words may indicate a breakdown at a
later stage in the naming process" (p. 152). Goodglass et al.'s study thus demonstrates that patients who quantitatively may not be
distinguished by an oral naming task nevertheless are differentiated
in their tacit knoweldge of the target words they cannot produce.
Goodglass (1980) interpreted the foregoing findings in the following
way: "there are two major paths to the emission of a word - one proceeding automatically from stimulus to oral response and based in a
one-to-one associative link between concept and output; the other
occurring when immediate association fails, involving a search process
and the mobilization of peripheral semantic and phonological associations" (p.653).

In the frame of a stage model approach Kremin (1981c) proposed
a method to discriminate semantic achievement from phonological failure in oral production with reference to naming. It has been pointed
out before that patients might achieve the concept of an item without
being able to access the phonological code of its name. In Kremin's
view the testing of gender assignment allows for the dissociation of
these two stages during the treatment of the stimulus word. In French, of course, every noun has a gender, masculine or feminine. In
fact, gender is sometimes the only key to the semantic representation
of spoken words. The phonological form of [$m\varepsilon r$], for example, corresponds to two different lexical entries, maire and mère, which
are auditorilly disambiguated only by different gender assignment:
la /mεr/ (the mother vs le /mεr/ (the mayor). Kremin, testing oral
naming plus gender assignment, found that even in patients who proved
incapable of evoking object names or gave altered and/or totally neologistic responses, the breakdown of word retrieval may occur only
after the arousal of its semantic representation. This seems to be
demonstrated by the patients' superior performances of oral production of gender (12, 18, 19 out of 20 items) in comparison with impaired production of the phonological form of the corresponding lexical
item (0, 4, 8 out of 20 itmes). We produce some of the patients'
oral productions for illustration:

    SPIRALE (spiral) :   UNE (feminine)

  ->mais c'est une ... ah ça ! c'est ... une ... /bou/...
    avec un R non plus ... il y a les escaliers qui sont comme
    ça mais je me rappelle plus ... c'est une ... non (which
    letter in the beginning? which sound?) je ne suis pas
    sûre... une... une (sp-) spirale.

ACCORDEON   (accordeon) : UN (masculine)

-> ça c'est un ... un ... un instrument de musique ... c'est
un ... un ... c'est un ... un... c'est un ... un ... il ne
marche plus ... un ... ah! ... un ... un ... c'est pas
le ... un ... un... (you know the first letter?) peut être ... /prese/ ... président (patient laughs) ... un...
peut être un F ... non! A! un A! un /mar/ ... /morică/
ça va pas... un... un abour... un /maksiño/ ... un amour
ah je sais! ... un... ça finit par O. N... /ame/ (it begins
with A and ends with ON?) oui... un million non pas un
million... un... un /amaksimom? non c'est pas ça... un
a... /aks/ ... non... (accordéon) oui un accordéon.

Gender assignment might also be a crucial variable to "locate"
a pathway (lexical vs non-lexical) in oral reading. Kremin (in press) recently pointed out that HAM, a patient who mainly produced phonological errors in oral reading of isolated words - thus being a
good candidate for using the non-lexical pathway which is assumed to
operate in surface dyslexia - often reproduced a written word (noun)
spontaneously with the corresponding article, definite or generic.
We skip the author's discussion of existing models concerning processes of reading and only report one of the pateint's oral misreadings
with simultaneous gender assignment: rhum [ram] (rum) -> du rhume
[rym] (a cold). This latter reading error is extremely interesting
because of its linguistic characterstics. In fact, both French words,
rhum (rum) as well rhume (cold), have masculine gender assignment.
But the French language permits the generic article only in the case
of rhum (rum) in expressions such as "du rhum? c'est bien!" (Rum?
That's great!), the construction "du rhume? c'est mauvais!" being
impermissible. The adequate construction in French would be "un
rhume? c'est mauvais!" (A cold? That's bad). As HAM never showed
any difficulties with grammar in any of the numerous tasks which are
part of our "Standard Examination" we propose the following explanation for this reading error : HAM correctly accessed the input logogen for rhum (rum) and treated the stimulus in her semantic system
where the adequate generic article to the target was generated (in
analogy to "du lait" (milk) or "de la bière" (beer) for example, and,
of course, in analogy to HAM's own production on onyx -> de l'onyx.
The actual reading error du rhume /rym/ might then have occurred for
the following reason: the adequate post-lexical phonological form
(output logogen) is not forthcoming; in order to spell out the word
- which has already been treated and understood - the patient utilizes the strategy of grapheme-to-phoneme conversion which is at her
disposal (as documented by her ability to read nonsense syllables).
In many cases this strategy is not reliable for the production of
real words from the phonological lexicon. Indeed, HAM almost exclusively produced non existant forms. There are but three exceptions
to this general pattern: two visual errors [anguille (eel) -> aigui-
lle (needle) and quotient -> continent and rhum (rum) -> rhume [cold].

We think that in the latter case grapheme-to-phoneme reading (combined with a partial failure in the application of grapheme-to-phoneme correspondence typical for HAM) results - somehow by chance - in the production of another word which actually exists in the phonological lexicon. This expalnation for HAM's reading error rhum -> du rhume [rym] seems to be reinforced by the fact that she read rhume [rym] (cold) -> un rhume [rym] (a cold), thus correctly "naming" the stimulus by assignment of the adequate indefinite article.

Unfortunately we did not ask the patient for her reading comprehension of these particular items. But there are other instances where we did so and which clearly show that the target word was immediately correctly understood in spite of an erroneous oral reading: toast [tost] (toast) -> /to-a/   /twal/ non....../twal/ qu'est ce que ça veut dire...... un /toast/ (what does it mean ?) on le mange .... un/toks/ non...... pas un /toks/ un/ taks/ non plus....... /toask/ ca se prononce pas comme ca......../to/....un/to-ast/.

As we mentioned before, on rare occasions the reverse pattern has been described: a patient might be able to correctly produce the name of an object or a written word but without "understanding" the reference. Heilman, Tucker and Valenstein (1976) mention such a case. Their patient (with mixed transcortical aphasia) correctly named 23 out of 25 different objects. But he correctly pointed to only 4 of the objects on auditory instruction. Since his repetition was excellent, the patient's failure in object designation cannot be accounted for by a failure to receive the auditory input. In fact, the patient's object designation stayed at the same low level when non-verbal instructions were given. Moreover, although the patient was capable of visually categorizing objects (37/78 trials correct in a multiple choice task) his performance stayed far below the normal range (69 out of 78 correct). - Finally, we saw a patient whose reading comprehension of isolated words, although less disturbed, seems to document a similar comprehension deficit. Patient PIG was able to read words and pseudowords (homophones of words, e.g. train (train vs trin) flawlessly. When his reading comprehension of the same items was tested in a multiple choice of four pictures the patient identified 80% of the real words and 70% of the pseudowords. Having, for example, correctly read aloud the word gant (glove) the patient hesitated a long time looking at the four pictures of the multiple choice (glove, shoe, mill, screw) - pictures he would correctly name! - and commented : "je devrais trouver ! qu'est-ce qu'ils veulent dire ces 4 lettres...." He finally points to glove and shoe and cannot make up his mind to decide which one corresponds to the written target.

WORD PRODUCTION : PARALLELS AND DIFFERENCES

It is evident from the possible dissociations found in pathology that there is no necessary parallelism in production performances

concerning speech, the reading of isolated words, their repetition,
and the naming of objects. It should be pointed out, however, that
- at least in group studies - such parallelism has often been remar-
ked. Indeed, Cappa, Cavalotti and Vignolo (1981) found an association between phonemic errors in naming and disruption of repetition,
and between lexical errors in naming and relatively preserved repetition.

Another group study of naming disturbances (Kremin and Koskas,
1982) suggested that the performances may be linked qualitatively as
well as quantitatively. In fact, Kremin and Koskas' comparison of
patient's naming performance and spontaneous speech showed significant correlations between the production of neologisms and of verbal
substitutions in both experimental tasks. The production of neologisms and substitutions thus seems to represent a general breakdown
of language, but at different stages. Yet another cross-modal study
has been carried out by Marshall and Newcombe (1977). Their analysis
of the (quantitative) performances of four patients in successive tests of object naming and word reading shows an impressive resemblance
in the shape of the patients' recovery curves in both tasks (see figure 6.1. p. 280-282, Marshall and Newcombe, 1977).

Another source of evidence that a deficit need not be modality-
specific comes from many cases with so-called deep dyslexia. One of
the constituent features of this syndrome is the production of semantic paralexias in the oral reading of isolated words (Marshall and
Newcombe, 1973; Schwartz, Saffran and Marin, 1977; Coltheart, 1980).
Kremin (1982), reviewing 20 patients who produced semantic paralexias
in reading, found that in the vast majority of these cases semantic
errors have also been observed in tasks other than reading. In fact,
Marshall and Newcombe (1977) explicitly mention that the presence of
"semantic errors or circumlocutions is consistent with the type of
word finding difficulties that are apparent in B. R.'s spontaneous
speech" (p.273); Marshall, Newcombe and Marshall (1970) mention the
parallelism between G. R.'s performances in reading and naming; Saffran et al. (1976) point out that their patients V. and H. "made
similar semantic substitutions in naming and writing to dictation"
(p. 257); etc. The recent study of yet another case (Nolan and Caramazza, 1982) revealed striking similarities in performance across
several modalities: indeed, B. L. produced semantic errors not only
in reading but also in object naming, and in the repetition and writing of isolated words. Finally, three recently-studied cases with
surface dyslexia are reported to suffer from a similar disturbance
(surface agraphia) in writing (Deloche, Andreewsky and Desi, 1982;
Kremin, 1980; in press).

Although the just-mentioned parallelism of patient's performance across various modalities is impressive, it should be stressed
that there are as many examples which contradict a unitary interpretation of aphasic disturbances. Indeed, LEC's spontaneous language,

recorded in different sessions, appeared normal in spite of semantic
errors in reading and repetition (Kremin, 1980). V. S. produced semantic errors in reading, naming, and writing, but not in the repetition of isolated words (Nolan and Caramazza, in press). (Indeed,
the syndrome of deep dyslexia was initially defined as such because
the patients could correctly repeat the words they were unable to
read). FRA produced many semantic errors in the repetition of words
(Goldblum, 1979 - patient B. F.). But none in oral reading in spite
of a selective reading impairment, i.e. surface dyslexia (Kremin,
1980). Two other patients, RIC (Kremin, 1981b) and HAM (Kremin, in
press) produced semantic errors in oral naming but not in the reading
of isolated words. Even more dissociations are to be found when writing and spelling are also considered. Thus R. G. could not read
nonsense syllables aloud (Beauvois and Dérouesné, 1979) but successfully wrote them to dictation (Beauvois and Dérouesné, 1981). HAM,
a patient with surface dysgraphia (that is spared phonological writing by phoneme-to-grapheme correspondence), demonstrated intact knowledge with regard to orthography when this variable was tested in a
recognition task (Kremin, in press). The well-known fact that patients with so-called pure (verbal) alexia are able to write (spontaneously and from dictation) words they cannot read should also be
mentioned in this context.

Although most patients with alexia and agraphia are incapable
of correctly spelling out loud, some cases with alexia and agraphia
have been reported who could spell out loud and comprehend orally
spelled words (Albert, Yamadori, Gardner and Hower, 1973; Rothi and
Heilman, 1981). Moreover, some patients show relatively preserved
oral reading and spelling but impaired written spelling (Hier, Mogil,
Rubin and Komros, 1980).

A patient, finally, may show a major deficit in oral language
(jargon in spontaneous language, impaired repetition and oral naming)
but written language (spontaneous writing, written naming, reading
aloud) may be preserved (Michel, 1979). A similar but not identical
case with impaired oral naming but preserved written naming was presented by Hier and Mohr (1977).

But parallels and differences in word production are not only
found in cross-modal or task comparisons. Dissociations also occur
within the same modality or task. Then they are to be accounted for
by the different linguistic properties of the stimuli. Patients may
read words but not isolated letters, they may read no graphematic
material at all but still read numbers and signs; or their reading
disturbance can selectively impair the reading of sentences (Hecaen
and Kremin, 1976); patients may read almost all words of the language
but are incapable of reading nonsense words (Patterson, 1982). The
same dissociation may be found in repetition (Beauvois, Dérouesné
and Bastard, 1980) and writing (Shallice, 1981). The part-of-speech
dimension (with nouns better than function words) can also be a

crucial variable for word production not only in reading (as in deep
dyslexia) but also in writing (Shallice, 1981; Nolan and Caramazza,
in press) and in repetition (Michel, 1979). The reverse pattern -
superior production of function words over nouns - has also been reported for oral reading (Kremin, 1980; Deloche, et al., 1982). Finally, the abstract/concrete dimension often plays a crucial role in
reading aloud (Coltheart, et al., 1980), writing (Nolan and Caramazza, in press) and in repetition (Michel, 1979). Usually concrete
words are more successfully produced than abstract words. It should
be underlined, however, that this pattern does not just reflect a general effect of abstract words being more "difficult" to produce,
since the reverse pattern - concrete words being more impaired - has
also been reported (for oral reading - see Warrington, 1981).

Now, how can these various dissociations possibly be accounted
for ? In fact, simultaneously with their taxonomy of reading errors
and the definition of three specific reading disorders, Marshall and
Newcombe (1973) proposed a theoretical model for reading. This model
allowed for word production via grapheme-to-phoneme correspondence
rules, if, as a consequnece of brain damage, the semantic pathway is
unavailable. Experimental research finally established that some patients suffer from an impairment of phonological reading (as shown
by their inability to read nonsense syllables - Shallice and Warrington, 1975). Thus it was possible to postulate the existence of a
(non-phonological) lexical route from print to meaning. Subsequently
most authors distinguished two routes by which a phonological output
might be obtained given a graphic visual input. Morton, too, tried
to integrate data from pathology into his logogen model of isolated
word recognition and production (Morton and Patterson, 1980). But
the relevance of this approach comes from outside neuropsychology,
as it is basically derived from experimental studies of normal subjects (Morton, 1979). The revised version of the logogen model has
been applied to account for symptoms found in particular forms of
acquired dyslexia (Morton and Patterson, 1980). Furthermore, the
model has been extended to account for other than reading performances, that is for repetition (Morton, 1980a) and writing (Morton,
1980b). The latter versions of the logogen model are based on the
assumption that there are three routes by which a phonological output can be obtained from visual or auditory input (see figure 6) :

1) after categorization of the stimulus in the input logogens
(visual or auditory), information flows directly to the output logogen system where the appropriate phonological code is produced:

2) the word is categorized in the input logogen systems (visual
or auditory) and information is sent to the cognitive system. Here
the semantics can be found and sent to the output logogen system where the appropriate phonological code could be obtained;

3) a) the visual stimulus is treated as sequence of graphemes

FIGURE 6. A simplified version of Morton's logogen model dealing
with the treatment of visual and auditory stimuli (according to Morton, 1980a, p. 190).

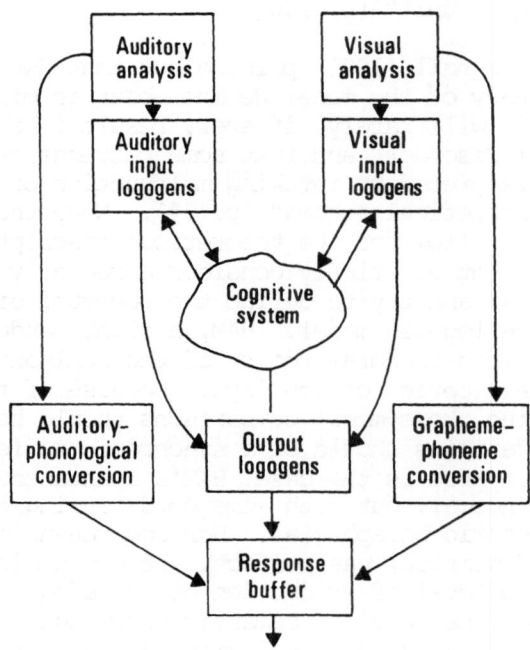

and converted by rule into a phonological code;
     b) the auditory stimulus is converted into a phonological code
by acoustic phonemic conversion.

     It should be noted that only pathway (1) is, in principle, error
free. It should furthermore be stressed that the logogen system

itself contains no semantic information (but only the notion of "word"
in terms of morphemes). Pathway (3) in contrast, has no concept of
"wordness", words and non-words being treated alike. It should furthermore be underlined that the same output logogens are operative
for different tasks (for example reading, repetition, naming, and
spontaneous output). With regard to the cognitive system Morton
(1980b) writes: "It contains everything which is not explicitly included else where....The only feature I will mention here is that in
contrast with most lexicons I do not see at all the information relevant to a particular word as located in the same "place" and accessed
simultaneously./ "Meaning" is something to be computed as necessary,
and not looked up as a unit" (p. 120).

    Newcombe and Marshall (1981) pointed out that "when assessing
the empirical adequacy of the model we must bear in mind that natural
lesions of the brain will rarely, if ever, result in absolutely "pure"
forms of behavioral disorder, and that some patterns of impairment
will have to be interpreted by invoking malfunction of more than one
component of the theoretical schema" (p. 34). Nevertheless, the logogen model seems to allow for the theoretical description of many
clinical symptoms. Let us briefly consider a recently described case (Kremin, in press) and try to define the reported disturbances in
the framework of the logogen model. HAM, a right-handed patient with
a lesion in the parieto-temporal region of the dominant hemisphere,
was examined within a period of ten days. Because of this relatively
short time of testing cross-modal comparisons should be possible,
because different deficits should be a synchronic reflection of underlying disturbances. Here is the case: HAM's spontaneous language
was fluent, almost normal, but with some word-finding difficulties
and (initially) phonemic paraphasias. Her comprehension of words and
sentences, oral and written, was perfect. Object naming was severely
impaired, but at the level of production of the adequate phonological
form, rather than at the level of semantic knowledge. (This is shown
by the patient's adequate gender assignment to the target words which
were omitted, or, when produced, semantically only in the sphere and/
or with phonemic errors). Repetition of isolated words and of nonsense syllables was preserved, but in sentence repetition HAM produced semantic and phonemic paraphasias. Furthermore, HAM could read
nonsense syllables correctly; but isolated words, although understood, were often reproduced as neoforms, the phonological errors being
due to her reading from left-to-right by graphemes-to-phoneme conversion. The reading of sentences was characterized by an important
number of whole word substitutions, some of them having a visual/se-
mantic relation to the target word. In sentence reading numerous
phonemic entanglements of the conduction type were also found. Kremin (in press) suggests that the patient's oral production (of words
and of strings of words) can be explained by just one underlying disturbance in spite of the various quantitative and qualitative differences in verbal production. The author, claims that HAM has a disturbance at the level of the output logogens. In this case, according

to the logogen model, the disturbance should be general and not modality specific.   Indeed, in all tasks where (supposedly) the cognitive
systems was engaged and/or where a phonological output is required
(spontaneous language, naming, repetition of sentences, reading aloud
of sentences) HAM's oral production of words was similar; phonemic
errors and semantically related responses characterize the patient's
output.   This pattern, however, does not hold for the repetition and
for the reading words in isolation.   Kremin suggests that in these
two tasks the patient, aware of his general output problems, adopts
compensatory strategies for word production : accoustic-phonemic conversion for auditorily presented words and grapheme-to-phoneme conversion for visually presented isolated words.   (That these two conversion sets are available is documented by the patient's ability to
read and to repeat nonsense syllables).   Words, regular and irregular,
ought to be successfully reproduced by acoustic-phonemic conversions.
The use of grapheme-to-phoneme conversion, however, does not guarantee the correct pronunciations of many words and results in the typical error pattern of surface dyslexia.   This is indeed the case for
HAM.

FIGURE 7.   Morton's version of the logogen model with extension to
            graphical output (from Morton, 1980b, Fig. 4, p. 123).

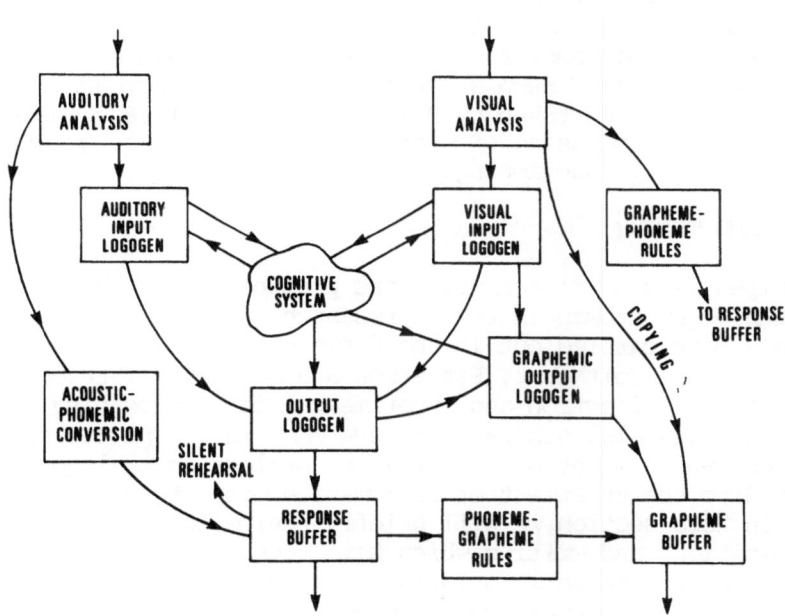

Figure 7 reproduces a version of the logogen model with extension to writing (from Morton, 1980b). Morton describes the following possibilities with respect to spelling and writing:

1) the visual input logogen "does not contain any accessible information with regard to spelling. It is responsible for recognizing that certain letter strings correspond to words and for passing information concerning the identity of these letter strings to the cognitive system and the output buffers" (p. 132);

2) the grapheme output logogen system "contains spelling patterns for words (or possibly morphemes). It is addressed by the cognitive system by means of a semantic code (by analogy with the output logogen system) and by the visual input logogen system by means of some simple one-to-one mapping procedures. Its output goes to the grapheme buffer" (p. 132);

3) the system of phoneme-to-grapheme rules treats words and non-words alike.

Morton's logogen model thus seems to be the most extensive version among theoretical approaches which deal with the processing of information. It indeed spurred researchers to study and define new syndromes by postulating the loss or malfunctioning of transmission pathways. Of course, we should bear in mind that the logogen model "locates" stages with regard to the treatment of information; it does not localize areas and/or connections in the brain correlated with pathological deficits. Such a neuropsychological approach, however, has recently been undertaken by Heilman and Rothi (1982) who propose a schema for the processing of written and spoken language with reference to cerebral functioning.

SYNDROMES AND THEORY

Acquired reading disturbances are probably among the most extensively studied syndromes in recent research. These investigations have mainly been carried out in the frame of an information processing approach (see Coltheart, Patterson and Marshall, 1980). Moreover, theoretical reflection and experimental data concerning reading behavior have revealed separable subsystems in the processing of informations which might operate in more-or-less an analogous fashion with regard to the treatment of information other than graphic and/or visual. In this section we will briefly review the syndromes in reading, repetition, and writing which have recently been described in the framework of such an information processing approach. We will also discuss some discrepancies between theoretical postulation and empirical experimental findings.

READING

Since visual word recognition and production has been given so much attention lately we will refer only to some points of the topic which remain open to discussion. [(The reader interested in more detail about acquired reading disorders should refer to the exhaustive reviews which exist in this field: Benson and Geschwind (1969), Hecaen and Kremin (1976), Albert (1979), Patterson (1981), Heilman and Rothi (1982), Kremin (1982)].

Research on reading disorders has become more and more a matter of theoretical concern. In spite of different approaches and interpretations two different models have been proposed to account for the processes implicated in the reading of isolated words: a two-route model (favored by numerous authors) and a three-way account (Morton's logogen model). Both theories assume that there is a visuo-semantic pathway of word production (bypassing pre-lexical phonology where phonology is retrieved post-lexically as a whole), and a non-lexical pathway in which words are processed by means of grapheme-to-phoneme conversion without prior semantic comprehension. Morton's logogen model is specific in that it proposes yet another way of reading aloud a written word, that is by means of a word recognizer (input logogen - - which contains no semantic information at all, merely translating a graphemic code into a phonological one (output logogens) by direct print-to-sound associations. Morton's model thus specifies separate systems for word recognition and for semantic processing. The lexical access theory is generally accepted since it has received support from experiments with both normal and pathological subjects. Indeed, studies of patients with so-called deep dyslexia and with phonological dyslexia showed that lexical reading is possible in spite of a disruption of phonological processing : these patients are incapable of using grapheme-to-phoneme conversion, as shown by their inability to read nonsense syllables. The reading impairment of both syndromes should thus reflect the characteristics of the spared non-phonological route(s). From the perspective of a two-route model phonological alexia is supposed to represent a "purer" syndrome than deep dyslexia, which has consequently been defined as a "multiple-component-syndrome" (Shallice and Warrington, 1980). The main variable that defines the two syndromes is production vs non-production of semantic errors during the reading of isolated words. In fact, the occurence of semantic paralexias is the constituent feature of deep dyslexia (Marshall and Newcombe, 1973). With the exception of semantic paralexias the descriptions of both syndromes are indeed quite similar, including visual and derivational errors and the part-of-speech effect with nouns being read more easily than function words. The latter dimension, however, seems to be a variable feature of phonological dyslexia since both have been described : phonological dyslexics who had a problem with functors (Beauvois and Dérouesné, 1979; Patterson, 1982) as well as patients who did not (Shallice and Warrington, personal communication, cited from Patterson, 1982). (All four published cases of phonological dyslexia, however, showed an impairment in reading affixes aloud).

Deep dyslexics and phonological dyslexics seem furthermore to
be distinguishable by the influence of the concrete/abstract dimension on oral reading : in contrast to deep dyslexics this variable
seems to be irrelevant for patients with phonological dyslexia.

The comparison of both reading impairments permits the conclusion that the occurence of semantic paralexias cannot be attributed
solely to the loss of phonological reading by use of grapheme-to-phoneme translation. Patterson (1982), however, considered the possibility that the phonological deficit might well account for the symptoms shared by the two syndromes: errors on grammatical bound morphemes (affixes and suffixes) and errors on function words.

Recent data from pathology, however, do not confirm Patterson's
theoretical reflections. Indeed, Funnell (1983) reports a patient
who read words, function words, and affixed words equally well although he was totally unable to read nonsense syllables. These findings suggest that the cases of so-called "phonological dyslexia" published to date ought in fact to be re-viewed as a multiple component
syndromes : they arise from a disruption of the direct pathway and
thus reflect various different malfunctionings of the semantic-lexical route as does deep dyslexia. Funnell's case who represents a
pure form of phonological (!) reading impairment furthermore suggests
that all types of words of the lexicon can be successfully read aloud in the absence of any use of grapheme-to-phoneme conversions, that
is, supposedly, by use of direct print-to-sound associations.

Confirmation for the psychological reality of direct print-to-
sound associations postulated in the logogen model, comes also from
other studies. Indeed, Schwartz, Saffran and Marin (1980) presented
a patient who could read aloud words (even with irregular spellings)
which he could not understand. Heilman and Rothi (1982) report similar findings with patients suffering from mixed or sensory transcortical aphasia. These patients could also use grapheme-to-phoneme
translation. But the use of this conversion set should only guarantee the correct pronunciation of many regular words. The empirical
finding that these patients correctly read words with irregular spelling patterns cannot be accounted for by the use of the peripheral
reading strategy. It rather suggests the use of a direct (non-semantic) pathway from print to sound the existence of which has been
postulated by the logogen model.

Morton's three-route approach has indeed the advantage of fur-
nishing an explanation for modality or task specific deficits and
non-specific deficits. In the frame of the logogen model it is possible to explain dissociations which a two-route model cannot account for. For example, patient RIC (Kremin, 1981b and this volume)
who suffers from a phonological impairment in oral reading (inability
to read non-sense syllables) reads words when they are in isolation
quite well and without any influence of the part-of-speech dimension.

This variable, however, becomes crucial when the same words are to be decoded in the frame of a sentence. The fact that in the latter task the patient's reading performance turns into "deep dyslexia at the level of sentences" suggests that, in this case, reading of isolated words is achieved by direct print-to-sound associations whereas words in a sentence are reproduced via the semantic pathway for reading aloud. Arguments in favor of a three-route model also come from outside the domain of reading; Patterson (1981) pointed out: "the finding that patients with impaired semantic memory (Warrington, 1975) showed significantly better memory span for words they could not comprehend than for non-words is particularly consonant with a model specifying separate recognition and semantic systems, i.e. the logogen model" (p. 171).

In contrast to phonological and deep dyslexia, reading aloud in surface dyslexia is not achieved by means of addressed phonology from a purely visual or graphemic code : misread words typically yield neologistic pronunciations and document the use of grapheme-to-phoneme conversion for the oral production of isolated words (Marshall and Newcombe, 1973; Holmes, 1978; Kremin, 1980; Deloche et al., 1982; Kremin, in press). It is a consistent theoretical claim as well as an empirical finding that no semantic paralexias are produced. Although surface dyslexic reading may include a partial failure in the application of grapheme-to-phoneme correspondence rules (Marshall and Newcombe, 1973) cases with a purer syndrome have now been described, one that is limited to the misapplication of a generally valid - but for the particular item inappropriate - grapheme-to-phoneme conversion. Indeed, the deficit may be limited to the reading aloud of irregular words (Shallice and Warrington, 1980).

In analogy to the oral reading of isolated words by grapheme-to-phoneme conversion it is usually assumed that in surface dyslexia lexical access depends on and takes place only after assembling phonology. The surface dyslexics' characteristic 'attempt after naming' (Marcel, 1980) - e.g. listen is read : liston...... the boxer (Marshall and Newcombe, 1973) - has been taken to "prove" the unavailability of semantic comprehension prior to phonological output and solely depending on orthographic specifications. Surface dyslexia has thus been defined as the mirror-syndrome of deep and/or phonological dyslexia. Recent investigations, however, revealed that surface dyslexic reading may be characterised by features which are not consonant with this interpretation:

- patients with surface dyslexia may show the influence of the part-of-speech dimension (Deloche et al., 1982; Kremin, 1980) which, with regard to deep dyslexia, is claimed to be a lexical (!) dimension;

- patients are able to read words and non-words, but the oral reading of both stimuli may yield different error patterns (Kremin,

1980), thus suggesting that both linguistic materials are not treated alike ;

   - although orthography seems to be unavailable for oral reading (and even writing) orthographic knowledge may be spared when tested in recognition tasks (Kremin, in press) ;

   - Finally, cases have been described where the semantic reading comprehension did not depend on the phonology of the erroneous read-ing response but on the orthography of the graphemic visual input (Deloche et al., 1982; Goldblum and Kremin, 1982; Kremin, 1980; in press).

   These findings suggest that, at least in some cases which exhi-bit the characteristic reading pattern of surface dyslexia in oral reading, comprehension of the graphic stimuli is achieved by the same pathway of orthographic whole word recognition as in deep dyslexia. For oral reading however these patients use a spelling out strategy by grapheme-to-phoneme conversion. Some patients with surface dysle-xia thus seem to be unable (or unwilling) to use the semantic-ortho-graphic information to activate the correct response in reading alo-ud. Goldblum (in press) discusses two possible accounts for this re-ading behavior: the first one is that the lexical/semantic route per se is not reliable for reading aloud. In this view even adequate se-mantic interpretation cannot guarantee the correct phonological out-put since only (a minimum of) phonological coding could help to ass-ign the correct sound with regard to the target in the cases for ex-ample, of close synonyms like small and little. Another account of surface dyslexic reading has to assume that in surface dyslexia (li-ke in deep dyslexia) patients suffer from response blocking from se-mantics to the phonological output. In both cases, however, rather than make a semantic error or an omission, surface dyslexics would use the intact (although non viable) grapheme-to-phoneme conversion for the oral production of words. This freely chosen reading stra-tegy in cases with spared semantic comprehension would, however, yi-eld the same oral productions as those produced by patients whose ph-onological output is not mediated by semantic reading comprehension. Kremin (1982) thus distinguished two different reading deficits in surface dyslexic patients, one at the level of the visual input lo-gogens (when "recognition" fails) and another at the level of the output logogens (with spared semantic comprehension). Since both types of disturbances should yield similar responses in reading alo-ud they can only be distinguished by their reading comprehension. The first type (with a disturbance at the level of the input logoge-ns) may show no comprehension at all or show the characteristic att-empt for meaning based on the phonological reading response, e.g. listen ->liston ......the boxer.

   In the second type (with a disturbance at the level of the out-put logogens and/or response blocking) semantic comprehension

correctly refers to the target, e.g. fuel [fjul] -> fy-el/ fyl/ comment on appelle ca.....du /fwal/ on pas du/fwal/ du /fyl/....(what
does it mean ?) pour chauffer....du /fyl/ du /fwal/ du /pwal/ on ne
l'appelle pas comme ca (Kremin, in press).

REPETITION

   In spite of their problems with word reading, deep dyslexic patients usually do not have problems with the repetition of words.
Patterson and Marcel (1977) reported deep dyslexic patients who were
able to repeat about 75% of the nonsense syllables they could not read at all. Referring to the symmetry of the logogen model with respect to modality of input, Morton (1980a) speculated as to "whether
patients can be found with roughly speaking, the mirror syndrome to
the deep dyslexics. This would constitute (1) no semantic paralexia,
(2) no problem with reading nonsense words, (3) semantic errors in
repetition of words, (4) inability to repeat nonsense words" (p. 189).
This pattern of theoretical reflection has indeed been experimentally
documented. Michel (1979) reported a case who could read any word
or nonsense syllable but who produced many semantic errors in word
repetition and was incapable of repeating nonsense syllables. And
Goldblum (1979) presented two cases with an analogue of deep dyslexia in word repetition, one of whom, B. F. was surface dyslexic in
reading aloud (Kremin, 1980 - patient FRA). This double dissociation
corresponds, in terms of the logogen model, to a disruption of the
auditory-phonemic conversion together with a disruption of the direct
route between the auditory logogen system and the output logogen system, and, with regard to the visual input, to a disruption of both
the direct and the semantic route (from visual input logogen to the
output logogen system) with the preservation of grapheme-to-phoneme
conversion. More cases with deep dyslexic features in the repetition
features in the repetition of words have been reported (Nolan and
Caramazza, 1982). As in reading, the number of the produced semantic
paraphasias varies considerably with the different patients (ranging
from 25% - 60% of total errors - Goldblum, 1979). The repetition of
nonsense syllables is impossible or severely disturbed. The concreteness of words has a facilitating effect and function words are more difficult to repeat than nouns (Michel, 1979; Nolan and Caramazza,
1982). Deep dyslexic repetition thus parallels deep dyslexic reading
and refers to the same general underlying disturbance, which has thus been documented with respect to two different input modalities,
auditory and visual.

   An "auditory parallel to phonological alexia" has also been described (Beauvois, Derouesne and Bastard, 1980). J. L. repeated words correctly but failed with nonsense syllables. But in contrast
to (some) described cases of phonological dyslexia, J. L. repeated
function words as well as nouns (and wrote them equally well from
dictation). If we compare J. L.'s performances in word repetition
with performances of patients having an auditory parallel of deep

dyslexia, we find the same differences that have been observed between reading in phonological dyslexia and reading in deep dyslexia:
overall performance is much better and, characteristically, no semantic errors are produced.

As to the possible parallelism between the treatment of auditory and of visual stimuli it can only tentatively be inferred that
J. L. used the direct pathway (input logogen -> output logogen) for
repetition as did Funnell's patient for reading (since J. L.'s repetition of affixed words was not formally tested) : J. L. repeated
87% correctly when single words were tested, but his performance dropped to 50% when words were to be repeated in the frame of a sentence. This pattern of performance, however, was characteristic for
another patient who - in reading - used direct associations for single items and the semantic-lexical pathway for sentences (see patient RIC, Kremin, this volume).

WRITING

Single case studies combined with an information processing approach not only documented the patients' behavior in reading, but spurred the study of components of writing as well. Thus, by analogy
to reading impairments, patients have been presented who suffer from
surface dysgraphia (Beauvois and Derouesne, 1981; Deloche et al.,
1982; Hatfield, 1982a; Kremin, 1980; in press), from phonological
dysgraphia (Shallice, 1981), and deep dysgraphia (Bub and Kertesz,
1982; Hatfield, 1982a; Nolan and Caramazza, 1982, in press).

In surface dysgraphia - which has also been called "lexical or
orthographic dysgraphia" (Beauvois and Derouesne, 1981) - the orthographic specifications of words seem to be lost for written production. Thus the patients are able to write nonsense syllables from
dictation and to orally spell these items, but the writing from dictation of real words (and their spellings) typically consists in productions which nearly always have the same sounds as the target words but lack adequate orthography of the actual words.

With regard to the structure of different languages Luria (1960)
predicted that such a pattern should emerge in English and French
"where the writing contains significant elements of conventional orthography, and in which the written word, resting on historically
stabilized conventional combinations, very often falls outside the
scope of the phonemic principle" (p. 18). Surface dysgraphia should
not be found in Russian and German where writing is "phonemic i.e.
constitutes a representation in conventional letters of the system
of consecutive phonemes of which a word consists" (p. 15). Indeed
surface dysgraphia to date has been reported for French and English.
Beauvois and Derouesne's (1981) patient is the most relevant case
for a dissociation of oral and written word production. R. G. suffered from an impairment of graphemic output without comparable

impairment of speech output: he suffered from surface dysgraphia,
his reading being characterized by phonological dyslexia (and not
surface dyslexia). We agree with Beauvois and Derouesne that this
case constitutes "further evidence to support the partial independence of the linguistic mechanisms used in the production of oral and
written language" (p. 34). In patients with surface dysgraphia the
impairment in writing and spelling refers to the particular orthography of a given word; the impairment does not affect the sound-letter
conversion as demonstrated by the patients' ability to write nonsense syllables. Surface dysgraphia thus reflects the disturbance of a
lexical process, with phoneme-to-grapheme conversion being spared,
e.g. photo -> fauto, nain -> nin, pigeon -> pijon (Beauvois and Derouesne, 1981); moelle -> moille, fuel -> fioul (Kremin, 1980); clef
-> clai, oeillet -> oeuillait (Kremin, in press); injury -> ingerry;
silhouette -> silluet, ghost -> goast (Hatfield, 1982a).

   This writing pattern might not be limited to writing from dictation but was also found in written naming (Beauvois and Derouesne,
1981; Kremin, in press) and spontaneous language (Beauvois and Derouesne, 1981). R. G.'s surface dysgraphic writing in all writing tasks
seems to demonstrate that the syndrome might be unrelated to the processing of auditorily presented words, i.e., acoustic-phonemic conversion. But in contrast to R. G., HAM (Kremin, in press) did not
employ this phonological writing strategy either in spontaneous writing or during the dictation of sentences (as opposed to isolated words): that is, when the cognitive system was (supposedly) engaged.
HAM's performances on these two tasks are not characterised by surface dysgraphia but rather total agraphia. Furthermore, HAM's production of the phonological form in written naming crucially depended on first having spelled out the target word. The patient thus
recreated, for written naming, a situation analogous to the repetition of isolated words. Only then did the patient seem to proceed
by acoustic grapheme conversion. Kremin discusses HAM's writing performances in terms of a possible compensatory strategy and suggests
that HAM had not yet acquired this compensatory strategy for all her
writing productions: spontaenous writing was still "spontaneous" -
that is, without preceding verbalization to create the condition (si-
ne qua non ?) for phoneme-to-grapheme conversion. (The same argument was advanced to account for HAM's writing to dictation of sentences: the patient understands them and wants to write them. Such a
task is usually executed without sounding out the target). Kremin's
interpretation remains, of course, with question marks. It is possible indeed, that there is more than one syndrome of surface dysgraphia (as there is more than one syndrome surface dyslexia). Still,
the factor "onset of testing period after accident" fits with Kremi-
n's tentatively-advanced hypothesis about surface dysgraphia as a
possible compensatory strategy (in the case of spared phoneme-to-grapheme conversion): HAM's writing was studied only one month after
cerebral accident whereas R. G.'s writing performances date from-one
to two (and five) years after surgical intervention.

The other two recently defined writing disturbances, phonological and deep dysgraphia, suffer from the opposite deficit: phonemic
information cannot be transformed into a graphemic code. These patients are unable to write nonsense syllables to dictation. In phonological dysgraphia this disturbance is unrelated to the repetition
of words. P. R. repeated 45/50 non-words correctly but successfully
wrote only 9/50 of the same items (Shallice, 1981). And even V. S.,
a case with deep dysgraphia, reproduced non-words much better in repetition (45%) than in writing to dictation (no correct reproduction
- Nolan and Caramazza, in press).

In analogy to the published cases of so-called "phonological
dyslexia", P. R. showed only a slight difficulty in writing words
from dictation. Indeed, he performed almost perfectly on the content words, but he made significantly more errors on function words
(Shallice, 1981). In the few instances "when nonsense material was
written correctly this nearly always depended upon P. R. using his
knowledge of the spelling of a related word as a mediator" (p. 422).
The patient's spelling capacity, oral and written, was fairly good
(83% and 72%). But P. R. also had a mild phonological alexia. Shallice (1981) pointed out that this parallelism is not a necessary
one. Indeed, Beauvois and Derouesne's patient R. G. (1979; 1981)
showed a double dissociation with nonsense syllable reading impaired
(phonological dyslexia) but nonsense syllable writing spared (surface dysgraphia). - In the light of the theoretical impact of Funnell's
(1983) case for reading we ought to doubt that P. R. represents a
pure disturbance of phonological (!) dysgraphia, that is of writing
words from dictation by using a direct connection between auditory
input logogen and graphical output logogen. P. R.'s problems with
the writing of function words from dictation rather suggests the use
of the semantic-lexical pathway. This argument is reinforced by the
finding that the (few) errors in P. R.'s spontaneous writing included omission of verbs, incorrect conjugation of verbs, and function
word substitutions. Moreover, Shallice (1981) observed: "it appeared that in order for the patient to write the word merely dictating
it to him was insufficient ; he needed to access its meaning"(p.421).

We are persuaded that by the time of writing this paper a case
of pure "phonological" dysgraphia has been detected, that is a patient capable of writing all types of words but no (or hardly any) nonsense syllables. At this moment, however, there is poor experimental
evidence for writing words from dictation by direct associations.
One observation in this direction is due to Morton (1980b) who mentions some particular features of Gail's writing performance.

This patient was able to use (and used) the acoustic phonemic
conversion strategy in writing words to dictation, e.g. cried->cride;
foam -> phome. Intriguing is that the patient spontaneously corrected these misproductions with regard to (even irregular) orthography. On another occasion the patient was asked to define the spoken

word plough. "She had no idea of its meaning but then wrote it down
correctly - not as PLOW, which would have been the obvious result of
a simple phoneme-grapheme conversion. She still seemed to have no
idea of what it meant and then said 'I've forgotten what it is -
(pause) see it in a field - using some sort of machine - something
to do with soil'" (Morton, 1980b, p. 131). The important thing about the example is that it demonstrates the use of the auditory input
logogen system rather than the acoustic phonemic conversion. This
example thus seems to be further evidence of direct associations ev-
en for writing (bypassing the cognitive system) as claimed by the
logogen model for reading repetition. In the case of the written word plough the spelling of the word could be obtained from the graphical output logogen via the (phonological) output logogen system.
But Morton also considers the possibility of a direct connection between the auditory input system and the graphical output system (although this connection exists only via the cognitive system in the
current version of the model).

In cases with deep dysgraphia (Hatfield, 1982a, b; Bub and Kertesz, 1982; Nolan and Caramazza, in press) the error pattern on words resembles that of deep dyslexia : semantic, derivational, and visual errors are produced, functors are substituted, and both abstractness and part-of-speech effects are observed. But in addition to
errors caused by a general lexical problem, the productions of deep
dyslexic writers are characterized by "spelling errors" which cannot
be accounted for by a central disturbance :

1. words are often written in non-linear order, e.g. knows ->
$\overset{23451}{CHERS}$; abode -> $\overset{14523}{ORGRE}$ (patient B. B. from Hatfield, 1982b);

2. words are often "tried out", e.g. west -> wele, weal, wear,
west (patient B. B. from Hatfield, 1982b);

3. in approximately $\frac{1}{2}$ of the words B. B.'s writing production
(to dictation) preserved the "general shape" of the target word, e.g.
(from Hatfield, 1982b) deep tump ; peace berrs ; power wanop;

4. More than $\frac{1}{2}$ of V. S.'s omission errors were "gap errors",
for example, when shown a picture of a bowl of alphabet soup, the
patient wrote alph let (Nolan and Caramazza, in press). Such gaps
were also characteristic for Gail (Morton, 1980b) who had to write
down at least the initial letter of a word before she could make any
spoken (!) response. Trying to retrieve the names of countries Gail
wrote :

In a (India); N Z (New Zealand); J p n (Japan); C na (China).
Gail claimed that she visualizes words she is trying to define. And
P. R., another patient who uses the lexical pathway for his writing
accounted for his ability to write words as transcribing from an

inner "screen" on which he sees the words (Shallice, 1981).

Nolan and Caramazza (in press) observed that V. S.'s spelling
errors (letter transpositions, omissions, substitutions) even occurred in tasks where, supposedly, lexical mediation was not involved
(such as copying from memory which did not show the deep dysgraphic
pattern but did show spelling errors). Since V. S. made similar spelling errors whether or not lexical mediation was involved, Nolan and
Caramazza (in press) conclude that "spelling errors do not result from an access problem but rather from a problem in output of a correct
representation", that is from a breakdown which occurs fairly late
in the writing process. Thus the presented cases of deep dysgraphia
might be accounted for by two independent disturbances, one central
(resulting in the "deep" pattern with semantic and derivational errors and functor substitutions or omissions) and one more peripheral
(resulting in spelling errors). Nolan and Caramazza think that the
latter writing errors are due to a problem at the level of the grapheme buffer : transposition errors would "reflect knowledge of item
information with loss of ordinal position information"; omission
errors should reflect "loss of specific item information"; letter
substitution errors (in which the substituted letter is similar in
shape) "may reflect retention of only partial identity information
of only some features of the intended letter, such as ascender or
curvilinear" gap errors, finally, "indicate that ordinal position
information has been retained for both the remaining letters and for
the omitted letter(s)". In Nolan and Caramazza's view these spelling errors arise from the deep dysgraphic impairment of phoneme-grapheme conversion (because information entering the grapheme buffer
decays rapidly and needs "refreshment" by input originating in the
response buffer). But these questions remain open to future research.

According to models of information processing deep dysgraphia
is supposed to reflect a central disturbance. In fact, Nolan and
Caramazza's patient produced semantic paragraphias not only in writing to dictation but also in written naming; and semantic errors
occurred in the reading of isolated words as well. Bub and Kertesz's
(1982) patient with deep dysgraphia, however, repeated and read words and nonsense syllables flawlessly. It can thus be inferred that
the patient used the corresponding peripheral pathways for the reading and repetition of isolated words. And indeed, when the cognitive system ought to be engaged (during the treatment of units larger
than the isolated word) "oral reading of sentences was markedly tele-
graphic, paralleling spontaneous output" (p. 155), and in repetition
"the response was halting and nonfluent with word-finding difficulty
and phonemic paraphasia" (p. 149).

Another point which merits consideration concerns the relation
between recognition and production of orthography. In fact, the written productions of both surface dysgraphic writers result in misspellings in spite of the different pathways which are used for

written production (acoustic-phonemic conversion and direct access from the semantic representations of words). Indeed, R. G., a patient with surface dysgraphia - when confronted with his own misspellings in a reading task - often (that is, in 62% of the cases) did not read anything and made remarks such as 'it's not a word', 'It's badly written', 'Oh what a mistake' (Beauvois and Derouesne, 1981, p. 32). HAM, another patient with surface dysgraphia (and surface dyslexia) recognized orthography (when this variable was tested in a lexical decision task) with an even higher degree of accuracy; she committed only 4% errors on real words, 7% errors on real nonsense syllables, and 13% errors on nonsense syllables which were homophones of words (Kremin, in press). Two other patients with surface dysgraphia (and surface dyslexia) did have problems with the recognition of orthography (Kremin, 1980; Deloche et al., 1982). This discrepancy in the performances of surface dysgraphic patients, however, indicates only that a general loss of orthographic representations can (but need not) occur in surface dysgraphia.

Good orthographic recognition has also been mentioned for a case with deep dysgraphia: V. S. made only 7/75 errors when she had to judge words and nonsense syllables - including her own spelling errors from writing - in a lexical decision task (Nolan and Caramazza, in press). Moreover, when asked to correct these mispelled items, V. S. was able to correct 76% of her initial writing errors. These results seem to indicate that V. S. "has access to intact orthographic representations of these words and that her inability to write these words correctly must be due to a breakdown in the process(es) involved in translating these representations to a form which is usable for writing" (Nolan and Caramazza, in press).

CONCLUDING REMARKS

We think that the usefulness of the information processing approach for the description of word-production and word-recognition in neurological syndromes need not be furthermore underlined. Studies carried out in this perspective may even change our notion of well established clinical pictures such as pure alexia without agraphia. In fact, a recent study by Friedman (1982) casts some new light on the underlying mechanisms of this syndrome. Friendman's case study demonstrates indeed that the pattern of impaired reading and intact writing and spelling (which is characteristic of alexia without agraphia) cannot be taken as evidence of intact visual word representations which - according to Geschwind (1965) - are just disconnected from the visual input. Friedman clearly demonstrates that patient M. C.'s spelling capacity coexists with an impaired orthographic lexicon: the patient's spelling of (regular) words and nonwords was extremely good, but exception words (such as island, does, beige) yielded only 56% correct spellings.

According to information processing models the spelling of

irregular words must depend upon a lexical route to the orthographic
representations. Since the patient's use of this route was disturbed (as shown by the high error score on exception words) Friedman
raises the possibility that M. C.'s spelling of regular words was
executed by using an indirect rule-guided mechanism. (That this mechanism was preserved is shown by the patient's successful spelling
of nonwords via the use of phoneme-grapheme rules. Friedman's interpretation is indeed consolidated by other experimental data. Thus
the patient's spelling of exception words showed a large frequency
effect. For regular words, however, there was no difference between
high and low frequency words. As the author pointed out "there is
no reason why a spelling mechanism based upon rules should show a
frequency effect" (p. 539). Moreover, some of M. C.'s cited spelling errors document indeed a rule-guided strategy, e.g. (gone) ->
G. O. N. ; (sure) -> S. H. O. U. R.; (chef) -> S. H. E. F.

Friedman's detailed study which was carried out in the frame of
information processing models raises indeed two main issues:

1) Again it is demonstrated that reading and writing/spelling can
depend on distinct mechanisms. The possible dissociations of these
mechanisms has already been ruled out by Beauvois and Derouesne's
(1979; 1981) case study of R. G.;

2) "The pattern of impaired reading intact spelling characteristic
of alexia without agraphia may in some cases reflect an impaired vi-
sual-orthographic lexicon and an intact "indirect" rule-guided spelling mechanism" (Friedman, 1982, p. 544).

We agree with Friedman that "more thorough examination of other
pure alexic patients may reveal that they are not as "pure" as they
first may seem" (p. 544). We think indeed that the information processing approach will help us to acquire more understanding with regard to the mechanisms that underly word-recognition and word-production in pathological and in normal performance.

REFERENCES

Albert, M. L. Alexia. In K. M. Heilman and E. Valenstein (Eds)
    Clinical Neurospychology, New York, Oxford University Press,
    1979.
Albert, M. L., Yamadori, A., Gardner, H. & Howes, D. Comprehension
    in alexia. Brain, 1973, 96, 317-328.
Beauvois, M. F. & Derouesne, J. Phonological alexia - Three disso-
    ciations. Journal of Neurology, Neurosurgery and Psychiatry,
    1979, 42, 1115-1124.
Beauvois, M. F. & Derouesne, J. Lexical or orthographic agraphia.
    Brain, 1980, 104, 21-49.

Beauvois, M. F.; Derouesne, J. & Bastard, V. - Auditory parallel to
    phonological alexia. Paper presented at the Meeting of the
    International Neuropsycholigical Society, Chianciano, Italy,
    June 1980.
Benson, D. F. & Geschwind, N. The alexias. In P. J. Vinken & G. W.
    Bruyn (Eds). Handbook of Clinical Neurology (Vol. 4), Amsterdam,
    North Holland, 1969.
Berndt, R. S. & Caramazza, A. A redefinition of the syndrome of
    Broca's aphasia: Implications for a neuropsychological model of
    language. Applied Psycholinguistics, 1980, 1, 225-278.
Bub, D. & Kertesz, A. Deep Agraphia. Brain and Language, 1982, 17,
    146-165.
Caplan, L. R. & Hedley-White, T. Cueing and memory dysfunction in
    alexia without agraphia : A case report, Brain, 1974, 97,
    251-262.
Cappa, S.; Cavalotti, G. & Vignolo, L. A. Phonemic and lexical err-
    ors in fluent aphasia: Correlation with lesion site. Brain and
    Language, 1981, 19, 171-177.
Coltheart, M. Deep dyslexia: a review of the syndrome. In M. Colt-
    heart, K. E. patterson & J. C. Marshall (Eds) Deep Dyslexia.
    London: Routledge and Kegan Paul, 1980.
Coltheart, M. ; Marshall, J. C. & Patterson, K. E. Deep Dyslexia.
    London: Routledge and Kegan Paul, 1980.
Deloche, G.; Andreewsky, E. & Desi, M. Surface dyslexia: A case
    report and some theoretical implications to reading models.
    Brain and Language, 1982, 15, 11-32.
Friederici, A. D.; Schoenle, P. W. & Goodglass, H. Mechanisms under-
    lying writing and speech in aphasia. Brain and Language, 1981,
    212-222.
Friedman, R. B. Mechanisms of reading and spelling in a case of
    alexia without agraphia. Neuropsychologia, 1982, 20, 533-545.
Funnell, E. Phonological processes in reading: new evidence from
    acquired dyslexia. British Journal of Psychology, 1983.
Gardner, H. & Zurif, D. Bee but not be: Oral reading of simple word
    in aphasia and alexia. Neuropsychologia, 1975, 13, 181-190.
Geschwind, N. Disconnection syndromes in animals and man. Brain,
    1965, 88, 237-294; 585-644.
Goldblum, M. C. Auditory analogue of deep dyslexia. In O. Cruetz-
    feld, H. Scheich & C. Schreiner (Eds) Experimental brain re-
    search, Supplementum II: Hearing mechanisms and speech.
    Berlin : Springer Verlag, 1979.
Goldblum M. C. Semantic processing of words in surface dyslexia.
    In J. C. Marshall, M. Coltheart & K. E. Patterson (Eds)
    Surface dyslexia, In press.
Goodglass, H. Disorders of naming following brain injury. Ameri-
    can Scientist, 1980, 68, 647-655.
Goodglass, H.; Kaplan, E.; Weintraub, S. & Ackerman, N. The "tip-
    of-the-Tongue" phenomenon in aphasia. Cortex, 1976, 12, 145-153.
Hatfield, F. M. Diverses formes de desintégration du langage écrit
    et implications pour la rééducation. In X. Seron and

C. Latterre (Eds). Rééduquer le cerveau ? Logopédie, psychologie, Neurologie. Brussels : Pierre mardaga. 1982 a.

Hatfield, F. M. Visual factors in acquired dyslexia. Paper presented at the Meeting of the International Neuropsychologocal Society, Deauvill, France, June 1982 b.

Hecaen, H. & Kremin, H. Neurolinguistic research on reading disorders resulting from left hemisphere lesions. Aphasic and "pure"
alexias. In H. Whitaker & H. A. Whitaker (Eds) Studies in neurolinguistics (Vol. 2) New York: Academic Press. 1976.

Heilman, K. M. and Rothi, J. Acquired reading disorders: A diagra-
mmatical model. In R. N. Malatesha and P. G. Aaron (Eds)
Reading Disorders: Varieties and Treatments, New York: Academic
Press, 1982.

Heilman, K. M., Tucker, D. M. & Valenstein, E. A case of mixed
transcortical aphasia with intact naming. Brain, 1976, 99,
415-426.

Hier, D. B. & Mohr, J. P. In congrenous oral and written naming.
Evidence for a subdivision of the syndrome of Wernicke's aphasia. Brain and Language, 1977, 4, 115-126.

Hier, D. B.; Mogil, S. J.; Rubin, N. P. & Komros, G. R. Semantic
aphasia: a neglected entity. Brain and Language, 1980, 10,
120-131.

Holmes, J. M. Regression and reading breakdown. In A. Caramazza &
E. Zurif (Eds) The acquisition and breakdown of language: Pa-
rallels and divergencies. Baltimore: John Hopkins University
Press, 1978.

Kremin, H. Deux stratégies de lecture dissociables par la pathologie
Description d'un cas de dyslexie profonde et d'un cas de dyslexie de surface. In Etudes Neurolinguistiques (issue of Grammatica). Université de Toulouse Le Mirail. 1980.

Kremin, H. Problèmes d'accès lexical et stratégies de lecture. In
Processus fondamentaux en oeuvre dans la lecture et la compré-
hension du langage écrit, spécial issue of Psychologie Fran-
çaise, 1981 a.

Kremin, H. On Broca's aphasia and agrammatic reading. Paper presented at the Meeting of the International Neuropsychological
Society, Bergen, Norway, June 1981 b.

Kremin, H. Naming disturbances and gender assignment. Paper presented at the Academy of Aphasia, 19th Annual Meeting, London,
Ontario (Canada), October 1981 c.

Kremin, H. Alexia: Theory and Research. In Malatesha R. N. &
P. G. Aaron (Eds) Reading Disorders: Varieties and Treatments.
New York: Academic Press, 1982.

Kremin, H. Routes and strategies - Data on acquired surface dyslexia and surface dysgraphia. In J. C. Marshall, M. Coltheart
and K. Patterson (Eds) Surface dyslexia. In Press.

Kremin, H. & Koskas, E. Naming and spontaneous language of subjects
with lesions of the left temporal lobe. Paper presented at the
Meeting of the International Neuropsychological Society, Deauville, France, June 1982.

Landis, T.; Regard, M. and Serrat, A. Iconic reading in a case of alexia without agraphia caused by a brain tumor: a Tachistoscopic study. Brain and Language, 1980, 11, 45-53.

Luria, A. R. Differences between disturbances of speech and writing in Russian and in French. International Journal of Slavic Linguistics and poetics, 1960, 3, 13-22.

Marcel, T. Surface Dyslexia and beginning reading - a revised hypothesis of the pronunciation of print and its impairments. In M. Coltheart, K. E. Patterson & J. C. Marshall (Eds) Deep Dyslexia. London: Routledge and Kegan Paul, 1980.

Marshall, J. C. & Newcombe, F. Patterns of paralexia: A psycholinguistic approach. Journal of Psycholinguistic Research, 1973, 2, 175- 199.

Marshall, J. C. & Newcombe, F. Variability and constraint in acquired alexia. In H. Whitaker and H. A. Whitaker (Eds) Studies in Neurolinguistics, (Vol. 3), New York: Academic Press. 1977.

Marshall, M.; Newcombe, F. & Marshall, J. C. The microstructure of wordfinding difficulties in a dysphasic subject. In G. B. Flores d'Arcais & M. G. M. Levelt (Eds) Advances in Psycholinguistics, Amsterdam, North Holland, 1970.

Michel, F. Préservation du langage écrit malgré un déficit majeur du langage oral. Lyon-Medical,1979, 241, (3), 141-149.

Morton, J. Word recognition. In J. Morton and J. C. Marshall (Eds) Psycholinguistic Series II. London: Elek Scientific Books, 1979.

Morton, J. Two auditory parallels to deep dyslexia. In M. Coltheart, J. C. Marshall and K. E. Patterson (Eds) Deep Dyslexia. London: Routledge and Kegan Paul, 1980 a.

Morton, J. The logogen model and orthographic structure. In U. Frith (Ed) Cognitive Processes in spelling. London: Academic Press, 1980 b.

Morton, J. & Patterson, K. E. A new attempt at an interpretation or an attempt at a new interpretation. In M. Coltheart, K. E. Patterson & J. C. Marshall (Eds) Deep dyslexia, London: Routledge and Kegan Paul, 1980.

Newcombe, F. and Marshall, J. C. On psycholinguistic classifications of the acquired dyslexia. Bulletin of the Orton Society, 1981, 31, 29-46.

Nolan, K. A. and Caramazza, A. Modality-Independent impairments in word processing in a deep dyslexic patient. Brain and Language, 1982, 16, 237-264.

Nolan, K. A. and Caramazza, A. An analysis of writing in a case of deep dyslexia. Brain and Language. In press.

Patterson, K. E. Neuropsychological approaches to the study of reading. British Journal of Psychology, 1981, 72, 151-174.

Patterson, K. E. The relation between reading and phonological coding: Further neuropsychological observations. In A. W. Ellis(Ed). Normality and Pathology in Cognitive functioning, London, Academic Press, 1982.

Patterson, K. E. & Marcel, T. Aphasia, dyslexia and the phonological coding of written words. Quarterly Journal of Experimental

Psychology, 1977, <u>29</u>, 307-318.

Rothi L. J. & Heilman, K. M. Alexia and agraphia with spared spelling and letter recognition abilities. *Brain and Language*, 1981, <u>12</u>, 1-13.

Saffran, E. M., Schwartz, M. F. & Marin, O. S. M. Semantic mechanisms in paralexia. *Brain and Language*, 1976, <u>3</u>, 255-265.

Schwartz, M. F., Marin, O. S. M. & Saffran, E. M. Dissociations of language function in dementia: A case study. *Brain and Language*, 1979, <u>7</u>, 277-306.

Schwartz, M. F., Saffran, E. A. & Marin, O. S. M. An analysis of agrammatic reading in aphasia. Paper presented at the International Neuropsychological Society, Santa Fe, February 1977.

Schwartz, M. F., Saffran, E. A. & Marin, O. S. M. Fractioning the reading process in dementia: evidence for word-specific print-to-sound associations. In M. Coltheart, K. E. patterson & J. C. Marshall (Eds) *Deep Dyslexia*, London: Routledge & Kegan Paul, 1980.

Shallice, T. Phonological agraphia and the lexical route in writing. *Brain*, 1981, <u>104</u>, 413-429.

Shallice, T. & Warrington, E. K. Word recognition in a phonemic dyslexic patient. *Quarterly Journal of Experimental Psychology*, 1975, <u>27</u>, 187-199.

Shallice, T. & Warrington, E. Single and multiple component central dyslexic syndromes. In M. Coltheart, K. E. Patterson & J. C. Marshall (Eds) *Deep Dyslexia*, London: Routledge & Kegan Paul, 1980.

Stachowiak, F. J. & Poeck, K. Functional dysconnection in pure alexia and color naming deficit demonstrated by facilitation methods. *Brain and Language*, 1976, <u>3</u>, 135-143.

Warrington, E. Concrete word dyslexia. *British Journal of Psychology*, 1981, <u>72</u>, 175-196.

Warrington, E. & Shallice, T. Semantic access dyslexia. *Brain*, 1979, <u>102</u>, 43-63.

Weigl, E. and Bierwisch, M. Neuropsychology and linguistics: topics of common research. *Foundations of Language*, 1970, <u>6</u>, 1-18.

Whitehouse, P., Caramazza, A. & Zurif, E. Naming in aphasia: Interacting effects of form and function. *Brain and Language*, 1978, <u>6</u>, 63-74.

Zurif, E. B.; Caramazza, A. & Myerson, R. Grammatical judgements of agrammatic aphasics. *Neuropsychologia*, 1972, <u>10</u>, 405-417.

COMMENTS ON PATHOLOGICAL READING BEHAVIOR DUE TO LESIONS
OF THE LEFT HEMISPHERE[1]

Helgard Kremin
Chargée de recherche au C. N. R. S.
Unité 111 de l' I. N. S. E. R. M.
2ter rue d'Alésia
75014 Paris - France

INTRODUCTION

Neuropsychological investigations of acquired reading disturbances have now been conducted for almost one century. Although the phonemena are the same, the interpretation of these impairments resulting from brain damage has recently been spurred by information-processing models which have been mainly proposed by psychologists. Recent assessment of lesion studies documents the trend to describe new cases (and to reformulate old data) in the perspective of "identifying components of behavior rather than localizing them" (Morton and Patterson, 1980; p. 96). Indeed, data from pathology have become determinant factors for the formulation of theoretical models concerning the mechanisms and/or processes involved in (normal) reading.

CLASSIFICATIONS AND LOCALIZATIONS

The first systematic approaches to the syndromes of the alexias, however, have been conducted from a neuropsychological perspective. The authors were concerned with the establishment of correlations between the localization of lesions and the corresponding syndromes. Thus Dejerine (1891, 1892) argued for the clinical reality of two different reading disorders : word blindness with agraphia produced by a lesion in the "center of visual images" (the left angular gyrus), and pure word blindness, produced by a subcortical lesion (in the lingual gyrus) that interrupted the connections between the angular gyrus and the visual cortex. In the latter variety both spontaneous writing and writing to dictation are preserved.

1. Part of this work was supported by an individual fellowship from the Foundation Fyssen, Paris.

Although subsequently there was a general agreement as to the
localization of pure word blindness, according to some authors, pure
alexia is best integrated in the general framework of the agnosias.
Thus pure alexia came to be known as "agnosic alexia" and alexia with
agraphia as "aphasic (or parietal) alexia". These classical types
of reading impairment have finally been complemented. In fact, Heca-
en(1967) distinguished three aspects of reading impairments, thus em-
phasizing the clinical existence of a third variety of reading disorders, that is alexia as part of sensory aphasia (arising from lesions
of the posterior part of the left temporal lobe). Finally, Benson
(1977) distinguished yet another type of reading impairment. This
impairment is seen in patients with Broca's aphasia and frontal lobe
pathology: these patients comprehended content words better than syntactic relations and appeared more letter than word blind.

But authors have also tried to establish classifications of the
alexias on criteria other than anatomoclinical. Thus it has been noted that reading disturbances may either be global in nature, relating to both letters and words, or they may affect them more or less
selectively. The distinction between literal and verbal alexia has
been standard since Dejerine. Most authors, however, interpreted this distinction only as different degrees of the reading impairment.
Hinshelwood (1900) can be cited as an early representative of the view that literal and verbal alexia are to be considered as distinct
forms of reading impairment which it is possible to come across in a
pure state. Hinshelwood based his views on extreme localization theories postulating different cerebral centers for letter, words, sentences, numbers and musical notes. His observations are interesting
though since his classification of reading impairments draws the attention to three basic disorders, letter-, word-, and sentence blindness: 1) patients with literal alexia can read words but they are
unable to name a letter in a word they have just read; 2) patients
with verbal alexia can name letters much better than they can read
aloud whole words and sentences; 3) some patients read letters and
words fairly well, but their performance deteriorates when confronted
with sentences.

Finally, it was established that two types of alexias may be distinguished on the basis of location of the lesion as well as on the
basis of different reading behavior. Alajouanine, Lhermitte and Ribaucourt-Ducarne (1960) stated that in "agnosic alexia" (with writing
intact) the reading of words and sentences is dramatically impaired,
but the reading of isolated letters only slightly affected. Words
are "deciphered" with great difficulty, letter by letter and syllable by syllable. The anatomically verified cases of agnosic (or verbal) alexia showed an occipital lesion. "Aphasic" (or literal) alexia with agraphia, in contrast, occured with lesions of the parieto-
temporal region. This reading disturbance - which is always (at least in the initial stage) accompanied by an impairment in oral language - is characterized by better word than letter reading. The

reading strategy is global, that is patients do not resort to a literal analysis of words (as they do in agnosic and/or verbal alexia).

Hecaen (1967) confirmed the distinction between alexia with and
without agraphia with reference to the role of localization of the
lesions and emphasized the possibility of a dissociation of the reading deficits with regard to the structural level of the linguistic
stimuli (isolated letters, words, sentences). In 1971, Dubois-Charlier assessed the structural independence of literal and verbal alexia, and furthermore suggested the presence of an additional type of
reading disturbance, that of "sentence alexia". Hecaen and Kremin
(1976) analyzed new cases of severely alexic patients without disorders of oral language and compared them with patients suffering from
left hemispheric lesions and associated syndromes. The study established that there was not only a quantitative difference between pure alexia and the other reading impairments, but also a qualitative
difference. Hecaen and Kremin maintained the classification of the
alexias according to the different linguistic levels (letters, words,
sentences) at which the disturbance was predominantly found, but they specified the varieties with regard to the three contrasts they
took into consideration that stem from the implicated cognitive processes or from the linguistic character of the presented material :
recognition vs reading, meaningfulness vs non-meaningfulness, and
analytical combination vs global apprehension of the stimuli.

With reference to cerebral localization Hecaen (1976) stated
that verbal alexia is always associated with occipital lesions of
the left hemisphere and can result in persistent syndromes without
any lesion of the corpus callosum. Literal alexia, in contrast, seems to result from a combined lesion in the occipital and parietal
or temporal region. For the published cases of sentence alexia there was clearly not enough information available to define the locus
of the lesion precisely. In fact, when difficulties with reading of
sentence occur (Dubois-Charlier, 1971; Hecaen and Kremin, 1976) the
difficulties seem to relate to the application of syntactic rules,
while letters and words are read well and relatively rapidly. Although other authors did not study "sentence alexia" from the perspective of an independent reading impairment, some recent investigations mention that the patient's reading behavior can crucially depend
in this variable: words may be read "differently" depending on whether they are presented in isolation or in the frame of a sentence
(see Andreewsky and Seron, 1975; Caramazza, Berndt and Hart, 1981;
Kremin, 1981).

With reference to localization, Geschwind's (1962, 1965, 1966)
disconnection theory for pure alexia should be mentioned. According
to his model, cases of pure alexia represent simply a deficit in the
verbalization of graphic symbols due to a lesion of the splenium :
the visual input does not go further than the right occipital lobe,
the right hemianopia preventing the visual stimuli from reaching the

language areas of the dominant hemisphere. Geschwind's interpretation would indeed explain the frequent association of pure alexia
with naming disorders for objects and colors. The disconnection theory has subsequently been widely accepted, particularly since the work of Sperry and Gazzaniga (1967) on patients who have undergone commissurotomy. These authors used a new technique limiting the access of the sensory input to just one hemisphere. They found that the
(isolated) right hemisphere, although capable of "understanding" letters and words (but not sentences or commands) is totally unable to
express orally what it is seeing.

It should be stressed however, that Geschwind's connectionist
model meets some important difficulties:

1) even if this concept may apply to global alexia, it is difficult to apply in cases where the deficit selectively affects certain graphemic ranks (letter, word, sentence);

2) there are (admittedly rare) cases in which alexia is present
without any problems in object and/or color naming (Quensel, 1927;
Ajax, 1964, 1967; Cummings, Hurwitz and Perl, 1970; Greenblatt, 1973;
Hecaen and Gruner, 1975);

3) although rare, observations have been made of pure alexia
without an associated visual field defect (Hinshelwood, 1900; Hoff
and Pötzl, 1937; Peron and Goutner, 1944; Alajouanine et al., 1960;
Ajax, 1967; Goldstein, Joynt and Goldblatt, 1971; Greenblatt, 1973);

4) Hecaen and Gruner (1975) presented an observation of pure
alexia where the post mortem examination showed that the corpus callosum was intact. In this case the (verbal) alexia had however pe-
rsisted for a period of four years.

From a non localizationist perspective Marshall and Newcombe
(1973) undertook an original approach to the classification of reading disturbances. They proposed a taxonomy of paralexic errors produced by aphasic patients, in whom the alexic component was predominant. The authors distinguished three dyslexic syndromes with reference to the relative distribution of each error type:

1) visual dyslexia, characterized by paralexias with visual
similarity to the target (e.g. dug -> bug; pamper -> paper.... could
be panzer);

2) deep dyslexia in which the errors are predominantly semantic (e.g. little -> small; entrance -> exit) and/or derivational
(truth -> true; height -> high);

3) surface dyslexia, in which the paralexias result mainly from a "partial failure" in the application of grapheme-to-phoneme

conversion rules (e.g. insect -> insist; guest -> just). As in (1)
semantic errors are absent from oral reading; moreover, the oral productions are characterized by numerous neologisms.

In 1975, Newcombe and Marshall tried to establish a relationship
between reading performance and localization of the lesion: visual
dyslexia occured with a very posterior parieto-occipital lesion; the
two cases of surface dyslexia had a combined temporo-parietal lesion;
for deep dyslexia, Newcombe and Marshall postulated a temporal lesion without any involvement of the occipital region.

ERRORS, PATTERNS, IMPAIRMENTS

Marshall and Newcombe (1973) proposing a theoretical frame to
account for the different types of paralexias (visual, semantic, phonological) pointed out that their model allows for the possibility
of "pure" visual dyslexia without other aphasic involvement. Cases
presented by Newcombe and Marshall (1973, 1975) produced indeed predominantly or exclusively visual errors. In a study by Gardner and
Zurif (1975) the difference between visual and other paralexias was
statistically significant for patients with alexia plus agraphia.
Hecaen and Kremin (1976) found that an average of 79% of the reading
errors produced by pure alexic patients was visual in nature. In this context it should also be mentioned that already Poppelreuther
(1917) stressed the predominance of visual reading errors in patients with lesions of the occipital lobe.

However, considering visual similarity between reading output
and target one should keep in mind that this similarity can result
from two different ways of reading: for SAL and CRO, patients suffering from pure verbal alexia (Hecaen and Kremin, 1976) it was rather a question of reconstruction, based on correct identification of
some letters in the stimulus word, by spelling out.

In contrast, this visual similarity was, for BLA and MAG (literal and sentence alexics, suffering also from a disturbance in writing -Hecaen and Kremin, 1976) and for Marshall and Newcombe's patients (1973, 1977) with visual dyslexia (and concomitant writing
problems) the result of an overall apprehension of the stimulus word by a global reading strategy.

It has furthermore been noted that visual (whole word) paralexias are usually accepted by the patients as correct readings (Patterson, 1978; Kremin, 1980). The target words yielding such visual
whole word paralexias have often been found to be relatively abstract (Morton and Patterson, 1980; Shallice and Warrington, 1980; Shallice and Coughlan, 1980; Kremin, 1980). But recently Warrington
(1981) reported a case whose visual paralexias occured predominantly
on concrete words. Such an influence of a linguistic stimulus dimension, however, has not been found with cases of "pure" (verbal)

alexia.

For some patients with pure alexia the "visual" difficulty may indeed be correlated with some perceptual problems (see Hecaen and Kremin, 1976, and Patterson, 1981, for a review). Such perceptual problems however do not necessarily occur in verbal alexia. It is clear that in some cases of word - without letter blindness visual errors are not due to a failure of visual analysis. One of Pötzl's (1928) patients could read all letters without being able to read the word. The same is true for a patient reported by Newcombe (19-79). Hecaen and Kremin (1976) mention that all their patients with verbal alexia were able to match letter strings up to eight letters in a multiple choice paradigm (where only one or two letters were varied). And Newcombe and Marshall (1981) reported that their pati- ent M. B. correctly spelled out over 60% of the stimulus letters, yet the patient could read only some 5% of the target words. (This case did not only have a reading impairment but also analogous diff- iculties in writing and spelling).

Some "spelling" readers, however, do not show a deficit in word production, provided they are given enough time (Warrington and Sha- llice, 1980). Sometimes this "spelling dyslexia" has been integra- ted into the more general impairment of simultanagnosia (Kinsbourne and Warrington, 1962). And it has often been pointed out that these letter-by-letter readers may reconstruct the whole word from their auditory (!) spelling.

In contrast to all other types of reading impaired patients re- ading aloud in (verbal) alexia without agraphia does not depend on linguistic dimensions of the stimuli: neither the part-of-speech di- mension (nouns vs function words) nor the meaningfulness (words vs nonsense syllables) plays a role for oral production. The length of the stimuli however does play an important role: short items are be- tter read than longer ones. A possible influence of the concrete/ abstract dimension of the stimuli is usually not assumed but remains controversial: Warrington and Shallice (1980) did not observe an in- fluence of this variable, whereas the (exceptional) case presented by Landis, Regard and Serrat (1980) seemed to read concrete nouns more easily.

Finally, the reading performance of patients with pure (verbal) alexia is characterized by a parallelism between reading aloud and comprehension. (Only for exceptions to this general pattern have been reported. Caplan and Hedley-White, 1974; Stachowiak and Poeck, 1976; Warrington and Shallice, 1979; Landis, Regard and Serrat, 19-80). The parallel performances in reading aloud and comprehension which are usually described for verbal alexics contrast with the di- ssociation of these processes in non "pure" cases.

Indeed, visual errors also occur in deep dyslexia, the second

variety of reading disorders defined by Marshall and Newcombe (1973).
The occurence of visual errors often even outnumbers the occurence
of semantic paralexias: Shallice and Warrington (1975) noted 61% visual errors but only 10% real semantic errors (opposed to 19% semantic derivational errors) produced by K. F., a patient similar to
G. R., the principal case of deep dyslexia (Marshall and Newcombe,
1966, 1973).

Nevertheless the occurrence of (at least some) semantic errors
is the condition <u>sine qua non</u> to define the syndrome of deep dyslexia (Marshall and Newcombe, 1973; Schwartz, Saffran and Marin, 1977;
Coltheart, 1980a).

With more cases being published it became apparent however that
deep dyslexia constitutes a symptom-complex. Most authors thus distinguish four main features :

1) The occurrence of semantic, derivational, and visual paralexias; omissions do also occur;

2) Severe or total impairment of grapheme-to-phoneme conversion as shown by poor reading of nonsense syllables;

3) Influence of the part-of-speech dimension: nouns are read
best, function words worst;

4) Influence of the concreteness/imageability dimension on
word reading.

It should be mentioned though that Coltheart (1980a) - reviewing 21 cases from the literature - listed 11 constituing features of
deep dyslexia. He claimed that the "occurrence of the semantic err-
or guarantees that the other eleven symptoms will occur" (p. 43).
This claim - however justified with reference to the cases Coltheart
reviewed - is false. Warrington and Shallice (1979) presented a case (of optic aphasia) who produced (some) semantic paralexias, but
A. R.'s reading deficit was relatively unaffected by word frequency,
word concreteness, word length or part-of-speech. Kremin (1982) mentioned more cases who had no major difficulty in reading function
words, although they produced (some) semantic paralexias. In this
context a study by Beauvois and Derouesne (1979) should also be mentioned : their patient R. G. was incapable of reading (long) nonsense syllables; while reading isolated words, he produced no semantic
error although his reading of function words and grammatical morphemes was impaired. (Again, frequency, concreteness and length of words had no main effect). The clinical existence of this syndrome of
"phonological alexia" has recently been documented by more case descriptions (Shallice and Warrington, 1980; Patterson, 1982). And it
now seems established that impairment of phonological reading by grapheme-to-phoneme conversion does not necessarily result in semantic

paralexias. Moreover, the production of semantic paralexias does
not necessarily co-occur with a reading deficit on function words.
Indeed, Caramazza, Berndt and Hart (1981) argued that an impairment
for reading function words rather co-occurs with the deep dyslexics'
difficulty to read abstract nouns. This hypothesis, however, cannot
account for R. G.'s reading either (Beauvois and Derouesne, 1979):
as mentioned before, this patient (with phonological alexia) had no
problem with the concrete/abstract dimension, although he did have
problems - in fact, the only ones - with function words and grammatical morphemes.

But let us go back to semantic paralexias. Semantic paralexias
have -(of course) - been produced before deep dyslexia was defined
as a clinical symptom complex. One of the most striking early descriptions of these errors is due to Beringer and Stein (1930) who
described a patient with so-called literal alexia.

A relationship between both literal and deep dyslexia has indeed been pointed out by some authors (Hecaen and Kremin, 1976; Marshall and Newcombe, 1977). Besides the global reading strategy which
is characteristic for both types, a certain resemblance of the reading disturbance is revealed by the occurrence of semantic paralexias
and the non-availability of phonological reading (Dubois-Charlier,
1971).

The number of semantic paralexias in word reading is subject to
a high degree of variation. Patients produced these errors within
a wide range from 69% (of total errors) to the occurrence of just
one isolated production (Kremin, 1982). The type of the semantic
relationship to the stimulus is subject to variation, too. The semantic relationship can be due to :
circumlocutions, e.g. beaver -> could be an animal, I have no idea
                                        which one
associative links, e.g. antique -> vase
adequate descriptions and/or synonyms e.g. uncle -> my father's bro-
                                                        ther;
                                    little -> small
and to shared feature responses e.g. tree -> bush;
                                    niece -> aunty.

Coltheart (1980b) examined the nature of the relationship between stimulus and semantic paralexia and tried to assess the relevance of these errors with respect to linguistic theories, that have
been proposed to explain how semantic paralexias may arise. Coltheart distinguishes two main types, associative semantic errors (merry
-> Christmas) and shared feature semantic errors, superordinates
(cattle -> animals) and co-ordinates (tulip -> crocus).

The inspection of semantic paralexias leads Coltheart to the
conclusion that "not only are there two distinct types of semantic

errors but also that the two error types require different explanations. Associative semantic errors arise via an associative link
between stimulus and response. Shared feature semantic errors arise
because some of the semantic features of the stimulus are lost or not
used during the process of deriving response from stimulus via semantic representation" (p. 156).

Coltheart discussed a possible third account of semantic errors
which has been mainly proposed by Richardson (1975) who studied G. R.
and three other deep dyslexics. According to Richardson imagery was
the prominent variable (over frequency and the concrete/abstract dimension) to account for the patients' reading errors. Richardson's
proposal clearly cannot account for many semantic errors produced by
deep dyslexics, but- following Coltheart - it may for some, especially abstract words, e.g. living room -> Oh, I know what that place
is, it is the place we go to after dinner to watch TV. - We think,
that these responses do not depend on imagery, but simply document
that the stimulus word was correctly understood and - the adequate
output logogen not forthcoming - the patient "commented" on that item. In fact some of our patients produced such adequate comments
for words which can hardly be accounted for in terms of imagery, for
example : sentimentalité -> l'amour est basé la dessus (Kremin, 1982).

Finally, it has been pointed out that semantic paralexias are
more frequently recognized as reading errors than are visual and derivational misreadings (Patterson, 1978). Marshall and Newcombe
(1977), however, noted about their initial patient G. R. (1966) :
"having made a semantic error G. R. usually considered that his response was correct, although occassionally such a response would be
preceded by the remark "I'm not sure" or succeeded by "Not quite right". He was not invariably confident about correct responses"
(p. 275).

Considering the influence of linguistic properties of the stimulus words yielding semantic paralexias, Patterson (1978) stated
that the (usually) good recognition (as opposed to erroneous production) fails when the words are close synonyms (e.g. gift -> present)
or highly abstract (oblivion -> infinity). Kremin (1980) stated yet
another relationship : patient LEC (who produced only 8 semantic paralexias) accepted the 6 semantic paralexias which had a (global)
visual resemblance with the stimulus, (e.g. flocon -> glaçon; locomotive -> automobile) as if they were visual paralexias (e.g. châtiment -> bâtiment; savoir -> ovaires). But the patient rejected the
two semantic errors without visual resemblance - and which in fact,
were comments rather than frank semantic paralexias (e.g. Raoul ->
homme.....homme; route -> ....c'est un itinéraire).

Semantic errors, finally, do not only occur on concrete words
but on abstract nouns, too (see Coltheart's review, 1980b ; Caramazza et al., 1981; Kremin, 1981b). Indeed, they also occur on

function words, since the responses of many deep dyslexic patients do not only stay within the grammatical category of function words but produce shared-feature substitutions, e.g. me -> him; her -> she; down -> up (from Coltheart, 1980b).

The relation between semantic paralexias and comprehension of the target word remains unclear (and somehow seems to depend on the perspective of the authors) : Morton and Patterson (1980) state that "in an auditory visual matching task - (one printed word, several spoken alternatives) - the patients can usually select the correct targets preference to their own semantic paralexias to these words" (p. 98). Conducting another test paradigm - (the patient had to point to the picture, from an array of 4 or 8 items, that matched a printed word) - Newcombe and Marshall (1981) noted that G. R. made a few semantic errors in this matching task which required no verbalization. The authors conclude: "we are thus compelled to invoke a central disturbance of lexical access or knowledge, although, in the case of G. R., the oral expression of this disorder is more marked in reading (and writing) than in the comprehension or expression of speech" (p. 39). In fact, Marshall and Newcombe claimed already in their initial paper (1973) that deep dyslexia cannot occur unless other aphasic features are present.

With regard to semantic paralexias we still feel like citing an earlier comment of concerned authors: "Whilst the predominance of semantic errors is fascinating, we find it difficult to state specific conclusions about their significance" (Marshall, Newcombe and Marshall, 1970, p. 421).

Errors which are phonologically similar to the stimulus seem to have merited attention only after the publication of the Marshall and Newcombe's paper (1973). Recently presented new cases (Shallice and Warrington, 1980; Deloche et al., 1982; Kremin, 1980) confirmed Marshall and Newcombe's claim that patients with surface dyslexia ought to produce a high number of neologisms. But these studies furthermore suggested that surface dyslexia can occur as a purer syndrome than the one initially described as a "partial failure" in the application of grapheme-to-phoneme correspondence rules. Indeed, the vast majority of the patients' "phonological" reading errors stemmed from a set of legal grapheme-to-phoneme candidates of the language which were assigned without context sensitivity and/or lexical knowledge (e.g. tiens /tjɛ̃/ -> /tjã/ - Deloche et al., 1982; chorus /kɔrys/ -> /ʃorys/ - Kremin, 1980).

In patient ROG (Shallice and Warrington, 1980) this reading disturbance was indeed limited to the reading of irregular words (and not due to a "partial failure" in the application of grapheme-to-phoneme correspondence rules as ruled out by Marshall and Newcombe in 1973).

Recent studies furthermore confirmed the absence of semantic
paralexias in surface dyslexic patients and the patients' possibility to read nonsense syllables. But some studies suggested that the
variable "part-of-speech" may well be a dimension in surface dyslexic reading as it is in deep dyslexia (Marcel, 1980; Kremin, 1980;
Deloche et al., 1982). (We will come back to this point later).

ROUTES, LOCATIONS, STRATEGIES

After Marshall and Newcombe's (1973) inspiring observations,
research on reading disorders became more and more a matter of theoretical concern. Deep dyslexia and surface dyslexia - both originally described as patterns of reading errors - served as prototypes
for the description of processes of reading. Indeed, most of the
authors concerned with reading assumed that there are two separate
routes for reading a given word, a direct route from print to meaning and a phonological route by grapheme-phoneme conversion. In the
framework of the information processing approach the direct route is
lexical, i.e. bypassing pre-lexical phonology and retrieving the phonology of words from the lexicon as a whole. In contrast, the phonological route is considered to be a non-lexical and rule governed
process: the letter string is pronounced by the application of grapheme-to-phoneme translation, thus treating words and non-words alike with reference to semantic access: phonological reading is supposed to allow access to the cognitive system only after the application of grapheme-to-phoneme correspondence rules, by checking procedures, (Marshall and Newcombe, 1973; Holmes, 1978; Morton and Patterson, 1980; Marcel, 1980; Patterson, 1981).

The major theoretical interest in surface dyslexia concerns the
issue of understanding a printed word from assembled phonology without intermediary semantic access. This issue remained unchanged in-
spite of the different interpretations proposed as to how phonology
may be assembled. There are indeed two main lines to account for
this procedure:

1) a non-lexical grapheme-to-phoneme algorithm would assign
the correct pronunciation of regular words; this process is abstract, even if the correspondence rules are, originally, derived from
knowledge about (the frequency of alternative pronunciations for)
words (Shallice and Warrington, 1980);

2) all orthographically allowed letter strings (words and nonsense syllables) would be read with lexical involvement. Marcel
(1980) thus rejects the distinction between lexical and non-lexical
routes: a segment will be assigned that pronunciation which most often occurs in real words. The left-to-right segmentation is over-
ridden by lexical knowledge for real morphemes. And surface dyslexic reading errors would thus occur because the orthographic specifications for some words are lost.

With reference to non-phonological reading it should be pointed out that, in contrast to other authors, Morton (1979; with Patterson, 1980) distinguishes two ways by which a phonological output can be obtained given a real word as visual input:

1) the "direct route": "after categorization of the stimulus in the visual input logogen system, information is sent directly to the output logogen where the appropriate phonological code is produced" (p. 94);

2) the "semantic route": "the word is categorized in the visual input logogen system and information is sent to the cognitive system. Here the appropriate semantics can be found and sent to the output logogen system where the appropriate phonological code could be obtained" (p. 94).

In Morton's view only (1) is, in principle, error free. This system of direct print-to-sound associations (input/output logogens) itself contains no semantic information. Recent research has indeed furnished arguments for the existence of such direct associations (Schwartz, Marin and Saffran, 1979; Schwartz, Saffran and Marin, 1980; Caramazza, Berndt and Hart, 1981; Kremin, 1981b). Especially the description of WLP's reading performance has influenced recent accounts of reading processes to be re-formulated in the frame of a three-route-model (Patterson, 1981; Newcombe and Marshall, 1981). The important observations about WLP are:

a) "That at a time when semantic knowledge was severely compromised and she was unable to access phonology for the purpose of naming or making reference, WLP retained the ability to read words aloud" (Schwartz, Saffran and Marin, 1980, p. 260);

b) "That her oral reading was not accomplished solely by the application of spelling rules" (p. 260) as shown by her successful reading aloud of exception words which do not confirm to regular spelling patterns.

Furthermore, Heilman and Rothi (1982) noted that patients (with a mixed or sensory transcortical aphasia) "can read aloud (including irregular words such as comb) almost flawlessly but are unable to comprehend what they have read"(p. 333). It thus seems that patients who supposedly have lost semantic (reading) comprehension do not (necessarily) use an a-lexical grapheme-to-phoneme route for oral reading (the use of which is claimed for surface dyslexic patients). These patients, rather, resort to using a "direct" route of word specific print-to-sound associations (visual input logogen/phonological output logogen) in accordance with the current version of the logogen model (Morton and Patterson, 1980).

If it is not patients with impaired semantic comprehension, who

then does use "phonological reading" ? Well, the patients with so-
called surface dyslexia: J. C. and S. T. (Marshall and Newcombe,
1973; Holmes, 1978), ROG (reported by Shallice and Warrington, 1980),
FRA (reported by Kremin, 1980), A. D. (reported by Deloche et al.,
1982), HAM (reported by Kremin, 1982 in press).

Especially the recently studied cases correspond to three of
the four features of surface dyslexia defined by Marshall (1976):

1) they can read even nonsense syllables,

2) they frequently produce non-lexical forms while reading
isolated words,

3) the majority of the reading errors are phonologically similar to the target word.

But HAM, FRA and even A. D. do not fulfill the fourth requirement, i.e. that their reading comprehension depends solely on the
erroneous reading response. Goldblum and Kremin (1982) studied this
problem in detail with their patient FRA. It turned out that the
patient's word comprehension was not affected by the dimension "successful vs unsuccessful oral reading". In fact, FRA understood 84%
of the target words with correct oral reading and she understood,
again, 82% of the target words in spite of an erroneous oral reading
response. These results are at variance with the postulated reading
comprehension (depending on oral output and not visual input) in surface dyslexia (Marshall and Newcombe, 1973; Holmes, 1978; Marcel,
1980).

The latter assumption, however, played the most important role
for the formulation of theoretical models with regard to reading.
Whether authors distinguished two main routes (Marshall and Newcombe, 1973; Coltheart, 1980; Shallice and Warrington, 1980) or three
possible ways to read (Morton and Patterson, 1980) their views coincided for the definition of a "Phonological" route where a phonological representation is achieved without intermediary semantic access. Indeed, all cases of surface dyslexia reported to date produced
reading errors which can mainly be accounted for by left-to-right
mapping of a phonetic value onto a graphemic item. But, what else
did the patients do ? How did they perform with reference to other
criteria of observation ? Marshall and Newcombe (1973) mention that
(only) approximately 25% of the reading errors of J. C. and S. T.
were neologisms (which seems to us a strong lexical tendency).

Holmes (1973) explicitly distinguished a "type of semantically
and/or syntactically related errors" (p. 122) for example, judgement
-> justice; govern -> governor; enlighten -> enlightening. Indeed,
J. C. confides ".... you see some of those words I recognize strai-
ght away....I don't read them, I recognize them...."(Holmes, 1973,

p. 116). If words are read (and treated) as logatomes, how do we
explain the part of speech effect found for A. D. and FRA. (function words were better read than nouns) and for J. C., too, (but in
the reverse direction) ? How do we deal with a Japanese surface dyslexic who committed semantic errors in reading kanji words (Sasanuma, 1980). How with HAM's "naming" of many written words by simultaneous gender assignment to the stimulus ? Why did FRA make many more visual errors in reading nonsense syllables than in reading real
words ? How do we deal with FRA's, A. D.'s, and HAM's preserved written word comprehension in (non-verbal) multiple choice paradigms
and lexical decision tasks ? HAM, obviously surface dyslexic and
surface dysgraphic, nevertheless showed a fair knowledge of orthography when this variable was tested in a lexical decision task: how does this result fit with the view that, "surface dyslexics have lost
those (orthographic) specifications for some words" in the input lexicon (Marcel, 1980, p. 249). Finally, how can we explain the over-
whelmingly numerous autocorrections of HAM, A. D. and FRA by an auditory access to the lexicon "by way of the intact auditory channel"
(Holmes, 1973, p. 111), especially in FRA's case whose auditory channel has been described as an "auditory analogue to deep dyslexia"
(Goldblum, 1979 and 1980 - patient B. F. being identical with FRA) ?

We mentioned elsewhere (Kremin, 1982; in press) that phonological reading (which constitutes the characteristic reading pattern of
surface dyslexic patients) might result from more than just one source of disturbance (total non availability of the semantic and/or
direct pathway). In fact, the disruption can be due to a failure of
"recognition" (at the level of the visual input logogens): the patient adopts a sounding out strategy by grapheme-to-phoneme mapping
which he disposes of; therefore words are not understood, even when
they are correctly read. This constellation occurred (but only in
some instances !) in FRA's case and in J. C. Both patients, however,
had an additional deficit to reading (and writing): they seem to have lost the orthographic specifications for (some) words. FRA had
problems discriminating real words from homophonic pseudowords (e.g.
étain (tin) vs éthin) and J. C.'s semantic comprehension of homophonic words (e.g. bee vs be) went one way or the other (Newcombe and
Marshall, 1981). Finally, the disruption can be due to a disturbance at the level of the output logogens: again, the patient opts for
phonological reading (instead of producing an omission or a vague
response "in the spere"). But in this case the written target word
is correctly understood in spite of reading errors on (at least) irregular words. This seems to be a freely chosen strategy for oral
production of (isolated) words by patients who are aware of their
general output problems: they adopt the one-to-one mapping of grapheme-to-phoneme conversion for reading aloud in order to overcome the
(aphasic!) deficit of phonemic combination. This seems to be true
for HAM.

These two levels of possible disruptions along the direct and/or semantic pathway(s) may account for phonological reading in oral production tasks. The two types of surface dyslexic patients should, however, be distinguishable by their different reading comprehension in spite of their common use of the spelling out strategy by grapheme-phoneme conversion.

The regular/irregular spelling of words does not impinge on the reading performances of patients with deep dyslexia or with phonological dyslexia. Nevertheless deep dyslexic reading cannot be accounted for solely by the nonavailability of phonological reading. Lexical variables such as the part-of-speech and the concrete/abstract dimension are also crucial features of the syndrome. As a consequence of the description of "phonological alexia" (Beauvois and Derouesne, 1979) deep dyslexia has been defined as a "multiple component syndrome" (Shallice and Warrington, 1980). In fact, already Marshall and Newcombe had claimed in their original description (1973) that deep dyslexia cannot occur unless other aphasic syndromes are present. A recent review of patients who produced paralexias in oral reading (Kremin, 1982) showed two constantly associated deficits: agraphia and the production of semantic errors in other tasks than reading aloud. Nolan and Caramazza (1982) go so far as to postulate that the defining symptoms of deep dyslexia will be observed in responses to any task which requires lexical mediation (naming, repetition, writing) since the underlying deficit is modality independent. Although we agree with Nolan and Caramazza's assumption of an underlying central deficit it should be stressed that the clinical observation of a given patient need not overtly document such a parallelism of performances. This is suggested by the relative independence of the peripheral routes and by their (possible) functioning without the lexicon. In fact, Nolan and Caramazza (in press) themselves reported another case of deep dyslexic reading, writing and naming but with relatively preserved repetition. Some other patients whose performances have been extensively investigated also show apparent dissociations with regard to the different modalities: R. G. cannot read nonsense syllables (Beauvois and Derouesne, 1979) but writes them almost perfectly to dictation (Beauvois and Derouesne, 1981). FRA, a patient with surface dyslexia (Kremin, 1980), produces numerous semantic paraphasias in word repetition (Goldblum, 1979). HAM, a patient with surface dyslexia and surface dysgraphia, produces semantic errors in oral naming and in the repetition and reading of sentences (Kremin, in press) as opposed to isolated words. The observation, finally, that deep dyslexic patients can generally repeat the words they cannot read is not necessarily a lack of thorough investigation but possibly reflects, in many cases, their possibility to use a non-lexical way for the reproduction of the same words in another modality.

Moreover the syndrome of deep dyslexia may well be the reflection of various disturbances along the semantic pathway. Indeed, different "locations" have been considered to be good candidates for

the occurrence of semantic paralexias. These errors can be due to
a central disturbance of the lexicon, but some authors (Patterson,
1978; Shallice and Warrington, 1980; Morton and Patterson, 1980) proposed that they may also occur at other levels during the treatment
of the (graphic) stimulus:

1) A. R. (Warrington and Shallice, 1979) had a selective difficulty which was limited to the visual modality. He could not access the precise meaning for words he could not read; but he could access broad categorical information about these same words. The patient produced only few semantic paralexias. Some of these errors
seem to show that the semantic error was potentially non-nominal in
nature, for example, the reading of thumb -> finger, no things, no
thimble. Shallice and Warrington (1980) comment that "such a deletion of a semantically related response for an unrelated one (things)
would not be expected for a nominal error, where the patient knows
what the word means. (A similar phenomenon occurred with KF, see
Shallice and Warrington, 1975). Overall it appears likely but by no
means conclusive that semantic errors can occur from difficulties in
semantic access" (p. 131).

2) Semantic errors can arise after semantic processing because
of problems in phonological retrieval: "the correct and full semantic code would be sent from the cognitive system to the output logogen system. The appropriate output not forthcoming and a response
being called for by the situation, the logogen nearest to threshold
activation would be selected. The printed word and the response word would thus be semantically similar" (Morton and Patterson, 1980;
p. 99). This "nominal" deficit should then be found in situations
other than reading and is in fact the most popular interpretation of
semantic errors in deep dyslexia.

3) Sometimes semantic errors are probably due to a disturbance
within the semantic system itself: some patients (see Kremin, 1982,
for review) fail to comprehend the words they cannot read. But a
general disturbance of the semantic system itself has not very often
been reported.

We think that the assumption that semantic errors can arise in
different ways might help to explain why they occur at extremely different rates in the different patients. Shallice and Warrington
(1980) distinguish indeed two types of patients and deficits with
regard to the occurrence of semantic paralexias: an "input" variety
(with relatively few semantic errors) and an "output" variety (with
abundance of semantic errors due to a "naming" deficit for the written word). "For one type an adequate semantic representation of
certain classes of visually presented words cannot be achieved, in
the other type, subsequent to adequate semantic processing, the appropriate verbal label cannot be obtained" (Shallice and Warrington,
1980, p. 138).

Visual errors might also be "located" at different levels:

1) Besides problems at the level of visual analysis, visual
errors can be due to the disruption of the visual word form itself
or of the access to it. This seems to apply for patients with pure
(verbal) alexia without agraphia. Patterson (1981) pointed out that
the functional deficit in this syndrome is not clear. Shallice and
Warrington (1980) argue that the visual input logogen system is damaged (and therefore bypassed by letter reading) whereas Patterson and
Kay (1980) argue for an impairment in the access from visual analysis
to the input logogen system. (It is clear that even the pure verbal
alexics' inability to discriminate words from non-words in lexical
decisions cannot be due to a failure in the visual analysis system:
they are capable of matching letter strings on the basis of physical
identity (Hecaen and Kremin, 1976). On rare occasions, however, this constellation occurs in "non pure" patients, too: thus A. R. (Warrington and Shallice, 1979), the patient with "semantic access dyselxia", A. R. (Deloche et al., 1982), a surface dyslexic, and RIC
(whose case study will follow) performed at (or just above) chance
level in lexical decisions on words vs non words. (It should be underlined, however, that, generally, deep dyslexics and surface dyslexics show good performance in lexical decision tests).

2) Mostly, however, visual errors occur at a "deeper" and more
central level as shown by the influence of lexical variables such as
the concrete/abstract dimension with regard to visual errors in deep
dyslexia. P. S., for example, whose phonological reading was impaired, produced significantly more visual errors on abstract than on
concrete words (Shallice and Coughlan, 1980). Moreover, the patient
has a selective comprehension deficit for abstract words which was
limited to the visual modality and not observed given auditory input.
In this respect it should be mentioned that abstract words cannot be
considered to be more "difficult" to read since the reverse error pattern (concrete words being more error prone) has recently been described, too. Indeed, Warrington (1981) presented a patient with writing and naming disturbance (object agnosia) who read abstract words
more successfully than concrete words (90/144 vs 49/144). There was
no part-of-speech effect and the concrete/abstract different was statistically more reliable than the effect of frequency. (The patien-
t's phonological reading was severely impaired). The observed pattern, again, reveals a deficit at the stage of accessing semantic representations of (some) written words. [Warrington (1981) concludes
that the concrete/abstract dimension reflects the categorical organization of semantic memory].

Yet another relationship between stimulus and response has been
established. In fact, not only did Warrington's (1981) patient read
abstract words more successfully, but it was also observed that "when
a visual error occurred the response tended to be more abstract than
the stimulus word" (p. 180); e.g. needle -> neither; Jelly -> jolly.

This abstracting tendency of the patient's visual errors responses was highly significant. Similarly, it has been observed that patients who have difficulties in reading abstract words tend to give a response word which is more concrete than the stimulus, e.g. univers -> un hiver; châtiment -> bâtiment (Kremin, 1980).

3) Visual errors may occur within the phonological route as well. FRA and HAM, our surface dyslexic patients, made indeed visual errors while reading nonsense syllables (39% and 31%) and words (10% and 30%). Both patients, however, often autocorrected those visual errors on both words and nonsense syllables. [This behavior of (at least some) surface dyslexic patients contrasts with the behavior of deep and phonological dyslexics who do not autocorrect their visual errors which arise along the lexical pathways]. Further evidence for the occurrence of visual errors along the phonological route can be drawn from misreadings where visual and phonological errors occur in combination on the same stimulus. One of our patients, for example, read steak (stɛk)-> stre-ak....ste-ak thus correcting the visual error but sparing the phonological error which is due to the left-to-right mapping by grapheme-to-phoneme conversion.

Let us go back to the two syndromes (deep dyslexia and phonological dyslexia) which are both characterized by a phonological reading deficit, that is inoperativity of grapheme-to-phoneme conversion as shown by the patients' inability to read nonsense syllables. Frank semantic paralexias have never been reported for phonological dyslexia but are a defining feature of deep dyslexia. Omissions are often reported for deep dyslexic patients but are negligible in phonological dyslexia. Derivational errors, in contrast, are produced by both varieties. [Shallice and Warrington (1980) stated 6% and 32% derivational errors for deep dyslexics; Beauvois and Derouesne (1979b) and Patterson (1982) reported 22% and 23% for their patients G. R. and A. M.].

The degree of abstractness of content words plays an important role in deep dyslexia but is irrelevant to phonological dyslexia. The part-of-speech effect, characteristic for both syndromes, is limited to the reading of function words in phonological dyslexia (verbs, nouns and adjectives being equally well read - see Patterson, 1982). Like deep dyslexics, phonological dyslexics mostly produce functor substitutions, generally on the basis of visual similarity, e.g. if -> it; with -> which. Like deep dyslexics they recognize function words in lexical decision tasks (Patterson, 1982). In phonological dyslexia the recognition and production of affixes and inflections can be selectively disturbed for written material without any impairment in oral comprehension and spontaneous production (Beauvois and Derouesne, 1979b). Indeed, the reading deficit in phonological dyslexia can be limited to the production of affixes in reading aloud, with function words spared. This is the case for GRN and BTT, two patients seen by Shallice and Warrington (1980).

It is clear from the comparison of the two syndromes that the occurrence of semantic paralexias does not result from an impairment of grapheme-to-phoneme reading since phonological dyslexics have no greater use of pre-lexical or non-lexical phonology than do (at least some) deep dyslexics. Patterson (1982) points out that "it remains a possibility however, that a deficit in assembling phonology from print is implicated in those symptoms shared by the two syndromes. Notable feature which A. M. shared with deep dyslexic patients were derivational paralexias and difficulty in reading function words". However, the following reservations ought to be made :

1) Bradley's (1978) results with regard to normal readers' performance on function words have not been confirmed by Gordon and Caramazza's recent investigation (1982). Gordon and Caramazza's failure to find a difference in reaction time in lexical decisions for open- and closed- class items thus leaves the question whether function words require a special treatment or status (in normal reading) open to future research.

2) Funnell (1983) reports a case of phonological dyslexia who read words (87%), function words (91%), and affixed words (87%) equally well in spite of the (total) unavailability of the peripheral reading by grapheme-to-phoneme conversion.

These findings from both normal and pathological subjects are of crucial impact for the description of the processes of reading. Funnell's study suggests indeed that there is only one (!) syndrome of "phonological" dyslexia: patients who are able to read all words of the language but no nonsense syllables. These patients (supposedly) use the direct pathway (visual input logogen -output logogen) .... as do the subjects without semantic reading comprehension we cited before. As a consequence of Funnell's case study all the other described cases of so-called "phonological dyslexia" (Beauvois and Derouesne, 1979; Shallice and Warrington, 1980; Patterson, 1982) ought to be re-viewed as multiple component syndromes which arise from a disruption of the direct pathway and thus reflect various different malfunctionings of the semantic-lexical route (as does deep dyslexia).

DYSLEXIA AND APHASIA : A CASE STUDY

Working on routes, locations, and isolated words only few of the authors concerned with theoretical models expect with Marshall and Newcombe (1977) "the nature of the dyslexia do vary with the degree and type of concomitant dysphasia and hence with the underlying anatomy" (p. 262). Clinical experience, however, often suggests that the difficulties in reading and in speech seem to reflect common underlying pathology. Indeed, patients with posterior and with anterior aphasia seem to be dissociable by relatively selective impairments in the comprehension of written material: patients with

anterior aphasias exhibit a syntactic disturbance in sentence comprehension (Zurif, Caramazza, and Myerson, 1972; Kolk, 1978; Berndt
and Caramazza, 1980) whereas patients with posterior aphasias show
an impairment of the semantic type (Von Stockert, 1972, 1976; Kremin
and Goldblum, 1975). This double dissociation has also been reported for the patients' oral reading performances. Thus, Marin, Saffran and Schwartz (1976) describe two asyntactic patients who, in reading sentences aloud, "made errors with precisely those kinds of
words which were absent or inappropriate in their spontaneous speech" (p. 877), e.g.
            Dinner is on the table -> dinner...dinner is.....the table.
            They walk to school -> this walking to school.

      This reading pattern was in sharp contrast with the performance
of a fluent aphasic "whose reading of sentences also reflected his
difficulties in spontaneous speech" (p. 877), e.g.
            Dinner is on the table -> Wendy is on the trip.
            They walk to school -> They work to school.

      Marin et al. furthermore investigated the reading of isolated
words in these patients. The results of this study supported the
authors' initial observations according to word type: "the two non-
fluent patients, H. T. and V. S., made three times as many errors on
functions words as on content words while the fluent patient, J. D.,
showed just the reverse pattern of errors" (p. 878).

      A study of two other cases by Friederici and Schoenle (1980)
confirmed Marin, Saffran and Schwartz's previous findings. Friederici and Schoenle furthermore observed that reading errors of the fluent aphasic mainly resulted in neologistic reproductions of content words whereas the non-fluent patient predominantly produced word
substitutions (on both vocabulary types). Even in one group study
the Broca's aphasics (n = 18) were worse in reading grammatical particles in comparison with concrete nouns (although the difference
was only about 10% - Gardner and Zurif, 1975). But from the latter
study it is not clear whether the spontaneous speech of the Broca
aphasics was defined only on a fluency scale or whether the patient's
speech was actually telegrammatic. If they had agrammatism in their
spontaneous speech Gardner and Zurif's results that the Broca' aphasics read about 75% of the function words correctly would be at variance with the other studies mentioned above.

      Indeed, the literature focussing on patients' acquired reading
disturbances often overlaps Broca's aphasia and the syndrome of deep
dyslexia. Although most of the studied cases presented a Broca's
aphasia as well, it seems now experimentally established that the
two syndromes need not occur in association : a study by Beauvois
and Derouesne (1979) showed that disturbance of the grapheme-to-phoneme conversion does not necessarily imply the other impairments
associated with deep dyslexia, Kremin (1980) presented a case with

typical features of deep dyslexia but normal spontaneous speech, and
Caramazza, Berndt and Hart (1981) reported one patient with the clinical syndrome of Broca's aphasia but who read content and function
words equally well (and, moreover, 57% of the nonsense syllables !).
So the empirical evidence concerning the relation between dyslexia
and aphasia remains contradictory, and the question is far from being
systematically explored. To present additional information concerning the complex of problems that remain open to question in this regard, we report a case study of a Broca aphasic with totally telegrammatic spontaneous speech.

CASE DESCRIPTION :

     Patient RIC, a 54 year old right-handed man (who has a degree
in philosophy) was hospitalized on March 7, 1980, because of the su-
dden onset of total hemiplegia and aphasia. The medical report mentions that there were no signs of agnosia, finger agnosia, ideomotor
apraxia, right-left indistinction, visuomotor ataxia or abnormal ocu-
lomotricity. But the patient was found to have a right homonymous
hemianopia, right hypoesthesis of the right side of the body, (apparently) a right sensitive extinction, a right Babinski, a right aste-
reagnosia, and a central facial paralysis. There was the impression
of a visual neglect, but when the patient had to check lines drawn
all over a sheet of paper he did satisfactorily. The patient showed
acalculia, but he could name isolated numbers. A CT Scan of March
17, 1980, showed a large lesion covering the totality of the left
Sylvian territory, due to a thrombosis of the left internal carotid
(Doppler effect).

     Assessment of general language functions:

     When we saw the patient at the end of March, 1980, his sponta-
neous speech was unchanged and telegrammatic, e.g. ".....alimentati-
on....faim......beaucoup faim......non non....euh.....trois heures
.....trois heures....coucher....trois heures....bien soucieux......
soucieux....paralysie....". ("...food....hunger....much hunger....
no no ...ah...three hours...three hours...(to) sleep....three hours
....very anxious.....anxious....paralysis...."). Articulatory difficulties was limited to the execution of simple commands. The patient named 14/20 objects correctly, half of the errors being semantic
paraphasias. Repetition of words (N = 90) was 71% correct, oral reading of words (N = 80) was 72% correct. In a written sentence arrangement test (cf. Kremin and Goldblum, 1975) the patient totally
failed when all elements of the surface structure were given (e.g.
le panier contient des pommes -> pommes panier le contient des;
l'homme ferme la fenêtre -> l' la ferme fenêtre homme). But he succeeded in rearranging half of the (short) sentences into the right
actor-action-object relationship when he was asked "to write a tele-
gram" with the lexical words exclusively (e.g. panier continent pommes; homme ferme fenêtre).

TABLE 1. Percentage of oral reading errors

```
Nouns (total N = 160)          32,25%
    High Freq.  (N = 40)       25%
    Low Freq.   (N = 40)       40%
    Concrete    (N = 60)       30%
    Abstract    (N = 20)       35%

Function words  (N = 40)       35%

Logatomes       (N = 60)       93%
```

SPECIAL TESTING

Oral reading of isolated words

The patient was given 260 stimuli to read (120 nouns, 40 function words, 60 nonsense syllables). The results of his oral reading
performance (see Table 1) indicate that the patient is totally incapable of proceeding by grapheme-to- phoneme correspondence rules, as
shown by his inability to read nonsense syllables. It can furthermore be seen that the patient, in spite of his agrammatic spontaneous speech, has no special problem with the reading of function words in comparison with nouns. The concrete/abstract dimension of the
stimuli does not seem to be a crucial variable either. Only nouns
with a low frequency of occurrence seem to be more difficult to read
aloud.

Complexity of the stimuli and oral output

As function words are usually shorter than content words we wanted to avoid an artifact in reading performances by controlling the
oral output. We therefore checked for a possible general articulatory problem in oral output by comparing the influence of the number
of syllables of the stimuli to be reproduced in two oral reproduction
tasks, repetition and reading of isolated words. As can be seen in
Table 2 the number of syllables is a crucial variable in both oral
reproduction tasks. We therefore constructed new lists of (short)
words for the patient to read, taking into account the complexity of
the stimuli : (1) abstract and concrete nouns with as much similarity as possible (e.g. âme : soul vs âne : donkey), (2) homophones of
lexical items and functors (e.g. lait : milk vs les : the, plural),
and (3) nouns and homophonic logatomes (e.g. coq : cock vs kok).
The patient's reading performance on these 160 new items is shown in
Table 3. Even with this controlled list the preliminary results
(cf. Table 1) are confirmed: patient RIC has no selective reading
disturbance on the variables tested, the only exception being his
difficulty in reading nonsense syllables. In fact, the patient was
able to read many words correctly that never occur in his speech,

TABLE 2.   Percentage of errors in two tasks of oral output

	Number of syllables			
	1	2	3	4+
Repetition (N = 90)	–	20%	33%	50%
Reading (N = 80)	16%	36%	27%	40%

TABLE 3.   Percentage of reading errors on items controlled for complexity

Nouns
       Concrete (N = 20)   25%
       Abstract (N = 20)   25%

Homophones I
       Lexical items (N = 30)   30%
       Function words (N= 30)   32%

Homophones II
       Nouns   (N = 30)   20%
       Logatomes (N = 30)   70%

especially grammatical particles (prepositions, conjunctions, and auxiliaries as well as pronouns and articles in the various forms that occur in French).

Analysis of reading errors

Combining the different lists of lexical items the patient made a total of 77 errors on 260 content words. In terms of error analysis the breakdown of patient RIC's reading performance is :

Visual (cigale - cigare)	44	(57.2%)
Neologism (flacon - flaclon)	16	(20.7%)
Derivational (douleus -douleureux)	10	(13.0%)
Semantic (punaise - puce)	5	(6.5%)
Other (album - chaud)	1	(1.3%)
Ommission	1	(1.3%)

This error pattern is close to those of deep dyslexic patients. But the occurrence of visual and of neologistic errors is rather high, and contrasts with a rather low incidence of semantic paralexias. The neologistic productions were, by the way, always visually close to the target.

We also checked whether the concrete/abstract dimension had an influence on the production of visual errors. Combining the lists

TABLE 4. Oral reading errors with reference to the concrete/abstract dimension

	Total errors	Visual errors Words	Visual errors Neologisms	Semantic errors	Omissions
Concrete Nouns (N = 80)	23	12	10	1	0
Abstract Nouns (N = 40)	12	6	5	0	1

(mentioned in Table 1 and Table 3), we analyzed the errors made on concrete and abstract words. It is evident from Table 4 that the concrete/abstract dimension has no influence on the production of visual errors, neither in terms of whole word reading errors nor in terms of (visually similar) neologistic productions.

It should be mentioned that the visual errors (criterion : at least 50% of the letters of the target word to be reproduced) do not show visual regularities: responses might be shorter than their stimulus (e.g. religion -> region) or longer (e.g. toit - toilette); most have only an "overall" resemblance with the stimulus (e.g. cidre -> cigare; acte -> acide; voeux -> veau). But there is a pronounced tendency of stimuli and responses to match at the beginning of the word.

Let us now have a look at the five "semantic" errors produced by RIC : punaise (bug) -> puce (flea); cigarette (cigarette) -> cigare (cigar); refrigérateur (refrigerator) -> friseur (freezer) ; pagaille (disorder) -> bagarre (scuffle); sang (blood) -> rouge (red) (Is that correct ?) sang ....hematome. It is evident that cigarette -> cigar, a visual-semantic error, could be just another instance of his numerous visual misreadings. This argument is strengthened by the fact that the patient misread both cigale and cidre as "cigare" (and this was not due to a simple perseveration effect). The misreading punaise -> puce has some visual elements as well as refrigerateur -> friseur, although not attaining the 50% cut-off criterion. But, again, the patient produced the same response to another word (pu -> puce), and a "telescoping" reading such as religion -> région might also account for régrigérateur -> friseur. The only "real" semantic error occured when we started asking the patient for the meaning of what he read; after having produced a neologism on the item richesse, and after having been asked whether he understood the target [he said he did not], RIC produced sang -> rouge. When asked whether his reading was right he corrected: sang.....hématome. These details of the patient's reading performance indicate that he actually produced less than the catalogued 6.5% of semantic errors,

TABLE 5. Oral reading errors on short items

Homophones	Number of errors	Production of words	Production of non-words
Nouns (N = 30)	10	9(90%)	1(10%)
Functors (N = 30)	9	8(91%)	1(9%)
Logatomes (N = 30)	21	16(73%)	5(27%)

probably none. We then looked at the distribution of reading errors
(in terms of real word and neologistic productions) on words and nonsense syllables (total of all lists). The patient produced 41% neologistic responses to real words and 42% real word responses to non-
word targets. It is impossible to conclude whether this almost
random difference in performance is due to a problem of the complexity of the visual input, the complexity of the oral output, or both;
we therefore compared the reading performances on the short words
exclusively. The results, shown in Table 5, indicate that reading
errors on short words result in the production of real words. They
furthermore indicate that there is no difference in the error pattern
for content and function words when complexity is controlled.
Reading errors on short logatomes, on the contrary, result in even
more real word productions than on complex ones (73% vs 42%).

Comprehension of written words

Unfortunately, we were unable to test this aspect of the patient's reading performance in full because of time pressure. On a
visual lexical decision task (10 words and 20 non-words) the patient
accepted all the words but, also, 13/20 logatomes. When we went through the list again item-by-item (we thought the patient had not
understood the task) he again accepted all the real words but also
9/20 logatomes apparently on the basis of some visual resemblance.
For example, when asked what stilotte, a non-word he had accepted,
means, the patient said "écrire" [probably referring to stylo (pencil)].

Comprehension of the words the patient read erroneously was not
tested systematically enough to present quantitative date. But it
can be mentioned that, whenever he produced a real word, his understanding of it coincided with his own misreading (e.g. acte -> acide
(?) chimie; tas -> tasse (?) café ; cigale -> cigare (?) fumer).
When the patient produced a neologistic form his reading comprehension did not show a systematic pattern: (a) comprehension could refer to the target (e.g. Moise -> /moisie/ ..../mouzon/ (?)bible);
(b) comprehension had no obvious relation to either target or response (e.g. fugue -> /fu/ (?) sobre; grue -> /kru/ (?) oiseau;

(c) the patient admitted that he did not understand (e.g. richesse
-> /rickop/ (?) non).

TABLE 6. Oral reading of semantically charged sentences.

	Correct	false	omission
Lexical items (N = 50)	25 (50%)	12 (24%)	13 (26%)
Function words (N= 37)	0	0	37 (100%)

Oral reading of sentences

     We constructed two lists of 10 sentences each: the first list
was "semantically overcharged" and controlled for syntactic complexity [NP + VP (V + NP + PP)], e.g. "le cambrioleus cache les bijoux
volés de la comtesse". The second list was "syntactically overcharged" and controlled for length e.g. "je le lui ai envoyé sans qu'il
le veuille". Patient RIC's reading performance of the first list is
represented in Table 6. Although we repeatedly insisted that he was
to read all the words of a sentence, the patient totally omitted function words (which in this list were limited to articles and the
preposition "de" of the French genitive construction). Half of the
lexical items were correctly read, one quarter were erroneously reproduced and one quarter were omitted. It should be noted that all
reading errors resulted in real word productions, all of them having
a derivational relationship to the target (e.g. cache -> caché ;
volés -> voleus; vitrier -> vitreaux]. No frank semantic paralexia
was produced. The patient's production in (semantic) sentence reading had a certain resemblance with his telegrammatic spontaneous speech: "caché ....bijoux...voleus...comtesse" (le cambrioleur chache
les bijoux volés de la comtesse); "piano....valse...rêver....réper-
toire" (le pianiste joue une valse rêveuse de son répertoire). Omissions and reading errors did not "favor" one of the grammatical categories of the lexical items (nouns, verbs, adjectives). It is worth mentioning that at first the patient did not want to read the
"syntactic" sentences of the second list. When he finally tried,
the quantitative pattern of performance (cf. Table 7) resembled that
of the first list: nouns were more easily read than functors, and
(with the exception of one neologism) the erroneous reading of lexical items led to visual and derivational relationships (e.g. expérience -> expert; rendre -> rendu; tardivement -> tard). Only two lexical items (8%) were omitted. Function words, by contrast, were
mostly omitted (62%). It is noteworthy though that in this second
list of sentences function words were, at least, produced and, in
28% of the instances, produced correctly. The false reproductions
of function words stayed within the grammatical category of functors. But these errors were only visually similar, i.e. without any

TABLE 7. Oral reading of syntactically charged sentences

	Correct	false	omission
Lexical items (N = 25)	17 (68%)	6 (24%)	2 (8 %)
Function words (N = 84)	23 (28%)	9 (10%)	52 (62%)

"semantic" relationship [e.g. ne (no) -> le (the) ; quoique(although)
-> quoi (that) ; sans (without) -> dans (in)]. The reproduction of
these (syntactic) sentences was merely telegrammatic, but totally de-
viant syntactically and semantically: "elle le fut mis elle courant
avant départ" (target: elle ne fut mise au courant qu'avant son
départ).

Comparison of reading and repetition

     We wanted to control whether the patient's "agrammatic" repro-
duction of sentences was specific to the visual modality. Hence a
list of (shorter) sentences was administered for oral repetition.
For the "semantic" sentences (N = 10) (e.g. la locomotive siffle dans la station) the pattern of performance turned out to be the same
as in reading: 28/40 lexical items were correctly repeated (there
were 11 omissions and 1 autocorrected semantic paraphasia), but only
4/40 function words were reproduced, the others being omitted. The
patient refused to repeat a list of "syntactic" sentences.

Comprehension of written sentences

     The above-mentioned "semantic" sentences of the first list were
combined with 20 other sentences of the same complexity: half of them were correct. French sentences but without any special semantic
cohesion (AA), while the other 10 sentences were impossible constructions (B) e.g.
                    (A) le cambrioleus cache les bijoux volés de la con-
                        tesse.
                    (AA) le promeneur aperçoit la vache immobile du voisin.
                    (B) le vétérinaire tond la chapelle poussiéreuse du
                        notaire.
The patient had to judge which of these were possible French sentences. He missed only one of the A-sentences and accepted only one
of the B-sentences; but he refused 7/10 of the possible AA-senten-
ces. These performances seem to indicate that the patient preserved
some (semantic) comprehension of written sentences: when the words
of a sentence were semantically "coherent" and "in the sphere", he
probably proceeded by associating the isolated words and accepted
the sentence. But without any strong semantic cues, such as in the
AA sentences, patient RIC judged possible sentence to be impossible.

Understanding of "syntactic" sentences was tested by a word-pronoun-paraphrase sentence test. The patient had a written target sentence with a multiple choice of 4 "paraphrases" (one correct; one possible but not correct in this context; two impossible), e.g. la mère lave le linge: Il la lave
                     Elle lui lave
                     Elle le lave
                     Le elle lave.
The patient succeeded in none of the 26 items tested.

SUMMARY

     Patient RIC's oral reading of single items bears some resemblance with the error pattern produced by deep dyslexic patients: a disturbance of the grapheme-phoneme conversion system (as shown by the patient's impaired reading of nonsense syllables) and the production of (rare) semantic paralexias. But the patient's reading performance also contrasts from those of deep dyslexics in several aspects:
1. There was no "agrammatism" with regard to the reading of isolated words: function words and nouns were of equal difficulty.

2. The patient's reading performance did not show any influence of the concrete/abstract dimension. This statement holds for the quantitative and for the qualitative error pattern, that is visual errors did not occur more often with abstract words than with concrete words;

3. The patient's written comprehension (when tested by lexical decisions) was very impaired;

4. All but one "semantic" paralexia reproduced visual elements of the stimulus as well. The only "real" semantic error was produced (and autocorrected) in a situation of reading comprehension. (Moreover, the production of semantic errors was not limited to concrete stimulus words but occured with abstract words, too).
However, the patient's oral reading of units larger than the isolated word shows a totally different pattern of performance. Indeed, the reading of sentences resulted in agrammatic productions where grammatical particles were mostly or totally omitted. This pattern thus contrasts with the patient's reading of isolated words. But it parallels spontaneous output (and the repetition of sentences). Erroneous reading of the lexical items of a sentence led to derivational errors exclusively (that is to errors with a semantic relationship to the stimulus, e.g. expérience -> expert), whereas the errors on isolated words were predominantly visual in nature, e.g. cigale (cicada) -> cigare (cigar).

     The patient's reading comprehension of isolated words was severely disturbed: he performed at chance level in lexical decisions, mainly by accepting nonsense syllables on the basis of some visual resemblance. Reading comprehension of sentences was also impaired. But at the semantic level there was some spared comprehension when the lexical items were semantically coherent and "in the sphere". Without such strong semantic cues possible sentences were judged to be impossible. Syntactic comprehension (in a word-pronoun-paraphrase test) was none. Moreover, the patient did not succeed in sentence arrangement when all elements of the surface structure had to be manipulated (lexical items and functors). But he demonstrated some comprehension of the actor-action-object relationship when the (same) sentences were to be arranged as "telegrams", that is without any grammatical items.

COMMENT

This case, again, demonstrates that the two syndromes, Broca's aphasia and deep dyslexia, need not occur in association. In fact, Kremin (1980) presented a case with normal spontaneous language but deep dyslexic reading of isolated words, and Caramazza, Berndt and Hart (1981) described a patient with Broca's aphasia but spared reading of isolated words (lexical items and function words) and, moreover, relatively good reproduction of nonsense syllables (57.5%). Our case furthermore demonstrates that not all Broca aphasia are agrammatic or deep dyslexic readers (when presented with isolated words). This seems to be true even for cases with a malfunction of the grapheme-to-phoneme conversion system as shown by patient RIC. In fact, RIC's reading of isolated words was not affected by any of the usually described lexical variables for deep dyslexia: there was neither an influence of the concrete/abstract dimension nor a part-of-speech effect nor did the patient produce frank semantic paralexias. (The only variable which affected the patient's reading of isolated words, frequency, is a general linguistic variable and not specific for reading and/or the presence of aphasia).

We already pointed out that RIC suffered from an impairment of the grapheme-phoneme pathway. He furthermore has a "lexical" reading strategy as shown by the fact that nonsense syllables were mostly read as real words. But does the patient read by a visuo-semantic pathway the use of which is usually claimed for deep dyslexic patients ? We think that he does not on the basis of the following arguments concerning his reading of isolated words:
 - as mentioned before, the patient did not produce any frank semantic paralexia;
 - no lexical variable intervened on his reading of isolated words in spite of his general agrammatic disturbance;
 - erroneous reading of functors did not result in omissions but in visual errors without any semantic relationship (most of them staying within the category of functors, but some of them were out of category).
 - his word comprehension was not superior to his reading performance.

    The patient's reading strategy was a guessing strategy, mainly
relying on the visual configuration of the beginning of the stimulus. So, besides his inability to use grapheme-to-phoneme correspondence rules, the patient sometimes did not achieve the correct visual word form. But his errors were not characterized by any lexical
dimension.

    This case would thus seem to provide strong evidence for the
role of word-specific print-to-sound associations in reading, the
existence of which was claimed by Morton on the basis of theoretical
reflections. According to Morton (1980) a direct reading mechanism
proceeds by automatically mapping the visual word-form (visual input
logogen) and a stored phonological representation (phonological output logogen). This direct pathway contains the notion of "wordness"
but no semantic information. And Schwartz, Marin and Saffran (1979)
presented indeed a case whose preserved oral reading could not be
semantically mediated because of a progressive dementia.

    We tentatively draw another argument for the existence of a di-
rect visuo-phonological pathway by comparing our patient's performances in word and in sentence reading: RIC's reading of isolated content words resulted in 77% of visual errors (words and neoforms) without any lexical relationship to the stimulus. But erroneous reading of content words presented in the frame of a sentence exclusively resulted in real word productions having a derivational relationship with the target. Word reading in sentences thus was lexical in
contrast with the reading of isolated words. We think, indeed, that
the reading of sentences is (almost) always mediated by a linguistic
processing system, whereas the reading of isolated words can be but
must not necessarily be mediated by the cognitive system.   The same argument might explain the dramatic dissociaton of reading performances with regard to grammatical words: in isolation none was omitted (1/3 being read mistakenly) but when they occur in sentences
2/3 or all of them were omitted. Reading of sentences (as well as
their repetition) usually (but not necessarily) implies treatment in
linguistic processing system....as does spontaneous production.
RIC's sentence reading thus reveals the agrammatism of Broca's aphasia. (By "agrammatism" we understand a general syntactic processing
deficit the existence of which has been shown by various authors for
the excessive as well as receptive faculties of Broca aphasics -see
Berndt and Caramazza, 1980).

CONCLUDING REMARKS

    We think that the implications from our case study with regard
to the information processing approach and to future research on acquired reading disturbances are clear: models concerned with processes of reading cannot be based solely on the reading of isolated
words. Because of this (initial) restriction we have been confronted with some puzzling and contradictory dissociations, but evidently

in appearance only. By extending the information processing approach to reading units larger than the isolated word, many divergencies disappear and the functional relation between reading deficits
and aphasic disturbances becomes apparent and understandable. With
some minor reservations the proposed models (Morton and Patterson,
1980; Newcombe and Marshall, 1981) are adequate to describe the empirical data when they are referred to in a frame of reference larger than the isolated word. It seems obvious to us that the reading
of sentences need not be in parallel with the reading of isolated
words. But the instances of such remarks are rare in the current
literature. The only recent investigation has been undertaken by
Caramazza, Berndt and Hart (1981) who studied word and sentence reading of four patients with Broca's aphasia. A reanalysis of their
data shows that two patients read function words better in isolation
than in the frame of a sentence, one patient made more errors on isolated nouns than on the same category of words in a sentence frame.
In fact, one patient did not have problems with single function words (as compared to single nouns) but was dramatically impaired while
reading function words in a sentence. Patient B. D. thus resembles
our patient RIC (but differs from the latter by relatively preserved
reading of nonsense syllables). Some more hints suggesting that sentence reading is not necessarily dependent on the same mechanisms
of information treatment can be found in the literature. Kremin (in
press) observed that HAM, a patient with surface dyslexia, produced
phonemic paraphasias as well as verbal and semantic substitutions
in the repetition and reading of sentences, that is when (supposedly) the cognitive system was engaged. Semantic treatment of sentences thus contrasted with a peripheral treatment of single items in
reading and in repetition. The same interpretation might be drawn
from data concerning a case of deep agraphia. Bub and Kertesz's
(1982) patient read and repeated words flawlessly when presented in
isolation. But the oral reading of sentences "was markedly telegra-
phic, paralleling spontaneous output" (p. 155); and when sentences
were used as stimuli in repetition, "the response was halting and
non-fluent with word-finding difficulty and phonemic paraphasia"
(p. 149).

     Moreover, Deloche and Andreewsky (in press) note (without givi-
ng more details) : "some deep dyslexic patients who do not produce
semantic errors while reading aloud single words (they do produce
them for sentences) are labelled "phonological alexics" (footnote
2). Even J. C. one of the two original cases with surface dyslexia
(Marshall and Newcombe, 1973) did not read single words in the same
way he read sentences: "when reading sentences or longer examples
of continuous text J. C. is able to use the syntactic and semantic
context quite well; he accordingly makes fewer errors and can produce many of the irregular words that he is unable to read as isolated items" (Newcombe and Marshall, 1981, p. 36). It seems to us that not only do we need to study reading disturbances in a frame larger than the reading of single items but we should also be (more)

concerned "with the additional dysphasic symptoms which seem to accompany the component features of an error taxonomy" (Marshall and
Newcombe, 1977, p. 257). Such an approach may even 'rehabilitate'-
from a different perspective however - the syndrome of "sentence dyslexia" which, somehow, remains neglected.

REFERENCES

Ajax, E. T. - Acquired dyslexia: A comparative study of two cases.
    Archives of Neurology, 1964, 11, 66-72.
Ajax, E. T. - Dyslexia without agraphia. Archives of Neurology,
    1967, 17, 645-652.
Alajouanine, T.; Lermitte, F. & Ribaucourt-Ducarne, B. De. Le ale-
    xies agnosiques et aphasiques. In T. Alajouanine (Ed.),
    Les grandes activités du lobe occipital. Paris: Masson, 1960.
Andreewsky, E. & Seron, X. - Implicit processing of grammatical ru-
    les in a case of agrammatism. Cortex, 1975, 11, 379-390.
Beauvois, M. F. & Derouesne, J. - Phonological alexia - Three disso-
    ciations. Journal of Neurology, Neurosurgery and Psychiatry,
    1979, 42, 1115-1124. a.
Beauvois, M. F. & Derouesne, J. - Data about phonological alexia
    (personal communication). 1979 b.
Beauvois, M. F. & Derouesne, J. - Lexical or orthographic agraphia.
    Brain, 1981, 104, 21-49.
Benson, D. F. - The third alexia. Archives of Neurology, 1977, 34,
    327-331.
Beringer, K. & Stein, J. - Analyse eines Falles von "reiner" Alexie.
    Zeitschrift für die gesamte Neurologie und Psychiatrie, 1930,
    123, 472-478.
Berndt, R. S. & Caramazza, A. - A redefinition of the syndrome of
    Broca's aphasia: Implications for a neuropsychological model of
    language. Applied Psycholinguistics, 1980, 1, 225-278.
Bradley, D. C. - Computational distinctions of vocabulary type.
    Unpublished Ph. D. thesis, MIT, Cambridge, Massachussets. 1978.
Bub, D. & Kertesz, A. - Deep Agraphia. Brain and language, 1982,
    17, 146-165.
Caplan, L. R. & Hedley-White, T. - Cueing and memory dysfunction in
    alexia without agraphia: a case report. Brain, 1974, 97,
    251-262.
Caramazza, A; Berndt, R. S. & Hart, J. - Agrammatic reading. In
    F. J. Pirozzolo and M. C. Wittrock (Eds) Neuropsychological and
    Cognitive Processes in Reading. New York: Academic Press, 1981.
Coltheart, M. - Deep Dyslexia: a review of the syndrome. In M. Colt-
    heart, K. E. Patterson and J. C. Marshall (Eds) Deep Dyslexia.
    London: Routledge and Kegan Paul, 1980 a.
Coltheart, M. - The semantic error: types and theories. In M. Colt-
    heart, K. E. Patterson and J. C. Marshall (Eds) Deep Dyslexia.
    London: Routledge and Kegan Paul, 1980 b.

Coltheart, M. - Reading, phonological recoding, and deep dyslexia. In M. Coltheart, K. E. Patterson and J. C. Marshall (Eds), Deep Dyslexia. London: Routledge and Kegan Paul, 1980 c.

Cumming, W. J. K., Hurwitz, L. J. and Perl, N. T. (1970) - A study of a patient who had alexia without agraphia. Journal of Neurology, Neurosurgery and Psychiatry, 1970, 33, 34-39.

Dejerine, J. - Sur un cas de cécité verbale suivi d'autopsie. Mémoires de la Société de Biologie, 1891, 197-201.

Dejerine, J. - Contribution à l'étude anatomo-pathologique et clinique des différentes variétés de cécité verbale. Mémoires de la Société de Biologie, 1892, 4, 61-90.

Deloche, G.; Andreewsky, E. & Desi, M. - Surface dyslexia: A case report and some theoretical implications to reading models. Brain and language, 1982, 15, 11-32.

Deloche, G. & Andreewsky, E. - From Neuropsychological data to reading mechanisms. International Journal of Psychology, in Press.

Dubois-Charlier, F. - Approche neurolinguistique du problème de l'alexie pure. Journal de Psychologie Normale et Pathologique, 1971, 1, 39-68.

Friederici, A. D. & Schoenle, P. W. - Computational dissociation of two vocabulary types: Evidence from aphasia. Neuropsychologia, 1980, 18, 11-20.

Funnell, E. - Phonological processes in reading: new evidence from acquired dyslexia. British Journal of Psychology, 1983, in press.

Gardner, H. & Zurif, E. - Bee but not be: Oral reading of simple word in aphasia and alexia. Neuropsychologia, 1975, 13, 181-190.

Geschwind, N. - The anatomy of acquired disorders of reading. In J. Money (Ed.) Reading Disability. Baltimore: Johns Hopkins Press, 1962.

Geschwind, N. - Disconnection syndromes in animals and man. Brain, 1965, 88, 237-294; 585-644.

Geschwind, N. & Fusillo, M. - Color naming deficits in association with alexia. Archives of Neurology, 1966, 15, 137-146.

Goldblum, M. C. - Auditory analogue of deep dyslexia. In O. Creutzfeld, H. Scheich & C. Schreiner (Eds) Experimental brain research, Supplementum II : Hearing mechanisms and speech. Berlin: Springer-Verlag, 1979.

Goldblum, M. C. - Un équivalent de la dyslexie profonde dans la modalité auditive. In Etudes Neurolinguistiques. Université de Toulouse, Le Mirail, Grammatica, 1980, 7, 157-177.

Goldblum, M. C. & Kremin, H. - Word comprehension in surface dyslexia. Paper presented at the Meeting of the International Neuropsychological Society, Deauville, France, June 1982.

Goldstein, M. N. ; Joynt, R. J. and Goldblatt, H. D. - Word blindness with intact cerebral visual fields: A case Report. Neurology, 1971, 21, 873-876.

Greenblatt, S. H. - Alexia without agraphia or hemianopsia: Anatomical analysis of an autopsied case. Brain, 1973, 96, 307-316.

Hecaen, H. - Aspects des troubles de la lecture (alexies) au cours des lésions cérébrales en foyer. Word, 1967, 23, 265-287.

Hecaen, H. - les problèmes des localisations lésionnelles des alexies. Languages, 1976, 44, 111-117.

Hecaen, H. & Gruber, J. - Alexie "pure" avec intégrité du corps calleux. In F. Michel and B. Schott (Eds) Les syndromes de disconnexion calleuse chez l'homme. Lyon, Hopital Neurologique, 1975.

Hecaen, H. & Kremin, H. - Neurolinguistic research on reading disorders resulting from left hemisphere lesions. Aphasic and "pure" alexias. In H. Whitaker & H. A. Whitaker (Eds). Studies in Neurolinguistics (vol. 2) New York, Academic Press, 1976.

Heilman, K. M. & Rothi, L. J. - Acquired reading disorders: a diagrammatic model. In R. N. Malatesha and P. G. Aaron (Eds) Reading disorders: Varieties and Treatments. New York: Academic Press, 1982.

Hinshelwood, J. - Letter-, word- and mind-blindness. London: H. K. Lewis, 1900.

Hoff, H. & Pötzl, O. - Reine wortblindheit beim Hirntmour. Der Nervenarzt, 1937, 8, 385-393.

Holmes, J. M. - Dyslexia: A neurolinguistic study of traumatic and developmental disorders of reading. Unpublished doctorate dissertation, University of Edinburgh, 1973.

Holmes, J. M. - Regression and reading breakdown. In A. Caramazza & E. Zurif (Eds) The acquisition and breakdown of language: Parallels and divergencies. Baltimore: Johns Hopkins University Press, 1978.

Kinsbourne, M. & Warrington, E. - A disorder of simultaneous form perception. Brain, 1962, 85, 461-486.

Kremin, H. - Deux stratégies de lecture dissociables par la pathologie: Description d'un cas de dyslexie profonde et d'un cas de dyslexie de surface. In Etudes Neurolinguistiques (special issue of Grammatica). Université de Toulouse Le Mirail, 1980.

Kremin, H. - On Broca's aphasia and agrammatic reading. Paper presented at the Meeting of the International Neuropsychological Society, Bergen, Norway, June 1981, b.

Kremin, H. - Alexia: Theory and Research. In R. N. Malatesha and P. G. Aaron (Eds) Reading Disorders: Varieties and Treatments. New York: Academic Press, 1982.

Kremin, H. - Routes and strategies. Data on acquired surface dyslexia and surface dysgraphia. In J. C. Marshall, M. Coltheart and K. E. Patterson (Eds) Surface Dyslexia, in Press.

Kremin, H. & Goldblum, M. C. - Etude de la comprehension syntaxique chez les aphasiques. Linguistics, 1975, 154-155; 31-46.

Landis, T, Regard, M. & Serrat, A. - Iconic reading in a case of alexia without agraphia caused by a brain tumor. A tachistoscopic study. Brain and Language, 1980, 11, 45-53.

Marcel, T. - Surface dyslexia and beginning reading - A revised hypothesis of the pronunciation of print and its impairments. In M. Coltheart, K. E. Patterson & J. C. Marshall (Eds) Deep Dyslexia. London: Routledge and Kegan Paul, 1980.

Marin, O. S. M., Saffran, E. M. & Schwartz, M. F. - Dissociations
   of language in aphasia: implications for normal function.
   Annals of the New York Academy of Sciences, 1976, 280, 868-884.
Marshall, J. C. - Neuropsychological aspects of orthographic representation. In R. J. Wales & E. Walker (Eds) New approaches to
   language mechanisms. Amsterdam: North-Holland, 1976.
Marshall, J. C. & Newcombe, F. - Syntactic and semantic errors in
   paralexia. Neuropsychologia, 1966, 4, 169-174.
Marshall, J. C. & Newcombe, F. - Patterns of paralexia: A psycholinguistic approach. Journal of Psycholinguistic Research, 1973,
   2, 175-199.
Marshall, J. C. & Newcombe, F. - Variability and constraint in acquired alexia. In H. Whitaker & H. A. Whitaker (Eds) Studies
   in Neurolinguistics (Vol. 3) New York: Academic Press, 1977.
Marshall, M, Newcombe, F. & Marshall, J. C. - The microstructure of
   wordfinding difficulties in a dysphasic subject. In G. B. Flo-
   res d'Arcais & M. J. M. Levelt (Eds) Advances in Psycholinguistics. Amsterdam: North-Holland, 1970.
Morton, J. - Word recognition. In J. Morton and J. C. Marshall (Eds)
   Psycholinguistic Series II. London: Elek Scientific Books,1979.
Morton, J & Patterson, K. E. - A new attempt at an interpretation
   or an attempt at a new interpretation. In M. Coltheart,
   K. E. Patterson & J. C. Marshall (Eds) Deep Dyslexia. London:
   Routledge and Kegan Paul, 1980.
Newcombe, F. - The processing of visual information in prosopagnosia
   and acquired dyslexia: Functional versus physiological inter-
   pretation. In D. J. Oborne, M. M. Gruneberg and J. R. Eiser
   (Eds) Research in Psychology and Medicine, Vol. 1, London: Academic Press, 1979.
Newcombe, F. & Marshall, J. C. - Traumatic dyslexia: Localization
   and linguistics. In K. J. Zülch, O. Creutzfeldt and G. C. Gal-
   braith (Eds) Cerebral localization, an Otfrid Forester Symposium. Berlin, Heidelberg : Springer, 1975.
Newcombe, F. & Marshall, J. C. - On psycholinguistic classifications
   of the acquired dyslexias. Bulletin of the Orton Society,
   1981, 31, 29-46.
Nolan, K. A. & Caramazza, A. - Modality-independent impairments in
   word processing in a deep dyslexic patient. Brain and Language, 1982, 16, 237-264.
Nolan, K. A. & Caramazza, A. - An analysis of writing in a case of
   Deep dyslexia. Brain and Language, In Press.
Patterson, K. E. - Phonemic dyslexia: Errors of meaning and the me-
   aning of errors. Quarterly Journal of Experimental Psychology,
   1978, 30, 587-601.
Patterson, K. E. - Neuropsychological approaches to the study of
   reading. British Journal of Psychology, 1981, 72, 151-174.
Patterson, K. E. - The Relation between Reading and Phonological
   Coding: Further Neuropsychological observations. In A. W. Ell-
   is (Ed) Normality and Pathology in Cognitive Functioning.
   London: Academic Press, 1982.

308 H. Kremin

Patterson, K. E. & Kay, J. A. - How word-form dyslexics form words. Paper presented at the British Psychological Society, Exeter, March 1980.

Peron, N. & Goutner, V. - Alexie pure sans hémianopsie. Revue Neurologique, 1944, 76, 81-82.

Poppelreuter, W. - Die psychischen Schädigungen durch Kopfschuss im Kriege, 1914-16. Leipzig: Voss, 1917.

Pötzl, O. - Die optisch-agnostischen Störungen. Vienna: F. Deuticke, 1928.

Quensel, F. - Die Alexie. In Kurzes Handbuch der Ophtalmologie. Berlin: Springer, 1931.

Richardson, J. T. E. - The effect of word imageability in acquired dyslexia. Neuropsychologia, 1975, 13, 281-288.

Sasanuma, S. - Acquired dyslexia in Japanese: clinical features and underlying mechanisms. In M. Coltheart, K. E. Patterson and J. C. Marshall (Eds) Deep Dyslexia. London: Routledge and Kegan Paul, 1980.

Schwartz, M. F., Saffran, E. A. & Marin, O. - An analysis of agrammatic reading in aphasia. Paper presented at the International Neuropsychological Society, Santa Fe, February 1977.

Schwartz, M. F., Marin, O. S. M. & Saffran, E. M. - Dissociation of language function in dementia: A case study. Brain and Language, 1979, 7, 277-306.

Schwartz, M. F., Saffran, E. M. & Marin, O. S. M. - Fractioning the reading process in dementia: Evidence for word-specific print-to-sound associations. In M. Coltheart, K. E. Patterson and J. C. Marshall (Eds) Deep Dyslexia. London: Routledge and Kegan Paul, 1980.

Shallice, T. and Coughlan, A. K. - Modality specific word comprehension deficits in deep dyslexia. Journal of Neurology, Neurosurgery and Psychiatry, 1980, 43, 866-872.

Shallice, T. & Warrington, E. K. Word recognition in a phonemic dyslexic patient. Quarterly Journal of Experimental Psychology, 1975, 27, 187-199.

Shallice, T. & Warrington, E. - Single and multiple component central dyslexic syndromes. In M. Coltheart, K. E. Patterson & J. C. Marshall (Eds) Deep Dyslexia. London: Routledge and Kegan Paul, 1980.

Sperry, R. W. & Gazzaniga, M. C. - Language following surgical disconnection of the hemispheres. In C. Millikan and F. Darley (Eds) Brain mechanisms underlying speech and language. New York : Grune and Stratton, 1967.

Stachowiak, F. J. & Poeck, K. - Functional dysconnection in pure alexia and color naming deficit demonstrated by facilitation methods. Brain and Language, 1976, 3, 135-143.

Stockert. Th. Von - Recognition of syntactic structure in aphasia. Cortex, 1972, 8, 323-334.

Stockert, Th. Von & Bader, L. Some relations of grammar and lexicon in aphasia. Cortex, 1976, 12, 49-60.

Warrington, E. K. - Concrete word dyslexia. British Journal of
    Psychology, 72, 175-196, 1981.
Warrington, E. & Shallice, T. - Semantic access dyslexia. Brain,
    102, 43-63, 1979.
Warrington, E. & Shallice, T. - Word form dyslexia. Brain, 103,
    99-112, 1980.
Zurif, E. B., Caramazza, A. & Myerson, R. - Grammatical judgements
    of agrammatic aphasics. Neuropsychologia, 1972, 10, 405-417.

CONSISTENCY AND TYPES OF SEMANTIC ERRORS IN A

DEEP DYSLEXIC PATIENT[1]

Christopher Barry
Department of Psychology
Dundee University
Dundee, DD1 4HN
Scotland

INTRODUCTION

Acquired dyslexias are varieties of reading impairments which may result when previously normal, adult readers suffer brain damage. In the last decade there has been a growing, and generally productive, interaction between the study of such patients and the development of information processing models of normal word recognition. Although this relationship is at its most fruitful when it is reciprocal, two separate directions of approach may be distinguished.

First, the pattern of preserved and impaired reading functions shown by a particular patient may be interpreted within models of normal word recognition. Typically, modular information processing (or computational) centers ("boxes") are functionally isolated or disconnected from other centers. This is achieved by the deletion of either the boxes themselves, or the information transmission lines between the boxes ("arrows" are severed). That coherent explanatory accounts of the reading performance of dyslexic patients can be obtained in this way often increases confidence in the validity of such models (see Coltheart, and Marshall, this volume, for some elegant examples of this approach).

Second, data from dyslexic patients can also be used to elaborate and refine the information processing models. For instance, if

1. This research was conducted while the author was working on a British Medical Research Council research to Dr. J. T. E. Richardson, at Brunel University, Uxbridge, England. I wish to sincerely thank John Richardson for his encouragement, G. R. for his patience, and both for their great help.

there exist patients who can perform reading function A but not function B, and other patients who can perform function B but not A,
then most models sensitive to neuropsychological data would be adapted to represent this functional independence, or double dissociation. Functions A and B would be given different boxes, although
interconnecting arrows between them would still be permitted, and
indeed would probably also be required, as they would need to be
functionally unified at some level in the normal intact system.

This theoretically generative type of approach usually stops,
however, at the postulation of assumed necessary functional separa-
tions (more boxes and/or more arrows). In this paper, I want to
advance and explore a claim for the greater and more detailed use
of the relevance of single-case studies of dyslexic patients to models of normal reading. The argument will be that data from such
patients may also be used to assist in the theoretical specification
of the precise nature of the processing intercommunication between
functionally separable components. The claim will be made that certain patient, in whom a particular reading "route" (a particular sequence of boxes and arrows) is assumed to be operating in functional
isolation, can aid the detailed specification of the normal operation
of this route (or at least stimulate plausible hypotheses concerning
its operation). For example, surface dyslexic patients (Marshall
and Newcombe,1973; Coltheart et al. 1983) have problems reading aloud
words with 'irregular' pronunciations (e. g. yacht and colonel), and
are assumed to be reading only by phonological recoding of print
prior to lexical access. However, there is a subset of psycholingui-
stically defined irregular words that all the patients studied by
Coltheart (personal communication) can read correctly. Inspection
of this set of words will therefore provide potentially useful information concerning the mechanism that is assumed to be responsible
for constructing prelexical phonological codes.

Deep dyslexia has probably been the most intensively studied of
the acquired dyslexias (see the recent volume edited by Coltheart,
Patterson and Marshall, 1980). Deep dyslexic patients show a fairly
complex pattern of reading impairments; they can read some words,
make no substantive response to others (called reading omissions),
and they make various types of paralexic reading errors. The interest of deep dyslexia for cognitive psychologists studying word recognition and production in reading lies in the opportunity that the
rich data-base collected from such patients presents for the critical
testing (and the possible elaboration) of models of normal lexical
processing.

In this paper I will present some new data from one such deep
dyslexic patient and use this to assist in the characterisation of
the nature of the functional interface between two separable subpro-
cesses (the semantic, or word comprehension system and the word
production system). Although the account offered here has as its

primary motivation the explanation of the reading of one patient
(and is therefore required to be self-consistent for that individual patient's reading; see Morton & Patterson, 1980), an attempt will also be made to generalise this account to processes operating in
normal readers.

The deep dyslexic patient to be described is the patient G. R.,
who has become quite famous in the acquired dyslexia literature, and
increasingly well known in the cognitive psychology literature also.
G. R. has been previously reported in the seminal papers of Marshall
and Newcombe (1966, 1973), (see also Marshall, Newcombe and Marshall,
1970, and Newcombe and Marshall, 1972, 1975, 1980a, 1980b), and also
by Richardson (1975a) and Barry and Richardson (notes 1 and 2).

G. R. has a very large left hemisphere lesion, which was caused by an accidental, through-and-through gun-shot wound in 1944, wh-
en he was 18 years old. The bullet entered the head in front of the
left ear and emerged in the superior parietal lobe of the left hemisphere. When the data to be reported here were collected in 1981,
he remained a non-fluent aphasic with a small upper-right heminopia
and a right hemiplegia. (See Marshall and Newcombe, 1966, for a full neurological report). He is also profoundly deep dyslexic.

G. R.'s Reading

G. R. shows all the major characteristics of deep dyslexic reading, which can be briefly summarised below. Barry and Richardson
(note 1) provide a more detailed description and analysis of his reading performance.

1. He has no print-to-nonlexical phonological recoding, and is totally unable to read aloud orthographically legal but meaningless
nonwords (such as mant). In fact, it is probably true to say that,
unlike many normal subjects in word recognition experiments, G. R.
hasn't read a nonword for over 38 years! He was also totally unable to judge that homophonic nonwords (such as burd) sound like real words, or to match simple printed and spoken nonwords.

2. He made various types of paralexic errors when reading individual words, including semantic (e.g. lion - "tiger"), visual (e.g.
sneak - "snake"), and derivational (e.g. cooking - "cook") errors.
He made very many semantic errors, and produced virtually as many
semantic errors as correct readings. Semantic errors constitute
around 50% of all his reading errors.

3. He displayed a clear and substantial effect of concreteness on
his reading success. As the stimulus word concreteness decreases,
his rate of correct reading decreased, and his rate of omissions
increased.

4.   There was also a part-of-speech (or syntactic class) effect, with nouns being read better than adjectives, which were, in turn, read better than verbs. He was very, very poor at reading grammatical
function words, correctly reading only 3 of a list of 138 function
words (she, is and a), and omitting 117. He made only 5 function
word substitutions (e.g. his - "she"), with the remainder of his errors being visual (e.g. while -"white"), semantic (e.g. her -"a woman, a girl") or unclassified. Further, G. R. appeared to appreciate his function word problem; shown the word that he said "that's
the trouble, this, those, these and this, all mixed-up together".

       These are G. R.'s impairments, but he has some preserved read-
ing functions. He can repeat spoken nonwords and words that he cannot read, and he shows quite good performance on the lexical decision (word/nonword discrimination) task. He correctly classified as
words over 80% of abstract words, and over 90% of function words that he was unable to read (Barry and Richardson, note 1).

       As mentioned in the introduction, the recent approach to the
explanation of the pattern of impaired and preserved reading skills
shown by acquired dyslexic patients has been to assume that their
reading reflects the operation of a restricted, but not qualitatively different, set of processes that are available to normal readers.
It will be assumed here that the only way that G. R. can make a reading response is via mediation of his semantic or conceptual system. It is highly unlikely that G. R. can read non-lexically, as his
ability to assemble phonological codes (as opposed to accessing them
lexically or semantically) is totally abolished. It is equally unlikely that he can read lexically but non-semantically, as he shows
a very large number of reading errors, a very large proportion of
which are semantically based. Within the model advanced by Morton
and Patterson (1980), G. R. would not appear to possess a grapheme-
to-phoneme correspondence reading route, or a direct visual input
logogen to output logogen connection; and, within the somewhat similar model advanced by Newcombe and Marshall (1981, and also see Marshall, this volume), G. R. does not have routes C or B. G. R.'s
reading appears to exclusively utilise the reading route shown in
Figure 1.

       Given G. R.'s very good lexical decision performance (he knows
that that is a word but thet is not), his word recognition system
must be working correctly and normally. Although G. R. makes visual paralexias in reading, these also show important effects of concreteness, indicative of involvement of processing stages in his
reading route that are later than the word recognition system. His
visual errors are made to words that are significantly less concrete than the words he reads correctly, and further, there is a significant tendency for his responses to be rated by independent judges as being more concrete than the target word (Barry and Richardson, note 1). His procedure for accessing (or computing)

FIGURE 1.   G. R.'s Reading Route

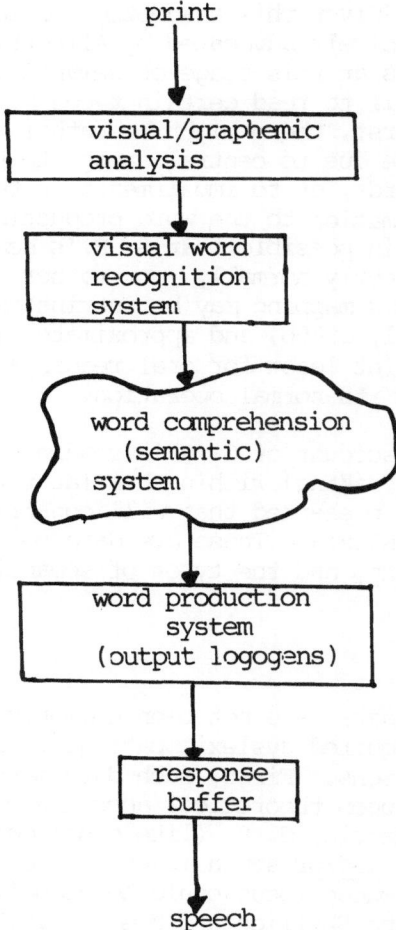

print

visual/graphemic
analysis

visual word
recognition
system

word comprehension
(semantic)
system

word production
system
(output logogens)

response
buffer

speech

the meaning of recognised words also appears to be essentially intact and normal. It is in the semantics-to-word production mapping
where his major reading difficulties appear to lie.

I will assume, with Allport (1982), that within the semantic
system "cognitive codes representing word-meanings are not, in any
way, language- or word-specific. [And that] there is no one-to-one
correspondence between cognitive codes and individual lexemes, or
words, in the language". Given this assumption of semantic independence of language (persuasively advocated by Allport), then logica-
lly, there are two reasons at this stage of semantics-to-word translation why G. R. could fail to read certain types of words and also
make semantic errors. First, there might be pathological changes at
this stage. This might be due to central damage to the semantic representations for some words, or to impairments in the normal transmission of semantic information to the word production system. Alternatively, however, it is possible that G. R.'s semantics-to-word
mapping is operating perfectly normally - or rather, normally but
imperfectly. That is, this mapping may be intrinsically unstable
(cf. Newcombe and Marshall, 1980b) and approximate, and that when
functioning in isolation (at least for oral reading) may be error-
prone as a consequence of its normal operation.

Before advancing an account of G. R.'s reading (and, in particular, his semantic error making) within this later type of approach, relevant data will be presented that will constrain any theoretical accounts of deep dyslexia. These are data concerning the consistency of G. R.'s reading, and the types of semantic errors that
he produced.

READING CONSISTENCY

Reading consistency data have not been commonly reported in
single-case studies of acquired dyslexic patients. This is unfortunate for at least two reasons. First, such data may place important empirical constraints upon theoretical accounts offered for deep
dyslexic reading. For example, G. R. (like other deep dyslexic patients) makes some visual and/or semantic errors (e.g. evil - "devil", and bake - "cake"), whose locus could be visual, semantic, or
an interaction of both (see Shallice and McGill, 1978). If it proved to be the case that the same words that produced such visual and/
or semantic errors, often produced visual errors but not semantic
errors, on repeated presentations, then the functional cause of these errors would be likely to be the same as that for pure visual errors. Second, they can also be used to test some emergent predictions from some accounts that have already been offered. For example, some explanations of semantic errors may suggest that they are
the result of a random loss or perturbation in the semantics-to-word
production mapping. An implication of such an account would be that
one would expect a large degree of interchange between correct

readings and semantic errors. Words read correctly on one occasion
might produce semantic errors on another occasion (and vice versa)
with equal frequency.

G.R.'s reading consistency was tested by presenting 643 single
words from the Brown and Ure (1969) word list twice. Repeated presentations of the same word were separated by at least two weeks (b-
ut often longer), and the words were presented in different random
orders on each testing session (with about 100 words being presented
each weekly testing session). The words were individually typed in
lower-case on plain white cards, and were presented 'across the desk'
for unlimited time. G.R.'s task was to simply read aloud the words.
Barry and Richardson (note l) have presented a full analysis of
G. R.'s reading responses to the first presentation of these words,
and they used the following twelve categories for response classification:

1. Correct responses; G. R. said the correct (or target) word, and
only that word.
2. Omissions; G. R. gave no response, other than "no", "don't know",
or even "I know it but I can't pronounce it".
3. Single word semantic errors; G. R.'s response (a single word)
was related in meaning (and only meaning) to the target (e.g. foot-
"shoe"; bitter - "pints").
4. Multiple semantic errors; the response contained more than one
word but was semantically related (e.g. person - "one bloke"; joy-
"happy, kids starting laughing, laugh").
5. Multiple errors that includes the target word; (e.g. village -
"small village"; black - "red, boots, black").
6. Single word visual errors; G. R.'s responses were semantically
unrelated but shared 50% of the letters with the target word, with
some account taken of their relative position (e.g. deep - "deer").
7. Multiple visual errors; these were fairly rare responses (e.g.
beating - "bed, bear").
8. Visual then semantic errors; these types of errors were first
observed by Marshall and Newcombe (1966) in their lovely example
sympathy - "orchestra". presumably via symphony (e.g. humour - "man,
all men", via human).
9. Visual and/or semantic errors; here the response was both visually and semantically related (e.g. evil - "devil").
10. Derivational errors; G. R.'s response word shared the same root
morpheme as the stimulus (e.g. farming - "farm").
11. Ambiguous errors; these were mainly nonverbal responses, and
some spoken responses accompanied by nonverbal gestures (e.g. shown
the word acorn, G. R. covered the first letter with his finger, and
said, "that one, wheat").
12. Unclassified errors; (e.g. errand - "tears").

The same classification system was applied to G. R.'s responses

to the second presentation of each stimulus word. G. R.'s reading
responses on the second presentation were then analysed as a function of his type of response on the first presentation. For the descriptive analysis shown in Table 1, some response categories were
combined if they were assumed to be indices of common underlying sources of impairment. Thus, single word and multiple semantic errors
(but excluding multiple responses that contain the target word) were
combined into a joint semantic error rate. Also, those errors where
the locus was assumed to be primarily visual (single and multiple
visual errors, and visual then semantic errors, but <u>not</u> visual and/
or semantic errors) were combined.

TABLE 1. G. R.'s reading consistency
          Contingency table showing, for each response category on
          the first presentation, the percentage of responses in
          each category on the second presentation.
          n = number of words producing responses in each category

		Second presentation					
	Cor.	Omis.	SEM	VIS	Der.	Other.	Unclass
n =	119	171	155	85	32	53	28
First presentation							
correct (n=133)	66	4	15	2	5	6	2
omission (n=228)	2	58	10	14	1	8	8
SEM errors (n=130)	11	7	64	5	5	6	3
VIS errors (n=58)	3	21	15	59	0	2	0
Deriv. errors (n=26)	8	0	27	4	54	4	4
Other errors (n=52)	13	10	25	15	4	31	2
Unclassified (n=16)	6	44	0	19	6	6	19

Notes.   SEM = single and multiple word semantic errors
         VIS = single and multiple word visual errors, and visual
               then semantic errors
         Other = semantic multiple errors that include the target
         errors word, semantic and/or visual errors, and ambiguous
                 errors.

     Table 1 shows, for each response category for the first prese-
ntation, the percentage (rounded-up to whole numbers) of those words
that produce responses in the various categories on the second presentation. The table should therefore be read by rows. For example,

of the 133 words G. R. read correctly on the first presentation, he
read 66% correctly on the second; he omitted only 4%, made semantic
errors to 15%, visually based errors to 2%, derivational errors to
5%, other errors to 6%, and unclassified errors to only 2%.

This table thus enables one to see which response categories
tend to cluster together in G. R.'s repeated reading of the same large sample of words. Barry and Richardson (note 2) report a full
analysis of G. R.'s reading consistency, and four main findings can
be briefly summarised here.

1. Of the words G. R. read correctly on the first presentation, most (66%) were also read correctly on the second presentation, and
although semantic errors were the next most common response category
(at 15%), they occured with less than a quarter of the frequency.
(Most of the 'other' errors for words read correctly on the first
presentation were multiple errors that included the target word).

2. Of the words G. R. omitted on the first presentation, most (58%)
were also omitted on the second, with the next most frequent type of
response being a visual error (14%). Notice also that unclassified
errors tend to cluster with reading omissions.

3. Words to which G. R. produced semantic errors on the first presentation also tended to produce semantic errors on the second presentation (64%). Of these words, 43% contained the same error in
both responses, and 57% contained different words (see later). His
next most common response was to read the word correctly, although
this occured (at 11%) with less than one fifth of the frequency of
semantic errors.

4. Of the words to which G. R. produced visually-based errors on
the first presentation, his most frequent response on the second
presentation was a visual error also. Further, there was a surprisingly high degree of consistency of the actual visual errors G. R.
produced. Of his double single word visual errors, the majority
(12/14) involved the production of the same error response on both
occassions (e.g. coward - "cow"; "cow"). This tendency also holds
for G. R.'s double visual errors that involve a visual then a semantic error. For example, the word sneak was read as "snake" on the
first presentation, and as "adder' (presumably via snake) on the
second. In fact, of all G. R.'s double visual errors, 28/34 contained the same error response (or presumed visually similar mediator).
This consistency of visual error making, coupled with the fact that
these errors also tend to be more concrete than the stimulus (Barry
and Richardson, note 1), therefore suggests that their functional
locus may be rather late in his reading route. Indeed, it is likely that they may reflect what Morton and Patterson (1980) call a
"second attempt" strategy to "produce an understandable outcome"
(p. 106), i.e. a candidate response in the word production system,

and/or what Coltheart (1980a) calls "approximate visual access", in an "effort to pronounce a word" (p. 366).

Finding 3 above suggests that semantic errors may be determined more by the nature of the <u>words</u> G. R. is trying to read, and not just the nature of the process underlying their reading. For instance, it cannot simply be the case that once the semantic representation of a word has been evoked, it is just a matter of luck whether it can then specify the correct pronunciation. As finding 1 above showed, some words seem to be consistently more successful than others in G. R.'s semantics-to-word mapping.

The words to which G. R. produced semantic errors have a mean concreteness that is intermediate between the means of those words he read correctly and those he omitted. For G. R.'s first reading of the 643 Brown and Ure words, there were significant differences (i) between words read correctly (mean Concreteness = 5.52) and words producing semantic errors (4.55) [$t(227)= 7.46$; $p < 0.00001$]; and [ii] between words omitted (4.16) and words producing semantic errors [$t(322)= 2.70$; $p < 0.01$].

SAME AND DIFFERENT SEMANTIC ERRORS

The nature of those words to which G. R. produced double semantic errors was then examined in more detail, and was compared with those words he read consistently correctly.

G. R. made 83 double semantic errors, and of these 36 contained the same word in both error responses, and 47 contained different words. Table 2 shows some examples of G. R.'s same and different semantic errors. For those double semantic errors that involved one or both responses as multiple semantic errors, 'same' errors were defined as those containing a common word in both responses. For example, responses to the word <u>eagle</u> were defined as 'same' as both responses contained the common word "hawk", but responses to the word <u>justice</u> was defined as 'different', as there was no overlap of response words. [Footnote 1]

An examination of the characteristics of the stimulus words to which G. R. produced these double semantic errors revealed that words to which he produced the same semantic error were significantly more concrete than those to which he produced different semantic errors. In fact, there were orderly differences between these two types of semantic errors, and the words which he either read consistently correctly or omitted on both presentations. These data are shown below, with the mean concreteness ratings taken from the Brown and Ure norms.

(a) Words read correctly on both presentations (n=88): 5.65;
(b) Words to which G. R. produced the same semantic error on both

TABLE 2. Examples of G. R.'s same and different double semantic
          errors

	Stimulus word	First response	Second response
SAME			
	seed	"wheat"	"wheat"
	eagle	"hawk"	"bird, hawk"
	fruit	"apple, pears, all types"	"apple"
	child	"boy, girl"	"a boy or a girl"
DIFFERENT			
	screen	"film"	"camera"
	justice	"lawyer"	"barrister or judge"
	religion	"mass, prayer"	"church"
	drink	"cheers, pub, I am thirsty"	"lemonade or orange juice"

       presentations (n=36): 5.05;
(c)   Words to which G. R. produced different semantic errors on re-
       peated presentations (n= 47): 4.19;
(d)   Words omitted on both presentations (n=132): 3.96.

       There were significant differences between (a) and (b) [t(122)
= 2.80; p < 0.01], and between (b) and (c) [t(81) = 3.17; p< 0.005].
The difference between (c) and (d), although showing a small trend,
failed to reach significance [t(177) = 1.24; p = 0.22, two-tailed
test].

TYPES OF SEMANTIC ERRORS

       Concreteness therefore seems to have clear and remarkably orde-
rly effects upon both the correctness of G. R.'s reading, and the
consistency of his semantic errors. There was also an effect of concreteness upon the nature of types of semantic errors that G. R.
produced. Coltheart (1980b) has distinguished between 'shared-feature' and 'associative' semantic errors, and like other deep dyslexic patients, G. R. makes both types of error. Table 3 shows some
examples of G. R.'s semantic errors in these two categories. Shared-
feature errors include synonyms and category super-ordinates and co-
ordinates (sub-ordinates were only very rarely produced). For these
errors, the response word shared very many semantic features with
the stimulus, and were often of the same syntactic class. Associative errors tended to be more loosely related, and often differed
from the stimulus both in terms of semantic and syntactic features.
Coltheart (1980b) has argued that the existence of "these two different forms of semantic error must be taken into account by theories

TABLE 3. Examples of G. R.'s shared-feature and associative
          semantic errors.

Shared - feature		Associative	
little	- "short"	faith	- "angel"
earth	- "world"	poetry	- "Shakespeare"
ocean	- "sea"	smell	- "perfume"
hand	- "arm"	yellow	- "paint"
beef	- "meat"	voyage	- "ship"
battle	- "war"	train	- "station"
blue	- "green"	guilty	- "crook"
lion	- "tiger"	rich	- "money"
cottage	- "house"	tobacco	- "money"

TABLE 4. Mean concreteness ratings for same and different shared-
          feature and associative semantic errors

	n	Mean con.
SAME Semantic errors		
shared-feature	13	6.10
associative	23	4.45
DIFFERENT Semantic errors		
both shared-feature	4	5.32
once shared-feat., once assoc.	11	4.44
both associative	32	3.96

of deep dyslexia" (p. 157), and implied that there existed no single,
parsimonious explanation to account for both.

When the nature of the stimulus words to which G. R. produced
these two types of error was examined, it was discovered that words
that produced shared-feature errors were significantly more concrete
than those that produced associative errors. Thus, for G. R.'s first reading of the Brown and Ure words, he made 96 single word semantic errors, of which 21 (22%) were shared-feature, and 75 (78%) were
associative. The mean concreteness values of the stimulus words that produced these errors were 5.74 and 4.22 respectively, and these
means were significantly differently [t(94) = 5.43; p< 0.0001]. This difference between shared-feature and associative errors was also
true for both G. R.'s same [t(34) = 4.51; p< 0.001] and different
semantic errors [t(34) = 2.40; p < 0.05], as can be seen in Table 4.

The difference between G. R.'s same and different semantic errors also held when separate comparisons were made for shared-feature
and associative errors, although, probably due to reductions in sample size, these effects were of only marginal significance [t(15) =
1.96; p = 0.069; and t(53) = 1.56; p= 0.125, both two-tailed tests].

There seem, therefore, to be two independent effects of concreteness. First, words that produced shared-feature semantic errors are more concrete than those that produced associative errors. Second, words to which G. R. produced the same semantic error on repeated presentations are more concrete than those to which he produced different semantic errors.

THE MODEL

How might one attempt to explain this pattern of results ? Following the work of Richardson (1975b, 1980), it is preferable to view concreteness as being a feature of lexical organization (or as a linguistic attribute), and not just as an alternative measure of a word's imageability. Richardson (1975b) has found that it is concreteness (and not imageability) that appears to determine performance in a semantic categorisation task, even where the task allowed the possible beneficial use of imagery. Although some attempts have been made to implicate a role of imagery in the mechanism underlying G. R.'s semantic errors (e.g. Richardson, 1975a), this now seems unlikely, for at least two reasons (see also Coltheart, 1980b). First, there are some semantic errors that G. R. makes that are very difficult to view as paraphasic misnamings of images, e.g. music - "orchestra", blue - "green", and spider - "snake". Second, some of G. R.'s semantic errors are made to relatively abstract words, e.g. alert - "fire", beauty - "handsome", and his - "she".

I would now like to offer a provisional model in which concreteness (or something that concreteness reflects, and is therefore very highly correlated with it) has important effects upon the nature of the interface between the semantic representation evoked by visual words and such semantically mediated access of words in the word production system. Specifically, it will be proposed that concreteness limits the range of semantic activation that a stimulus word produces, but that it also increases the degree of that activation for particular "units" within that range that may ultimately map-onto words in the word production system. These "units" will ultimately correspond to the stimulus word itself and words related to it.

If one considered the pattern of semantic activation evoked by stimulus words of various levels of concreteness (as such activations are used to locate and select words in the word production system), then (i) the range of activation is the number of different units (that ultimately map-onto words) that receive some activation, and how "close" in semantic space they are to the stimulus: and (ii) the degree of activation of those units is the likelihood of certain units "capturing" substantial and appropriate amounts of that activation.

It is further proposed that only units activated to a sufficient degree (i.e. whose value exceeds some threshold) could then ultimately map-onto (or specify) a word as a candidate response to be emitted in the word production system. It is from this <u>set</u> of candidate responses (it is proposed) that G. R. selects in order to make a reading response.

Consider the word <u>small</u>. Its semantic representation, in terms of evoked semantic features and by 'spreading activation', would also activate units that ultimately would correspond to words such as 'little', 'short', 'tiny', 'wee', 'minute', etc., and also perhaps words such as 'large', 'big', 'tall', and even 'size', 'height' etc. The number of units that receive some activation is what I have called the <u>range</u> of activation, and how much activation particular units receive is what I have called the <u>degree</u> of activation. Also, not all the units within the range would be activated to a degree sufficient to exceed the hypothetical threshold device, and so only a subset would be considered as candidate responses.

For very concrete words, there will be a very narrow range of semantic activation, and only a very small number of units that are activated to degree that they could be considered as candidate responses. It will be assumed that the unit corresponding to the target word itself will be maximally activated for very concrete words, although there may also be a small number of synonyms and close category coordinates activated as well. [Footnote 2]. G. R. selects one unit from this very small and semantically compact set of candidate responses, and then emits it as his reading response. The smaller this set is, the more likely it is that G. R. will select the same and correct word on a repeated presentation, or the same and very closely related shared-feature semantic error (e.g. <u>mother</u> -"mum").

For somewhat less concrete words, there will be a larger range of activation, with a larger set of units activated above the hypothetical threshold. If G. R. selected from this set, he might well choose the wrong (but of course semantically related) response, and the smaller this set is, the more likely he would be to choose the same wrong one on a repeated presentation (hence, same semantic errors).

For words that are even less concrete, there will be a greater range still, and a larger and more varied set of units activated above threshold (although to a lesser degree), and including many associatively related units. Selecting from this set, G. R. would be very likely to choose an incorrect response, and the larger the set is, the greater the likelihood of his choosing a different incorrect response on a repeated presentation (hence, different semantic errors).

For very abstract words, the range is assumed to be really

quite large, but with no clearly distinguished units within the range being activated to a sufficient degree to uniquely specify any word as a candidate response. When this situation arises, G. R. will make no reading response.

As mentioned in the introduction, any account offered for the reading performance of acquired dyslexia must primarily be self-consistent for individual patients. In an attempt to explore the implications of this model for G. R.'s reading, 187 of his single word semantic errors (taken from both his first and second readings of the Brown and Ure words) were given to 13 independent judges who rated the "semantic relatedness" between the stimulus word and his response to it. A five-point rating scale was used, which had the following labels: 1 = unrelated, 2 = only a little related, 3 = quite related, 4 = related, and 5 = very related. The model presented here would expect that G. R.'s errors would be closer in meaning to more concrete words than to more abstract words. Correlations were performed between the mean ratings of semantic relatedness for each error and the concreteness value of the stimulus word. Shared-feature and associative semantic errors were analysed in separate correlations.

The correlation for the shared-feature semantic errors was meagre [r= +0.027; t(50) < 1]. However, the correlation for the associative semantic errors, while also being small, was positive and significant [r = + 0.186; t(133) = 2.19; p< 0.05]. As stimulus word concreteness increases, so does the mean rated semantic relatedness of G. R.'s associative semantic error to it. There are a number of points to make about these correlations. Their small size may be due to two limiting factors. First, the range of concreteness values of the stimulus words was quite restricted due to the fact that G. R. tended to make semantic errors to words intermediate in concreteness between those he read correctly and those he omitted. Also, there was a large and significant difference [t(185) = 6.12; p < 0.0001] between the mean concreteness values of the words that produced shared-feature and associative semantic errors (5.57 and 4.39 respectively, on this sample). Second, the range of semantic relatedness was also restricted, or at least skewed to the high end, as all the word pairs were semantically related (they were all semantic errors). This was especially true for the shared-feature semantic errors, which were (by definition) clearly and categorically related. Indeed, the mean ratings of semantic relatedness was significantly different for shared-feature (3.99) and associative errors (3.03) [t(185) = 6.59; p< 0.0001].

Thus, finding a significant and positive correlation between concreteness and semantic relatedness for G. R.'s associative errors (especially in the absence of any a priori prediction for such an effect) is self-consistent with the reading performance of G. R. and therefore supports the theoretical model advanced here.

But why should concreteness apparently be the crucial dimension of the interface between a word's semantic representation and the word production system? It is plausible that it is not concreteness as such, but some propositional dimension which concreteness reflects.

In a recent paper, Jones (note 3) showed that normal subjects' ratings of how easy it is to think of factual statements (or predicates) describing a word, correlates very highly with the word's rated concreteness (and, indeed, with its rated imageability also). The more concrete a word is, the more semantic predicates subjects can think of to describe it. Consider the words dog and idea; there are clearly more predicates that can be easily adduced to describe the word dog than for the word idea. However, it would appear that one must also consider the generality of the underlying predicates describing (or evoked by) these words. Whereas the word dog might produce both general predicates (e. g. IS AN ANIMAL) and very specific predicates(e. g. BARKS AND CAN BE A DOMESTIC PET), the word idea might produce fewer but only fairly general predicates (e. g. IS AN INTERNAL OR EXTERNAL EVENT). The generality of these predicates, that is, the number of words to which they might apply, would correspond to what has been called the range of semantic activation. The larger the number of predicates, then the more likely they are to be specific to particular words, and this would correspond to the degree of activation. Further, the more specific predicates there are, the more likely they are to apply to a set of categorically related words or synonyms; that is, to words related in a shared-feature fashion.

Jones (note 3) presented 125 words (fortunately all taken from the Brown and Ure list) to 30 normal subjects to rate of their ease of predication. The mean ratings for G. R.'s reading consistency for this set of words is shown below. It can be seen that the orderly pattern of results is essentially identical to that for the concreteness values presented earlier.

(a) Words read correctly on both presentations (n=34): 5.76;

(b) Words to which G. R. produced the same semantic error (n=11): 4.70;

(c) Words to which G. R. produced different semantic errors (n=11): 4.02;

(d) Words omitted on both presentations (n=11): 2.93.

The difference between (a) and (b) was significant [$t(43) = 3.02$; $p < 0.005$]; the difference between (b) and (c), although showing a small trend, failed to reach significance, probably due to the reduction in sample size [$t(20) = 1.26$; $p = 0.2$, two-tailed test]; but the difference between (c) and (d) was significant [$t(20) = 2.63$; $p < 0.05$]. [Footnote 3].

DISCUSSION

The model advanced above claims that G. R.'s reading is mediated by the following sequence of processing. After preliminary
visual and/or graphemic analysis, words are categorized as such
(recognized) in the word recognition system (or visual input logogens). These words then access, or compute, their corresponding
semantic representations, which are structured in terms of propositional, non-linguistic semantic predicates. These predicates
are then used to create a set of units, from which G. R. selects
one (or, in the case of multiple word semantic errors, a number)
in order to emit a reading response from the word production system
(or output logogens). This set will be determined by both the generality of the semantic predicates (which will effect the number,
and semantic compactness, of the units within the set), and also
by the number of predicates (which will effect the degree of activation, or probability of certain units being produced).

The model is an attempt to describe the information transcoding operation (the functional interface) between the semantic
and the word production systems. There are at least two possibilities that may describe the precise nature of this intercommunication. First, semantic activation could be sent to the word
production system directly. In terms of Morton's logogen model
(Morton, 1979, 1980, 1981; Morton and Patterson, 1980), semantic
information could directly increment the level of activation in
output logogens. The logogen that exceeds its threshold (i. e.
the logogen with the highest level of activation) would then fire
and the word be emitted as a reading response.

Second, there may be an intermediate level of processing
(if not a functionally separate stage) at which the activated
units generated by the semantic system are assembled, and from
which, one is selected to be sent to the word production system
(output logogens). According to this second possibility, what has
been called the degree of activation would be a measure of the
relative probability of certain units being selected to proceed
to the word production system. (According to the first possibility, degree would correspond to activation levels within the
output logogen system.) Recently, Saffran (1982) has proposed a
view of semantically generated word production in language which
is similar to this second possibility. She suggested a "three-
tiered conceptualization of lexical function", which consists of:
(i) a conceptual system, which corresponds to what has been

called the semantic (or word comprehension) system here, and in
which"meaning elements are not necessarily in one-to-one correspondence with word units"; (ii) a "lexical/semantic system", which
consists of a system of units "each of which corresponds to a word
in the language" that are "organized with respect to semantic relations". Interestingly, for its implication for deep dyslexia,
she argues that "it is this level that is accessed when we 'know'
a word but cannot realize its phonological form"; and (iii) the
output logogen system, or word production system, where "each word
in the language is represented in the form of a phonological code
that can be utilized by the speech production system" (all quotes:
p. 327).

It is not clear whether it is necessary to maintain that
Saffran's "lexical/semantic system" exists as a functionally separate modular <u>stage</u> sandwiched between, and mediating, the two
others, or whether it is simply useful tool to describe a <u>level</u>
of processing. At the present, there exists no convincing evidence
to arbitrate between these two options, although the possibility
which suggests that activation is sent directly to the word production system has two points in its favor: (i) parsimony, as
only two 'levels' need to be postulated, and not three; and
(ii) the fact that G. R. sometimes produces multiple responses
may be easier to explain within such a model.

It is now time to address some difficulties with both the
model, and some of its assumptions and implication. I will limit
discussion to only four major issues.

1.   It might be argued that the semantics to word production system route is the usual mechanism for the articulation of thoughts,
ideas, etc. into words in normal spontaneous speech. If the operation of this route is assumed to be the cause of G. R.'s semantic
errors and difficulty in reading abstract words, then, one may ask,
why do normals apparently not show these characteristics in spontaneous speech? There are two responses to this objection. First,
the explanation advanced above was primarily for G. R.'s oral
reading of individual words presented devoid of any context. It
might be that the semantics obtained from a single printed word
are somewhat impoverished relative to the more integrated cognitive intentions that we endeavour to produce in speech. It might
also be that in normal speech production, the semantic specifications sent to the word production system are more detailed, and/
or guided by higher-order (and interactive) pragmatic, contextual,
prosodic, grammatical and systactical constraints.

Second, having admitted this, it is plausible that semantic "errors" (or, perhaps, more appropriately, semantic approximations) are frequently made in spontaneous speech, especially when using abstract words, but pass undetected by both listener and speaker. Indeed, some readers may feel that I have made such an "error" in writing the previous sentence, in my selection of the word plausible in preference to possible. Our speech (like G. R.'s reading) may be littered with second attempts to overcome the experience of "knowing" that there exists a more precise or appropriate word, but not being able to pronounce it, and we may often use instead a more general term for a concrete object (a shared-feature "error), or a semantically similar word for an abstract concept (an associative "error").

2.   The model advanced here attempts to propose a unitary mechanism (in terms of semantic predicates) for the processing of all words. [Footnote 4]. This basic approach may be compromised by data, recently reported by Warrington (1981a), of an acquired dyslexic patient, C. A. V. Like deep dyslexic patients, C. A. V. has a very impaired ability to read nonwords (although this was not totally abolished, as he read 14% correctly), but unlike deep dyslexic patients, C. A. V. was able to read abstract words more successfully than concrete words. Warrington interprets the data from C. A. V. as demonstrating the functional separability of concrete and abstract semantics (see also Warrington, 1975, 1981b). C. A. V.'s reading was characterised by numerous visual errors, which showed the opposite tendency to those shown by deep dyslexic patients; they were made to fairly concrete words, and the responses were more abstract than the stimulus word (e. g. moon - "mood"). However, C. A. V. made virtually no semantic errors (apart from the single hand - "hip"), and the concrete word impairment also tended to diminish during the later stages of his illness, when his overall reading success also improved. For example, on the first testing session , he correctly read 41.7% of abstract words but only 13.9% of concrete words. When tested a mere eight days later, however, he correctly read 80.6% of abstract words and 72.2% of concrete words.

Nevertheless, if one concluded from this data (and/or for other reasons) that it is necessary to functionally separate concrete and abstract semantic systems (e.g. Warrington, 1981a, 1981b; and Morton and Patterson, 1980), then I would want to maintain that the notions of range and degree of semantic activities would still be characteristics of the concrete semantic system. Moreover, there are conceptual problems associated with proposed separate concrete and abstract semantic systems. Primary among these is the question of how a binary system is to deal with the apparently continuous dimension of concreteness. There exist many words with intermediary concreteness values (and some with both concrete and abstract meanings or senses, e.g. Nice). In the Paivio, Yuille and Madigan (1968) norms, in which words were rated for concreteness on a 1-to-7 scale, the clearly concrete word ambulance has a mean rating of 7.00, and the very abstract word shame has a rating of 1.1. However, the word reflex has a rating exactly half way between two extreme values. Which separated semantic system would 'comprehend' this word ? The problem of the overlap (i.e. the duplication) of semantic representations for words is left unresolved in models proposing separate concrete and abstract semantic systems (as is the issue of whether the two systems would have similar or qualitatively different organisations).

3. It has been argued that whereas most acquired dyslexias may be explained by the functional dissociation of components subserving normal word recognition, the complexity, and integrity (cf. Coltheart, 1980c), of the symptoms shown by deep dyslexic readers demands the postulation that they are reading by a completely different system, in particular one located in the right cerebral hemisphere (Coltheart, 1980a; Saffran, Bogyo, Schwartz and Marin, 1980). There are two points to make here. First, the account offered here actually reduces the complexity of postulated functional impairments responsible for deep dyslexia. Indeed, the model presented here maintains that there are only two such functional "lesions"; one which isolates (or destroys) the box responsible for phonological recoding, and one which severes the direct arrow between the word recognition system and the output logogen system. In this account, the only remaining reading route available to G. R. (the semantically mediated route) is assumed, as a consequence of its normal operation, to be the cause of semantic errors and difficulties with reading abstract words.

Second, the account offered here may actually be compatible with the right hemisphere hypothesis, should it prove to be correct, although this may be unlikely (cf. Shallice and Warrington, 1980), or, at least, with a certain interpretation of it. The semantics-to- words mapping account advanced here may prove to be a general (or universal) description of how semantics used in natural language must be represented, and not simply a particular psychological mechanism proposed to account for such processing (i.e. it may

reflect an inherent, and necessary, property of how meaning is expressed in words). If this were true, then the model advanced here
would hold for <u>any</u> system in which non-linguistic semantic representations (irrespective of the hemisphere presumed to be responsible
for their storage) are mapped onto words in a speech production system.

4. General criticisms have been made of the research assumption adopted here that acquired dyslexic patients read using a restricted
(but not necessarily qualitatively different) set of processes that
are available to normal readers; or, what has been called the "sub-
traction" account (Henderson, 1981). There are three particular variants of this assumption that warrant discussion here. The first
is the issue of whether G. R.'s reading route is working in isolation. As was argued above (and see also Barry and Richardson, note 1),
this seems to be undeniably true. The facts that G. R. has no phonological recoding ability, and displays a very large proportion of
semantic errors in his oral reading, demand the conclusion that he
is reading <u>only</u> via semantic mediation.

Second, there is the issue of whether G. R.'s reading route is
really working without impairment. This assumption needs to be addressed both empirically and conceptually. Empirically, in so far as
it can be tested, it would appear that both G. R.'s word recognition
stage, and the stage that accesses or computes the correct (and reasonably full) meanings of recognised words, are intact and operating
normally. His lexical decision performance is very good, and his
semantic errors clearly demonstrate a good deal of appropriate (if
not totally accurate) comprehension. It certainly appears not to be
the case that G. R. fails to achieve semantic access. [Footnote 5].
Conceptually, the presumed cause of semantic errors must be examined.
Apart from the cause advanced here (namely, one at the output stage
of semantics-to-word mapping), two other possible causes may be considered. First, errors such as <u>lion</u> - "tiger" may result from damage to the semantic system itself. However, one must then explain
how this damage could produce such errors, and in doing so, further
examine one's views of the relationship between brain damage and consequent cognitive change. For example, one might explain semantic
errors by assuming that the stimulus word accesses incorrectly the
full semantic representation of response word; e.g. <u>lion</u> would activate the full entry for the word <u>tiger</u>. However, in so doing, one
has also implicitly suggested that brain damage has had the effect
of <u>creating</u> new functional cognitive connections, which, perhaps, is
<u>harder</u> to countenance than the possibility that brain damage destro-
ys or impairs such connections. Second, one might explain semantic
errors by assuming that the stimulus word accesses only <u>part</u> of the
normally full semantic representation; e.g. <u>lion</u> might activate only
the general semantic features LARGE PREDATORY CATS, which would correspond to a <u>set</u> of words. The deep dyslexic patient might then
either use this incomplete information to make the best of a bad job,

or somehow fill-in any missing information. Whereas this possibility may be true for some deep dyslexic patients (see Shallice and Warrington's, 1980, discussion of 'input' and 'output' types of deep dyslexic patients), such an account is less likely for G. R.; if it was, then one would also need to implicate concreteness as an important dimension (or limiting factor) of this semantic deterioration, as G. R. reads very concrete words correctly, and tends to make semantic errors to words with intermediate concreteness values. Finally, it may be argued that even if G. R.'s reading system is re-organized as a result of brain damage, then its operation may still show similarities with subsystems of normal reading because both systems need to cope with similar task (and language) demands, and may therefore reveal similar operational features in their functional solutions. On this line of reasoning, the study of acquired dyslexia would still be informative about normal reading.

     Third, Patterson (1981) has succinctly (and, perhaps, rather too eloquently) stated the following objection to the research strategy adopted here that a sceptic might raise: even if one accepted that "component A of the patient's reading system is the same as A in the normal system, and [is] further willing to agree that the damage to other components of the patient's system yields a privileged view of how A operates when uninfluenced by B, C and D. [Then one] might still object that the operation of A in isolation may be different from (and therefore not informative about) its function when in its normal context of B, C and D" (p. 170-171). It is indeed true that normal readers do not frequently make semantic errors or have any severe difficulties reading abstract words. It is further true that this is undoubtedly because the semantically mediated route is both interacting with, and being stabilised by, other reading routes available to the normal reader (namely the direct input to output logogen connection, and the mechanism responsible for the assembly of phonological codes). Although there is no simple rebuttal to this objection, Patterson makes the realistic argument that "if the performance of neurological patients can reveal separable subsystems in the reading process, then that is useful information whether or not those subsystems operate in quite the same way in patients and normal readers [....] it is useful information because it changes our models" (p. 171). Also, a semantically mediated route is necessary for word comprehension in normals, and if (as has been argued here) this route is operating in an undamaged way in G. R., then the study of his reading may be instructive when considering performance in tasks where these other, reading-specific routes are assumed not be involved. On this line of reasoning, the study of G. R.'s reading route may then afford a privileged insight into processes involved in word comprehension and tasks requiring the analysis of word meaning.

     In an attempt to explore this possibility, I had 30 normal subjects produce discrete free-associations to 20 concrete and 20 abstract nouns (matched for word frequency and, as far as was possible, meaningfulness ratings from the Paivio et al. norms). The model advanced here would predict two things: (i) that there should be more responses given to abstract words (i.e. a greater range of responses), and (ii) that there should be more shared-feature than associative types of responses produced to the concrete words. Although there were, on average, more different words produced as free-associates by the 30 subjects to the abstract words (16.3) than to the concrete words (15.35), this difference failed to reach significance [t(38) = 0.75]. However, when I examined the nature of the semantic relationship between each stimulus word and the most commonly produced free-associate to it, and classified these in the same way as I classified G. R.'s semantic errors, I found that there were 16 'shared-feature' and 4 'associative' relationships produced to the concrete words, and only 5 'shared-feature' but 13 'associative' relationships produced to the abstract words (2 were antonyms, e.g. life - "death"). The difference between the relative rates of these two types of relationships was significant [chi square (1) = 8.44; p < 0.005]. The model advanced here therefore has made predictions that have been supported by data collected from normal subjects.

Finally, on a note of radical scientific factitiousness, one might perhaps suggest that once a theoretical model has been launched into the uncertain and murky waters of empirical accountability, there is a possibility that it might prove sea-worthy (if not completely water-tight) despite any great decay of the principles guiding and nurturing its epistological superstructure. The model will now sink or float on its own terms. With life-jacket readily to hand, I await the approaching storm.

CONCLUSION

The large proportion of semantic errors in G. R.'s reading (coupled with his total abolition of nonword reading), suggests that G. R. reads exclusively via his semantic/conceptual system. In this paper I have argued that in the word comprehension system, stimulus words activate non-linguistic and propositional representations, in terms of semantic predicates. The generality of these evoked predicates determines the range of possible words to which they might apply. The number of more specific predicates determines the likelihood of particular words that are included in this set, and their degree of plausibility. It is from this set of highly activated or candidate responses that G. R. selects in order to emit a reading response. More concrete words tend to evoke a small but specific set of items related in a shared-feature fashion, whereas abstract words tend to evoke a larger but more amorphous set, containing many looser and associatively related words.

I would like to think that G. R.'s semantics-to-word mapping mechanism is the normal process, and that his brain-damage has allowed a privileged view of this system working in functional isolation.

I have proposed that his reading performance is not the result of
damage to his word comprehension system. G. R. may be simply relying upon his extant normal system that is intrinsically approximate,
potentially error-prone, yet orderly.

FOOTNOTES

1. N.B. Multiple semantic errors that included the target word
were not included in this analysis.

2. In its present form, the model does not specify the time course
of this activation. It is therefore conceivable that synonyms could
achieve higher degrees of activation before the stimulus word itself
achieves its maximal activation.

3. The fact that there were significant differences in ease-of-pre-
dication values between the words G. R. read correctly and those to
which he produced semantic errors indicates that the account of semantic errors in deep dyslexia offered by Jones is inadequate as a
general explanation.

4. At least for all content words. For the moment, I would like to
keep open the possibility of differential storage for, and processing
of, function words. G. R. has a notably severe problem with reading
function words, and displays only a relatively low rate of function
word substitution errors, which may make such a separation necessary.
Note, however, that the semantic predicate argument is in principle
extendable to function words, most of which are semantically quite
barren.

5. G. R.'s procedure for accessing the semantics of pictures, however, may not be working perfectly. He both makes some semantic paraphasias when naming pictures, and some errors in a task requiring
single words to be matched to an array of semantically related pictures; Newcombe and Marshall (1980a) report that 32.5% semantic errors were made in such a task devised by D. Bishop. However, when
the task is one of matching a picture to one of two semantically related words (Barry, note 4), where the related distractors included
G. R.'s own word reading of picture naming errors to the targets used, his error rate was considerably less (10.5%), which indicates
that his problems with pictures are greater than his problems with
words.

REFERENCES

Allport, D. A. Language and cognition. In R. Harris (ed.), Aspe-
     cts of Language. Oxford: Pergman press, 1982.
Brown, W. P. & Ure, D. M. J. Five rated characteristics of 650 word
     association stimuli. British Journal of Psychology, 1969, 60,
     233-249.

Coltheart, M.   Deep dyslexia: a right-hemisphere hypothesis.   In
     M. Coltheart, K. Patterson & J. C. Marshall (Eds.)   Deep Dy-
     slexia.   London: Routledge & Kegal Paul, 1980a.
Coltheart, M.   The semantic error: types and theories.   In M. Colt-
     heart, K. Patterson & J. C. Marshall (Eds.) Deep Dyslexia.
     London: Routledge & Kegal Paul, 1980b.
Coltheart, M.   Deep dyslexia: a review of the syndrome.   In M. Colt-
     heart, K. Patterson & J. C. Marshall (Eds.) Deep Dyslexia.
     London: Routledge & Kegal Paul, 1980c.
Coltheart, M.   This volume.
Coltheart, M., Patterson, K. E., & Marshall, J. C. Deep Dyslexia.
     London: Routledge and Kegal Paul, 1980.
Coltheart, M. et al.   Surface dyslexia.   London: Routledge and Ke-
     gal Paul, 1983.
Henderson, L.   Information processing approaches to acquired dysle-
     xia.   Quarterly Journal of Experimental Psychology, 1981, 33,
     507-522,
Marshall, J. C. This volume.
Marshall, J. C. & Newcombe, F.   Syntactic and semantic errors in pa-
     ralexia.   Neuropsychologia, 1966, 4, 169-176.
Marshall, J. C. & Newcombe, F.   Patterns of paralexia: a psycholin-
     guistic approach.   Journal of Psycholinguistic Research, 1973,
     2, 175-199.
Marshall, M., Newcombe, F., & Marshall, J. C.   The microstructure of
     word-finding difficulties in a dysphasic patient.   In G. B.
     Flores d'Arcais & W. J. M. Levelt (eds.) Advances in Psycholi-
     nguistics.   Amsterdam: North Holland Publishing Company, 1970.
Morton, J.   Facilitation in word recognition: experiments causing
     change in the logogen model.   In P. A. Kolers, M. E. Wrolstad
     & H. Bouma (Eds.) Processing of Visible Language.   New York:
     Plenum Press, 1979.
Morton, J.   The logogen model and orthographic structure.   In
     U. Frith (Ed.) Cognitive processes in spelling.   London: Aca-
     demic Press, 1980.
Morton, J.   The status of information processing models of language
     Philosophical Transactions of the Royal Society of London,
     1981, B 295, 387-396.
Morton, J.   & Patterson, K. E.   A new attempt at an interpretation,
     or, an attempt at a new interpretation.   In M. Coltheart,
     K. Patterson & J. C. Marshall (Eds.) Deep Dyslexia.   London:
     Routledge & Kegal Paul, 1980.
Newcombe, F. & Marshall, J. C.   Traumatic dyslexia: localization
     and linguistics.   In K. J. Zulch, O. Creutzfeldt & G. S. Gal-
     braith (Eds.) Cerebral localization: an Otfrid Foerster Sym-
     posium.   Berlin: Springer-Verlag, 1975.
Newcombe, F. & Marshall, J. C.   Response monitoring and response
     blocking in deep dyslexia.   In M. Coltheart, K. patterson &
     J. C. Marshall (Eds.) Deep Dyslexia.   London: Routledge &
     Kegal paul, 1980a.
Newcombe, F. & Marshall, J. C. Transcoding and lexical stabilization

in deep dyslexia. In M. Coltheart, K. Patterson & J. C. Marshall (Eds.) Deep Dyslexia. London: Routledge & Kegal Paul, 1980b.

Newcombe, F. & Marshall, J. C. On psycholinguistic classifications of the acquired dyslexias. Bulletin of the Orton Society, 1981, 31, 29-46.

Paivio, A., Yuille, J. C. & Madigan, S. Concreteness, imagery, and meaningfulness values for 925 nouns. Journal of Experimental Psychology, 1968, 76, (1, pt. 2).

Patterson, K. E. Neuropsychological approaches to the study of reading. British Journal of Psychology, 1981, 72, 151-174.

Richardson, J. T. E. The effect of word imageability in acquired dyslexia. Neuropsychologia, 1975, 13, 281-288, a.

Richardson, J. T. E. Concreteness and imageability. Quarterly Journal of Experimental Psychology, 1975, 27, 235-249, b.

Richardson, J. T. E. Mental imagery and stimulus concretenss. Journal of Mental Imagery, 1980, 4, 87-97.

Saffran, E. M. Neuropsychological approaches to the study of language. British Journal of Psychology, 1982, 73, 317-337.

Saffran, E. M., Bogyo, L. C., Schwartz, M. F., & Marin, O. S. M. Does deep dyslexia reflect right-hemisphere reading ? In M. Coltheart, K. Patterson & J. C. Marshall (Eds.) Deep Dyslexia. London: routledge & Kegal Paul, 1980.

Shallice, T. & McGill, J. The origins of mixed errors. In J. Requin (Ed.) Attention and Performance VII. Hillsdale, New Jersey: Lawrence Erlbaum, 1978.

Shallice T. & Warrington, E. K. Single and multiple component central dyslexic syndromes. In M. Coltheart, K. Patterson & J. C. Marshall (Eds.) Deep Dyslexia. London: Routledge & Kegal Paul, 1980.

Warrington, E. K. The selective impairment of semantic memory. Quarterly Journal of Experimental Psychology, 1975, 27, 635-658.

Warrington, E. K. Concrete word dyslexia. British Journal of Psychology, 1981, 72, 175-196. a.

Warrington, E. K. Neuropsychological studies of verbal semantic systems. Philosophical Transactions of the Royal Society of London, 1981, B 295, 411-423. b.

REFERENCE NOTES

1. Barry, C. & Richardson, J. T. E. "I know it, I can't pronounce it": reading in a deep dyslexic patient (Submitted for publication).

2. Barry, C & Richardson, J. T. E. Reading consistency in a deep dyslexic patient. Paper presented at the Experimental Psychology Society meeting at St. Andrew, July, 1982. (Also, in preparation for publication).

3. Jones, G. V. Ease of prediction: implications for imagery, categorizability, retreival asymmetry, and deep dyslexia. Paper presented at the Experimental Psychology Society meeting,

    Cambridge, March, 1982.
4. Barry, C. Processing of pictures and words in deep dyslexia.
    (In preparation).

PHONOLOGICAL DYSLEXIA: A REVIEW[1]

Giuseppe Sartori
Department of Neurology,
U. S. L. 10, Regione Veneto,
Treviso, Italy, and Institute
of Psychology, University of
Padova, Italy

Christopher Barry
Department of Psycho-
logy, Dundee University
Scotland

Remo Job
Institute of
Psychology,
University of
Padova, Italy

INTRODUCTION

Normal readers are able to read aloud both real words and ortho-graphically legal but meaningless nonwords (such as mant). How they achieve these two feats, and in particular whether they normally use different processes to do so, is an important issue for both the co-gnitive psychology and neuropsychology of reading. Patterson (1982) has made a distinction between "accessed" and "assembled" phonology. By the former, she means phonological codes that are retrieved from some hypothetical internal (or mental) lexicon. This procedure could be used for all words, but not for nonwords (which, by definiti-on, have no representation in the internal lexicon).

By assembled phonology, she means the procedure for ascribing a phonological code to a letter-string that does not entail the di-rect retrieval of that string's lexical phonology (if any). This is the procedure that would be used for reading nonwords, as well as also being able to be used for those real words with orthographically 'regular' spelling-to-sound correspondences (i.e. this system would not be accurate for 'irregular' or 'exception' words, such as yacht and colonel).

---

1. We are grateful to Doctors Bardin, Bruno, Cusumano, and Serena of the Neurology Department of Treviso Hospital for neurological and neuroradiological assistance in interpreting the data from Bea-trice, Lucrezia, Leonardo, and Raffaella, and to Roberta Francesco-tto for her help in testing Beatrice.

At present, there are two competing theories as to how such assembled phonological recoding occurs. Within "dual-route" theories (e.g. Coltheart, 1978, 1980a), nonwords are read by the application of abstract and non-lexical grapheme-to-phoneme correspondence (GPC) rules. Within the more recent "lexical analogy" family of theories (Glushko, 1979, 1981; Marcel, 1980; Kay and Marcel, 1981; Henderson, 1982), nonwords are read by analogy with the way graphemic segments contained therein are pronounced in words. For example, the nonword mant might be pronounced by analogy with the phonology of corresponding segments in the words man, ant, mint, etc. The experimental task of reading aloud nonwords is therefore an important one for investigating the psychological procedure used for the constructing non-lexical phonological information [Footnote 1], the possible role of phonological recoding in normal word recognition, and for revealing how assembled phonological recoding may break-down in acquired dyslexic patients.

In the literature on acquired dyslexia (disorders of reading following brain damage), an impairment of reading nonwords is often reported. Apart from the case of phonological dyslexia (the major subject of this paper), this symptom has been described in three other varieties of acquired dyslexia: deep dyslexia, semantic access dyslexia, and concrete word dyslexia.

Deep dyslexia has been described elsewhere in this volume (see the papers by Coltheart, and by Barry), and such patients show a very severely impaired, and often totally abolished, ability to read aloud nonwords, although they may correctly read some words and display comprehension of others, which is seen clearly in the occurence of semantic errors in these patients (e.g. lion - "tiger").

Semantic access dyslexia (Shallice and Warrington, 1979) is similar to deep dyslexia, although only one patient with this variety of dyslexia has been reported (A. R.). This patient could read aloud only 27% of 3-letter nonwords correctly. Like deep dyslexic patients, A. R. also made some semantic errors in reading words (e.g. month - "week"), although these constituted only a small proportion of his errors, and he also showed a small, but significant, effect of word concreteness. Unlike deep dyslexic patients, A. R. showed no major impairment in the reading of function words, or any syntactic class effect on his reading success, and, further, his word comprehension and lexical decision performance fairly poor.

There has also been only one patient reported as having concrete word dyslexia (Warrington, 1981). This patient, C. A. V., was able to read aloud only one of a list of 20 nonwords, and was further impaired in both the naming and cross-case matching of letters (i.e. judging that R and r have the same name). C. A. V. made many visual word reading errors (e.g. moon - "mood"), but only one semantic error (hand - "hip"). Further, and in a pattern of results that is completely the opposite of deep dyslexic patients, C. A. V. was able to read correctly more abstract than concrete words.

Two conclusions may be drawn from this brief consideration of these three dyslexic syndromes. First, an impairment of nonword reading can exist with substantially better word reading performance; i.e., an impaired ability to assemble phonological codes does not necessarily lead to a total abolition of word reading. Second, there is no uniform pattern of word reading impairments that accompanies an impairment of nonword reading. For this reason, the varieties of acquired dyslexia briefly reviewed above have been classified by Warrington and Shallice (1980) and by Shallice (1981) as being "multi-component central" dyslexias. That is, they are assumed to have at least two non-peripheral functional impairments: one to the system assumed to be responsible for reading nonwords and, in addition, damage to other functional reading systems.

PHONOLOGICAL DYSLEXIA

Phonological dyslexia, on the other hand, has been classified by Shallice and Warrington (1980) as a "single-component central" dyslexia, in that it has been assumed to reflect damage to the system responsible for nonword reading only. This variety of acquired dyslexia was first described (in the French patient R. G.) by Beauvois and Dérouesné (1979). This patient showed a clear and selective impairment in reading nonwords (although not a total abolition) coupled with a reasonably preserved (but not perfect) ability to read aloud words. R. G. did not make any semantic errors and showed no effect of word concreteness on his reading success. However, he did make some derivational errors, and also made some function word substitutions, characteristics which are also shown by deep dyslexic patients.

Derivational errors (e.g. applaud - "applause") and function word substitutions (e.g. this - "these") have also been observed by Patterson (1982) in her extremely detailed, scholarly, and elegant study of the English patient A. M. Patterson argued that these word reading problems were a consequence of a grossly impaired system assumed to be responsible for the assembly of phonological recoding. That is, she argued that such recoding was normally (and necessarily?) used for the recognition of the affixed forms of words and grammatical function words.

Before addressing the theoretical issues raised by these two seminal reports, we shall attempt to provide a review of phonological dyslexia. Our purpose in doing so is to broaden the empirical data-base on which one may establish and test theoretical accounts of both the role of, and the mechanism underlying, the system responsible for assembling phonological codes. Such a review is especially pertinent now as a substantial number of patients have been discovered in the last eighteen months, including a number of unpublished cases of phonological dyslexia in readers of the very regular orthography of Italian.

A REVIEW OF 16 PATIENTS

We have information (of various degrees of detail) from 16 patients who may, at least to a first approximation, be classified as phonological dyslexics. Apart from R. G. and A. M., there are other published reports: the patients J. A., P.H. and M. F., by Dérouesné and Beauvois (1979); R. O. G. and B. T. T., by Shallice and Warrington (1980); A. L., by Allport and Funnell (1981); W. B., by Funnell (1983); and J. S., by Martin (1982) and Marin and Caramaza (1982). Some patients have been reported at recent neuropsychological conferences: the patients L.B., by Dérouesné and Beauvois (note 1); 'Leonardo', by Job and Sartori (note 2); and A. M. M., by De Bastiani, Barry and Carreras (note 3). There are also three (as yet unreported) cases that we have recently tested in Treviso: the patients 'Raffaella', 'Beatrice' and 'Lucrezia' (Sartori and Barry, note 4)[Footnote2].

Although the data from these patients that are directly comparable is fairly low, there are enough to allow a fairly coarsely grained sketch of the main features of this syndrome. Table 1 presents these patients (by the language they read) with some basic neurological information, and each patient's nonword and word reading success rates.

All these patients developed their dyslexia following a C. V. A. or a head injury, and most also show concomitant aphasic symptoms. However, there does not seem to be any straightforward relationship between type of aphasia and phonological dyslexia, as 5 patients are non-fluent aphasics, 5 are fluent, 2 have aphasia that was not specified in the reports, and 2 were reported as having no aphasia at all (R. G. and P. H.). Three patients developed their dyslexia following right hemisphere damage, and among these one is right handed with no history of familial sinistrality (Leonardo). Probably all were dysgraphic, although the severity and form of their writing impairments were not generally reported.

In the last columns of Table 1, we have signalled (using arbitrary limits) those patients who (a) read less than 10% of nonwords correctly, and (b) read more than 75% of words correctly. There are only four patients who show both these features (G. R. N., A. M., W. B., and A. M. M.). Thus, there exist only a few patients with a cleanly dissociated pattern of impaired nonword reading and preserved word reading. There is also a great deal of variation in the patients nonword and word reading, which we shall now explore.

NONWORD READING IN PHONOLOGICAL DYSLEXIA

Very few patients classified as phonologic dyslexic showed a

TABLE 1. Phonological Dyslexic Patients.   Patients are shown by language, with their sex, hemisphere damaged, handedness, aphasia and dysgraphia.

Patient	Sex	Hem.	Hand	Aphas.	Dysgr.	Reading (% correct) Nonword	Words	a	b
French									
R. G.	M	L	R	–	+	10–25	80	–	+
L. B.	M	R	L	F	+	48	95	–	+
J. A.	M	L	R	+	+	55	100	–	+*
P. H.	M	?	R	–	+	80	100	–	+*
M. F.	F	L?	R	+	+	42	100	–	+*
English									
B. T. T.	F	L	R	?	+	50	90	–	+
G. R. N.	F	L	R	?	+	5–8	95	+	+
A. M.	M	R	L	F	+	0–26	86	+	+
A. L.	M	?	?	F	?	can't	12–65	+	–
W. B.	M	L	R	NF	+	0	87–93	+	+
J. S.	M	L	R	F	+?	15–20	38	–	–
Italian									
Raffaella	F	L	R	F	+	15–30	83	–	+
Beatrice	F	L	R	NF	+	0	62	–	–
Leonardo	M	R	R	NF	+	0–10	50	+	–
Lucrezia	F	L	R	NF	+	0–6	55	+	–
A. M. M.	F	L	R	NF	+	2–6	88	+	+

Notes for Table 1.

Hem. = hemisphere damaged   Hand = handedness of patient

Aphas. = Aphasia. F = fluent; NF = non-fluent; + = present but not specified

Dysgr. = Dysgraphia. + = present; ? = not reported

a: + = nonword reading is less than 10% correct

b: + + of which word reading is above 75% correct

* = these patients appeared to be tested only on their reading of 40 nouns. These patients are thus excluded from any following tables.

total abolition of their ability to read nonwords, and further, there is also a good deal of variability in the quality of their residual nonword reading performance. Most phonological dyslexics would appear to generally attempt to give some response to nonwords (irrespective of whether the patients know the letter-string is a nonword or not). [Footnote 3]. These responses may include visually similar words (e.g. brooze - "booze") and some incorrect nonwords (e. g. brait - "brack"). For example, the patient A. M. (Patterson, 1982), on a sample of 40 nonwords, read 17.5% correctly (and a further 5% were corrected), omitted only 5%, produced visually similar words to 52.5%, and incorrect (but usually visually similar) nonwords to 20%. This contrasts quite markedly with some deep dyslexic patients. For example, the patient G. R. (Barry and Richardson, note 6), on a sample of 99 nonwords, read none correctly, omitted 85.9%, and produced visually similar words to the remaining 14.1%. G. R. never produced a nonword as a reading response.

The Italian phonological dyslexic patient A. M. M. also showed a very low rate of reading omissions, a high degree of visually similar word responses, and some incorrect (but usually visually similar) nonwords. In contrast, the patient W. B. (Funnell, 1983), on a sample of 30 nonwords, omitted 56.7%, read only 3.3% correctly, produced visully similar words to 26.7%, other words to 10%, and incorrect nonwords to only 3.3%. Unfortunately, however, it is often the case that reports of phonological dyslexia do not provide a sufficiently detailed analyses of the non-correct responses to nonwords. It is also unfortunate that many reports do not investigate the reading of different types of nonwords, in particular nonwords that are homophonic to real words (e. g. burd and bloo). Both Beauvois and Dérouesné (1979) and Patterson (1982) have reported that their patients are more successful at reading homophonic nonwords than pronounceable but non-homophonic nonwords (e.g. durd and ploo), although this difference may well be confounded with visual similarity to real words (see Martin, 1982, and Patterson, 1982). [Footnote 4].

There would therefore appear to be both a quantitative difference between deep and phonological dyslexic patients in their phonological impairment, and some qualitative differences in their attempts to read nonwords. Figure 1 shows, in diagrammatic form, the relative distribution of noncorrect responses to nonwords by both types of patient.

WORD READING IN PHONOLOGICAL DYSLEXIA

Phonological dyslexic patients make visual errors, some derivational errors, and (sometimes) omissions in reading individual words. It is also true for at least some patients (e.g. A. M. M.) that nonwords are also occassionally produced to words. Unlike deep dyslexic patients, semantic errors are totally absent in all but the patient W. B. (Funnell, 1983), who made only 2 or 3 such errors that were

Relative
proportion
of nonword
reading

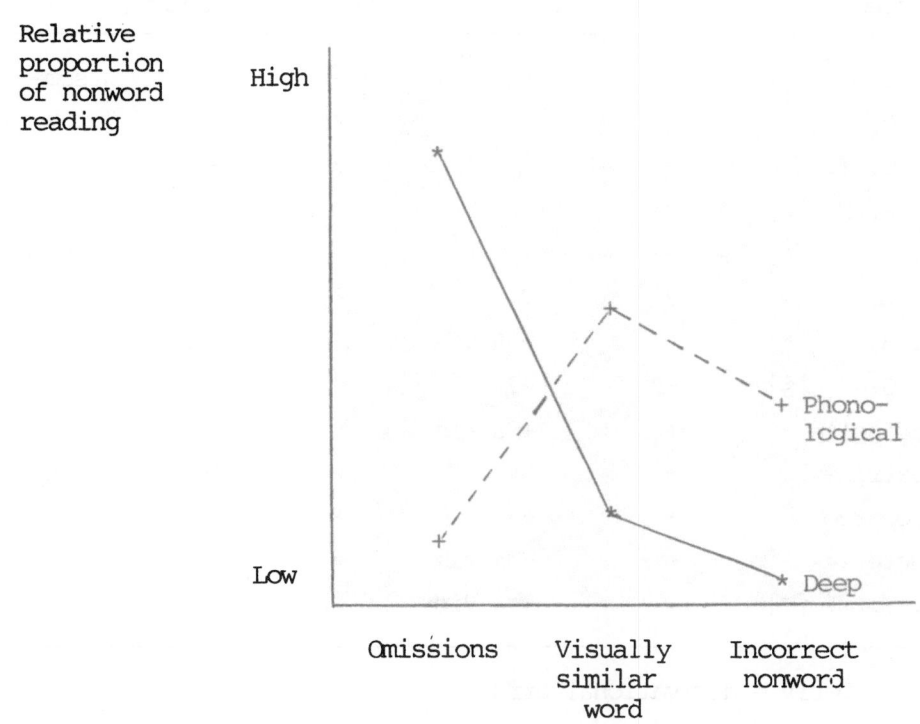

FIGURE 1. Nonword reading in phonological and deep dyslexic patients.

not also visually similar (e.g. girl - "boy"; protein - "bone").
[Footnote 5]. Function word substitutions are also generally observed, although in many patients these show some visual similarity
also (e.g. W. B.'s errors an - "and", any - "many", and A. M.'s
neither - "either", and is - "his"). The patient Beatrice, however,
makes many visually dissimilar function word substitutions (e. g.
per - "con", and il - "un"). There exists no patient who makes function word substitutions but no visual errors (see Table 2). It
is therefore possible that such errors (and also derivational errors)
really represent a sub-class of visual errors. As yet there has
been no research that has attempted to disentangle these possibilities. Possible research strategies to do so might be, as have been
applied to deep dyslexic patients, the examination of confidence
ratings and auditory-visual matching (cf. Patterson 1978, 1980),
reading consistency (cf. Barry, this volume), and reading the same
words individually and in text (cf. Kremin, this volume).

Table 2 shows that only one patient (Beatrice) among the 16

TABLE 2. Types of word reading errors in phonological dyslexia

Patient	Deriv.	F.W.S.	Visual	Semantic	Omission
R. G.	+	+	+	-	some
L. B.	?	?	?	-	?
B. T. T.	?	?	?	-	?
G. R. N. [*]	?	?	?	-	?
A. M. [*]	+	+	+	-	some
A. L.	?	?	?	-	some
W. B. [*]	+	+ & Vis	+	some	few
J. S. [§]	-?	-?	-	-	?
Raffaella	+	+ & Vis	+	-	few
Beatrice	-	+	+	-	most
Leonardo	+	-	+	-	few
Lucrezia	+	+ & vis	+	-	some
A. M. M. [*]	+	+ & Vis	+	-	few

Deriv = derivational errors

F. W. S. = Function word substitutions

[*] = the 4 patients with the clearest dissociation of non-
       word impairment and preserved word reading

[§] = this patient was reported as having mainly neologisms
       as incorrect word readings (Martin, 1982).

+ = present   - = not present

? = not tested/reported/clear from report

&Vis = most errors were also visually similar

phonological dyslexics made visual errors but no derivational errors.
Beatrice showed a very high rate of word reading omissions (82% of
all her non-correct responses), and many visual errors. However, she
did make 14 errors that may be classified as derivational (in that
they had the same root morpheme), but only to verbs (e.g. entrerò -
"entro"). In contrast, the patient Leonardo made both visual and
derivational errors with a fairly high degree of frequency. We compared these two patients on their reading of regular and irregular
Italian verbs. Regular verbs can be easily decomposed into a root
morpheme and affix, whereas irregular verbs are not so easily decom-
posable in this way. Therefore, one would expect that a patient who

makes 'true' derivational errors should be more accurate in reading
irregular verbs than regular one. We presented Leonardo and Beatrice
with 33 regular and 33 irregular Italian verbs (matched for word frequency, length and concreteness) individually for oral reading. Leonardo read 15/33 irregular verbs but only 6/33 regular verbs (a difference which reached significance). However, Beatrice showed no
significant difference (11/33, and 6/33). Furthermore, Leonardo
made more derivational errors in to the regular verbs (10) than to
the irregular one (3), while Beatrice showed a lower rate of derivational errors that did not distinguish between regular (4) and irregular (3) verbs [Footnote 6]. These data suggest that Beatrice is
not impaired in processing affixed words when such variables as length, frequency and concreteness are controlled. This therefore supports our notion that her 14 derivational errors are thus likely to
be instances of visual errors [Footnote 7]. As yet no reports have
analysed possible differences between 'inflexional' (e.g. farming -
"farmer") and 'derivational' (e.g. go - "went") errors in English.

All patients for whom data exist make some visual errors. However, these errors appear to be qualitatively different from those
made by deep dyslexic patients, whose visual errors are both made to
words that are less concrete than those read correctly, and where the
response word tends to be more concrete than the stimulus word. These results have been found for many deep dyslexic patients, including
the patients K. F. (Shallice and Warrington, 1975), G. R. (Barry and
Richardson, note 6), and B. L. (Nolan and Caramazza, 1983), whose
reading (in terms of relative proportions of semantic and visual errors, and preserved word comprehension ability) and associated symptoms (such as oral repetition) are fairly different.

These features do not appear to be generally true of phonological dyslexia, however. First, most patients show no effect of concreteness on their reading success. Table 3 shows the reported effects of various psycholinguistic variables (or word dimensions) that
affect word reading success in these patients, and one can see that
there are no variables which have a consistent or general effect.
If these patients did produce visual errors to abstract words, then
a concreteness effect should be detected. Second, although no reports have formally analysed the relative concreteness ratings of the
stimulus and response in phonological dyslexic patients, inspection
of the error corpuses provided by Patterson (1982) and Funnell (1983)
suggest that the error responses are not strikingly or generally more
concrete (e.g. A. M.'s contemplate - "compensate", and W. B.'s pen -
"open"). De Bastiani et al. (note 3) had five independent judges
rate 23 of A. M. M.'s visual errors on a 3-point scale (stimulus is
more concrete than the response, stimulus and response are of equal
concreteness, and response is more concrete than the stimulus). Only
13 of the 23 errors had a majority of ratings in the final category,
an effect that is much smaller than that found for deep dyslexic patients, and which may also be confounded by possible differences in

TABLE 3. Variables affecting word reading in phonological dyslexia

Patient	Content/ Function	Noun/ Verb	Concrete/ Abstract	Length	Frequency
R. G.	+	-	-	-	-
L. B.	-	verbs	-	-	-
B. T. T.	?	?	?	?	?
G. R. N. [*]	-	-	?	?	?
A. M. [*]	+	-	-	-	-
A. L.	+	+?	+?	?	?
W. B. [*]	-	-	-	-	-
J. S.	?	?	?	?	?
Raffaella	-	verbs	-	+	-
Beatrice	+	verbs	+	if > 8	+
Leonardo	-	verbs	-	+	-
Lucrezia	-	-	-	-	-
A. M. M. [*]	-	verbs	-	-	-

[*] = the 4 patients with the clearest dissociation of nonword
      impairment and preserved word reading.
 - = no effect
 + = effect present
 ? = not tested/reported/clear
verbs= verbs worse than nouns

the relative word frequencies of stimulus and target word. It would
not be too surprising if phonological dyslexic patients produced as
a visual error a word that was more frequent than the stimulus.

    The patients performance on some relevant tasks other than or-
al reading are shown in Table 4. Generally, patients are capable
of performing the lexical decision (word/nonword discrimination) task, and of comprehending visually presented words. It is interesting that at least one patient has been reported as being able to correctly classify in the lexical decision task those very nonwords
that produced a visually similar word error in oral reading (De Ba-
stani et al., note 3). This may not be true for all deep dyslexic
patients. For example, Barry and Richardson (note 6) found that the
patient G. R. showed virtual chance performance in the lexical decision task for those nonwords to which he produced a visually similar
word response in reading (5/9 were incorrectly classified as words),
whereas he was virtually perfect at correctly rejecting those non-
words he omitted in reading (41/42 were correctly classified as non-
words). However, it is unfortunate that oral reading and lexical
decision data have not often been frequently reported for the same
sample of stimuli presented in the same testing session, for either
phonological or deep dyslexic patients.

TABLE 4. Phonological dyslexic patients performance on other tasks

Patient		Lexical decision	Synonym matching	Word/ picture matching	Oral repeti- tion	Auditory compre- hension
R. G.		?	?	?	+	+
L. B.		?	?	?	?	?
B. T. T.		?	?	?	?	?
G. R. N.	[*]	?	?	?	?	?
A. M.	[*]	+	+	+	+	+
A. L.		?	?	?	?	+
W. B.	[*]	?	+	+	+	+
J. S.		+ ($)	?	+	?	-
Raffaella		+	+	+	+	+
Beatrice		-	-	-	+	+
Leonardo		+	+	+	+	+
Lucrezia		-	+	+	+	+
A. M. M.	[*]	+	?	+	+	+

[*] = the 4 patients with the clearest dissociation of nonword impairment and preserved word reading.

($) = this was reported as being good only for visual lexical decision. Note that this patient also had very poor audi- tory comprehension.

+   = preserved ability

-   = impaired ability

?   = not tested/reported/clear

PHONOLOGICAL VS. DEEP DYSLEXIA

Within those characteristics that this review has found to be common to both phonological and deep dyslexics (nonword reading im- pairment and visual errors in word reading), there are two main di- fferences of potential theoretical significance. First, in reading responses to nonwords, phonological dyslexics make relatively few omissions, very many visually similar words, and some incorrect non- words. One may also note that some patients may also produce some nonwords when attempting to read words. Second, the visual reading errors to words made by phonological dyslexics are not made to abst- ract words, and show no substantial tendency for the response to be more concrete than the stimulus.

These facts lead us to re-examine the view that the functional
impairments responsible for deep dyslexia can be seen as being exactly those presumed to be responsible for phonological dyslexia, plus
some (one or more) others. Phonological dyslexics may have a phonological deficit that is similar to, but less severe than that in deep dyslexia. However, if this is so, then such an impairment manifests itself in a qualitatively different pattern of reading responses
to nonwords. Newcombe and Marshall (1980) have suggested that the
reading disturbances (and particularly the presence of semantic errors) in deep dyslexia are caused by a total functional loss of any
(non-lexical or assembled) graphemic to phonological conversion.
Such recoding, they argue, serves to 'stabilise' semantically mediated reading. The fact that R. G. (the only phonological dyslexic patient known to them at the time of their writing) could read some
nonwords correctly suggested to Newcombe and Marshall that "very minimal phonological re-coding can block the overt expression of semantic errors in reading" (p. 185). This argument, however, cannot explain either the concreteness effect or the presence of visual errors in deep dyslexic word reading.

However, the possibility that phonological dyslexic reading reflects a sub-set of those functional impairments that are present in
deep dyslexia (irrespective of their extent) cannot be entirely dismissed. It is perfectly possible that a damaged but not destroyed
procedure for assembling phonological codes could produce the qualitatively different pattern of responses to nonwords shown by phonological dyslexics. (It is also open to suppose that a similar reading disturbance shown by two patients could be due to different,
and perhaps multiple and interacting functional impairments). It is
also possible that deep and phonological dyslexia represent points
along some continuam of functional impairment.

We have studied the development of dyslexic symptoms in the patient Leonardo (Sartori et al., note 5). Very soon after his C. V.A.
Leonardo made some semantic errors in his word reading, and indeed
showed all the characteristics of deep dyslexia (except for any great impairment in reading function words). His semantic errors consisted of only a small proportion of his errors (about 5%), and some
were visually similar also. At this time he was completely unable
to read nonwords, his only response to them being to name the first
couple of letters. This pattern of reading changed quite quickly.
Within one month, he ceased making semantic errors, showed no concreteness effect, and his reading performance (as detailed in this review) approximated to the pattern of phonological dyslexia. A somewhat similar change has also been observed in an English patient studied by Christine Temple and John Marshall (personal communication),
who showed a decreasing proportion of semantic errors in reading (although they are still present). It is interesting to note that their
patient made more semantic errors than Leonardo in his short-lived
'deep' phase, tantilisingly indicative of the possibility that

Leonardo's dyslexia was somehow 'less severe' than their patient and
so more open to change.

THEORETICAL ISSUES

The fact that visual errors would appear to occur in word reading in all these phonological dyslexic patients, raises two important issues. First, it questions the assumption of whether phonological dyslexia can be seen as a "single component" dyslexia. If one
assumes that the system responsible for assembling phonological codes is damaged, then word reading dysfunctions may be due either to
additional functional impairments (if one also assumes that phonological recoding is not commonly used in word recognition; Coltheart,
1980a) or to the fact that the phonological is somehow involved in
normal word reading, or at least some aspects of it. This later approach was invoked by Patterson (1982) in her explanation of derivational errors in phonological dyslexia. She observed that, at the
time of her writing, all patients (deep and phonological) who showed
an impairment of nonword reading also made derivational errors, and
suggested that phonological recoding is implicated in the normal process of recognising affixes to root morphemes. Such an argument was
bolstered by data from normal readers that root and bound morphemes
may be segmented in the recognition process.

However, it is clearly less tenable to apply a similar argument
to visual errors in word reading. Whereas it is true that all patients who have a nonword reading impairment also make visual errors
(phonological and deep dyslexics, and the patients A. R. and C. A.-
V.), the differences between phonological and deep dyslexic patients
in the concreteness effects on these errors strongly suggests that
they arise from damage to different functional systems (with damage
'later' in the reading process in deep than in phonological dyslexia). It is also possible that some visual errors may reflect either the interaction of more than one partially damaged system or some
compensatory strategic change.

Second, phonological dyslexia has been previously interpreted
within dual-route models of word recognition, in which only the non-
lexical phonological recoding route is selectively damaged. Recently, however, De Bastiani, Barry and Carreras (note 3) have attempted
to interpret it within a lexical analogy (or a "one process, not
two") theory of reading. Within this account, the functional impairment can be seen in terms of damage to the functions of orthographic segmentation and phonological assembly. De Bastiani et al.
argued that the reading of their patient (A. M. M.) reflected major
damage to the assembly of lexically activated phonology, which would
explain both the presence of her visual word errors to nonwords (e.g.
funvo -- "fungo"), and to the fact that she often produced strings
of such responses (e.g. ralog - "salgo, salvo"), which, further sometimes included hesitantly pronounced (and usually incorrect) nonwords

(e.g. tampo - "tango, tan-po"). Such an account may also be extended to visual errors to words, if it was assumed that there was also a slight impairment to the process of orthographic segmentation.

This is a far from settled possibility, however. De Bastiani et al. discussed how a dual-route model (by adjustments to the assumption concerning the word reading route) might be modified to also account for this finding; one would need to posit strategic lowering of word detector thresholds and some lack (or loss) of specificity and/or accuracy of such detectors. Also, Funnell (1983) has argued that an orthographic segmentation and phonological assembly model is unable to explain her data. W. B. was able to find and pronounce words embedded in nonwords (e.g. alforsut), which indicated that orthographic segmentation was intact. Funnell further argued that W. B.'s phonological assembly function was intact because he could repeat separately two syllables of an auditorily-presented word (e.g. "forget" - "for", "get"). However, W. B. was also able to orally repeat letter-strings that he could not read; it is possible, therefore, that Funnell's phonological assembly tasks were performed by an auditory "arm" of a model of phonological recoding, and not one that is necessarily involved in the assembly of phonology obtained from print.

THE SYNDROME OF PHONOLOGICAL DYSLEXIA

We have therefore shown that the reading performance of phonological dyslexic patients does not present a very neat pattern. As Coltheart (1980b) has noted, a neuropsychological syndrome may be characterised in a number of different ways. Two of these are: (i) a given set of symptoms is always observed. Some of these symptoms may also occur in other syndromes but another subset not. Furthermore, the existence of one or more key symptoms ensures that all the others are observed; and (ii) a given set of symptoms is always observed, but each individual symptom may also form part of other syndromes.

Coltheart (1980a) argued that deep dyslexia is an example of the first type of syndrome; the presence of semantic errors in oral reading ensures that the other symptoms (concreteness effect, part of speech effect, derivational, visual, and function word substitution errors, and problems reading nonwords) will also occur. Phonological dyslexia, however, cannot be such a syndrome. A selective impairment of nonword reading is seen in a variety of dyslexic syndromes as well as phonological dyslexia; that is, other word reading symptoms can be dissociated. A "pure" case of a nonword reading impairment has yet to be discovered, and by "pure" we mean both selective , in that only nonword reading is impaired and that word reading is perfect, and total, in that no responses at all are produced to nonwords. [Footnote 8]. However, as Max coltheart has counselled, one always needs /pashentz/ (patience and patients).

Phonological dyslexia appears to be an example of the second type of syndrome. Table 5 presents our concluding summary of this syndrome as it appears at the present. The question of whether it represents a single component syndrome, at the moment, depends upon one's theoretical preference for dual-route or lexical analogy models of reading. At the present it remains an open question of whether phonological dyslexia is to be adequately explained within either the dual-route or the lexical analogy reading model. Whatever the outcome of the debate between these two models, more detailed data from patients with impaired nonword reading will be necessary both as fuel for the controversy and, perhaps, as oil for troubled waters.

TABLE 5. Phonological dyslexia

Critical symptoms (seen in all patients).

> Nonword reading is impaired relative to word reading. Visual (or orthographic) errors in word reading, but no semantic errors, or concreteness effect.   Dysgraphia.

Associated symptoms (seen in most patients)

Nonword reading	- few omissions
	- many visually similar words
	- some incorrectly produced nonwords
Word reading	- derivational errors
	- nouns > verbs [in French and Italian]
Aphasia.	

FOOTNOTES

1. Some early researchers believed that assembled phonological were necessary to access word representations in the internal lexicon. As a general account of word recognition, this now seem unlikely [see Coltheart, 1980a]. Also, in some languages, such as Italian, pre-lexical phonological recoding could be successfully applied to all words. However, as Marshall and Newcombe [1981] argue, this may not demand that such recoding is necessarily used in word recognition.

2. Note the stylish Italian way of using as pseudonyms for the Treviso patients, names of important Italian cultural and historical figures.

3. Comparisons of the reading of words and nonwords presented in blocks, and the same stimuli presented randomly intermixed either have had no great effect, or have not been reported.

4. Due to its spelling-to-sound regularity, it is impossible in Italian to create nonwords that are homophonic to single words.

5. Funnell [1983] classified 5 errors as being "semantic", and 2 as "visual/semantic". Apart from the two errors given in the text, the other "semantic" errors were: <u>light</u> - "night", <u>truck</u> - "tractor, no", and <u>train</u> - "plane", the first two of which are clearly visually similar also. The visual/semantic errors were: <u>pen</u> - "pen no pencil", and <u>arm</u> - "armchair".

6. An irregular form of a verb in Italian <u>may</u> be decomposed in root morpheme and suffix, but its root morpheme <u>is</u> associated with substantially fewer suffices than the root morpheme of infinite verbs. This is the reason why some derivational errors may be observed as responses to irregular verbs.

7. This comparison, using two Italian patients, shows the advantages to be accrued from studying readers of languages other than English. Different languages may permit different [and perhaps more sensitive] experimental manipulations. Such cross-cultural (or cross linguistic) neuropsychology may thus assist in resolving theoretical possibilities.

8. This situation would be similar to a person who has learned to read some (but not all) Chinese ideographic characters. Such a person would not be able to make any response (other than one of total frustration) to totally novel characters.

REFERENCES

Allport, D. A. & Funnell, E. Components of the mental lexicon. <u>Philosophical Transactions of the Royal Society of London,</u> 1981 <u>B 295</u>, 397-410.

Beauvois, M. F. & Dérouesné, J. Phonological alexia: three dissociations. <u>Journal of Neurology, Neurosurgery, and Psychiatry</u> 1979, <u>42</u>, 1115-1124.

Coltheart, M. Lexical access in simple reading tasks. In G. Underwood (Ed.), <u>Strategies of Information Processing</u>. London: Academic Press, 1978.

Coltheart, M. Reading, phonological recoding and deep dyslexia. In M. Coltheart, K. Patterson & J. C. Marshall (Eds.), <u>Deep Dyslexia</u>. London: Routledge & Kegal Paul. 1980 a.

Coltheart, M. Deep dyslexia: a review of the syndrome. In M. Coltheart, K. Patterson & J. C. Marshall (Eds.), <u>Deep Dyslexia</u>. London: Routledge & Kegal Paul. 1980 b.

Dérousné, J. & Beauvois, M. F. Phonological processing in reading: data from alexia. <u>Journal of Neurology, Neurosurgery, and Psychiatry</u>, 1979, <u>42</u>, 1125-1132.

Funnell, E. Phonological processes in reading: new evidence from acquired dyslexia. <u>British Journal of Psychology,</u> in press. 1983.

Glushko, R. J. The organisation and activation of lexical knowledge in reading aloud. <u>Journal of Experimental Psychology</u>: Human

Perception and Performance, 1979. 5, 674-691.

Glushko, R. J. Principles for pronouncing print: the psychology of phonography. In A. M. Lesgold & C. A. Perfetti (Eds.), Interactive processes in reading. Hillsdale, New Jersey: Lawrence Erlbaum Associates, 1981.

Henderson, L. Orthography and word recognition in reading. London: Academic Press. 1982.

Kay, J. & Marcel, A. One process, not two, in reading aloud: lexical analogies do the work of non-lexical rules. Quarterly Journal of Experimental Psychology, 1981, 33A, 397-413.

Marcel, A. Surface dyslexia and beginning reading: a revised hypothesis of the pronunciation of print and its impairments. In M. Coltheart, K. Patterson & J. C. Marshall (Eds.), Deep Dyslexia. London: Routledge & Kegal Paul. 1980.

Marshall, J. C. & Newcombe, F. Lexical access: A perspective from pathology. Cognition, 1981, 10, 209-214.

Martin, R. C. The pseudohomophone effect: the role of visual similarity in non-word decisions. Quarterly Journal of Experimental Psychology, 1982, 34A, 395-409.

Martin, R. C. & Caramazza, A. Short term memory performance in the absence of phonological coding. Brain and Cognition, 1982, 1, 50-70.

Newcombe, F. & Marshall, J. C. Transcoding and lexical stabilization in deep dyslexia. In M. Coltheart, K. Patterson & J. C. Marshall (Eds.), Deep Dyslexia. London: Routledge & Kegal Paul, 1980.

Nolan K. A. & Caramazza, A. Modality-independent impairments in word processing in a deep dyslexic patient. Brain and Language, in press. 1983.

Patterson, K. E. Derivational errors. In M. Coltheart, K. Patterson & J. C. Marshall (Eds.), Deep Dyslexia. London: Routledge & Kegal Paul. 1980.

Patterson, K. E. Phonemic dyslexia: errors of meaning and the meaning of errors. Quarterly Journal of Experimental Psychology, 1978, 30, 587-601.

Patterson, K. E. The relation between reading and phonological coding: Further neuropsychological observations. In A. W. Ellis (Ed.), Normality and Pathology in Cognitive Functioning. London: Academic Press, 1982.

Shallice, T. Neurological impairment of cognitive processes. British Medical Bulletin, 1981, 37, 187-192.

Shallice, T. & Warrington, E. K. Word recognition in a phonemic dyslexic patient. Quarterly Journal of Experimental Psychology, 1975, 27, 187-199.

Shallice, T. & Warrington, E. K. Single and multiple component central dyslexic syndromes. In M. Coltheart, K. patterson & J. C. Marshall (Eds.), Deep Dyslexia. London: Routledge & Kegal Paul, 1980.

Warrington, E. K. Concrete word dyslexia. British Journal of Psychology, 1981, 72, 175-196.

Warrington, E. K. & Shallice, T.   Semantic access dyslexia.
    Brain, 1979, 102, 43-63.

REFERENCE NOTES

1. Dérouesné, J. & Beauvois, M. F.   Phonological alexia.   Paper
    presented at the Fifth I. N. S. European Conference, Deauville,
    France.   June, 1982.
2. Job, R. & Sartori, G.   Affix processing in a phonological
    dyslexic patient.   Paper presented at the Fifth I. N. S. Euro-
    pean Conference, Deauville, France.   June 1982.
3. De Bastiani, P., Barry, C., & Carreras, M.   Phonological dysle-
    xia in an Italian reader.   Paper presented at the European Bra-
    in and Behavior Society, Parma, Italy.   September, 1982.
4. Sartori, G. & Barry, C.   Impairments of nonword reading in three
    Italian dyslexic patients.   In preparation.
5. Sartori, G., Barry, C., & Job, R.   "Leonardo": deep or phonolo-
    gical dyslexic, or both ?   In preparation.
6. Barry, C. & Richardson, J. T. E.   "I know it, I can't pronounce
    it": Reading in a deep dyslexic patient.   Paper submitted for
    publication.

SOURCES OF REFERENCE FOR THE PATIENTS

R. G.	Beauvois & Dérouesné (1979)
L. B.	Dérouesné & Beauvois (note 1)
J. A.	Dérouesné & Beauvois (1979)
P. H.	"
M. F.	"
B. T. T.	Shallice & Warrington (1980)
G. R. N.	"
A. M.	Patterson (1982)
A. L.	Allport & Funnell (1981)
W. B.	Funnell (1983)
J. S.	Martin (1982)
Raffaella	Sartori & Barry (note 4)
Beatrice	"
Leonardo	Job & Sartori (note 2)
Lucrezia	Sartori & Barry (note 4)
A. M. M.	De Bastiani, Barry & Carreras (note 2)

ACQUIRED DYSLEXIAS AND NORMAL READING

Max Coltheart
Department of Psychology
Birbeck College,
University of London
Malet Street, London WC1E 7HX
U. K.

MODELLING READING

One of the tasks of experimental psychology is to attempt to discover what the procedures are by which we are able to read - that is, to develop theories which explain how we might proceed from print to meaning (in the case of silent reading for comprhension) or from print to speech (in the case of reading aloud). A variety of such theories has emerged over the past fifteen years. These theories have been concerned solely with the reading of single words, rather than with the reading of continous text; furthermore, they share a particular pretheoretical perspective in that reading is viewed as an information-processing activity. I mean by this that the various processes which go on during reading are characterised as involving the transformation of information from one form of representation to another. Reading for meaning is viewed as transforming an orthographic representation of a word into a semantic representation. Reading aloud is the transformation of orthography into phonology.

Numerous different types of transformation of mental representations are involved in reading, apart from the examples already given. In an information-processing framework, each of these transformations is assumed to be accomplished by a specific information-processing component. The system we use when we read, then, is assumed to be made up of a number of separate information-processing components, each with its own particular information-processing job, i.e., each responsible for transforming one kind of representation into another, with different transformations depending upon different components.

This description of information-processing theories of reading makes it clear that such theories are modular, in that they conceive of the reading system as a collection of independent information-processing modules. Any specific information-processing theory of reading will, therefore, take the form of an explicit description of each one of a set of information-processing modules, plus an account of what pathways of communication exist between these modules.

When one considers how theories of this kind have developed, one can discern at least three different influences at work. The first of these is evidence from laboratory studies of normal skilled reading: data from such studies are used to guide the development of theories after they have been developed. The second influence comes from investigations of abnormalities of reading. Data from such investigations are relevant to theories of reading for the following reason. Suppose it is possible to demonstrate close parallels between a) the ways in which a patient with a reading impairment due to brain damage reads and b) the ways in which a particular model of reading would read if the functioning of one of its modules were impaired or abolished, with the remaining modules performing normally. Any such parallels, if demonstrated, provide evidence in support of the model, because its modules appear "psychologically real" (as well as anatomically distinct). Such parallels also provide economical theoretical descriptions of the patterns of reading impairment exhibited by brain-damaged patients. Research involving this kind of interplay between the modelling of normal reading and the study of acquired disorders of reading is currently a flourishing enterprise: reviews of this work may be found in Coltheart (1981), Newcombe and Marshall (1981), Patterson (1981), and Shallice (1981).

The third influence upon theory development has been non-empirical: a priori considerations of the nature of the English writing system and its relationships to English pronunciation lead naturally to the formulation of certain theoretical ideas about how the reading of English might be accomplished. Consider, for example, what might happen when you read aloud the word van. Here you have derived a phonological representation from a printed one. How did you do it ? One obvious possibility is that you simply recognised the letter string van as a familiar visual configuration, one you have seen before and whose phonological equivalent you have previously learned. Here reading van aloud has much in common with naming a picture of a van: one gains access to a store of previously learned visual/verbal correspondences.

This is not the only possibility, however. An alternative, which would account equally well for your ability to read van aloud, is that you use a system of rules for deriving a sequence of phonemes from a sequence of letters. You might know, for example, how each of the letters of the word is usually pronounced, and so could use such letter-sound rules to read the word aloud. On this account, the fact that <u>van</u> is a real word which you have seen before, and about which you may have learned much, is irrelevant. A completely unfamiliar letter string - a non-word such as <u>vam</u> - would be read aloud just as well by this rule-based procedure as would a familiar word such as <u>van</u>.

Let us refer to these two possible ways of reading aloud as <u>lexical</u> and <u>non-lexical</u> procedures. All I mean by the term "lexical procedure" is that this procedure depends crucially upon the pre-existing storage of the whole letter string in some kind of mental lexicon: without the existence of a lexical entry for the letter string, the lexical procedure must fail. All I mean by the term "non-lexical procedure" is that the procedure is indifferent as to whether the letter string to be read aloud does or does not exist as an entry in the mental lexicon.

If there are two entirely adequate procedures by which <u>van</u> can be read aloud, how can one decide which (if either) procedure a reader actually uses ? This question can only be explored by defining the two procedures in more detail; that is, only by offering theories as to the nature of the lexical and non-lexical procedures for deriving phonology from print.

The non-lexical procedure for reading aloud

Consider first the non-lexical procedure - that is, the method used when one reads aloud letter strings such as <u>vam</u>, strings which do not possess lexical entries. At least three accounts of such non-word reading have been offered: lexical analogy theory, orthographic-phonological correspondence theory, and grapheme-phoneme correspondence (GPC) theory.

According to lexical analogy theory, it is misleading even to use the term "non-lexical procedure" in discussing how non-words are read aloud, because on this theory non-words are read aloud via reference to lexical entries, even though non-words do not possess lexical entries. The basic idea is that a non-word such as <u>vam</u> results in the retrieval from the lexicon of information about words orthographically similar to <u>vam</u>: <u>van</u> and <u>ham</u>, for example. Analysis of the phonological forms of these words into components corresponding to va- and to -am, and subsequent synthesis of these components, permits the reader to produce the appropriate phonological representation for the non-word <u>vam</u>: he has achieved this, however, by consultation of a lexicon which contains entries only for words, and not for non-words. Accounts of this kind may be found in Glushko (1979, 1981), Marcel (1980), Kay and Marcel (1981), and Henderson (1982).

According to what I have termed "orthographic-phonological correspondence theory", non-words are read aloud by using knowledge of correspondences between orthographic segments of various sizes and

their appropriate phonological forms. With vam, for example, the
reader might possess pre-existing knowledge not only about the pronunciation of v, a, and m, but also about how va, am, and perhaps
even vam are pronounced. This knowledge is non-lexical in the sense
that it is possessed regardless of whether or not the orthographic
segments whose phonological forms are known are words or not. This
theory has been formulated by Shallice (1981) and extended by Shallice, Warrington and McCarthy (1983).

The third theory, GPC theory, is a special case of orthographic-
phonological correspondence theory, in the sense that it does not
permit various sizes of orthographic unit, but only one size of unit
- this unit being the grapheme. The term grapheme is used to refer
to any letter or letter-cluster which corresponds to a single phoneme. Thus the word cherry possesses six letters, but only four graphemes, these graphemes being ch, e, rr, and y. By definition, the
number of graphemes in the orthographic form of a word is equal to
the number of phonemes in its phonological form. When used in this
way, grapheme is synonymous with the term "functional spelling unit"
as used by Venezky (1970). According to GPC theory, non-words are
pronounced by application of a system of grapheme-to-phoneme correspondences; orthographic units larger than the grapheme (e.g., the
va in vam) are not used. This kind of theory has been discussed in
some detail by Coltheart (1978).

Efforts are currently being devoted to experimental adjudicati-
ons between these three competing theories. Nothing decisive has
yet emerged, although data provided by Funnell(1983) are not easy to
reconcile with the first or second theories; on the other hand, data
provided by Glushko (1979) pose problems for the third theory. This
third theory is more precisely defined, and postulates simpler mechanisms, than the other two; moreover in my view it receives stronger
support than the other two from studies of reading disorders. It is
GPC theory, then, that I will be using as an account of how we read
non-words aloud, i.e., of how the non-lexical procedure works; and
hence I will have a little more to say about what mechanisms might
be involved in the use of GPCs to read aloud.

It was argued by Coltheart (1978) that, before one could assign
the phoneme /tʃ/ to the relevant letters of a non-word like cheeth,
one must first establish that a single phoneme is to be assigned to
the two-letter cluster ch, rather than using the assignation c ->
/k/ and h -> /h/, which would obviously produce an error. Consequently, the first stage of a GPC procedure must be graphemic parsing:
analysing a letter string into its constituent graphemes, as in
cheeth -> [ch] + [ee] + [th]. Once these graphemes have been identified, the appropriate phoneme can be assigned to each grapheme in
accordance with the system of grapheme-phoneme correspondences. This second stage Coltheart [1978] referred to as phoneme assignment.
A final stage, not discussed by him but nevertheless essential, is

blending: converting a string of individual phonemes into a single
coherent whole. This view of the nature of the GPC procedure is described in Figure 1.

Figure 1. Reading aloud via grapheme-phoneme correspondences

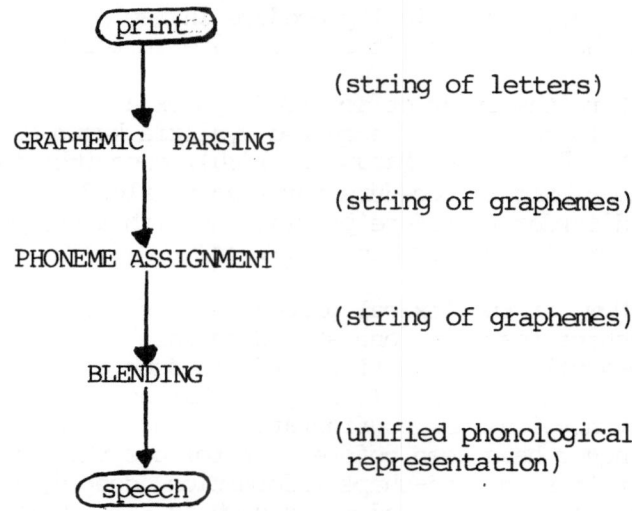

(string of letters)

GRAPHEMIC PARSING

(string of graphemes)

PHONEME ASSIGNMENT

(string of graphemes)

BLENDING

(unified phonological
representation)

One of the ways of exploring the plausibility of this particular account of the non-lexical procedure is to study reading in patients
with an acquired dyslexia - specifically, an acquired dyslexia in
which there is impairment of the non-lexical procedure and hence impaired reading of non-words. This type of dyslexia exists; it is
known as phonological dyslexia and is described in more detail later,
where it will be argued that patients with this dyslexia do indeed
provide evidence in favor of the theory of the non-lexical procedure
set out in Figure 1.

The lexical procedure for reading aloud

     A vague definition of the lexical procedure for reading aloud
was offered earlier: it is that procedure which relies on being able
to recognise a letter string as a configuration whose pronunciation
has previously been learned (i.e., which is represented as an entry
in the mental lexicon).

     There are two ways in which this definition is vague. Firstly,
it is not clear what is meant by "familiar visual configuration".
Secondly, it is not clear how one proceeds from the orthographic representation of a word to its phonological representation, i.e., not
clear exactly how the mental lexicon permits this. These two issues

will be considered in turn.

When referring to the "familiar visual configuration" of a word like ham, one might have in mind something like overall word shape. Perhaps ham is recognized in terms of a bundle of visual features such as [initial ascender + closed loop in central letter + three verticals in last letter]. If we could somehow prevent a reader from using the non-lexical procedure for reading aloud, which would allow us to study the lexical procedure in isolation, we might be able to learn whether or not it does operate in terms of word-shape features.

Here the study of acquired dyslexia makes a decisive contribution. In the form of acquired dyslexia known as deep dyslexia (Coltheart, Patterson, Marshall, 1980), described in more detail later, the non-lexical procedure for reading aloud is entirely abolished. This disorder therefore provides us with a unique way of studying the lexical procedure in isolation.

Now, if the lexical procedure does recognize words in terms of word-shape features, one should be able to prevent it from being used successfully by distorting words in such a way that word-shape features are destroyed. If we print ham as HaM, we have produced an entirely novel visual configuration, a new word-shape which readers will never have seen before. It follows that if the lexical procedure relies on word-shape information, deep dyslexics will be unable to read case-alternated words such as HaM. They cannot use the non-lexical procedure (since it is abolished in deep dyslexia) and they cannot use the lexical procedure if the latter procedure depends upon word shape.

This prediction was tested and refuted by Saffran (1980): she showed that deep dyslexics could read case-alternated words. Indeed, deep dyslexics can read words which are shown to them one letter at a time, a condition in which word shape could not be perceived (Patterson, 1981). It follows that word shape is not the sole basis for word recognition via the lexical procedure (though it may contribute to such recognition).

An alternative to the word-shape hypothesis is that words are recognized via their constituent letters, and that this letter recognition is abstract in the sense that A and a are identified as the same letter (not as two letters having the same name). Word recognition mediated by abstract letter identification would succeed even for words printed in alternating case.

Is there any evidence in support of this concept of abstract letter identification? Once again, the study of acquired dyslexia assists us. Certain patients are impaired at making any kinds of phonological judgments about single letters: their letter naming is poor, and even their ability to make silent judgements about whether

letter rhyme or not is poor. Such patients can perform perfectly,
however, when asked to judge whether A and a represent the same letter (Coltheart, 1980; Caramazza and Martin, 1982). They could not be
making this judgment using a visual encoding of the letters (since
in terms of visual encoding A and a are not the same); they could
not be making the judgment using a phonological encoding, since they
are so poor at phonological encoding of single letters; a third code
must therefore be available, and this is the abstract letter identity.

It will be assumed, then, that the "visual recognition" involved
in the lexical procedure actually consists of recognizing words in
terms of the abstract identities of their individual letters. This
assumption deals with one of the sources of vagueness in the concept
of the lexical procedure. The other source has to do with how the
reader, having identified a word in terms of its orthography, uses
this orthographic representation to obtain the phonological form of
the word in order to read it aloud.

One could argue along the following lines. The reader must be
able to proceed from orthography to semantics (since this is how he
comprehends print). He must also be able to proceed from a word's
semantic representation to its phonological form (since this is the
essence of speech production in spontaneous speaking). Therefore,
one can account for the reader's ability to proceed from orthography
to phonology using a lexical procedure by proposing that the route
is an indirect one: orthography is converted to semantics, and then
semantics to phonology. This is a parsimonious account of the lexical procedure for reading aloud, because the two steps involved must
exist anyway.

Suppose that such semantic mediation were always a necessary
part of the lexical procedure for reading aloud. A patient who,
because of brain damage, has lost the non-lexical procedure entirely
would therefore be compelled to read via semantic mediation. Funnell (1983), however, has shown that this is not the case. Her patient could not read any non-words aloud at all (and so had lost the
non-lexical procedure entirely). He was also poor at comprehending
printed words (and so had a serious inability to gain access to semantics from orthography). Nevertheless, his reading aloud of words
was excellent: about 90% correct for all classes of word. It follows
that, although there must be an indirect route from orthography to
phonology via semantics (since both the part of this route must exist) there must also be a direct route, a mapping directly from the
orthographic form of a word to its phonological form. Thus the lexical procedure for reading aloud is actually two procedures: a direct orthographic-to-phonological route plus an indirect route via semantics. Two other quite different kinds of neuropsychological observations also support the view that this direct link from the orthography of a word to its phonology exists (Schwartz, Saffran and Marin, 1980; Coltheart, Masterson, Byng, Prior and Riddoch, 1983).

A dual-route model of reading

Arguments given above lead to a model of reading in which the output of an abstract letter-identification stage serves as the input to two reading procedures: a non-lexical procedure based upon grapheme-phoneme rules and a lexical procedure whose first stage is orthographic word-recognition. The output of this stage proceeds both to a semantic system (responsible for comprehension) and to a phonological system (responsible for producing spoken words). This model is displayed in Figure 2; it is essentially that of Coltheart (1981) whose model in turn differs only in minor ways from models proposed by, for example, Morton and Patterson (1980) and Newcombe and Marshall (1980).

FIGURE 2. A dual-model of reading

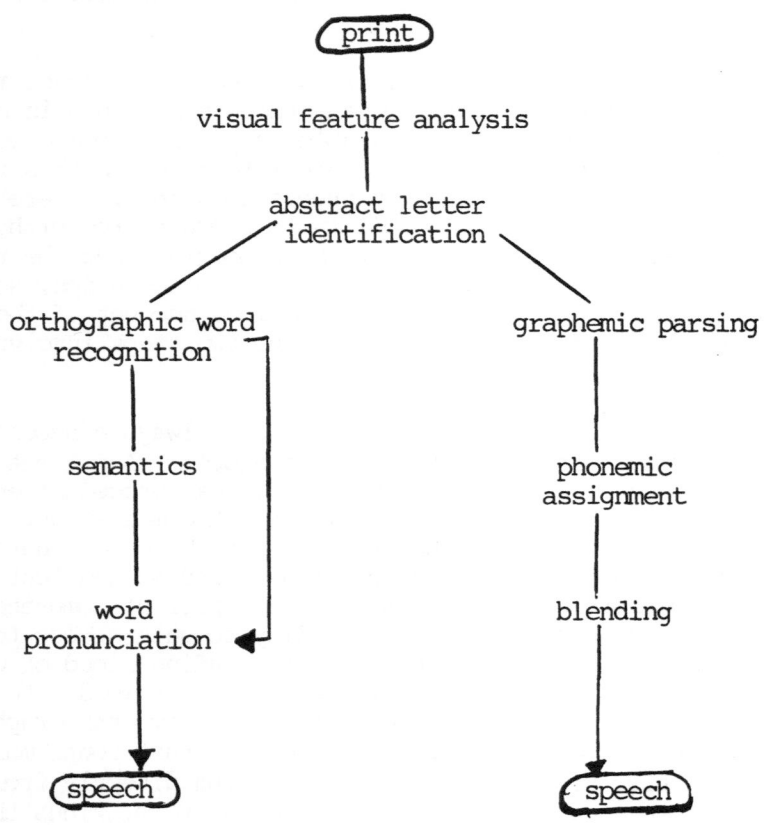

Certain features of this type of model need emphasis:
a) the Orthographic Word Recognition module contains devices for recognising each word in the reader's sight vocabulary, but does not respond to non-words or to words outside the reader's sight vocabulary.

b) the Word Pronunciation module, analogously, contains devices for producing each word in the reader's output vocabulary, but does not play any part in the speaking of non-words (as occurs, for example, when non-words are read aloud).

c) The pathway from Semantics to Word Pronunciation in the model is assumed to be identical to the route used during spontaneous speech to convert semantics to phonology.

Regular words, irregular words and non-words

Earlier in this paper a distinction was drawn between two procedures by which one might read aloud correctly the word van. Particular views were then offered as to how each of these procedures actually operated. A consequence of these views is that, although either procedure would succeed in reading van correctly, it would not be the case that every kind of letter-string could be read correctly by both procedures.

The lexical procedure is by definition mute when confronted with a letter-string which is not a word - vam, for example. This is so because, in terms of Figure 1, the first stage of the lexical procedure is the Orthographic Word Recognition module, and this system does not respond to non-words.

Conversely, there is a stimulus class which the non-lexical procedure by definition fails to handle successfully: the "irregular" or "exception" words of English. When this procedure, assumed to operate by using GPCs, is applied to words like new, mew or few, it assigns the phoneme /u/ to the grapheme ew. It must do the same with the irregular word sew, thus producing an incorrect pronunciation. In general, then, any word in which the phoneme associated with a particular grapheme is not the phoneme most commonly assigned to that grapheme - any irregular word, that is - will be read wrongly by the non-lexical procedure, because the GPC principle assumed to underlie that procedure depends upon assigning to each grapheme the phoneme which most often corresponds to it in English.

In terms of the model shown in Figure 1, therefore, regular words can be read by either the lexical procedure or the non-lexical procedure, whereas non-words can only be read by the non-lexical procedure, and irregular words can only be (correctly) read by the lexical procedure.

This is a crucial property of the model as far as its application to reading disorders is concerned, because it allows one to use specific types of stimuli to assess the intactness in patients of specific components of the model. A patient who can read non-words correctly must have an intact non-lexical procedure. A patient who can read irregular words correctly must have an intact lexical procedure.

This leads us to a consideration of disorders of reading and their interpretations within the framework offered by the model described in Figure 2. I will describe four varieties of acquired reading disorder and consider for each of these how it might be interpreted within the context of this model.

FOUR VARIETIES OF ACQUIRED DYSLEXIA

Letter-by-letter reading

This form of acquired dyslexia is known under a number of equivalent names: pure alexia, alexia without agraphia, word-form dyslexia, word blindness, and spelling dyslexia. It was first described in the nineteenth century, but very little systematic investigation of the syndrome was carried out until very recently. Two extensive studies have, however, recently been reported (Warrington and Shallice, 1980; Patterson and Kay, 1982).

Although there have been reports of this disorder in which the patient is said to have been unable to read any words at all, the patients studied by Warrington and Shallice and by Patterson and Kay could read some words promptly. For those words which could not be read aloud promptly, a slow left-to-right letter-by-letter identification procedure is used: this normally takes the form of naming each letter aloud. If all of the letters are correctly identified the word itself can usually be read. The use of this slow serial letter-identification procedure means that the time between when a word is presented and when it is read aloud increases steeply as a function of the number of letters in the word. For long words, time before correct reading can be very long - several minutes on many occasions. Non-words are also read aloud using the letter-by-letter procedure.

This is the only form of acquired dyslexia in which writing and spelling can be unimpaired. Many letter-by-letter readers can write fluently and accurately, but then cannot read what they have written-especially if they have written in cursive script, as letter-by-letter readers have more difficulty in reading cursive script than block print.

Identification of single letters is often rather imperfect, and patients characteristically will trace letters in the air or on the desk with their fingers when having difficulty in naming them. Copying of letters is often poor and "slavish", the patient behaving as if he is copying unfamiliar forms : indeed, patient L. D.

expalined that, to him, "copying" was an inappropriate term, and that he considered that the term "drawing" was a more appropriate description of what he did when asked to copy letters, except on those
occasions when he immediately recognised a letter.

It is frequently reported that the reading of Arabic numerals
is relatively preserved in letter-by-letter readers.

Explanations of this disorder in terms of Figure 1 have so far
been rather sketchy. One possibility (Patterson and Kay, 1982) is
that the abstract letter identification (ALI) stage can no longer
operate simultaneously upon several letters at once, but can only
operate singly, one letter at a time. Another possibility is that
communication from the ALI stage to the orthographic word recognition
and orthographic-phonological conversion stages is sometimes completely impossible, whilst communications from the ALI stage to a system
for naming letters (a system not shown in Figure 1) is possible, and
the ability to understand what a word is when it is spelled aloud is
one which is intact. The first interpretation offers no explanation
of why naming the letters aloud is so frequent when letter-by-letter
readers are trying to read words. The second interpretation confli-
cts with evidence (Coltheart et al., 1983) suggesting that the task
of understanding a spelled-aloud word is achieved via the route letter names -> abstract letter identities -> orthographic word recognition. If this indeed is the appropriate route, it could not be regularly used by the letter-by-letter reader if access from ALIs to
orthographic word recognition is impaired.

Phonological dyslexia

The patient with phonological dyslexia shows rather good reading
of words coupled with extremely poor reading of non-words. The first
studies of this disorder were by Beauvois and Dérouesné (1979) and
Dérouesné and Beauvois (1979) and other cases are described by Shallice and Warrington (1980), Patterson (1982) and Funnell (1983).
The patient studied by Patterson showed some systematic impairments
in reading words: some errors were made in reading function words and
inflected or derived words. It appears that such errors are not a
necessary feature of phonological dyslexia, however, since neither
type of error with words was shown by the patient studied by Funnell (1983). Similarly, some phonological dyslexics can read some non-
words, but it is possible to find cases where non-word reading is
completely abolished (Funnell, 1983).

The interpretation of this disorder in terms of Figure 2 is straightforward. The patient has lost the use of the GPC procedure.
Words can be read via the (intact) lexical procedure, but non-words,
of course, cannot.

Now, malfunctioning of the non-lexical route might arise, if we adopt the scheme given in Figure 1, at any one or more of the three stages: bad non-word reading would be produced if graphemic parsing were defective, or if phoneme assignment were defective, or if the patient had difficulty in blending. Relevant evidence is available only in connection with the first of these possibilities, that is, graphemic parsing. Dérouesné and Beauvois (1979)studied this by using two types of non-word. For one of these types, there was a one-to-one mapping of <u>letters</u> to phonemes (e.g., <u>iko</u>). For the other type of non-word, two-to-one letter-phoneme mappings occured (e.g., <u>zou</u>). If graphemic parsing cannot be performed, and so phonemes are therefore assigned to <u>letters</u> rather than graphemes, this would not harm reading for non-words like <u>iko</u>, but would affect reading of non-words like <u>zou</u>. Results from four phonological dyslexics studied by Dérouesné and Beauvois (1979) are shown in Table 1. Three of them were

TABLE 1.   Evidence for an impairment of the graphemic parsing stage in phonological dyslexia (Data from Dérouesné & Beauvois, 1978).

Percentage Correct Oral Reading

	Non-words requiring graphemic parsing	Non-words not requiring graphemic parsing	
	(e.g., <u>zou</u>) (N=40)	(e.g., <u>iko</u>) (N=80)	
Subject			
A	50	89	$x^2 = 21.7$ p < .001
B	65	93	$x^2 = 14.4$ p < .001
C	62	80	$x^2 = 4.32$ p < .05
D	55	68	$x^2 = 1.76$ p < .25

significantly worse at reading non-words which required graphemic parsing than non-words which did not. This suggests that in at least
some cases of phonological dyslexia, the impairment of the non-lexical procedure which is a defining characteristic of this disorder
arises at the graphemic parsing stage. Hence studies of phonological
dyslexia provide evidence in support of the particular theoretical
characterisation of the non-lexical procedure set out in Figure 1.

Surface dyslexia

    In this disorder, regularly-spelled words are read much better
than irregular words. Misreadings of irregular words often take the
form of regularisations - that is, assigning the most common phonological correspondence to orthographic segments of the irregular word.
Such assignment must of course produce an incorrect pronunciation,
since by definition an irregular word is one in which at least some
orthographic-phonological correspondences are not the most common.
Examples of regularisation errors made by surface dyslexics are pint
-> "/Pᴜnt/", sew -> "/su/", and bear -> "beer". Stress errors are
also observed in surface-dyslexic reading: all the phonemes of a polysyllabic words are produced correctly, but stress is assigned incorrectly (e.g., oboe - "/əbоѡ/"). Printed words are often comprehended
via their pronunciations, so that the surface dyslexic may not be able
to decide whether the printed word I means "me" or means "an organ of
sight", and may define bear as "a drink". Spelling and writing are
impaired: the majority of spelling errors are phonologically correct
(such as spelling "search" as surch or "hydraulic" as highdrolic).
This disorder was first discussed by Marshall and Newcombe (1973) and
subsequent reports include those by Coltheart et al. (1983) and Shallice, Warrington and McCarthy (1983).

    This disorder, like phonological dyslexia, can be readily inter-
preted within the theoretical framework of Figure 2. The surface dyslexic is sometimes unable to read aloud via the routes from the Orthographic Word Recognition stage of Figure 2, and so must sometimes
use the GPC route. This route permits correct reading of regular words, but produces regularisation errors in the reading of irregular
words, since the GPC stage uses the most common orthographic-phonological correspondences of English. Stress errors will also result from the use of the GPC route because, for many English polysyllabic
words, there is no rule which correctly predicts stress: knowing what
stress to use depends on knowing what the word is, and such word-specific knowledge is not available when the GPC route is used to read
aloud.

Deep dyslexia

    The most prominent symptom of this disorder is the semantic error
in reading aloud: a deep dyslexic, given the single word tulip to read, might read it as "crocus". These patients also make visual errors

(sword -> "words), derivational errors (runner -> "running") and omissions (failures to respond) when asked to read aloud. Abstract words
are less likely to be read aloud than matched concrete words. Function words are less likely to be read aloud than content words (whether this is genuinely an effect of part-of-speech or a consequence of
differences in concreteness between the two classes of word is as yet
unclear). Non-words cannot be read aloud at all. Writing and spelling is severely impaired or almost abolished. Aphasia has been present in all cases of deep dyslexia so far described: usually, but not
always, Broca's aphasia.

     Whether one can interpret deep dyslexia in terms of the model
given in Figure 2, as I have attempted to interpret the other three
dyslexias, is in dispute. An interpretation of this kind was offered
by Morton and Patterson (1980). In contrast, Coltheart (1980) and
Saffran, Bogyo, Schwartz and Marin (1980) argued that deep dyslexia
does not reflect reading by a partly-damaged and partly-preserved reading system in the left hemisphere (a reading system of the kind represented in figure 2). They suggested that instead the deep dyslexic's left-hemispehre reading system cannot be used at all, and that
reading in deep dyslexia is the product of a right-hemisphere reading
system. This account of deep dyslexia was attacked by Warrington
(1981) and by Patterson and Kay (1982), and defended by Coltheart
(1983).

FUTURE DIRECTIONS

     I have described four syndromes of acquired dyslexia and consi-
dered how each might be interpreted within a particular model of normal reading. The concept of the syndrome has been a useful one in
developing work relating dyslexic syndromes to reading models. However, its usefulness is likely to be short-lived. The reason is that,
if a dyslexic syndrome is a specific pattern of preservations and
impairments of reading abilities which reliably co-occur, and if a
modular model of reading of the type shown in Figure 2 is appropriate,
it follows that there are many different possible dyslexic syndromes.
Any unique pattern of impairments to the boxes and arrows of Figure 2
will produce a unique syndrome; since Figure 2 has enough boxes and
arrows to produce a large number of different unique patterns of impairments, it generates a large number of different syndromes.

     We might, therefore, expect a rapid multiplication of syndromes
as information-processing studies of acquired dyslexia continue. We
might also expect fractionation of syndromes that is, demonstrations
of the same syndrome with different underlying causes. For example,
a patient will exhibit phonological dyslexia if he has either a) an
impairment of graphemic parsing, or b) an impairment of phoneme assignment, or c) an impairment of blending. Similarly, surface dyslexia
(defined as disproportionate difficulty in reading irregular words)
will occur if either a) there is impairment of orthographic word

recognition, or b) there is impairment of the word pronunciation module, or c) there is impairment of communication between these two
modules.

If there are going to be very many different syndromes, and if
syndromes are themselves going to split into sub-types, thinking about acquired dyslexia in terms of syndromes will become very unwieldy:
this is why I have suggested that the concept of the syndrome may soon be seen to have outlived its usefulness in the study of acquired
dyslexia.

To abandon this concept may seem an alarming step, because thinking in terms of syndromes allows one to generalise from previous to
future patients. If a basic set of syndromes has been developed from
past work, assigning future patients to one or other of the syndrome
categories and so using them as subjects for research aimed at telling
us more about the nature of that syndrome appears to be a way of allowing one's knowledge of acquired dyslexia to cumulate. If one does
not work in terms of syndromes, what alternative is there to treating
every patient as unique - and if one does this, how could there be a
universally applicable body of knowledge about acquired dyslexia ?
A solution, it seems to me, is to use models of reading to make universal statements. Even if every patient exhibited a unique reading
disorder, it might still be possible to interpret every patient's behavior in the context of a single model of reading. The assumption
that a single model should be applicable to all patients allows each
new patient to be an appropriate source of data for testing the model:
and this permits one to generalize from previous to future patients
even if one has rejected the policy of thinking in terms of syndromes.

REFERENCES

Beauvois, M. -F., and Dérouesné, J. Phonological alexia: three dis-
     sociations. Journal of Neurology, Neurosurgery and Psychiatry,
     1979, 42, 1115-1124.
Caramazza, A., and Martin, R. Short-term memory performance of pho-
     nological coding. Brain and Cognition, 1, (in press). 1982.
Coltheart, M. Lexical access in simple reading tasks. In Under-
     wood, G. (Ed.), Strategies of Information Processing. London:
     Academic Press. 1978.
Coltheart, M. Deep dyslexia: a right hemisphere hypothesis. In
     Coltheart, M, Patterson, K. E., and Marshall, J. C. (Eds.),
     Deep Dyslexia. London: Routledge and Kegan Paul, 1980 a.
Coltheart, M. Visual information-processing. In Dodwell, P. C.
     (Ed.), New Horizons in Psychology. 2nd ed. London: Penguin
     Books. 1980 b.
Coltheart, M. Disorders of reading and their implications for models
     of normal reading. Visible Language, 1981, XV(2), 245-286.

Coltheart, M., Masterson, J., Byng, S., Prior, M., and Riddoch, J.
    Surface dyslexia. Quarterly Journal of Experimental Psycholo-
    gy, (in press). 1983.
Coltheart, M., Patterson, K. E., and Marshall, J. C. (Eds.) Deep
    Dyslexia. London: Routledge & Kegan Paul; 1980.
Dérouesné, J., and Beauvois, M. -F. Phonological processing in
    reading: data from alexia. Journal of Neurology, Neurosurgery
    and Psychiatry, 1979, 42, 1125-1132.
Funnell, E. Phonological processes in reading: new evidence from
    acquired dyslexia. British Journal of Psychology, (in press)
    1983.
Glushko, R. J. The Organisation and activation of orthographic know-
    ledge in reading aloud. Journal of Experimental Psychology
    (Human Perception and Performance), 1979, 5, 674-691.
Glushko, R. J. Principles for pronouncing print: the psyhcology of
    phonography. In Lesgold, A. M., and Perfetti, C. A. (Eds.),
    Interactive Processes in Reading. Hillsdale: Lawrence Erlbaum
    Associates, New Jersey, 1981.
Henderson, L. Orthography and Word Recognition in Reading. Academic
    Press, London. 1982.
Kay, J., and Marcel, A. J. One process, not two, in reading aloud:
    lexical analogies do the work of non-lexical rules. Quarterly
    Journal of Experimental Psychology, 1981, 33A, 397-415.
Marcel, A. J. Surface dyslexia and beginning reading: a revised hy-
    pothesis of the pronunciation of print and its impairments. In
    Coltheart, M., Patterson, K. E., and Marshall, J. C. (Eds.),
    Deep Dyslexia. London: Routledge & Kegan paul, 1980.
Marshall, J. C., and Newcombe, F. Patterns of paralexia: a psycho-
    linguistic approach. Journal of Psycholinguistic Research,
    1973, 2, 175-199.
Morton, J., and Patterson, K. E. A new attempt at an interpretation,
    or, an attempt at a new interpretation. In Coltheart, M.,
    Patterson, K. E., and Marshall, J. C. (Eds.), Deep Dyslexia.
    London: Routledge & Kegan Paul, 1980.
Newcombe, F., and Marshall, J. C. Transcoding and lexical stabili-
    sation in deep dyslexia. In Coltheart, M., Patterson, K. E.,
    and Marshall, J. C. (Eds.), Deep Dyslexia, London: Routledge
    & Kegan Paul, 1980.
Newcombe, F., and Marshall, J. C. On psycholinguistic classificati-
    ons of the acquired dyslexias. Bulletin of the Orton Society,
    1981, 31, 29-46.
Patterson, K.E. Neuropsychological approaches to the study of rea-
    ding. British Journal of Psychology, 1981, 72, 151-174.
Patterson, K. E. The relation between reading and phonological co-
    ding: further neurological observations. In Ellis, A. W. (Ed.),
    Normality and Pathology in Cognitive Function. London: Acade-
    mic Press, 1982.
Patterson, K. E., and Kay, J. Letter-by-letter reading: Psychologi-
    cal descriptions of a neuorlogical syndrome. Quarterly Journal
    of Experimental Psychology, (in press). 1982.

Saffran, E. M. Reading in deep dyslexia is not ideographic. Neuropsychologia, 1980, 18, 219-223.

Saffran, E. M., Bogyo, L. C., Schwartz, M. F., and Marin, O. S. M. Does deep dyslexia reflect right-hemisphere reading ? In Coltheart, M., Patterson, K. E., and Marshall, J. C. (Eds.), Deep Dyslexia, London: Routledge & Kegan paul, 1980.

Schwartz, M. F., Saffran, E. M., and Marin, O. S. M. Fractionating the reading process in dementia: evidence for word-specific print-to-sound associations. In Coltheart, M., Patterson, K. E., and Marshall, J. C. (Eds.), Deep Dyslexia, London: Routledge & Kegan Paul, 1980.

Shallice, T. Neurological impairment of cognitive processes. British Medical Bulletin, 1981, 37, 187-192.

Shallice, T., Warrington, E. K., and McCarthy, R. Reading without semantics. Quarterly Journal of Psychology, (in press) , 1983.

Warrington, E. K. Concrete word dyslexia. British Journal of Psychology, 1981, 72, 175-196.

Warrington, E. K., and Shallice, T. Word-form dyslexia. Brain, 1980, 103, 99-112.

NEUROPSYCHOLOGICAL ASSESSMENT OF CHILDREN AND ADULTS WITH DEVELOPMENTAL DYSLEXIA[1]

Ian Q. Whishaw and Bryan Kolb
Department of Psychology
The University of Lethbridge
Lethbridge, Alberta

As many as ten percent of children have great difficulty learning how to read, and many of these may never acquire adequate reading skills. Since there is no obvious cause for their disability, it has been called developmental dyslexia, to contrast it with acquired dyslexia that results from brain damage to reading adults (Critchley, 1970). The clinical descriptions of developmental dyslexia are now quite comprehensive (cf. Malatesha and Dougan, 1982) and have led to many theories regarding their etiology (cf. Benton and Pearl, 1978). One explanation of developmental dyslexia is that it results from brain abnormalities that are acquired genetically or result from some type of perinatal trauma. Little is known, however, about the possible forms of brain abnormalities or their location, although the most frequently suggested brain site is the posterior neocortex of the left hemisphere. This suggestion derives by analogy from anatomical and behavioral studies of acquired dyslexia (Benson, 1974; Geschwind, 1962), from an architectonic study on a deceased dyslexic (Galaburda and Kemper, 1979), from electroencephalographic recording studies (Ahn et al., 1980), evoked potential studies (Preston et al., 1977; Symann-Lovett et al, 1977), and from computerized brain tomography (Hier et al., 1978). As compelling as these data may be in

1. This research was supported by grants from the Alberta Mental Health Research Fund. The authors thank Barbara Wilson and Sandra McKay for their assistance in testing the subjects, Jo-Ann Zaborowski for help with data analysis, Richard Dyck for making figures, Adria Allen for typing, the Lethbridge Separate and Public School System, the Lethbridge Community College, and Lethbridge Mental Health services for referring the subjects, and the special education staff of the Lethbridge Separate School System for their aid in various aspects of the study.

implicating left posterior neocortical abnormalities in developmental dyslexia, they do not exclude the possibility that similar abnormalities can be found in the right hemisphere or elsewhere in the left hemisphere. In fact, the results of studies using neuropsychological tests have led to suggestions that different forms of developmental dyslexia may be found that result from abnormalities of either the left or right hemisphere, or even both hemispheres (cf. Gaddes, 1980; Knights and Bakker, 1978; Malatesha and Aaron, 1982). Although we are in sympathy with the notion that there may be various etiologies for developmental dyslexia, we feel that the psychological studies have a serious flaw in that they have not utilized test batteries that have been demonstrated to be capable of discriminating patients with circumscribed cortical lesions. A battery of tests validated at the Montreal Neurological Institute meets this condition.

Since 1950, over 1,000 patients at the Montreal Neurological Institute undergoing a cortical excision for the relief of intractable epilepsy, the removal of small indolent tumors, or the repair of vascular abnormalities such as angiomas or aneurysms have been given an extensive battery of psychological tests prior to surgery. They have been retested postoperatively over intervals ranging from 2 to 3 weeks to, in some cases, 5 to 20 years. From these studies it has been possible to identify psychological tests that reveal consistent impairments in patients with localized cerebral damage in the frontal, temporal, or parietal lobes of each hemisphere (cf. Kolb and Whishaw, 1980; Milner, 1975; Taylor, 1969; 1979), and to identify discrete areas of dysfunction or damage. Furthermore, the performance of people with different disorders such as learning disabilities can be compared directly to the published data on patients with surgical excisions. Impaired performance on individual tests cannot be taken as evidence of brain injury or dysfunction, as normal control subjects often perform poorly on individual tests; however, impaired performance on clusters of tests known to be associated with localized cortical areas permits valid inferences about cerebral injuries, rather than on patients with ill-defined zones of damage, such as strokes, tumors, and closed head injuries, among others. Also, the reassessment of patients over periods of up to 20 years has permitted the refinement of the tests. Tests have also been added which have proven useful with other patient populations, such as the war veterans studied extensively by Teuber, Semmes, and their colleagues (Semmes et al., 1963). Finally, information has been accumulated about very localized areas of the cortex as additional patients with particular areas of localized damage became available for assessment (cf. Corkin, 1980; Milner, 1975; Taylor, 1979).

We report the results obtained from 38 reading disabled subjects who varied in age from 6 to 38 years. By way of comparison we tested 12 subjects, ages 9 to 15 years, who were referred because of poor grades but who had average reading scores and 30 subjects, from the same classes as the reading disabled group, whose school performance was strictly average. The reading disabled group was comprised of successive referrals who had no other neurological diagnosis and who had had a medical, a vision, and a hearing examination.

SUBJECTS

The dyslexic group consisted of 38 Caucasian subjects aged 6 to 38 years who were referred for testing because they were having trouble learning to read. Referrals were from the Lethbridge Public and Separate Systems and from the Lethbridge Community College. Prior to referral, all of the primary and secondary school students had been placed in remedial reading programs and were found to have made little or no progress despite additional instruction. The adults were referred by the Lethbridge Community college because they had been unable to pass an English competency exam and were not profiting from remedial language instruction. Upon referral the medical records of the subjects were obtained to ensure that they had never been diagnosed as having any other neurological or psychological disability, to ensure that they had not been diagnosed as hyperactive or received medication for hyperactivity, and to ensure that they had received a medical examination that included vision and hearing tests. The subjects were then given the Wide Range Achievement Test (WRAT). Subjects who had reached grade 4 or higher in school were included in the study if they scored two years below their age norm on reading. The performance of the reading retarded group was compared with two other groups. The first group consisted of 12 children, aged 9 to 15 years, who were referred for testing because their parents were concerned about their poor school marks. None of the subjects had ever been placed in a remedial reading class, none had failed a grade, and all achieved normal scores on the WRAT. The second group consisted of 30 subjects, matched for age and sex, and who were selected from the same classes as the reading disabled group. The home room teacher was asked to identify students who, based upon their classroom performance and school grades, were average students; that is, they received neither outstanding nor failing grades in any subject.

The tests used in the current study are described in Table 1. Wechsler Intelligence Tests (WISC-R, WAIS) were given to provide a reference point for other test data that may be influenced by general intelligence.

BEHAVIORAL TESTS

Speech Lateralization

A dichotic listening test was used to infer speech lateralization (Kimura, 1973). Two different words were presented simultaneously, one to each ear, and the subject's task was to recall as many words as possible after listening to three pairs of words. Since the ear contralateral to the hemisphere containing speech has a preferential input to that hemisphere, more words will be recalled from this ear, and the dominant hemisphere for speech can be inferred.

TABLE 1. Summary of neuropsychological tests used in the study

Theoretical function	Test name	Basic references
1. General intelligence	Wechsler Adult Intelligence Scale	McFie (1975)
	Wechsler Intelligence Scale for Children-Revised	
2. Speech lateralization	Dichotic words	Kimura (1973)
3. Memory	Wechsler Memory Scale	Milner (1967)
	Delayed Recall of Wechlser Stories	Milner (1967)
	Delayed Recall of Wechsler Figures	Milner (1967)
	Delayed Recall of Paired Associates	Milner (1967)
	Delayed Recall of Rey Complex Figure	Taylor (1979)
4. Visual perception	Mooney Closure Figure	Milner (1980)
	Copy of Rey Complex Figure	Taylor (1979)
	Draw-a-bicycle	McFie and Zangwill (1960)
5. Spatial orientation	Right/Left differentiation	Semmes et al. (1963)
	Semmes Body Placing Test	Semmes et al. (1963)
6. Frontal lobe	Wisconsin Card sorting Test	Milner (1964)
	Chicago Word Fluency Test	Milner (1964)
	Gotman-Milner Design Fluency	Jones-Gotman and Milner (1977)
7. Language	Token Test	de Renzi and Vignolo (1962)
	Newcombe Word Fluency Test	Newcombe (1969)

Memory

All subjects were given Form-I of the Wechsler memory Scale
and the memory quotient (MQ) was calculated. In addition, Milner's
extensive studies linking certain memory functions with the temporal
lobes have provided several tests useful in assessing memory functions. Milner (1975) and Taylor (1979) have found that delayed recall of the stories (Logical Memory) and paired associates (Associate
Learning) of the Wechsler Memory Scale are particularly sensitive
to the function of the left temporal lobe, and the delayed recall of
the simple designs of the Wechsler Memory Scale and the delayed recall of the Rey Complex figure are sensitive to the function of the
right temporal lobe. For the Rey figure test, the subjects were
presented with a printed copy of the Rey Figure (see Fig. 7) and
were asked to copy the figure as exactly as they could. Forty-five
minutes later the subjects were asked (without advance warning) to
reproduce as much of the figure as they could remember.

Visual Perception

Visual perceptual functions were inferred from the copy of the
Rey Figure and from performance on the Mooney Closure Faces Test
(Mooney, 1956). In the closure test, a series of 26 incomplete representations of faces were presented to each subject (see Milner,
1980, for an example). The task was to state the sex and approximate age of the person depicted. In the Rey Figure the task is to
copy the figure displayed (see Fig. 7).

Spatial Orientation

Two tests of spatial orientation were drawn from the extensive
studies of Semmes et al. (1963). In the right/left differentiation
test the subject was shown a series of pictures of body parts and
clothing (see Fig. 8) and asked to determine if each was of the left
or right. In the body placing test the subject was shown a series
of drawings of a person that had a series of numbers on various body
locations (see Fig. 9) and the task was to point to the location of
the numbers on the subject's own body. The left-right differentiation test is thought to be sensitive to left parietal function, whereas the body placing test is thought to be more sensitive to left
frontal than parietal cortex function.

Card Sorting

Milner and her colleagues have described the Wisconsin Card
Sorting Test as particularly sensitive to frontal lobe function.
In the test the subject was presented with four stimulus cards bear-
ing designs that differed in color, form and number. The subject's
task was to sort a pack of cards that varied along these dimensions.
The correct sorting strategy was changed, without warning the

subject, every time 10 consecutive cards were sorted correctly.

Language

Three tests of language function were given in addition to the WRAT. In the Chicago Word Fluency Test, the subject was asked to write down as many words as possible beginning with a particular letter ("S") in 5 min., and as many words beginning with another letter and having only 4 letters ("C _ _ _ ") in 4 min. This test is sensitive to left frontal and left posterior cortex function. The Token Test (de Renzi and Vignolo, 1962) was given as aphasia screening test to only those subjects in which language comprehension problems were suspected. In the Newcombe Word Fluency Test (Newcombe, 1969) the subject was asked to give as many objects, and then animals, as possible in 1 min. The test differs from the Chicago Word Fluency Test in that more structure is provided for the subjects, which allows frontal lobe patients to perform the test within normal limits.

Analysis

The results were assessed using Analysis of variance procedures and follow-up t-tests. Since the tests differed slightly for different age groups (the coding test in the WISC-R changes for children reaching the age 8, and the WAIS was used for intelligence assessment after age 15) the analysis included subgrouping the dyslexic and control groups into 3 groups each: 1) children under eight; 2) adolescents under 16; and, 3) adults. For the comparison with the group of students who had poor grades, the analysis (t-tests) was done comparing only the adolescent-dyslexic group with the poor-grades group. Finally, for some tests we compared the performance of the dyslexic group to the control group using cut-off scores, which were one standard deviation below the norm on that test or else were scores which would be unlikely for a normal subject to obtain. Design fluency and draw-a-bicycle tests are not reported in this paper because data collection was incomplete.

RESULTS

A summary showing age, sex, handedness, ear dominance on the dichotic listening tests, as well as some features of performance on the Wechsler I. Q. and Memory Tests is shown in Figure 1. The dyslexic group differed from the normal population in that there were more males than should occur by chance (73%), and there were more left-handers (as judged by writing hand) than should have occurred by chance (14/38 in the dyslexic group vs. 2/3 in the control group). Twenty-three of the 38 dyslexic children had a higher performance than verbal I. Q. as compared with 16/30 in the control group; neither this difference nor the magnitude of the difference was significant. Figure 1 also displays the "scatter" displayed on the intelligence and memory tests. In this figure large dots

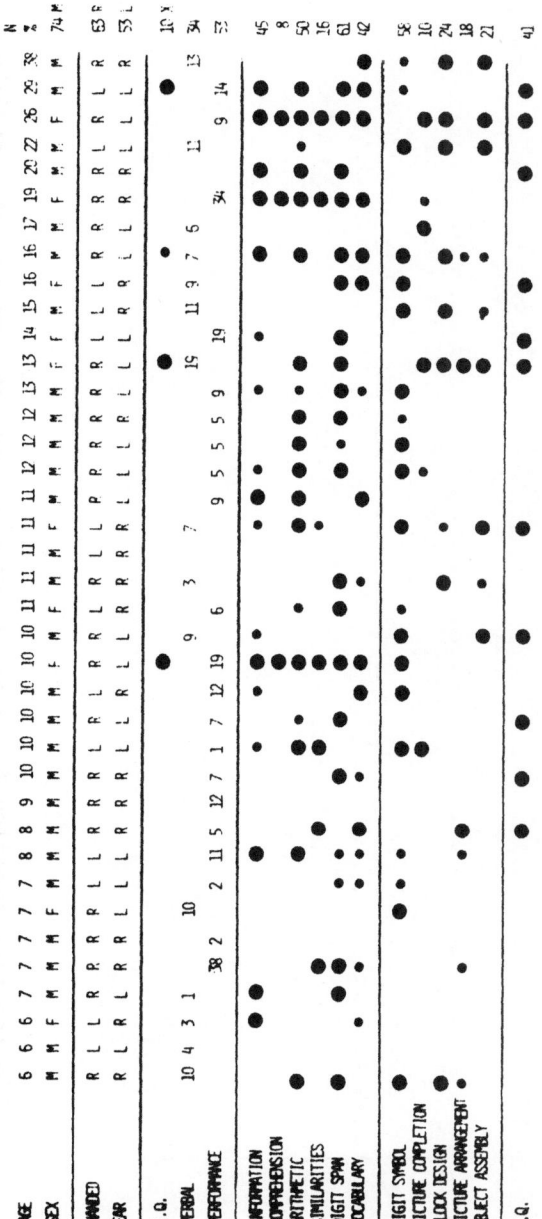

FIGURE 1. Developmental dyslexic subjects, age, sex, handedness, dominant ear in dichotic
listening, intelligence test subscores and MQ. Large dots show scores one standard
deviation below population norm, small dots, scores three quarters of a standard
deviation below the population norm.

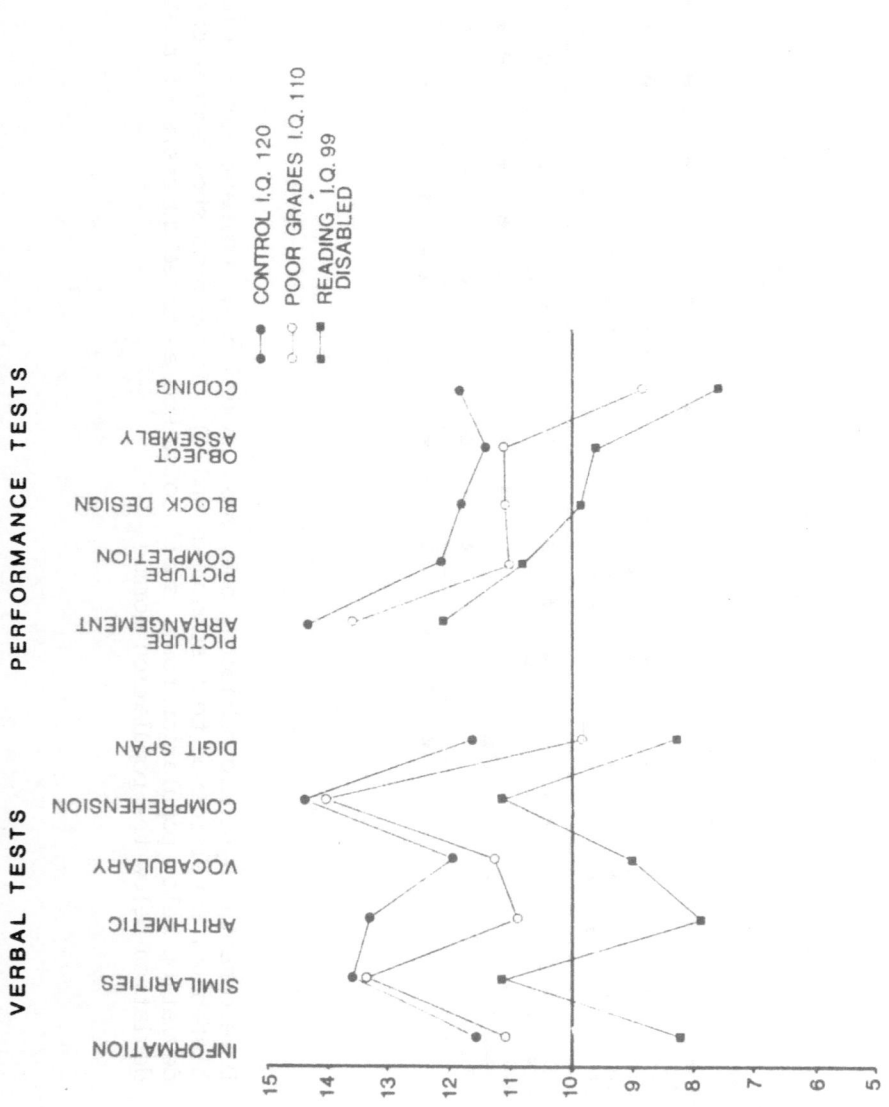

FIGURE 2.   Intelligence test profiles for control, poor grades and developmental dyslexic groups.

represent scores that fall one or more standard deviations below the
population norm, and smaller dots represent scores that fall three-
fourths of a standard deviation below the population norm. A central point illustrated by the scatter is that it is difficult to classify the dyslexic group into meaningful subgroups on the basis of
any of these measures. Nevertheless, it can be noted that only three subjects had full-scale I. Q. scores less than 85. None had an
I. Q. less than 80. It can also be seen that performance was worse
on some subtests than on others. More than 45% of the dyslexic subjects registered poor performance on the Information, Arithmetic,
Digit Span, and Digit Symbol subtests, whereas fewer subjects had
poorer performance on the other subtests. Finally, it can be seen
from Figure 1 that 41% of the dyslexic subjects received M. Q. scores of less than 85.

Intelligence

    Figure 2 contrasts the profiles of the I. Q. subtests for the
three test groups. The mean full scale I. Q.'s were: dyslexic group, 99 (Verbal IQ [VIQ] = 96.5, performance IQ [PIQ] = 100), poor
grades group, 110 (VIQ = 112, PIQ = 108), and normal group, 120 (VIQ
= 120, PIQ = 119). An analysis of variance showed that there were
significant differences among groups (F = 49, p < .001). Follow-up
t-tests (p's < .01) showed that each of the three groups differed
from the others.

    The profile on the subtests is noteworthy. For the dyslexic
group, on the verbal subscale it has the shape of an "M" whereas on
the performance of subscale it has the shape of an "\". The profile for the poor-grades group was the same though displaced upwards.
The profile for the normal group was not quite the same, note especially the difference in the arithmetic and coding scores. Characteristically, as noted above, the lowest scores for both the dyslexic and poor grades groups were on information, arithmetic, digit
span and coding tests.

    To determine if the I. Q. scores and profiles of our dyslexic
group were characteristic of those of other studies, we prorated
and combined the scores from 25 different studies reviewed by Rugel
(1975). The result is illustrated in Figure 3. The mean full scale I. Q. score of the 1,521 dyslexics was 100, a value that is almost the same as that reported here. Moreover, the profile of the
subtest scores for the dyslexic group was also the same as that shown by our 38 dyslexic subjects. The control groups reviewed by
Rugel (1974) had a somewhat lower full-scale I. Q. score than our
control group, and the profile of subtest scores in his control group was not the same as that of his dyslexic group.

    We subdivided our dyslexic group into three subgroups by age:
ages 6-8 (n = 10); ages 8-15 (n = 19); and ages 16 and up (n = 9).

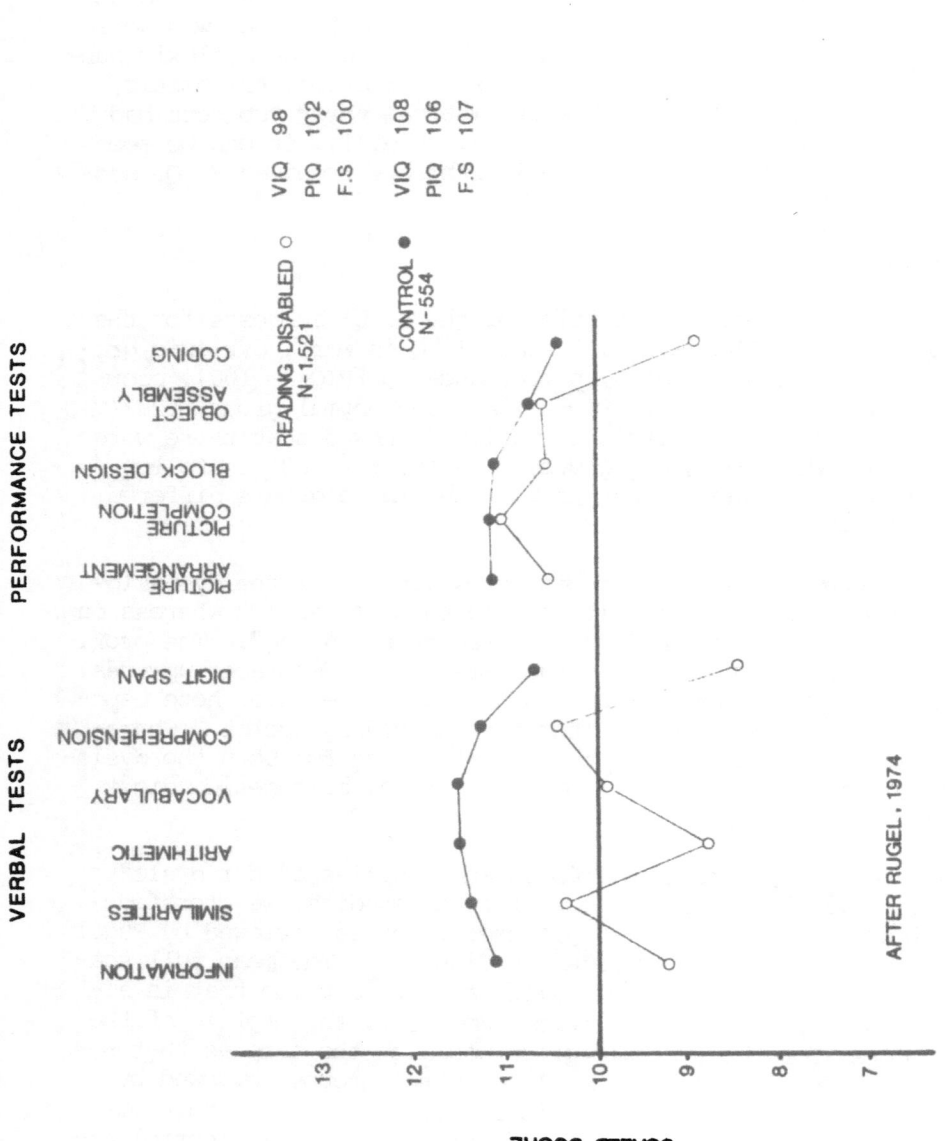

FIGURE 3.   Intelligence test profiles of the developmental dyslexic and control subjects
              summarized by Rugel (1974).

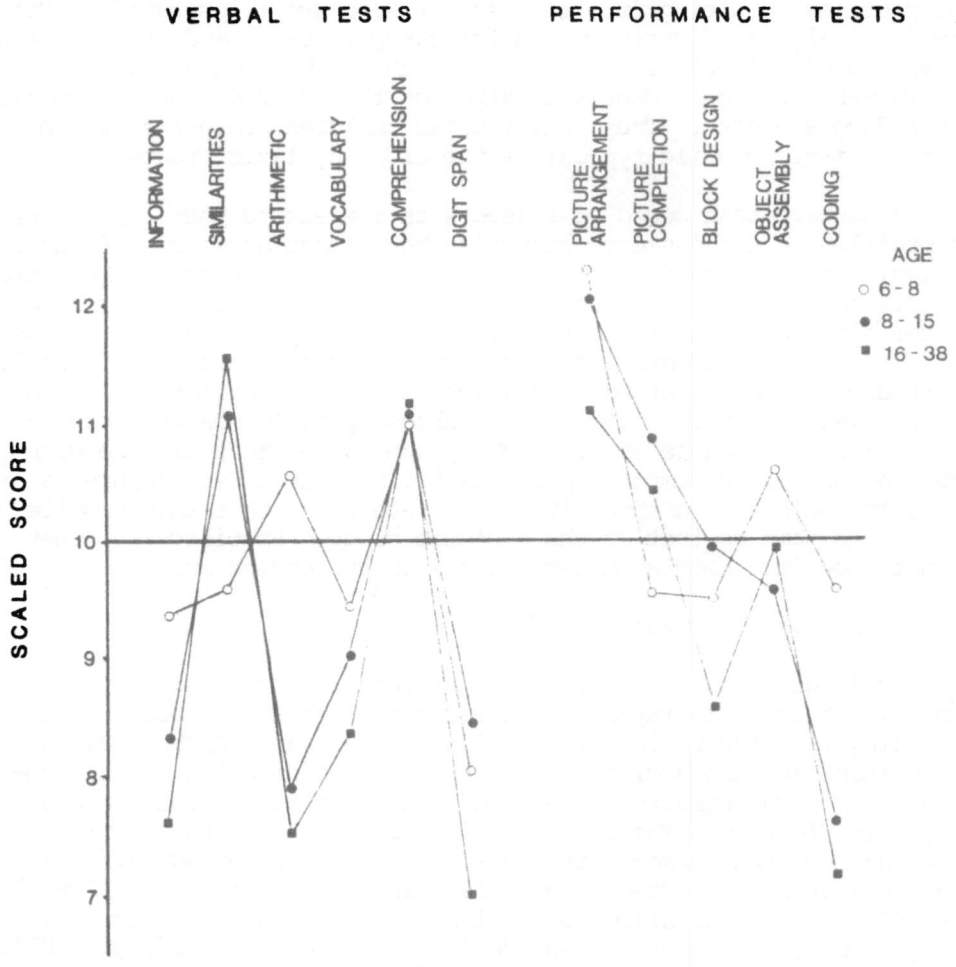

FIGURE 4. Intelligence test profiles for developmental dyslexic
groups of three different ages.

The profiles resulting from this subdivision are illustrated in Figure 4. Analysis of variance and follow-up tests showed that the two older groups did not differ from each other. The younger group, however, was not significantly impaired on the information, arithmetic and coding subtests. Thus, the younger children did not show the characteristic profile typical of the older dyslexic groups.

A concern that could be raised with respect to the I. Q. subtest profiles of the dyslexic group is that almost any group of neurological patients would display a similar profile. Since we have previously collected data on children and adults with Gilles de la Tourettes disease (Sutherland et al., 1982) we computed their I. Q. subtest profile for comparative purposes. It is displayed in Figure 5. There are two important ways in which the profile differs from that of the dyslexic group. The verbal subtest profile has the shape of an "N" and performance appears to improve rather than decline with age. We have also computed profiles for a group of schizophrenia patients (Kolb and Whishaw, 1983) and have found that this profile is not the same as that of the dyslexic group. Specifically, they do not show impairments on the digit span and coding subscales.

Speech Lateralization

As illustrated in Figure 1, significantly more dyslexic than control subjects displayed a left ear effect on the dichotic word listening task (20 of 38 vs. 2 of 30). We summarized the results by dominant and non-dominant ear, irrespective of which was the dominant ear. The results for each of the three age groups are displayed in Figure 6. The analysis of variance on the total number of words reported showed that there was a significant age effect; the older groups reported more words than the younger group (F = 31, p < .01). There was also a significant group effect; the control group reported more words than the dyslexic group (F = 23, p < .01). Comparisons of the total number of words reported from each ear showed that in children the control group reported more words from the dominant ear than the dyslexic group (t = 2.7, p < .05), and the adolescent control group reported more words from the dominant ear than the adolescent dyslexic group (t = 3.3, p < .05), but the difference between the adult dyslexic and control group was not significant. Just the opposite effect was obtained from the nondominant ear. Only the adult control group reported more words than the dyslexic group (t = 2.8, p < .05). The results suggest a trend in the dyslexic groups to show a continued improvement in age in the number of words reported from the dominant ear, whereas little improvement appears to occur in recall from the nondominant ear. In the poor-grades group only 1 of 10 subjects showed a left-ear effect. In terms of total number of words reported the poor-grades group was intermediate to the dyslexic and control groups, and the group effect was significant (dyslexic mean = 46; poor grades, 52; control, 62; F = 9.2, p < .01). The results of the dichotic liste-

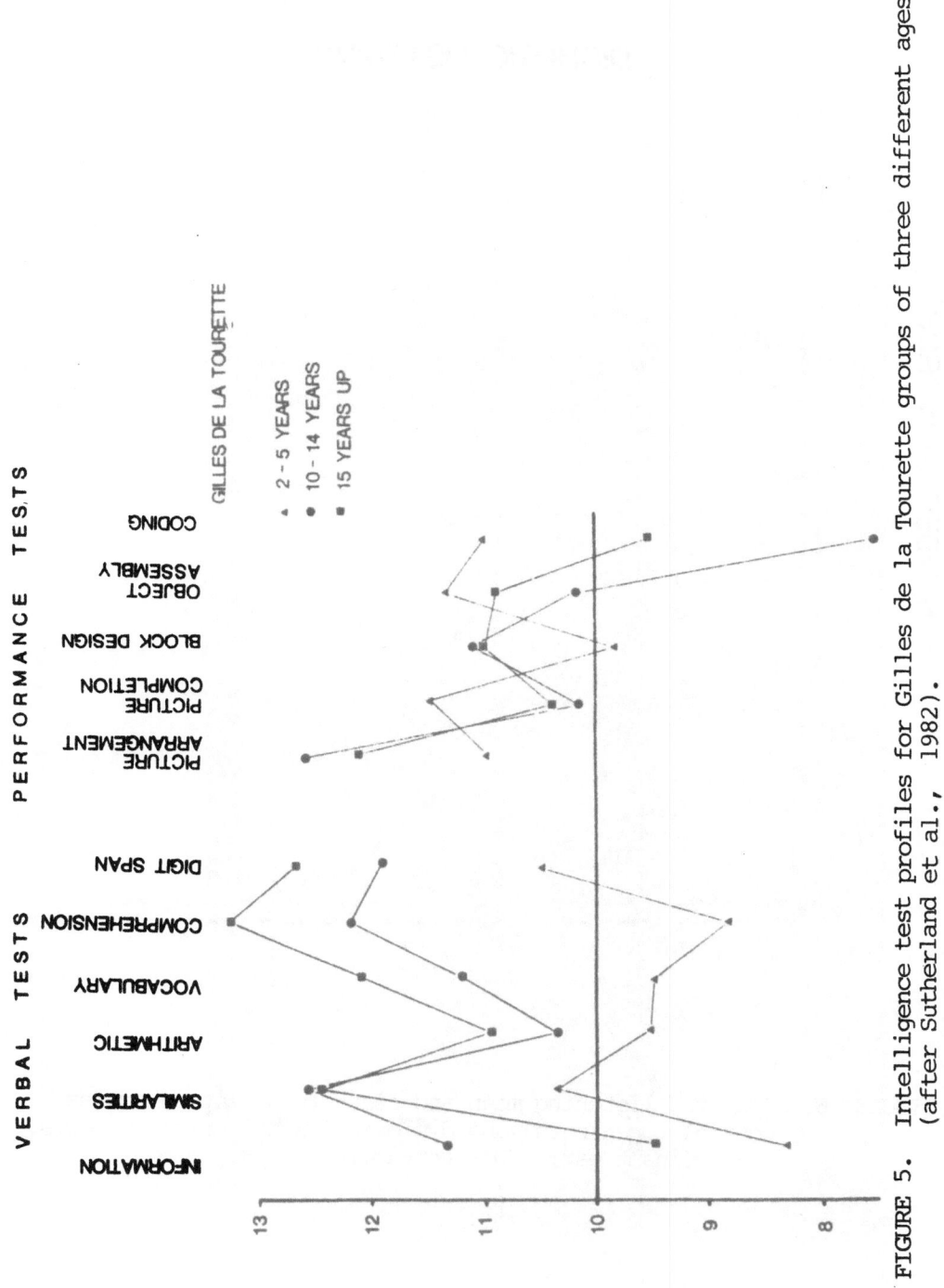

FIGURE 5.   Intelligence test profiles for Gilles de la Tourette groups of three different ages (after Sutherland et al., 1982).

I. Q. WHishaw and B. Kolb

DICHOTIC LISTENING

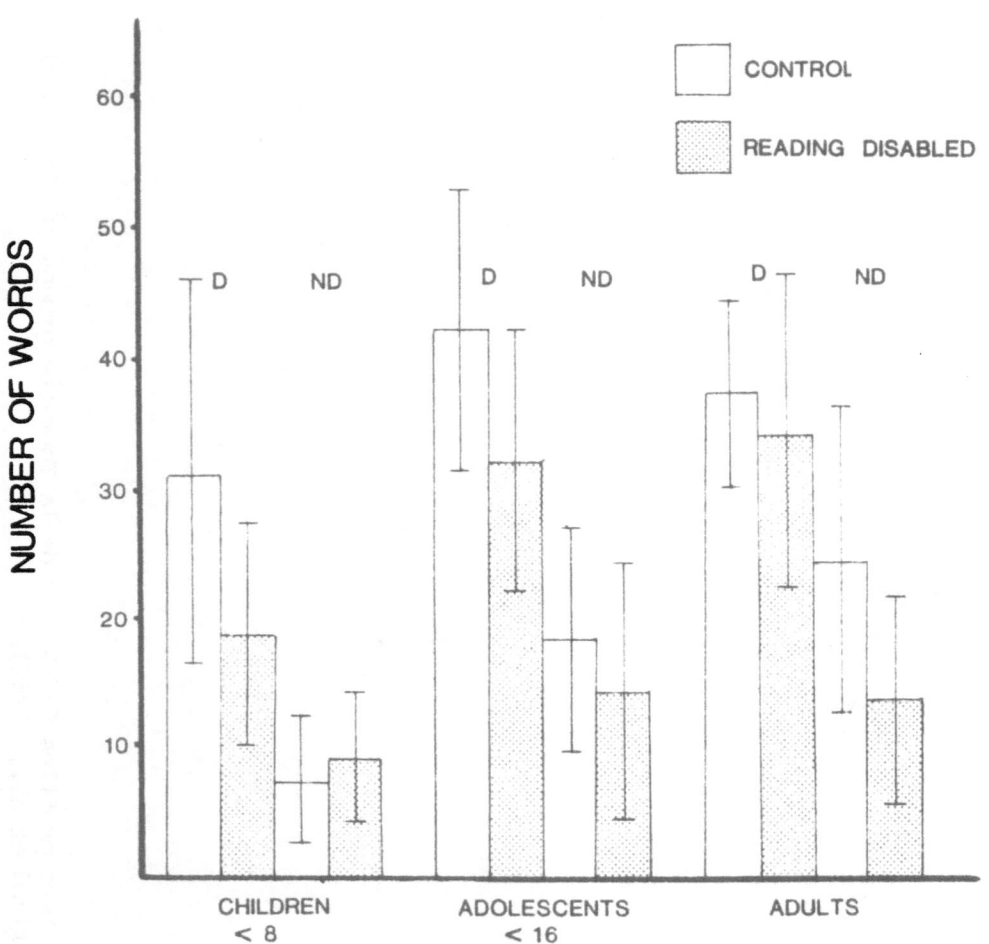

FIGURE 6. Dichotic listening mean and standard deviation scores control (open bars) and dyslexic (shaded bars) subjects. D - dominant ear; ND - non-dominant ear.

ning task are consistent with the early work of Sparrow and Satz (19-70) which shows that a left ear advantage is common in dyslexic but not control children. The results are also consistent with other studies which show that in dyslexic groups, as contrasted with individuals, a reduced right ear advantage is common (cf. Satz, 1976).

Memory

Wechsler memory quotients were computed for only the adolescent and adult dyslexic and control groups. Analysis of variance revealed a significant group effect ($F = 4.7$, $p < .05$). The dyslexic group had significantly lower memory quotients (mean = 91) compared with the control group (mean = 112). The age effect was not significantly presumably because the scaled score is corrected for age. A comparison between the dyslexic-adolescent group and the poor-grades group showed the dyslexic group to have significantly lower scores (dyslexic mean = 92, poor grades = 104, $t = 3.1$, $p < .05$). In addition to overall low group means, 11 of 28 dyslexic adolescent and adult subjects had M. Q. scores one standard deviation below the population mean of 100 (Wechsler, 1945). There were no subjects in the control and poor grades group with scores equally low.

The performance of the dyslexic group was significantly poorer on both immediate and delayed recall of logical memory, ($F = 19.3$, $p < .01$; $F = 17$, $p < .05$). There was no significant age effect (scores were converted to percentages to allow comparisons between the children and older groups who received different stories). The dyslexic group was not significantly worse than the poor-grades group on either immediate ($t = 0.7$, $p < .05$) or delayed recall ($t = 1.7$, $p < .05$), but the poor-grades group had scores intermediate to the dyslexic and control group. We calculated the number of scores falling one standard deviation below the population norm (Wechsler, 1945) and found that 20 of 38 dyslexic subjects had low scores on both immediate and delayed recall, whereas only 3 of 30 and 1 of 12 poor-grades subjects had low scores. Analysis on the performance of paired associate learning showed that performance on acquisition was impaired in the dyslexic group ($F = 57$, $p < .01$). The impairment was present at all age levels. There was no significant difference in performance on retention. A comparison of the performance of the adolescent dyslexic group to the poor-grades group also showed an impairment on acquisition ($t = 2.08$, $p < .05$), but no difference on retention ($t = 0.7$, $p < .05$). The difference in acquisition performance between the dyslexic and control group was large (Fig. 12), nevertheless only 3/20 adolescent and adult dyslexic subjects, and no control or poor-grades subjects, performed lower than one standard deviation below the Wechsler (1945) norms.

The dyslexic group had a significantly poorer performance than the control group on both immediate recall ($F = 8.5$, $p > .05$) and delayed recall ($F = 17$, $p > .05$) of the Wechsler visual reproductions,

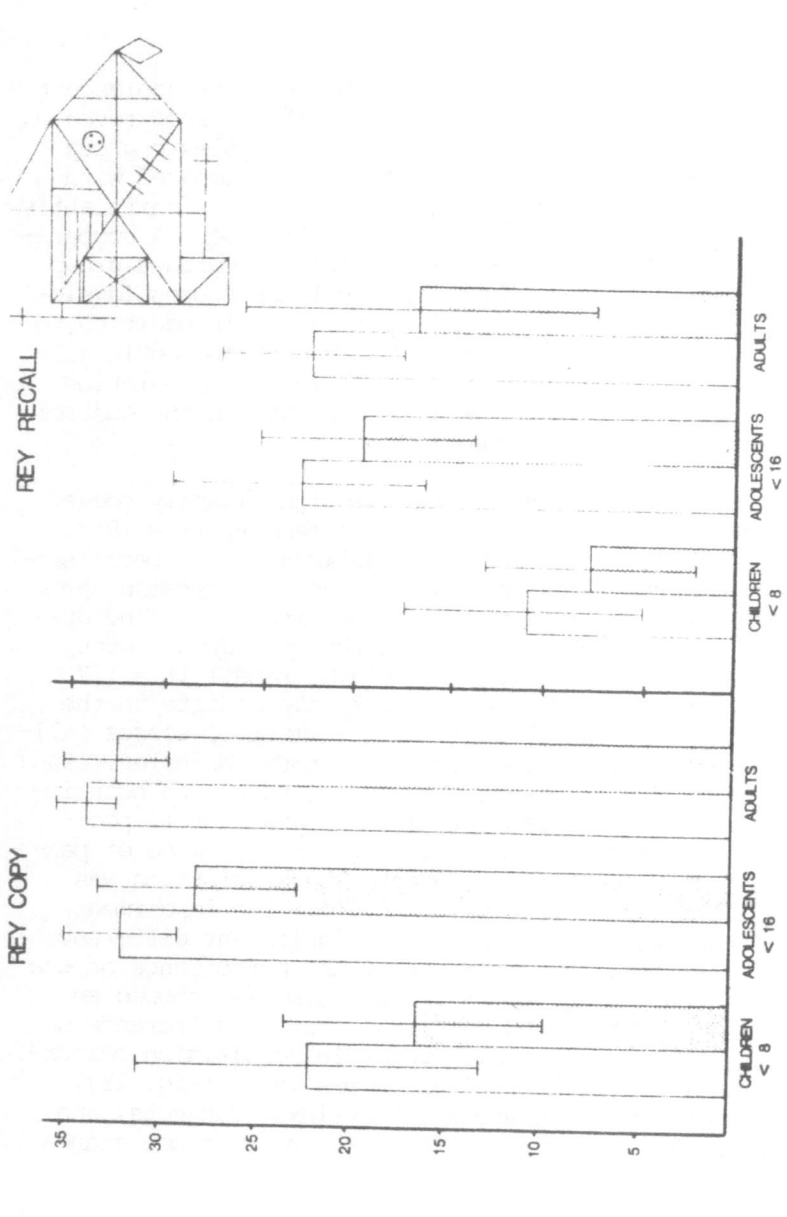

FIGURE 7. Copy and recall (means and standard deviations) on the Rey Complex Figure Task by control (open bars) and dyslexic (shaded bars) subjects.

but not on the delayed recall of the Rey figure (F = 1.14, p < .05). Performance on the Rey recall is illustrated in Figure 7. There was a significant age effect in all of the tests, but follow-up t-tests showed the impairments between the dyslexic and control subjects were present in all age groups on the Wechsler visual reproductions. Comparisons between the dyslexic and control group showed no significant differences (p > .05) on the different tests. Among adolescent and adult groups, 13/28 dyslexic vs. 3/23 control and 3/12 poor-grades subjects had scores one standard deviation below the population average on immediate recall (Wechsler, 1945), and for delayed recall the values were 7/28, 5/23 and 0/12 subjects, respectively, one standard deviation below average.

The results of the memory tests show impaired M. Q.'s, logical memory, and paired associates, which are thought to measure left temporal and parietal function, and impaired visual reproductions, which is thought to measure right parietal function (Fig. 12). Unambiguous interpretation of the delayed logical memory and visual reproductions, which are thought to be sensitive to temporal lobe function, is not possible since there was such poor memory for these items in the dyslexic group on the immediate test. However, performance on delayed paired associates and Rey recall, tests sensitive to left and right temporal lobe function respectively, was within normal limits.

Visual Perception

Analysis of variance on the performance on the Mooney closure test and the Rey figure copy (Fig. 7) showed no difference between the dyslexic and control group or between the dyslexic and poor-grades group. Both tests are thought to be sensitive to right parietal lobe function.

Spatial Orientation

The dyslexic group was impaired relative to the control group on both the left/right differentiation test (Fig. 8) and the Semmes Body Placing Test (Fig. 9); however, the patterns of the deficits were quite different on the two tests. On the left-right test the dyslexic group did little better than chance at all ages, whereas the performance of the control group improved from chance performance below eight years of age to excellent performance in adults (F = 30, p < .01). For the body placing test the group difference (F = 9.9, p < .05) was shown by follow-up tests to be attributable to better performance by the adult control group relative to the adult dyslexic group. When performance on the two tests was compared to cut-off scores, 22 of 28 adolescent and adult dyslexic subjects and 3/23 control subjects were impaired on the left/right task, 7/28 and 4/23 were impaired on body placing. In fact, by these measures all of the adult dyslexic group were impaired at left-right but none at body placing. Furthermore, virtually all the errors made on body

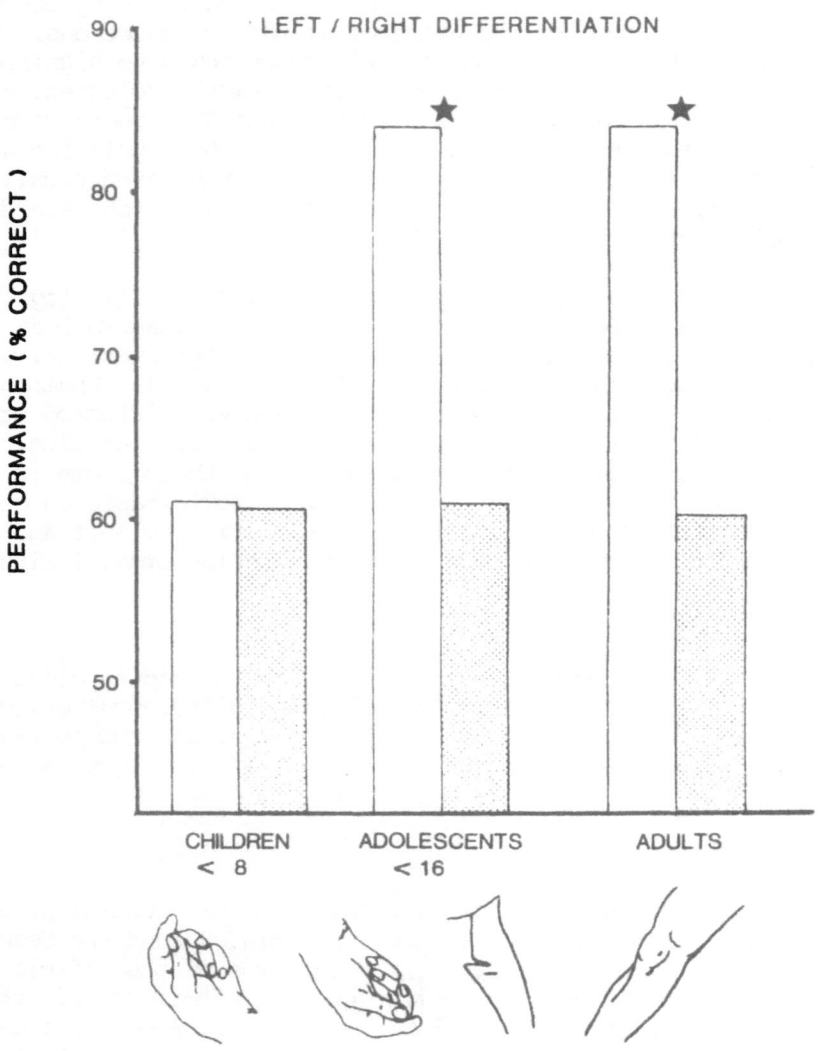

FIGURE 8. Performance on the left-Right Differentiation test by
            control (open bars) and dyslexic (shaded bars) subjects.
            Stars signify significanct group differences.

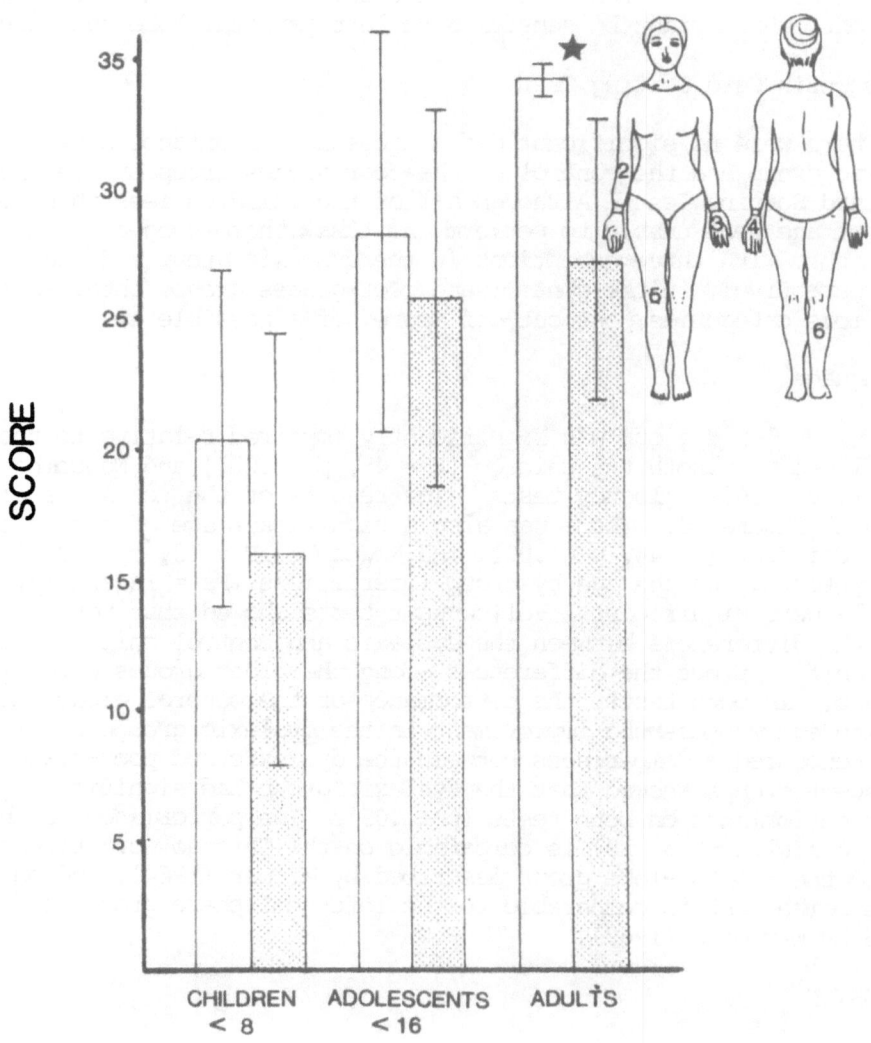

FIGURE 9. Performance (mean and standard deviations) on the Semmes
            Body Placing Test by control (open bars) and dyslexic
            (shaded bars) subjects. Star signify significant group
            differences.

394   I. Q. WHishaw and B. Kolb

placing by the dyslexic group were left/right reversals rather than
body part identifications. In the poor-grades group 5 of 12 were impaired on the left/right task and 2/12 were impaired on the body placing task. As is shown in Figure 12 the left/right task is thought
to be sensitive to left parietal-lobe function and the body placing
task largely to left frontal-lobe function, excepting the left/right
component, which might be sensitive to left parietal-lobe function.

Wisconsin Card Sorting Test

There were no significant differences in performance between the
dyslexic group and the control or the poor-grades group on the Wisconsin Card Sorting Test. Although all of the children less than eight
years of age were unable to perform the task, those subjects older
than eight, with three exceptions in the dyslexic group and two and
none respectively in the control and poor-grades group, obtained four or more categories, our cut-off score, of a possible six.

Language

The dyslexic group was significantly impaired relative to the
control group on both the Chicago (F = 45, p < .001) and Newcombe
(F = 41, p < .001) fluency tests. The results of the tests are displayed in Figure 10. There was also a significant age effect in both the Chicago (F = 44, p < .001) and Newcombe (F = 13, p < .001)
fluency tests, and the age by group interactions (Fs = 12 and 13,
p < .01) were significant. Follow-up t-tests showed that for both
tests the differences between the dyslexic and control children was
not significant but the differences among the older groups were significant. In both tests, the performance of the control group improved with age whereas the improvement in the dyslexic groups was much
less pronounced. Comparisons between the dyslexic and poor-grades
adolescent groups showed that the dyslexic group had significantly
poorer performance on both tests (p < .05). The performance of the
dyslexic adults (Fig. 10) is comparable on the Chicago word fluency
test to the frontal-lobe group described by Milner (1964), and on
the Newcombe test is comparable to the left-hemisphere group as described by Newcombe (1969).

DISCUSSION

Our comparison of the performance of normal control and dyslexic children on a battery of tests, which are differentially sensitive to atrophic lesions of the left or right frontal, temporal or parietal cortex, revealed that the dyslexic children performed particularly poorly on tests sensitive to left posterior cortex damage.
Thus, these children performed significantly more poorly on tests
of left/right discrimination, verbal fluency, short-term and long-
term verbal memory, and digit span than did normal children or children with poor grades. These results imply that developmental dysle-

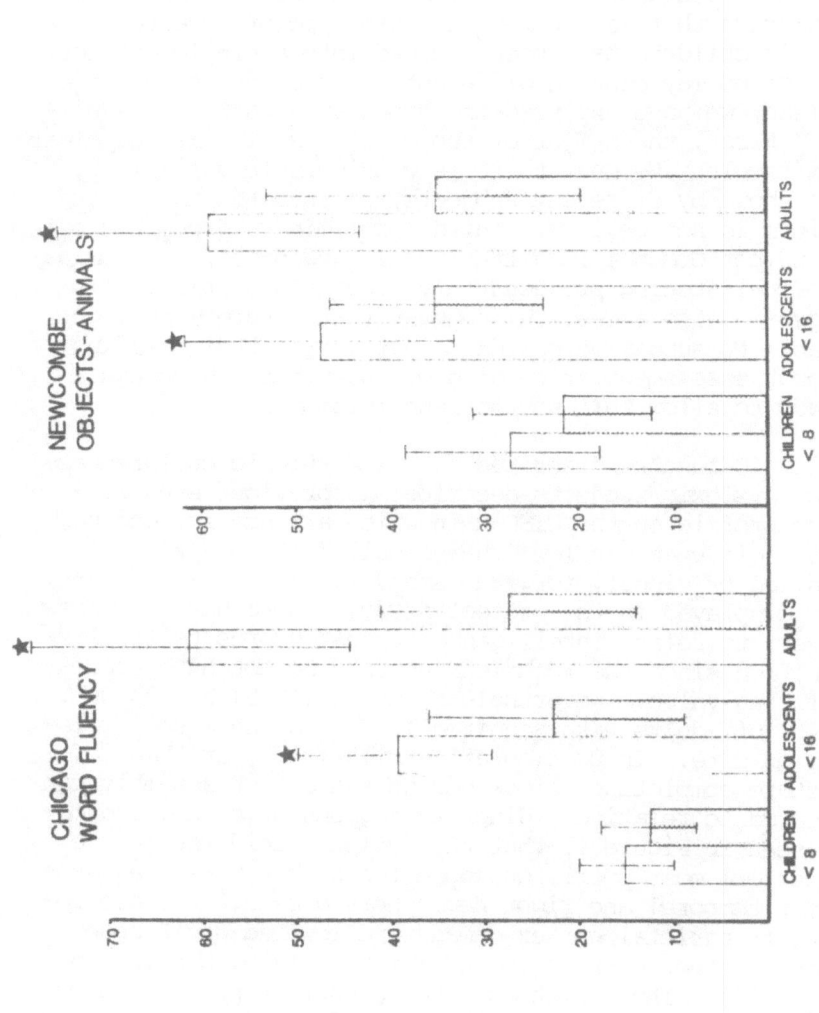

FIGURE 10. Performance (mean and standard deviation) on chicago Word Fluency and Newcombe objects and Animals Fluency tests by control (open bars) and dyslexic (shaded bars) subjects. Stars signify significant group differences

xia is associated with a dysfunction of the left temporal-parietal
cortex. Nevertheless, the dyslexic group also failed some individual
tests sensitive to left frontal lobe function (verbal fluency) and
right hemisphere function (Wechsler figures).

We recognize that the evaluation of the performance of our dyslexic children is compromised to some extent by two different problems. First, we have assumed that our tests can in fact be validly used to infer cerebral dysfunction in dyslexic children. This is, of
course, an assumption that is inherent in this type of research. Second, our dyslexic children have been grouped into a single category
even though the group may contain different types of dyslexic subjects. Nevertheless, we have analyzed the group as a whole for a number of reasons. First, the number of subjects is small, making clear-
cut division difficult. Second, there is considerable variability
in the deficits shown by different subjects, so that the basis for
subclassifications is not obvious. Third, preliminary groupings based on verbal and performance IQ differences, handedness, and dominan-
nt ear on dichotic listening produced only minor and statistically
insignificant group differences. We suggest that future work might
find it profitable to subdivide children in terms of their reading
deficits, although assessment of reading was not thorough enough in
the current study to allow this sort of subdivision.

The Wechsler IQ results described for our dyslexic children appears typical of dyslexic subjects described in previous studies.
For example, the profile on the WISC-R in which arithmetic, coding,
information and digit span are low (the so-called 'ACID' profile)
has been recognized previously (cf. Huelsman, 1970), and it is particularly clearly displayed in the present study. There have been few
attempts, however, to relate intelligence subtest scores to localized brain dysfunction since the Wechsler subtests do not have especially good localizing value. Nevertheless, McFie (1975) has shown
that the subtests of adults with acquired lesions do show some relationship to lesion site. In particular, similarities, arithmetic,
digit span, picture completion, block design and object assembly can
be reliably related to relatively discrete regions of cerebral damage. It can be seen in Figure 11 that the dyslexic chidlren in the
present study perform most poorly on those tests that McFie has associated with left temporal and right hemisphere damage. A close relation between left parietal cortex damage and lowered digit span
is also reported in other work (Kolb and Whishaw, 1980; Warrington
and Weiskrantz, 1973). Thus, although the IQ subtest profile in our
dyslexic children cannot be taken as evidence of a left parietal dysfunction, it is atleast consistent with such an interpretation. Furthermore, the lower full scale IQ of the dyslexic children is also
a characteristic of patients with left parietal lesions (e.g. Teuber, 1975).

We evaluated the deficits displayed by the dyslexic group on the tests comprising the neuropsychological test battery in three ways. First, individual scores were compared to "cut-off" scores usually used for individual assessment. These scores are usually one standard deviation below a control mean, or else they are a score that would be unusual in control subjects. Second, we compared group scores from the dyslexic subjects to scores of students who were referred because of poor grades. The Wechsler intelligence scores of this group approximate the scores of control groups typically used for comparative purposes in studies on reading disabilities (Rugel, 1974). Third, we compared the performance of the dyslexic group with the performance of a control group of students who had no school problems. Understandably this group had quite high I. Q. scores. For the latter comparison the magnitude of the difference between the two groups was used to define an impairment. A summary showing the latter comparison is given in Figure 12. The figure shows tests of left and right hemisphere performance, the most probable cortical site sensitive to the test, and a bar graph of the difference in performance in standard deviations. All three methods of comparison showed that the dyslexic group was impaired at tests of left/right differentiation, Newcombe word fluency, logical memory, paired associate learning, verbal I. Q., Wechsler memory quotient, and Chicago word fluency. All of these tests are at least partly sensitive to left parietal cortex function. Impairments were much less severe or absent altogether on tests of left hemisphere frontal or temporal lobe function. The dyslexic group was also impaired on some tests of left hemisphere parietal function including visual reproductions and performance I. Q., but not on the Mooney closure test or the copy of the Rey Complex figure. Deficits were mild or absent on tests of right temporal lobe function.

It should be noted at this point that many tests seem diagnostically useful for dyslexic individuals are not useful for children under eight. Part of the problem here is that some of the tests are different for children below and above eight years of age (coding, logical memory, dichotic listening). More importantly, the abilities that the tests measure are either absent or so poorly developed in the younger children that the tests have no assessment value. Consequently, deficits on some of the tests emerge with age and increase with increasing age. This was particularly true for left-right discrimination, verbal fluency, and arithmetic. Rourke (1976) has reviewed similar patterns of developing deficits reported in studies on dyslexia. The presence of such an emerging deficit is thought to have diagnostic utility for developmental dyslexia.

A complicating factor in interpreting the deficit in dyslexia is that many different symptoms may occur in any individual, e.g., left handedness, altered lateralization for dichotically or tachistoscopically presented stimuli (Satz, 1976), I. Q. subtest scatter, etc. Each symptom could be indicative of different underlying deficits, which may occur in different combinations in different indivi-

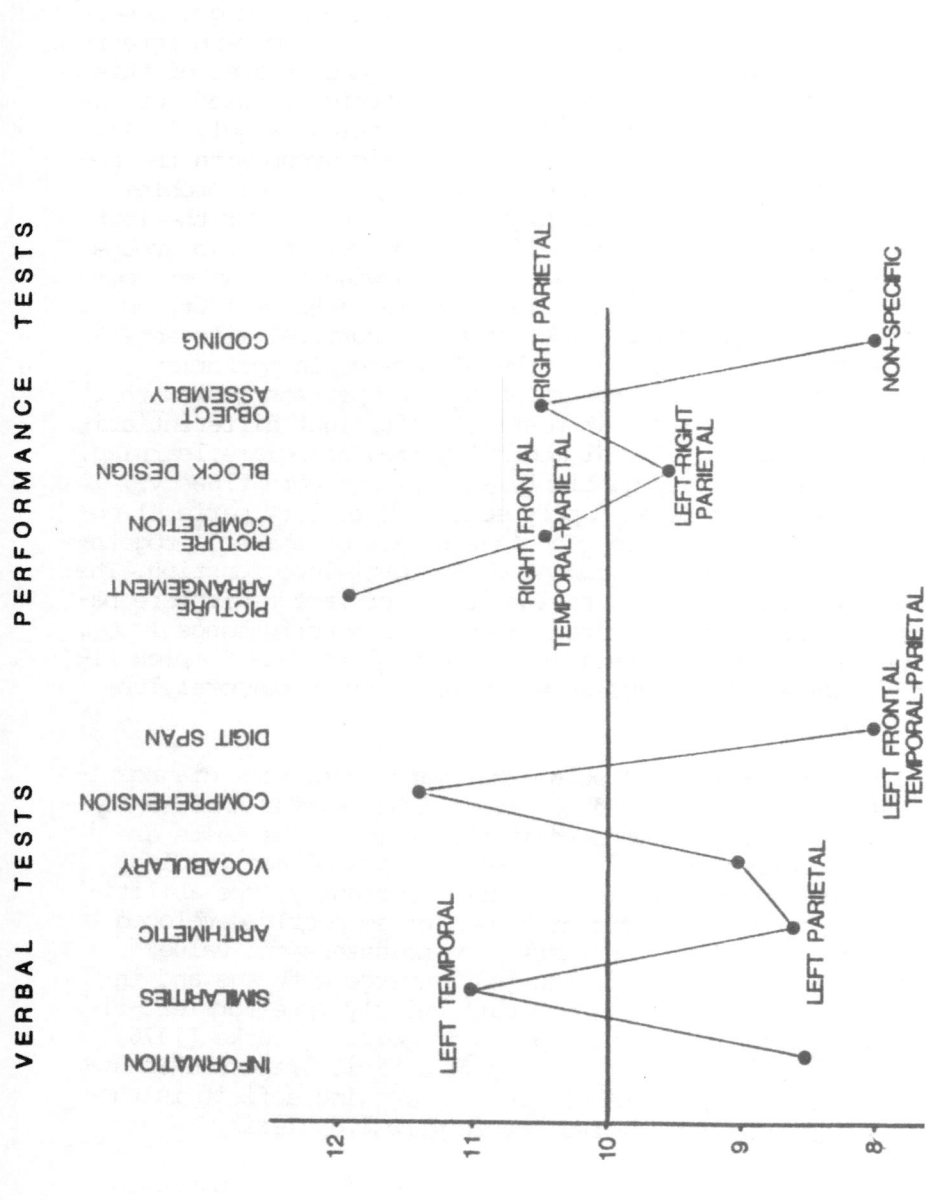

FIGURE   11.   The relation between the Intelligence test profiles of developmental dyslexic
              subjects and sub-test-lobe relations described by McFie (1975).

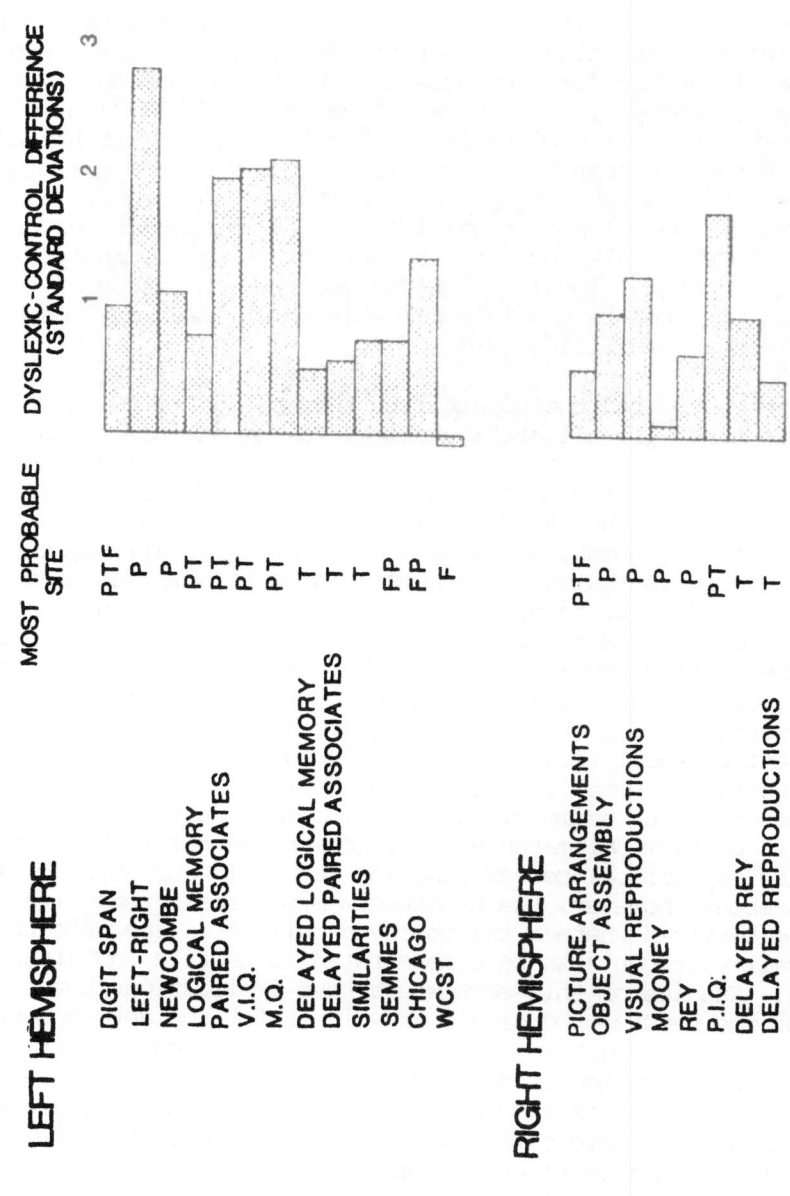

FIGURE 12. Summary of performance of developmental dyslexic and control groups Left: theoretical relation between tests and hemisphere; Middle: theoretical relation between tests and lobes; Right: deficit (standard deviations) in dyslexic as contrasted with control groups on the different tests.

duals. They may, however, also be diagnostic of one common underlying deficit. Based on the present work we favor the idea that the
deficit is in the left parietal cortex in systems that usually play
a special role in language (Geschwind, 1968) or movement (Kimura, 19-
79). Since the abnormality is likely present before maturation is
complete, the inherent plasticity of the developing cortex may provide a number of avenues for accommodating shifts in handedness, language dominance, eyedness, etc. Bakan, Dibb and Reed (1973) have explicitly suggested such an explanation for some types of left handedness, although they suggest the abnormality may lie in the pyramidal
tract rather than in the left parietal cortex as we suggest. Such
alternations in the focus of control for different aspects of behavior would, however, also complicate neuropsychological analysis, for
the rules for cortical localization derived from the study of normal
adults would not then be easily applicable to children with developmental learning disabilities.

We have considered the possibility that the deficits shown by
the dyslexic group are all attributable to a common underlying deficit. There is, however, no clear cut answer to what the deficit is.
Jorm (1979) has suggested that developmental dyslexia is attributable
to an abnormality in the inferior parietal lobule which produces an
auditory short-term memory deficit, whereas Frith (1981) suggests it
has its origin in speech motor systems. There is some appeal to the
idea that a key deficit in dyslexic subjects is in certain types of
'short-term memory'. Many of the tests on which learning disabled
children are impaired could be seen to have short-term memory components (e.g. digit span, coding, arithmetic, recall of dichotically
presented words, etc.), whereas other tests on which dyslexic subjects do relatively well (e.g. Rey Figure, Mooney closure test, WISC-R
picture arrangement, etc.), appear to make little requirement on short-term memory. Furthermore, short-term memory must be particularly
important in cross-modal matching, a function thought to be importantly related to parietal cortex function (cf. Kolb and Whishaw, 19-
80). At present, however, the hypothesis must remain tentative until
it can be determined whether the observed deficit is specific to auditory modality or can also be demonstrated in tactile and visual
modalities. Studies of this sort would have implications both for
theories of the nature of dyslexia as well as for the development of
effecitve remedial programs. Finally, it will be necessary to determine how a short-term memory deficit can be related to the observations of poor language skills in dyslexic children. It may prove to
be the case that dyslexic children suffer both from a short-term memory deficit in addition to an abnormality in one of the underlying
linguistic-motor systems.

REFERENCES

Ahn, H., Prichep, L., John, E. R., Baird, H., Trepetin, M. and Kaye, H. Developmental equations reflect brain function. Science, 1980, 210, 1259-1262.

Bakan, P., Dibb, G. and Reed, P. Handedness and birth stress. Neuropsychologia, 1973, 11, 363-366.

Benson, D. F. Towards a pathology of reading disorders. Paper presented at the Hyman Blumberg Symposium on Research in Early Education, Baltimore, 1974.

Benton, L. and Pearl, D. (Eds.), Dyslexia: An appraisal of current knowledge, New York: Oxford, 1978.

Corkin, S. A prospective study of cingulotomy. In E. S. Valenstein (Ed.), The psychosurgery debate. San Francisco: W. H. Freeman, 1980.

Critchely, M. The dyslexic child. London: William Heinemann Medical Books Ltd., 1970.

de Renzi, E. and Vignolo, L. A. The token test: a sensitive test to detect disturbances in aphasics. Brain, 1962, 85, 665-678.

Frith, U. Experimental approaches to developmental dyslexia: An introduction. Psychological Research, 1981, 43, 97-109.

Gaddes, W. H. Learning disabilities and brain function. New York: Springer Verlag, 1980.

Galaburda, A. M. and Kempers, T. L. Cytoarchitectonic abnormalities in developmental dyslexia: A case study. Annals of Neurology, 1979, 6, 94-100.

Geschwind, N. The anatomy of acquired disorders of reading. In J. Money (Ed.), Reading disability: Progress and Research Needs in Dyslexia. Baltimore: John Hopkins Press, 1962.

Geschwind, N. Neurological foundations of language. In H. R. Myklebust, (Ed.), Progress in learning disabilities VI. New York: Grune & Stratton, 1968.

Hier, D., LeMay, M., Rosenberger, P. and Perlo, V. P. Developmental dyslexia. Archives of Neurology, 1978, 35, 90-92.

Huelsman, C. B. The WISC subtest syndrome for disabled readers. Perceptual and Motor Skills, 1970, 30, 535-550.

Jones-Gotman, M. and Milner, B. Design fluency: the invention of nonsense drawings after local cortical lesions. Neuropsychologia, 1977, 15, 653-674.

Jorm, A. F. The cognitive and neurological basis of developmental dyslexia: A theoretical framework and review. Cognition, 1979, 7, 19-33.

Kimura, D. The asymmetry of the human brain. Scientific American, 1973, 222, 70-78.

Kimura, D. Neuromotor mechanisms in the evolution of human communication. In H. D. Steklis and M. J. Raleigh (Eds.), Neurobiology of social communication in primates: An evolutionary perspective. New York: Academic Press, 1979.

Knights, R. M. and Bakker, D. J. (Eds.), The Neuropsychology of Learning Disorders: Theoretical approaches. Baltimore: University

Park Press, 1976.

Kolb, B. and Whishaw, I. Q. Fundamentals of human neuropsychology.
    San Francisco: W. H. Freeman, 1980.

Malatesha, R. N. and Aaron, P. G. Reading Disorders: Varieties and
    Treatments, New York: Academic Press, 1982.

Malatesha, R. N. and Dougan, D. R. Clinical subtypes of developmen-
    tal dyslexia: Resolution of an irresolute problem. In Malate-
    sha, R. N. and Aaron, P. G. (Eds.), Reading Disorders: Varieti-
    es and Treatments. New York: Academic Press, 1982.

McFie, J. Assessment of organic intellectual impairment. New York:
    Wiley & Sons, 1975.

McFie, J. and Zangwill, O. Visual-constructive disabilities associa-
    ted with lesions of the left cerebral hemisphere. Brain, 1960,
    83, 243-260.

Milner, B. Some effects of frontal lobectomy in man. In J. M. Warr-
    en & K. Akert (Eds.), The frontal granular cortex and behavior.
    New York: McGraw Hill, 1964.

Milner, B. Brain mechanisms suggested by studies of the temporal
    lobes. In F. C. Darley (Ed.), Brain mechanisms underlying spee-
    ch and language. New York: Grune & Stratton, 1967.

Milner, B. Psychological aspects of focal epilepsy and its neurosur-
    gical management. Advances in Neurology, 1975, 8, 229-321.

Milner, B. Complementary functional specializations of the human
    cerebral hemispheres. Pontificae Academiae Scientiarum Scripta
    Varia, 1980, 45, 601-625.

Mooney, C. M. Age in the development of closure ability in children.
    Canadian Journal of Psychology, 1957, 2, 219-226.

Newcombe, F. Missil wounds of the brain. London: Oxford University
    Press, 1969.

Preston, M. S., Guthrie, J. T. and Childs, B. Visual evoked respon-
    ses (VERs) in normal and disabled readers. Psychophysiology,
    1977, 14, 8-14.

Rourke, B. P. Reading retardation in children: Developmental lag or
    deficit. In R. M. Knights and D. J. Bakker (Eds.), The Neuro-
    psychology of learning disabilities: Theoretical approaches.
    Baltimore: University Park Press, 1976.

Rugel, R. D. WISC subtest scores of disabled readers: A review with
    respect to Bannatyne's recategorization. Journal of Learning
    Disabilities, 1974, 7, 48-64.

Satz, P. Cerebral dominance and reading disability: An old problem
    revisited. In Knights, R. M. and Bakker, D. J. (Eds.), The
    Neuropsychology of Learning Disorders. Baltimore: University
    Park Press, 1976.

Semmes, J., Weinstein, S. Ghent, L. and Teuber, H. L. Correlates of
    impaired orientation in personal and extra-personal space.
    Brain, 1963, 86, 747-772.

Sparrow, S. and Satz, P. Dyslexia, laterality and neuropsychologi-
    cal development. In D. J. Bakker and P. Satz (Eds.), Specific
    reading disability: Advances in theory and method. Rotterdam:
    Rotterdam University Press, 1970.

Sutherland, R. J., Kolb, B., Schoel, W. M., Whishaw, I. Q. and Davies, D. Neuropsycholgoical assessment of children and adults with Tourette Syndrome: A comparison with learning disabilities and Schizophrenia. In T. N. Chase and A. J. Friedhoff (Eds.), Gilles de la Tourette Syndrome. New York: Raven Press, 1982.

Symann-Lovett, N., Gascon, G. G., Matsumiya, Y. and Lombroso, C. T. Wave form difference in visual evoked responses between normal and reading disabled children. Neurology, 1977, 27, 156-159.

Taylor, L. B. Localization of cerebral lesions by psychological testing. Clinical Neurology, 1969, 16, 269-287.

Taylor, L. B. Psychological assessment of neurosurgical patients. In T. Rasmussen and R. Marino (Eds.), Functional Neurosurgery. New York: Raven Press, 1979.

Teuber, H. L. Recovery of function after brain injury in man. In Outcome of severe damage to the nervous system. Ciba Foundation Symposium 34. Amsterdam: Elsevier-North Holland Publishing Co., 1975.

Wechsler, D. A standardized memory scale for clinical use. The Journal of Psychology, 1945, 19, 87-95.

A DIAGNOSTIC SCREENING TEST FOR SUBTYPES OF DYSLEXIA:

THE BODER TEST OF READING - SPELLING PATTERNS[1]

Elena Boder
Department of Pediatrics
Division of Pediatric Neurology
School of Medicine
University of California
Los Angeles, California

Sylvia Jarrico
Research Psychologist
Los Angeles, California

In the last fifteen years there has been a remarkable growth of awareness among physicians, psychologists and educators that many normal healthy, well motivated and intelligent children have unusual difficulty in learning to read by standard methods of reading instruction that are adequate for their peers. Such unexpected reading failure is referred to as specific reading disability, developmental dyslexia or simply dyslexia.

The objects of this paper are (1) to describe the Boder Test of Reading-Spelling Patterns, a newly published diagnostic screening test for subtypes of developmental dyslexia based on systematic analysis of reading and spelling performance alone, and (2) to show how this test is related to the prevailing diagnostic criteria for developmental dyslexia in the fields of medicine, psychology, and education.

High levels of reliability and validity have been obtained for the results of the Boder Test in four doctoral dissertations (Ginn, 1979; Menken, 1981; Rosenthal, 1980; Sporn, 1981) and a number of post-doctoral studies (Aaron, 1978, 1980; Fried et al, 1981; Hanley, 1974; Malatesha and Dougan, 1982; Whiting and Jarrico, 1980) in psychology, education, neuropsychology, and electrophysiology. Thus, the current evidence suggests that the three clinical dyslexic subtypes identified by the Boder Test represent three distinct neuropsychological syndromes identified on the basis of reading and spelling performance alone.

---

1. Adapted by the authors from Chapters 1 and 8 of the manual of the Boder Test of Reading-Spelling Patterns (Boder & Jarrico, 1982), with the permission of the publisher.

PREVAILING DIAGNOSTIC APPROACHES

Diagnosis by exclusion: Dyslexia has generally been defined in
negative terms, i.e., in terms of what it is not, and diagnosed by
exclusion. Being essentially a differential diagnosis, diagnosis
by exclusion is the approach most widely used by physicians. It relies on ruling out all nonspecific factors - physical, mental, emotional, sociocultural and educational- that may interfere with the
child's ability to learn to read. Diagnosis by exclusion does indeed provide a reliable diagnosis of dyslexia, but it has the critical
shortcoming of identifying far too few children. In fact, it exclu-
des from diagnostic consideration all the dyslexic children in whom
dyslexia coexists with and is aggravated by one or more nonspecific
contributory factors. Dyslexia tends to be viewed as a rarity, therefore, by those who rely exclusively on definitions by exclusion.
It is regarded as virtually nonexistent by those who will diagnose
it only in the absence of emotional factors, because dyslexic readers characteristically have emotional problems that are secondary
and reactive to the dyslexia. This emotional overlay tends to be
interpreted as the primary cause of the inability to read.

In recent years, definitions of dyslexia by exclusion have been
extended to include a positive statement recognizing that cognitive
disabilities underlie developmental dyslexia (Critchley, 1970), and
diagnosis by exclusion has been increasingly challenged (Blank, 1978;
Rosenthal, 1980; Rutter, 1978; Taylor et al, 1979). These cognitive
disabilities are generally regarded as representing a specific neu-
rodevelopmental lag or deficit that is usually of constitutional and
genetic origin, rather than due to brain damage (Bender, 1975; Benton, 1975; Critchley & Critchley, 1978). The impressive familial
incidence of developmental dyslexia and its marked predilection for
boys (in a ratio of about 4 boys to 1 girl) are amply documented in
genetic studies (Finucci et al, 1976).

Indirect Diagnosis: With the recognition that a variety of cognitive deficits, predominantly in the language function (Duane, 1974;
Myklebust, 1978), may underlie developmental dyslexia, it became apparent that developmental dyslexia is not a homogeneous clinical entity, and attempts to identify subtypes within the population of dyslexic readers have steadily increased. The growing interest in the
typology of developmental dyslexia has been enhanced by the expectation that identifying subtypes with differing cognitive strengths
and weaknesses will offer a rationale for new approaches to prescriptive remediation.

The cognitive disabilities associated with dyslexia, both cau-
sative and concomitant, have been elucidated through psychological,
psycholinguistic and neuropsychological test batteries. Such indirect diagnostic approaches, sometimes combined with direct analysis
of reading and spelling, have identified a variety of syndromes or

subtypes of dyslexia (Myklebust & Boshes, 1960; Kinsbourne & Warrington, 1963; Bannatyne, 1966; Bateman, 1968; Mattis et al, 1975; Friedman et al, 1976; Denckla, 1977; Doehring & Hoshko, 1977; Gordon & Harness, 1977; Bakker, 1979; Petrauskas & Rourke, 1979; Pirozzolo, 1979). The subtypes vary with the criteria used to delineate them. There is considerable overlap, however, since it is the same general population that is being studied, i.e., children who are poor readers for no apparent reason. In fact, the subtypes identified are mainly of two types, giving evidence of cognitive deficits in either the visual or the auditory channel functions. Though invaluable in exploring the cognitive deficits that underlie dyslexia and in identifying dyslexic subtypes, the specialized neuropsychological test batteries used diagnostically are too specialized and time-consuming to be practical for general interdisciplinary application.

The most common method of indirect diagnosis relies on eliciting the typical neurological concomitants ("soft signs") and psychometric concomitants of developmental dyslexia. Although this approach is essential to a diagnostic evaluation, it is insufficient by itself for the diagnosis, since most of these concomitants can occur independently of dyslexia.

Direct Diagnosis: The most widely used method of direct diagnosis is based on the analysis and classification of so-called dyslexic errors in the reading and spelling performance and relating them to deficit functions. This classic and practical direct approach succeeded in demonstrating that dyslexic children read and spell differently from normal readers qualitatively as well as quantitatively. This qualitative difference proved to be a reliable diagnostic criterion and pointed the way toward further direct studies of dyslexia in terms of the specific cognitive disabilities reflected in reading and spelling behavior.

Studies of reading and spelling errors alone have failed, however, to identify clear-cut subtypes of dyslexia through replicable studies. The main reason is that this approach tends to focus on the cognitive deficits reflected in reading and spelling errors to the exclusion of cognitive strengths with which the deficits may be associated. A complicating factor in any attempt to identify dyslexic subtypes on the basis of reading and spelling errors alone is that different kinds of dyslexic children may make the same kinds of errors for different reasons (Boder, 1971b; Gjessing, 1980). In addition, except for visuospatial reversals, it is often not at all obvious whether a given error in reading or spelling should be classified as a "visual" or an "auditory" error.

A NEW APPROACH TO DIRECT DIAGNOSIS

It is now widely accepted that developmental dyslexia frequently underlies academic underachievement and school behavioral problems. To promote successful remediation and to prevent school failure with its concomitant resulting emotional problems and loss of self-esteem, it is crucial to ensure that children with reading disabilities are identified early. In addition, the educational remediation of specific reading disability calls for specialized techniques that are not required for nonspecific reading retardation. There is therefore a widely felt need for a practical, direct, diagnostic screening procedure that will differentiate developmental dyslexia from nonspecific reading retardation and identify reading disability subtypes with differing remedial implications. The Boder Test of Reading-Spelling Patterns is designed to fill this need.

The Boder Test is an interdisciplinary instrument that can be administered, scored and interpreted by a variety of professionals who are concerned with the early identification and remediation of reading disability: teachers, who usually are the first to discover that a child has a reading problem; psychologists and physicians, who usually are the first to be consulted; reading specialists, who are involved in both diagnosis and remediation; and speech therapists, who have become increasingly aware of the interdependence of spoken and written language.

A Definition of Dyslexia

The Boder Test is based on the premise that the dyslexic reader has a characteristic pattern of cognitive strengths and weaknesses in two distinct components of the reading process: the visual gestalt function and the auditory analytic function. The visual gestalt function underlies the ability to develop a sight vocabulary through visual perception and memory for whole words; the auditory analytic function underlies the ability to develop phonic word-analysis skills. This test is designed to elicit evidence of the child's characteristic pattern of cognitive strengths and weaknesses in the reading and spelling performance itself.

The Boder Test thus provides an operational definition of developmental dyslexia as a reading disability in which the reading and spelling performance give evidence of cognitive deficits in either the visual gestalt or auditory analytic function, or in both. A corollary of this definition is that when the reading-spelling pattern of poor readers gives no evidence of such cognitive deficits, their reading disability is regarded as nonspecific rather than dyslexic.

Purposes of the Test

The diagnostic purposes of the Boder Test are (1) to differentiate specific reading disability, or developmental dyslexia, from nonspecific reading retardation through reading and spelling performance alone, (2) to classify dyslexic readers into one of three subtypes on the basis of their reading-spelling patterns, each with its

own prognostic and remedial implications, and (3) to provide guidelines for the remediation of each of the four reading disability subtypes identified by the test - the nonspecific subtype and the three
dyslexic ones.

A Unique System of Analysis

In the presence of significant reading retardation - which is
usually defined as two or more years below normal expectancy for age-
grade level or mental age, although a reading retardation of even
one year may be diagnostically significant - the Boder Test makes it
possible to diagnose developmental dyslexia by jointly analyzing reading and spelling as interdependent functions. The system of analysis used in the Boder Test identifies diagnostic reading-spelling
patterns not through errors alone - which reflect only what the dyslexic reader cannot do - but through the reading and spelling performance as a whole - which reflects what the dyslexic reader can as
well as cannot do. By thus evaluating cognitive strengths as well
as cognitive weaknesses, the test offers a fuller range of prognostic
and remedial implications than can traditional direct diagnosis through reading and spelling errors alone.

Through a systematic sequence of simple reading and spelling
tasks, the Boder Test offers an essentially qualitative analysis of
the ability to learn to read and spell, for which quantitative criteria are provided. It is the analysis of how the child reads and
spells, as well as at what grade level, that enables the examiner to
identify the child's pattern of cognitive strengths and weaknesses
in the reading and spelling performance.

The main procedural innovations are: (1) using a set of word
lists with equal numbers of phonetic and nonphonetic words graded
for both reading and spelling from the preprimer to the adult level;
(2) determining the reading level exclusively on the basis of the
child's sight vocabulary, that is, on the words recognized instantly
as whole-word configurations, or gestalts; (3) administering a written spelling test based on the results of the oral reading test;
(4) dictating two separate spelling tests, each composed of equal
numbers of phonetic and nonphonetic words - a list of words that are
in the child's sight vocabulary ("Known Words") and a list of words
that are not ("Unknown Words") - in order to assess strengths and
weaknesses in the visual and auditory channel functions; and (5) scoring the spelling lists in terms of the percent of Known Words spelled correctly and the percent of Unknown Words spelled as good phonetic equivalents.*

---

* The rationales for these procedural innovations are discussed in
Chapters 2, 3 and 6 of the Boder Test Manual (Boder & Jarrico, 1982).

The two basic components of the reading-spelling process thus explored by the Boder Test (visual gestalt function and auditory analytic function) are, in fact, the two cognitive functions that are basic to the two standard methods of initial reading instruction: the whole-word method and the phonics method. The whole-word ("look-say") method relies on the child's ability to experience the written word globally as a visual gestalt, and the phonics method relies on the child's ability to analyze words into their phonemic components. In addition, these two cognitive components of the reading process correspond to the gestalt-simultaneous processing and the analytic-sequential processing that, according to current neuropsychological evidence are mediated by the right and left brain hemispheres, respectively (Aaron, 1978; Bogen, 1977; Dalby & Gibson, 1981; Gordon & Harness, 1977; Wittrock, 1978).

A READING DISABILITY TYPOLOGY

The strengths and deficits in the gestalt and analytic functions of dyslexic children are manifested in three atypical reading-spelling patterns not found among good readers who are at or above grade level in both reading and spelling. These patterns are the dysphonetic, the dyseidetic, and the mixed dysphonetic-dyseidetic.** A fourth, normal, reading-spelling pattern is exhibited not only by good readers and spellers but by poor readers whose reading retardation is secondary, or nonspecific. Within each reading-spelling pattern, the pattern of reading and the pattern of spelling are mutually predictive. Fig. 1 shows how the four reading-spelling patterns are related to strengths and weaknesses in the gestalt and analytic functions. The characteristics of the three dyslexic subtypes are summarized in Table 1.

Each of the three dyslexic subtypes identified by the reading-spelling patterns has differing prognostic and remedial implications (Boder, 1968, 1971a, b, 1973). Group I, the dysphonetic group, is by far the largest of the subtypes. Dysphonetic dyslexics have difficulty in integrating written symbols with their sounds, with resulting disability in developing phonic word-analysis decoding skills but without gross deficit in visual gestalt function. (Their typical misspellings are dysphonetic, or phonetically inaccurate, e.g., "sleber" for scrambled. Their typical misreadings are word substitutions based on minimal clues, e.g., "diesel" for dress, and gestalt substitutions, e.g., "horse" for house. Their most striking misreadings are semantic substitutions, e.g., "funny" for laugh and "planet" for moon.)

** The terms dysphonetic, dyseidetic and mixed dysphonetic-dyseidetic were coined by Boder (1968) as descriptive clinical terms that designate the three dyslexic subtypes and have remedial implications. Dyseidetic derives from the Greek word eidos, meaning "form", "shape" or "gestalt".

FIGURE 1. The four Reading-Spelling Patterns: Identifying the Normal
Reader and Four Reading Disability Subtypes

ANALYTIC FUNCTION

	STRONG	WEAK
STRONG	Normal Pattern Normal Reader and Nonspecific Reading Retardation	Dysphonetic Pattern Dyslexic Group I
WEAK	Dyseidetic Pattern Dyslexic Group II	Mixed Dysphonetic-Dyseidetic Pattern Dyslexic Group III

GESTALT
FUNCTION

WEAK

Figure 1 shows the four combinations of relative strengths and
weaknesses in the gestalt and analytic function. Each combination
corresponds to a reading-spelling pattern. The four reading-spelling
patterns include the normal pattern, which reflects strength in both
the gestalt and analytic functions, and the three dyslexic patterns,
which reflect weakness in either gestalt or analytic function, or in
both. The normal pattern identifies both the normal reader and the
poor reader whose reading retardation is nonspecific.

Group II, the dyseidetic group, manifests deficits in visual
perception and memory for letters and whole-word configurations, or
gestalts, with resulting disability in developing a sight vocabulary.
Dyseidetic dyslexics have no disability in developing phonic skills.
(Their typical misspellings are phonetically accurate and decodable,
e.g., "laf" for laugh and "toc" for talk. Their typical misreadings
are phonetic renditions of nonphonetic words, e.g., "talc" for talk.
Visuospatial letter and word reversals in both reading and writing
are also typical of this group, e.g., "bib" for did, "no" for on.)

Dyslexics in Group III, the mixed dysphonetic-dyseidetic group,
combine the cognitive deficits of the first two subtypes, with resul·
ting disability in developing both sight vocabulary and phonic skills; some are virtually nonreaders and nonspellers. (Their typical
misreadings are wild guesses from minimal clues. Their typical misspellings are phonetically inaccurate, as in Group I, but usually
more bizarre, often only a single wrong initial letter, e.g., "R"
for "stop". Visuospatial letter and word reversals, as in Group II,
and letter-order reversals, as in Group I, are also typical).

Each of the diagnostic reading-spelling patterns that identify

TABLE 1.   Subtypes of Developmental Dyslexia based on Three Diagnostic Reading-Spelling Patterns

Group I Dysphonetic	Reading-spelling pattern indicates cognitive deficit in integrating letters with their sounds, with resulting disability in developing phonic word-analysis decoding skills. (Dysphonetic dyslexics have no gross deficit in visual gestalt function).
Group II Dyseidetic	Reading-spelling pattern indicates a cognitive deficit in visual memory and perception for letters and whole-word configurations, or gestalts, with resulting disability in developing a sight vocabulary. (Dyseidetic dyslexics have no gross deficit in analytic function, i.e., no disability in developing phonic skills).
Group III Mixed dysphonetic-dyseidetic	Reading-spelling pattern indicates a combination of the cognitive deficits of the dysphonetic and dyseidetic subtypes, with resulting disability in developing both sight vocabulary and phonic skills. (Dysphonetic-dyseidetic dyslexics may be virtually alexic, that is, "nonreaders" and "nonspellers").

the four reading disability subtypes has its own prognostic and remedial implications.   In addition to these guidelines, the Boder Test Provides a broad sample of the child's current reading and spelling skills, and a quick assessment of the reading level, both of which can be helpful to teachers and reading specialists in developing
prescriptive remedial programs.

USES AND LIMITATIONS OF THE TEST

Assessing Reading Achievement

The quick assessment of reading level provided by the Boder Test correlates well with the reading-level assessment obtained with
the Wide Range Achievement Test (WRAT) and is more sensitive than the
WRAT to early reading and spelling difficulties (Ginn, 1979).   The
Boder Test does not, however, supplant the WRAT or other standard

tests of reading and spelling achievement when widely standardized
scores are sought.

The cognitive functions evaluated by the Boder Test are essential in the learning-to-read process and are precursors of reading comprehension, but neither the reading level nor the reading-spelling
pattern established by the test should be regarded as indices of a
child's level of reading comprehension. The reading level determined
by the test can, however, indicate the grade level at which reading
comprehension testing, with graded paragraphs, can begin.

Developing an Informal Inventory of Reading and Spelling Skills

The results of the Boder Test can provide a useful informal inventory of what the child has learned and failed to learn through reading and spelling instruction from grade to grade. The remedial reading teacher or reading specialist will want to supplement this information, however, with testing that uses instructional materials
to which the child actually has been and will be exposed.

Screening for Developmental Dyslexia

As a screening instrument, the Boder Test should not be used
alone in making a definitive diagnosis of developmental dyslexia.
It should be used as an integral part of a multidisciplinary "neuro-
psychoeducational" evaluation and in conjunction with other diagnostic test instruments, as required. This is essential for comprehensive diagnosis and management, and for fully effective remedial education (Boder, 1976, 1980). Although the test can make a reliable
early diagnosis of reading disability and identify the child's preferred modality, visual or auditory, in learning how to read, a formal diagnosis of dyslexia should be made with great caution in children between 5 and 8 years of age. Developmental dyslexia in its
milder and transient forms, found in young children, may represent
a normal variation in reading readiness, a maturational lag that may
be spontaneously overcome by the age of 8.

Although a definitive diagnosis of developmental dyslexia must
await a coordinated multidisciplinary evaluation that takes all of
the existing causal and contributory factors into account, such an
evaluation may not be immediately available. The teacher or reading
specialist, however, can begin immediately to use educational strategies based on the remedial implications of the child's reading-
spelling pattern as revealed by the Boder Test.

MULTIDISCIPLINARY VALUE

Common Ground for the Team Approach

As a direct diagnostic instrument based on reading-spelling

patterns, the Boder Test yields results that are equally meaningful
to physicians, psychologists and educators. The Boder Test thereby
provides a common ground for the multidisciplinary team approach that is essential to the comprehensive diagnosis and management of reading disabilities. Moreover, the test may enable the teacher to
play a more knowledgeable role in the early identification of children with reading-spelling disabilities who are in need of further
diagnosis evaluation and remedial instruction.

Common Ground for the Study of Subtypes

The Boder Test provides a convenient interdisciplinary research
tool for the study of subtypes. It is generally assumed that there
must be considerable overlap among the increasingly numerous reading
disability subtypes reported in the literature, but there have been
no systematic studies to document the basic similarities among the
subtypes. The Boder Test would allow researchers to compare their
results by relating the subtypes, identified on a diversity of criteria, to the basic cognitive components of the reading process -
gestalt and analytic - reflected in the reading-spelling patterns.

OTHER RESEARCH APPLICATIONS

Most research on dyslexia has been done by comparing undifferentiated groups of poor readers with good readers in an effort to establish significant correlates of reading disability - psychometric,
psycholinguistic, neurological, psychiatric, or pedagogic. The oft-
en conflicting or inconclusive findings of such studies may reflect
a failure to recognize not only the heterogeneity of the general category of poor readers but the heterogeneity of dyslexia itself (Benton, 1975). In the overall results obtained for undifferentiated
groups of poor readers, the significant differences that exist among
unrecognized clinical subtypes will be masked or distorted.

By providing a direct approach to differentiating developmental
dyslexia from nonspecific reading disability and identifying three
dyslexic subtypes, the Boder Test offers a fresh point of departure
for undertaking new studies on dyslexia and for reevaluating the findings of earlier studies. By combining diagnosis by exclusion with
direct diagnosis through the Boder Test, the investigator can obtain
relatively homogeneous clinical samples of the three dyslexic subtypes, thereby providing purer experimental groups than have hereto-
fore been used in research on dyslexia. Clearly, such homogeneous
groups are essential in a wide range of needed research efforts on
dyslexia, including the following:
  Etiological and genetic studies
  Systematic trials of a variety of remedial pedagogic techniques
  Transcultural studies of the effects of varying linguistic structures on the incidence, clinical manifestations, and remediation
of developmental dyslexia.

Neuropsychological research relating the cognitive strengths and deficits that underlie the three dyslexic subtypes to brain mechanisms and to subtypes of reading disability that have been delineated on a variety of other criteria, including psychometric, psycholinguistic, and neuropsychological test batteries.

With respect to transcultural studies, the Boder Test is adaptable for use in any written language that uses an alphabetic system. In the area of neuropsychological research, the pioneering studies of Sperry et al. (1969) on the specialized gestalt and analytic functions of the right and left hemispheres have in recent years engendered a marked increase of interest in studying reading disabilities as related to the cognitive processes of the brain (Bogen, 1975; Dalby & Gibson, 1981; Doehring et al, 1981; Gaddes, 1980; Hynd & Obrzut, 1981; Witelson, 1977; Wittrock, 1978; Zaidel & Peters, 1981; Zangwill, 1982).

In addition, the Boder Test provides a systematic way to study reading and spelling behavior in alexia, or acquired dyslexia, and thus a basis for determining the similarities and differences between the various subtypes of acquired and developmental dyslexia.

REFERENCES

Aaron, P. G. Dyslexia, an imbalance in cerebral information-processing strategies. Perceptual and Motor Skills, 1978, 47, 699-706.

Aaron, P. G. and Baker, C. The neuropsychology of dyslexia in college students. In R. Malatesha & L. C. Hartlage (Eds.), Neuropsychology and Cognition, Vo. I. Hague, Holland: Martinus and Nijhoff, 1982.

Bakker, D. Dyslexia in developmental neuropsychology: hemisphere-specific models. Paper presented at the International Conference on Psychology and Medicine, Swansea, Wales, July 1979.

Bannatyne, A. Visual and spatial abilities and reading. Paper presented at the First International Reading Association Congress, Paris, France, August 1966.

Bateman, B. Interpretation of the 1961 Illinois Test of Psycholinguistic Abilities. Seattle: Special Child Publications, 1968.

Bender, L. A fifty-year review of experiences with dyslexia. Bulletin of the Orton Society, 1975, 25, 5-23.

Benton, A. Developmental dyslexia: neurological aspects. In W. Friedlander, Ed., Advances in Neurology, Vol. 7 New York: Raven Press, 1975.

Benton, A. Some conclusions about dyslexia. In A. Benton and D. Pearl, Eds.,Dyslexia: An Appraisal of Current Knowledge. New York: Oxford University Press, 1978.

416   E. Boder and S. Jarrico

Blank, M. Review of "Toward an understanding of dyslexia: psychological factors in specific reading disability". In A. Benton and D. Pearl, Eds., Dyslexia: An Appraisal of Current Knowledge. New York: Oxford University Press, 1978.

Boder, E. Developmental dyslexia: a diagnostic screening procedure based on three characteristic patterns of reading and spelling. In M. Douglass, Ed., Claremont Reading Conference 32nd Yearbook, Claremont, Calif.: Claremont University Center, 1968.

Boder, E. Developmental dyslexia: a diagnostic screening procedure based on three characteristic patterns of reading and spelling. In B. Bateman, Ed., Learning Disorders, Vol. 4. Seattle: Special Child Publications, 1971 (a).

Boder, E. Developmental dyslexia: prevailing diagnostic concepts and a new diagnostic approach. In H. Myklebust, Ed., Progress in Learning Disabilities, Vol. 2. New York: Grune & Stratton, 1971 (b).

Boder, E. Developmental dyslexia: a diagnostic approach based on three atypical reading-spelling patterns. Developmental Medicine and Child Neurology, 1973, 15, 663-687.

Boder, E. School failure - evaluation and treatment. Pediatrics, 1976, 58, 394-403.

Boder, E. Reading disorders. In S. Gellis and B. Kagan Eds., Current Pediatric Therapy, 9th ed. Philadelphia: W. B. Saunders Co., 1980.

Boder, E. and Jarrico, S. The Boder Test of Reading-Spelling Patterns: A Diagnostic Screening Test for Subtypes of Reading Disability. New York: Grune & Stratton, 1982.

Bogen, J. Some educational implications of hemispheric specialization. In M. Wittrock (ed.), The Human Brain. Englewood Cliffs, N. J. : Prentice-Hall, 1977.

Critchley, M. The Dyslexic Child, 2nd ed. Springfield, Ill.: Charles C Thomas, 1970.

Critchley, M., and Critchley, E. Dyslexia Defined. Springfield, Ill.: Charles C Thomas, 1978.

Dalby, J., and Gibson, D. Functional, cerebral lateralization in subtypes of disabled readers. Brain and Language, 1981, 14, 34-48.

Denckla, M. Minimal brain dysfunction and dyslexia: Beyond diagnosis by exclusion. In M. Blaw, J. Rapin, & M. Kinsbourne (Eds.), Child Neurology. New York: Spectrum, 1977.

Doehring, D., and Hoshko, I. Classification of reading problems by the Q-technique of factor analysis. Cortex, 1977, 13, 281-294.

Doehring, D., Trites, R., Patel, P., and Fiedorowicz, C. Reading Disabilities. New York: Academic Press, 1981.

Duane, D. A neurologic overview of specific language disability for the non-neurologist. Bulletin of the Orton Society, 1974, 24, 5-36.

Finucci, J., Guthrie, J., Childs, A., Abbey, H., and Childs, B. Genetics of reading disability. Annals of Human Genetics, 1976, 40, 1-23.

Fried, I. Cerebral dominance and subtypes of developmental dyslexia. Bulletin of the Orton Soceity, 1979, 29, 101-112.

Fried, I., Tanguay, P., Boder, E., Doubleday, C., and Greensite, M. Developmental dyslexia: Electrophysiological corroboration of clinical subgroups. Brain and Language, in press.

Friedman, M., Guyer, B., and Tymchuk, R. Cognitive style and specialized hemispheric processing in learning disabilities. In R. Knights and D. Bakker, eds. The Neuropsychology of Reading Disorders. Baltimore, Md.: University park Press, 1976.

Gaddes, W. Learning Disabilities and Brain Function. New York: Springer-Verlag, 1980.

Ginn, R. An Analysis of Various Psychometric Typologies of Primary Reading Disability. Unpublished doctoral dissertation, University of Southern California, Los Angeles, March 1979.

Gjessing, H. Functional analysis of reading and writing behavior. In R. Knights and D. Bakker, eds., Treatment of Hyperactive and Learning Disordered Children. Baltimore, Md.: University Park Press, 1980.

Gordon, H., and Harness, B. A test battery for the diagnosis and treatment of developmental dyslexia. Dash: Speech and Hearing Disorders, 1977.

Hanley, J. Optimizing Manpower Selection, Report No. 1974 H11. Air Force Office of Scientific Research, 1974.

Hynd, G., and Obrzut, J. Neuropsychological Assessment and the School-age Child. New York: Grune & Stratton, 1981.

Ingram, T., Mason, A., and Blackburn, I. A retrospective study of 82 children with reading disability. Developmental Medicine and Child Neurology, 1970, 12, 271-281.

Kinsbourne, M., and Warrington, E. Developmental factors in reading writing backwardness. British Journal of Psychology, 1963, 54, 145-156.

Malatesha, R. and Dougan D. Clinical subtypes of developmental dyslexia: Resolution of an irresolute problem. In R. N. Malatesha and P. G. Aaron (Eds.), Reading Disorders: Varieties and Treatments. New York: Academic Press, 1982.

Mattis, S., French, J., and Rapin, I. Dyslexia in children and young adults: three independent neyropsychological syndromes. Developmental Medicine and Child Neurology, 1975, 17, 150-163.

Menken, G. A Comparison of Auditory Disabled and Non-Auditory Disabled Children on a Time/Speech Compression Task. Unpublished doctoral dissertation, University of Southern California, June 1981.

Myklebust, H. Development and Disorders of Written Language: Picture-Story Language Test. New York: Grune & Stratton, 1965.

Myklebust, H. Toward a science of dyslexiology. In H. Myklebust, Ed., Progress in Learning Disabilities, Vol. 4, New York: Grune & Stratton, 1978.

Myklebust, H., and Boshes, B. Psychoneurological learning disorders in children. Archives of Pediatrics, 1960, 77, 247-156.

Orton, S. Reading, Writing, and Speech problems in Children. New York: Norton, 1937.

Petrauskas, R., and Rourke, B. Identification of subtypes of retarded readers. Journal of Clinical Neuropsychology, 1979, 1, 17-37.

Pirozzolo, F. The Neuropsychology of Developmental Reading Disorders. New York: Praeger Publishers, 1979.

Rosenthal, J. Neuropsychopathology of Written Language. Chicago: Nelson Hall, 1977.

Rosenthal, J. Neuropsychological Studies of Primary Developmental Dyslexia. Unpublished doctoral dissertation, University of California. San Francisco, 1980.

Rosenthal, J., Boder, E., and Calloway, E. Typology of primary developmental dyslexia: Electrophysiological evidence for its construct validity. In R. N. Malatesha and P. G. Aaron (Eds), Reading Disorders: Varieties and Treatments. New York: Academic Press, 1982.

Rutter, M. Prevalence and types of dyslexia. In A. Benton and D. Pearl, Eds., Dyslexia: An Appraisal of Current Knowledge. New York: Oxford University Press, 1978.

Sperry, R. W., Gazzaniga, M., and Bogen, J. Interhemispheric relationships: the neocortical commissures; syndromes of hemisphere disconnection. In P. Vinken and G. Bruyn, Eds., Handbook of Clinical Neurology, Vol. 4. Amsterdam: North-Holland, 1969.

Sporn, E. Personal communication, 1980. Is Dyslexia a Middle-class Disability? A Critique of Some Definitions. Unpublished doctoral dissertation, Yeshiva University, 1981.

Taylor, G., Satz, P., and Friel, J. Developmental dyslexia in relation to other childhood reading disorders: significance and clinical utility. Reading Research Quarterly, 1979, XV 84-101.

Whiting, S., and Jarrico, S. Spelling patterns of normal readers. Journal of Learning Disabilities, 1980, 13, 40-42.

Witelson, S. Neural and cognitive correlates of developmental dyslexia: age and sex differences. In C. Shagass, S. Gershon and A. Friedhoff, Eds., Psychopathology and Brain Dysfunction. New York: Raven Press, 1977.

Wittrock, M. Education and the cognitive processes of the brain. In Education and the Brain, 77th Yearbook of the National Society for the Study of Education, Part II. Chicago: University of Chicago Press, 1978, Ch. III, pp. 61-102.

Zaidel, E., and Peters, A. Phonological encoding and ideographic reading in the disconnected right hemisphere. Brain and Language, 1981, 14, 205-234.

Zangwill, R. Cerebral dominance. In R. N. Malatesha & L. Hartlage (Eds.), Neuropsychology and Cognition, Vol. I, Hague, Holland: Martinus & Nijhoff, 1982.

DYSLEXIA: A DIAGNOSTIC PROFILE FOR A "SPECIAL-EDUCATIONAL NEED"

Margaret Newton
Applied Psychology Department
The University of Aston in Birmingham
Birmingham, United Kingdom

This paper seeks to trace the emerging recognition of a special
group of children, whose literacy and fluency problems can be appropriately designated by the scientific term "dyslexia". Implicit in
the term's usage is that the difficulty is most probably primary,
constitutional and developmental; but can also in a minority of cases be traumatic in origin. The paper will describe how, over the
last fifty years or so, patterns of differential functioning in perce-
petual, motor and lexical mechanisms have been observed, which do
not apparently favor the acquisition of symbolic skills based upon
the linear ordering of ciphers; and how, in addition, a related set
of epi-phenomena is continuously being observed and reported by sci-
entists and clinicians. These differential functions would appear
to yield behavioral markers - or as Dr. Money in 1962 wrote "a pattern of signs which appear in contiguity". It is the writer's contention that sufficient evidence of such a learning syndrome is now
present; and strong enough to form the basis for early diagnosis,
leading to appropriate identification and teaching in the class-room.

A brief history, then, of the emergence of an educational problem; but linked to medical/neurological factors - the context of
"language and the brain". In the United Kingdom during the late
40's, the 50's and the 60's, the term "the under-functioning child
in the class-room" had replaced the earlier descriptor, "dull and
backward" for educational failure. Schonell in his text "Backwardness in the Basic Subjects (1942) had put forward the notion that
failure to read, write and spell (and to acquire numeracy also), was
not necessarily due to low intellectual capacity. He introduced the
term "retardation" to describe a situation in which a child of ordinary, average - and indeed above average - innate ability was failing to acquire basic literacy skills. "Retardation" referred to the

discrepancy between so-called "mental-age" on the one hand and "attainment age" on the other. Thus the notion of the "underfunctioning"
child. This concept could be graphically represented a "profile" -
a "thumb-nail sketch" so to say, of a child's attainment and ability
levels, graphically presenting the discrepancies between both chronological age and attainment; and so-called "mental-age and attainment". For example:- Professor Schonell in the 1930's and 40's had
uncovered the overwhelming nature of environmental stresses in the
backgrounds of many children which, it was hypothesised, could prevent them from acquiring formal language-learning in school settings. Amongst these, as described by Vernon (1967) were socio-economic deprivations, ill-preparing a child for a formal, verbally-based
education; emotional trauma within the family with consequent inhibiting anxiety effects; and inadequate school situations. These observed inhibiting features, together with obvious signs of neurological deficit, were the accepted and approved "barriers to learning"
in educational psychology practices at that time.

    By 1964 however, several authorities in the United Kingdom -
mainly medical - were beginning to attribute other causation to literacy failure. Ingram (1964) in his paper "The Dyslexic Child",
used the term "dyslexia" to describe the reading difficulties of a
distinct group of children. This special group had emerged in the
course of a survey of some Scottish schools. Critchley (1964) in
his seminal work "Developmental Dyslexia", had described a learning
phenomenon of an apparent constitutional origin, with well defined
identifying features within the individual; and linked to possible
variants in differential hemispheric functioning. Zangwill (1960)
had described possible neuropsychological factors operating in reading failure, including the term "cerebral dominance" as an underlying mechanism of importance and the apparent pre-eminence of the left brain hemisphere for language. The eminent neuro-psychologist
Stuart Dimond (1974) was also beginning his studies into relationships between "language and the brain". Kimura (1961) a neuro-psychologist working in Canada was researching cerebral dominance and the
perception of verbal stimuli, and the role of the right hemisphere
in visuo-spatial encoding.

    In the United States of America, the significance of differen-
tial functioning in the C. N. S. for the easy acquisition of literacy and fluency had been recognised much earlier by Orton (1925) (the
term he first used "word blindness" had in fact been employed by the
Scottish ophthalmologist Hinshelwood (1895) to describe the paradoxical situation in which "boys" of good intelligence, ordinary school opportunities, stable personalities and normal vision were failing to learn to read). Hinshelwood had related the failure to deficits in the angular gyrus region of the left hemisphere on the brain
- to so called "language area", a concept recognised by neurologists
since the time of Broca (1856) and Berlin (1887); but Orton introduced the concept of competing hemispheres, "lack of cerebral

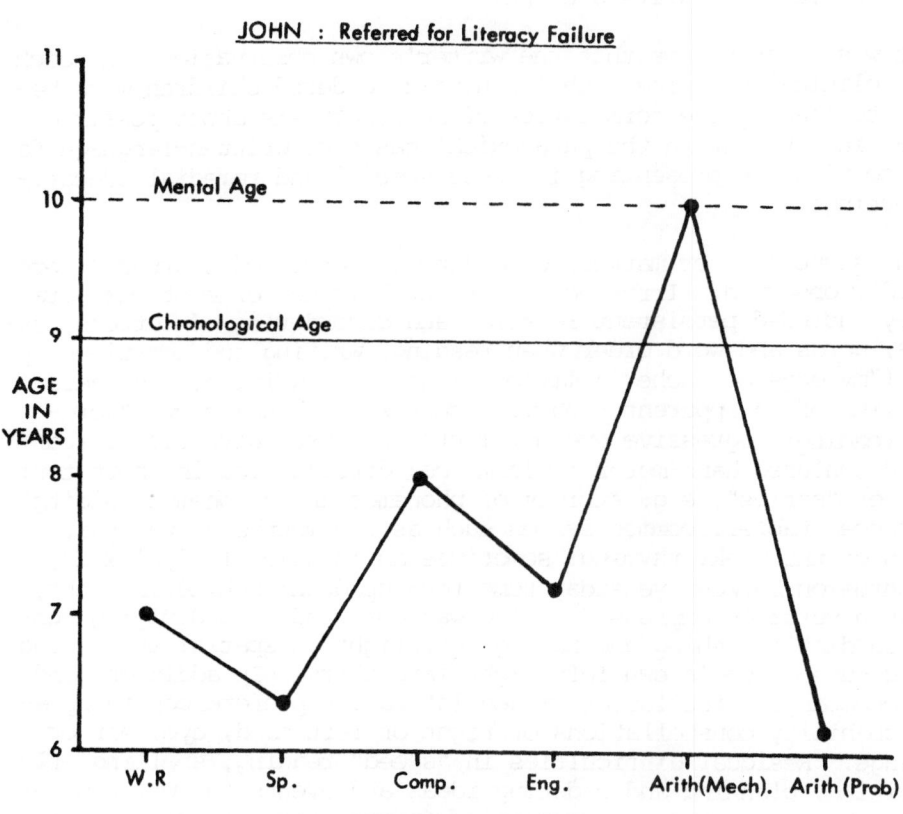

JOHN : Referred for Literacy Failure

TEST SCORES (In attainment-ages)

KEY :

W.R.	Word Recognition	Eng.	English
Sp.	Spelling	Arith(Mech).	Mechanical Arithmetic
Comp.	Comprehension	Arith(Prob).	Problem-solving Arithmetic

FIGURE 1.

dominance, mirror-imaging, failure to acquire series and other asymmetric functions". Sperry (1964) had also begun his work in America
on "lateral specialisation in the surgically separated hemispheres".

In neurology, and neuro-psychology then, by 1964 research had
begun into the relationships between brain and language and their possible consequences for developmental, constitutional difficulties
in learning to read, write and spell.

It was at this time that the writer's own observations in teaching and clinical practice with learning-disordered children were beginning to lead to the formulation of an hypothesis about possible
C. N. S. involvement in the paradoxical cases of written-language failure, continually presenting in these special and remedial educational settings.

The signposts, or markers of a "special group of learners" were
repeatedly observed. Irrespective of intelligence or emotional trauma they included persistent reversal and disordering of letters, syllables, words and word order when reading, writing and sometimes speaking ("my eggs do lache"); mirror images when writing; disorders
in spelling of an apparent random, inconsistent kind; slow, "word-
bound" reading; regressive eye movements; confused directional scanning and confused hand-motor performance; difficulties in short term
memory for "series", e.g. strings of phonemes and graphemes; digits
in sequence: tables: common series such as the months of the year
and days of the week: rhyming: sometimes an ideational "dyslexia",
e.g. confusion between yeserday/tomorrow; up/down; behind/in front,
etc., when verbally expressed. Also was observed an underlying confusion in distinguishing and naming left/right in spatial events and
in being sure of one's own left/right laterality. In addition, and
often accompanying the latter, mixed laterality preferences in apparent probability constellations of right or left hand, eye, ear or
foot usage. Residual difficulties in "speed" reading, spelling, fluent writing, planning and ordering ideas and events for written te-
xts; and the ability to skim passages of prose for meaning, persist-
ed into adulthood in those persons who experienced the acute dyslexic delays in early childhood.

These patterns of differential functioning in perceptual, motor
and lexical mechanisms have since been reported by many authorities:
Newton et al (1979); Critchley (1981); Miles (1981); Rawson (1981).
But in 1964 educational policy in the United Kingdom was influenced
by authorities such as Tizard (1972) who failed to acknowledge a
"syndrome" - and pursued the earlier diagnostic features as described by Vernon (ibid); in spite of Money's (1962) statement "it is
not at all rare in psychological medicine ....that a disease should have no unique identifying sign, that uniqueness being in the
pattern of signs that appear in contiguity".

The Aston work began therefore to test the hypothesis of individual differences in cognitive style affecting acquisition of literacy skills, and identifiable by the above "marker variables", with special reference to "language and the brain". Experimental work has included the three following investigations, all concerned with examining hemisphere-differentiation, linked to cerebral-dominance theories of language.

1. A neuro-psychological Investigation in Dyslexia, using the techniques of electro-encephalography. Newton et al. (1979).

The hypothesis for the research was: There is a difference in cortical lateral organisation between successful readers and children with the form of severe disability described as dyslexia, and that this difference can be manifested by using the techniques of electro-encephalography.

Fifty children between the ages of eight and thirteen took part in the study. The experimental group consisted of 25 diagnosed dyslexics (mean reading age = 6.4 years), referred to as 'cases'. They were compared with a similar number of matched controls whose reading ability was within the normal range (mean RA = 10.3 years). The groups were matched for age, intelligence : IQs ranging from 80-125 as measured by the WISC, socio-cultural background and school opportunities.

The experimental group comprised of children referred to child guidance clinics and a university child study centre for written language difficulties. They had received an average of 18 months therapy and remedial tuition but their reading failure had proved resistive to this treatment, and their average reading retardation at the time of testing was 4.1 years. Pre-, peri-, and postnatal histories of the group were recorded together with information on genetic familial factors. Where relevant, the cases were classified in terms of pregnancy or birth complications (possible neurological impairment) and genetic predispositions.

The EEG recordings were made either in the school (controls) or in the Child Guidance Clinics (cases). The procedure was standardised for both groups. All readings were bi-polar, using silver stick-on electrodes placed according to the 10-20 international system. An Elther eight-channel portable electroencephalograph machine was used. A full routine record was taken for visual interpretation and in addition, tape recordings were made from right and left tempero-parieto-occipital derivations on a frequency modulated tape recorder. The tapes were subsequently replayed through the standar eight-channel Offner machine. Analysis was carried out on the tap recorder derivations, using a four-channel low frequency BNI wave analyser. The filter trays in use for this study covered the frequencies 8, 9, 10, 11, 12 and 13 c/sec. The analyser was modified to provide a digital output of the abundance of each alpha frequency, which was automatically encoded and punched on to paper tape for processing by an Elliott 803 computer. The statistical analyses carried out by the computer on the frequency analyses were as follows:

1. Harmonic Mean, a statistical procedure which is used to calculate the mean of data which are in rates, in this case cycles per sec.

2. Mean Abundance, the arithmetic mean of the abundances of all frequencies.

3. Kendall's Concordance, a measure of the variability of the ranked analyser abundances from epoch to epoch. The score varies between zero and one, a score of one indicating no variability.

In general the findings of the present study suggest the presence of lateral dominance and cortical organisation in the control group of normal readers. There appears to be no comparable resolution of dominance in the group of dyslexics, a feature of both genetically and neurologically determined cases.

A significant difference (p < .02) was found between the groups in the amount of alpha activity present in the two cortical hemispheres, cases showing almost exact symmetry of alpha rhythm or slightly greater dominant hemisphere activity. The controls, on the otherhand, showed more alpha activity on the non-dominant side - the alternation being on the dominant where, according to Raney (quoted by Vernon 1957), 'the "central excitatory state" and the peripheral nerve sensitivity (a) greater than those of the non-dominant side since the alpha rhythm is less', i.e. where cerebral activity is at its greatest. These findings, therefore, could have implications for the facilitation or inhibition of learning in the areas of the cortex most commonly associated with the acquisition of language, and especially of reading.

From the results of the automatic analysis of the EEG data, a more detailed comparison was made. In the cases of reading failure there appeared to be a smaller lateral difference occipitally in cortical organisation (Kendall's Concordance) but with a right sided predominance. Temporally there appeared firstly a smaller asymmetry of alpha and theta rhythms, indicating no defined cortical dominance, and secondly a lateral equivalence in cortical organisation (Kendall's Concordance). In the control group, however, the variability of cortical organisation showed greater laterality differences. In the temporal regions there was asymmetry of alpha rhythm indicating cortical dominance, with an asymmetry of theta abundance also. (As the subjects were children, theta rhythm would be a normal developmental characteristic). There was greater concordance in the right hemisphere. These findings again appear significant if we consider that the temporal regions are associated with the development of language skills, long-term memory, and auditory organisation, three critical prerequisites for the acquisition of reading skill.

Of subjects showing immature, unstable records, 80% were 'cases' where ante- or peri-natal neurological impairment was suspected. This result is compatible with the view held by many neurologists that some of the reading disorders in childhood may be dependent upon minimal cerebral injury. Kawai and Pasamanick (1959) for example, postulated 'a continuum of reproductive casuality' extending all the way from death in utero and in the neonatal period to minimal cerebral damage resulting in minor behavior dysfunction. Reading disorders would constitute one component of this continuum.

In all, 88% of the experimental group showed evidence of unresolved dominance in the EEG recordings, as compared with 16% of the controls. Of the 'cases', 35% were in the 'possible genetically determined' group and a further 40% in the 'possible neurological impairment' group (20% of the cases figuring in both groups). These results support the writings of Critchley (1970) and Reitan (1964) amongst others, and in this small sample at least, unresolved dominance is a critical feature of dyslexia and would appear to be concomitant with both genetic and neurological symptoms.

2. A Comparison of Laterality Effects in Dyslexics and Controls using Verbal Dichotic Listening Tasks.

Dyslexic children and a control group were presented with dichotic listening task involving digits, words, reversible words (saw/was), similar words (big/pig) and reversible nonsense syllables (mag/gam). The task involves presenting the stimuli at exactly the same time over stereo-headphones, and this is interpreted in terms of hemisphere dominance for the processing of the particular stimulus, there being a direct neurological connection between right ear and left hemisphere and vice versa. The control group showed the right ear superiority effect for digits, words, reversible and similar words. The dyslexic group showed no difference or a left ear superiority for these tests, and a right ear effect for the nonsense syllables.

The results were related to the possible mechanisms involved in terms of hemispheres, and it was suggested that the dyslexic group showed a less well established dominance of hemispheric function. Individual differences of this nature were suggested as being less efficient for processing written language which is serial, sequential and directional.

3. Visual Identification of Words in Dyslexics and Controls, using Tachistoscopic Techniques.

The use of 'mediated' and 'immediate' identification, based

in Smith's feature analytic model of the reading process is investigated in dyslexic and control children. High and low redundancy letter triplets were presented tachistoscopically and the light intensity levels required for the children to identify the letters was recorded, as well as any errors made. It was found that the dyslexics
failed to make use of sequential redundancy in the identification of
letters, and made many types of confusion error compared to controls.
The results were interpreted as indicating the use of 'mediated' letter identification in the dyslexics, using similar processes to
'normal' beginner readers, whereas the control used 'immediate' recognition, being fluent readers. The results were related to linguistic and perceptual features of the learning to read process, suggesting difficulties with sequence and order within words.

All these three studies would appear to support neurological
findings of left hemisphere pre-eminence for both serialisation and
lexical encoding. In a series of studies using the noo-tropil drug
piracetam, Wilsher (1979) found sequencing and short term memory effects related to both left-hemisphere specialisation, and a differential effect between experimental group ("dyslectics") and control
group. Clinical observation has continued into the incidence of confused laterality patterns and serial order difficulties. These
epi-phenomena of dyslexia have also been tested in field-work - comparing such patterns in experimental and control groups in school
settings. Both in the clinical and school situation findings have
supported the links between literacy delay and failure on the one
hand and confused laterality and directionality on the other; Newton
et al (1979). Most marked has been the evidence of difficulties in
processing symbolic information which is sequential in nature. Again, observed clinically, and supporting the evidence brought forward
by Critchley (1970) has been the strong familial and constitutional
aspect of such behavioral functions, linked to reading, writing and
spelling difficulties. Newton, Bate (1979) have also noted the evidence of specific spatial and perceptuo-motor aptitudes in the population under review - again suggesting a difference in cognitive processing rather than a defect per se. Most recent work at Aston is
in this field of differential skills, including a current research
program into the subtests of the WISC and BAS tests of "intelligence" and the repeated emergence of the so called A. C. I. D. profile
in the records of dyslexic persons, i.e. depressed scores in items
which present tasks analogous to those of reading and spelling in
that they require consistent and fluent tracking and serialisation
- Thomson and Grant (1979).

Thomson and Hartley (1979) described the emotional stresses linked to literacy failure; and a present study at Aston conducted by
Roberts (1982 continuing) is examining the self-concept of special
educational-need children and the phenomenon of teacher expectation
- the "Pygmalion in the classroom" effect.

In addition to an intense study of the behavioral and functional differences in dyslexia, attention has been drawn to the key features of an alphabet script, which could present so much difficulty
to the above kind of "learner"; reading a phonetic-alphabetic script
- or as Liberman (1979) writes, "ciphers on the phonemes of language".
The work of Frank Smith (1971) in the psycho-linguistic aspects of
reading - especially his observation of the "immediate versus the
mediated" reading styles - and how the dyslexic learner would appear
to remain always in the latter mode. Newton and Thomson (1979) describe the "inter-face" so to say of child and written system and note the possible break-down points which continued research findings
would indicate.

Reference has often been made to the clumsy child syndrome and
its relationship with dyslexia. In fact some confusion has existed,
diagnostically, upon this issue. Whitsell (1965) has helped to clarify the situations by his hypothesis that three types of dyslexia
could be described: first a "pure elective" type, constitutional and
developmental in origin characterised by confusions in perceptual,
motor and lexical functions, and acute difficulties in reading, writing and spelling, but no other apparent 'stigmata'; secondly a learning disability caused by brain trauma - pre, peri or post-natal -
and marked also by attentional deficits, motor clumsiness, hyper-activity, aphasias and general linguistic delays; and thirdly an interactive condition of the two. Marth Denkla's work, first in Boston
and now in New York, has specialised in the neurological deficit child and has described the three to four hour or so battery of tests
which can establish the diagnostic profiles of such children. This
battery includes the Halstead psychological assessment schedules in
addition to a series of neurological items devised by Marth Denkla
herself. From this data, a profile of neurological deficit with implications for special teaching is drawn - Hospital personnel then
liase with schools. Her work in Boston has been taken over by
Dr. Jane Holmes. A crucial aspect of their work of course, is its
dependence on 'language and the brain' - in this case "brain deficit" rather than "brain difference" as seems to be the case in the
"pure" constitutional types. Dr. Holmes quotes the interesting mo-
tor-perceptual differences related to left or right hemisphere damage, shown so graphically in the childrens' drawings of a bicycle; -
left brain damage leading to a wholistic, impressionist drawing of a
bicycle, lacking specificity and detail, whereas right brain damage
leads to drawings characterised by fragmented series of detail -
handlebar, bell, wheels, etc., in isolated sections with no unit or
"gestalt". These findings underline again the key role of intrinsic,
C. N. S. involvement in representational skills.

Eventually it was the overwhelming evidence of the differential
patterns of cognitive functioning which led to the beginnings of
applied research at Aston. International evidence and support were
growing for the existence of a "special group of learners", who by

differential functioning in key aspects of C. N. S. organisation could be described and identified by the term "dyslexia". Rutter et
al (1975); Geschwind (1980); Tarnopol (1976); Klasen (1978); Bakker
(1972); Satz (1975) and Blank (1981 - personal communication during
Aston Course "Dyslexia: Diagnosis and Teaching).

The first task at Aston therefore, appeared to be that of providing for teachers in the classroom identification "markers", based
on research findings, in order that the presently described "special
educational-need child"- Warnock (1978) - could be recognised and
diagnosed as early as possible. Consequently an Index of 16 sub-tests was devised, yielding a learning and behavioral profile, linked
to the sub-skills of literacy and indicating individual areas of weakness and strength. This measure is known as the ASTON INDEX, Newton and Thomson (1976). The index seeks to sample, in the simplest
and most direct way possible, the sub-skills and behaviors which seem essential if the young learner is to make the "conceptual leap"
into written, symbolic, lexical representations of reported events.
The results of the 16 sub-tests yield a learning profile.

The second task was to devise a set of activities and techniques for creating individual teaching programs to match the profiles
drawn up by the Aston Index. This work, the Aston Portfolio - Aubr-
ey, Hicks, Eaves and Newton (1981) is now completed. During the background research for the Portfolio, various interesting features of
teaching and remedial teaching were recorded, e.g. it was found during teaching trials that "teaching to the strength" (i.e. choosing
a reading scheme based on a child's better abilities) and remediati-
ng the weaknesses in special tutoring sessions, was the most effective strategy. Difficulties within the "general" dyslexic profile
were recognised as being visual or auditory (corresponding to Boder's
(1982) dys-eidetic and dys-phonetic categories) graphomotor and ideational; and various combinations of these "modes". The Portfolio
contains over 500 teaching techniques - mnemonics; rules; auditory,
visual and kinaesthetic "perceptual anchors"; ideas for reinforceme-
nt, novelty, motivation, etc. The aim of such "mediational" teaching
is to present the linguistic element in such graphic, clear and unambiguous form, that a child with inherent perceptuo-lexical confusions can perceive its nature and make the necessary conceptual leap. Such teaching not only enables the linguistic signal to be assimilated in meaningful form, but also provides links and associations which make appropriate retrieval possible. The supporting mnemonic devices can include rhythm, doggerel, pictorial enhancement of
letters and morphemes (e.g. Wendon, 1977), acronyms (e.g. I Go Home
To-night and fight); narrative based on etymology (e.g. "gh" words
with the "ghosts" of the old vikings); and alliterative sound patterns (e.g. the Swiss swan swam sweetly into the swamp; King Kong
had a game of ping pong; The knight knocked his knuckle on the kn-
ob). The Aston Portfolio provides examples of such "perceptual anchors" and memory aids in order that appropriate teaching programs

can be created for individual learners.

In summary then, a specific learning profile has emerged during the course of teaching/clinical observation and scientific research; a profile based on the theory of probabilistic differences in C. N. S. development. These individual differences appear linked to organisational possibilities in hemispheric specialisation for language, sequencing and analytic skills; and related to familial, constitutional factors.

Specific behavioral markers can be identified in children which provide diagnostic clues to establishing a "dyslexia" syndrome. Such learning profiles guide the teacher to appropriate teaching techniques: diagnosis leading to prescriptive teaching. Some profiles appear "pure", elective and linked to developmental lexical, perceptual and motor mechanisms, others indicate "the clumsy-child syndrome" in which neurological deficits rather than just "differences" appear to inhibit easy learning. The latter cases would seem to be associated with pre, peri or post-natal trauma, and include attentional deficit, hyper-activity, perceptuo-motor difficulties and organic speech defects. These results of C. N. S. trauma interacy in some cases with the pure, constitutional features causing grace school learning problems.

The outcome of such pure and applied research could enable the teacher, in Margaret Rawson's words (1981), "to teach language as it is to the person as he is". In present terms, to identify the special-educational need child in the classroom, recognise his problems, draw his diagnostic profile and plan appropriate, mediational teaching programs for the very earliest days of "first-school".

REFERENCES

Bakker, D. J. A set of brains for learning to read. In K. C. Diller (Ed.), Individual differences and universals in language learning aptitude, Newbury house, 1978.
Berlin, R. Eine besondere art der wortblindheit, Wiesbaden, 1887.
Broca, P. Sur la faculte du language articule. Bulletin de la Societe d'Anthropologie, 1856.
Critchley, M. Developmental dyslexia, London: William Heinemann, 1964.
Dimond, S. and Beaumont, J. Hemisphere function in the human brain, Elek, 1974.
Geschwind, N. The anatomical basis of hemisphere differentiation, In Dimond S & Beaumont, J. Hemisphere function in the human brain, 1974.
Geschwind, N. Brain "miswired" in dyslexics? Med. News, 1980.
Hinshelwood, Word-blindness and visual memory, Lancet, 2, 15-64.

Ingram, T.   The dyslexic child, Bulletin I, 4, 1964, 1.

Kimura, D.   Cerebral dominance and the perception of verbal stimuli,
    Canadian Journal of Psychology,   1961, 15, 156-165

Klasen, E.   The syndrome of specific dyslexia, Lancaster: Medical and
    technical co.,   1972.

Money, J.   Reading disability, Baltimore: Johns Hopkins, 1962.

Newton, M. et al.   Readings in dyslexia, Learning developmental aids,
    Cambs. 1979.

Orton, S. T.   Word-blindness in school children, Arch. Neur. Psych-
    iat.,   1925, 14, 581-615.

Pavlidis, G. and Miles, T. R.   Dyslexia: Research and its application
    to education, John Wiley, 1981.

Rutter, M. et al. The concept of specific reading retardation,
    J. Child Psychol. Psychiat., 16. 181-197.

Satz, P.   Specific reading disability, Rotterdam University Press,
    1970.

Schonell,   Backwardness in the basic subjects. Oliver & Boyd, 1942.

Smith, F.   Understanding reading, Holt, Rinehart & Winston, 1971.

Sperry, R. W.   The great cerebral commissure. Sci. American, 1964.

Tarnopol, L.   Reading disabilities: An international perspective,
    Baltimore: University Park Press, 1976.

Tizard, J. D. E. S. report of the advisory committee on handicapped
    children. HMSO, 1972.

Vernon, M. D.   Backwardness in reading, Cambridge University Press,
    1957.

Warnock report, Special educational needs, HMSO, 1978.

Whitsell. Neurological aspects of reading disorders, Philadelphia:
    Davis, 1965.

Wilsher, C. Piracetam as an aid to learning in dyslexia, Psycho-
    pharmacology, 1979, 65, 107-109.

Zangwill, O. L. Cerebral Dominance and its Relation to psychologi-
    cal Function. Edinburgh: Oliver Boyd, 1960.

AN EXPERIMENTAL STUDY OF MULTI-SENSORY TEACHING

WITH NORMAL AND RETARDED READERS[1]

Charles Hulme   and
Department of Psychology
University of York
Heslington, York
YO1 5DD, U. K.

Lynette Bradley
Department of Experimental
Psychology
South Parks Road
Oxford, OX1 3UD U. K.

INTRODUCTION

It is now well established that there are a number of children who, despite adequate general intelligence, experience inordinate difficulties in learning to read and to write (Rutter, Tizard, & Whitmore, 1970; Clark, 1970). A considerable amount of research in recent years has been directed towards defining and understanding the nature of these children's reading difficulties (for reviews, see Vellutino, 1979; Hulme, 1981; Rutter & Yule, 1973). It is clear from this body of research that in many cases reading retardation is associated with subtle impairments of language function and deficits in verbal memory. In contrast to this, however, deficits in visual perception and memory can be ruled out as a cause in the majority of cases.

A major goal of research into reading retardation must be the improvement of ways in which to treat the disorder. Research into the cognitive deficits associated with the condition (e.g., perceptual abilities, verbal memory problems) is undoubtedly useful in this respect; but by itself it is insufficient. Many findings concerning psychological processes in these children are essentially neutral with regard to the question of how they are best taught to read. This is well illustrated by the traditional educational debate as to whether to teach to a child's strengths or weaknesses. A concrete example may clarify this. It appears that retarded readers are particu-

1. We wish to thank Mrs. U. Pearce of the East Oxford Reading center, and Miss J. Abbs of Badger Hill Infants School, York, for their permission to conduct this research. We also thank the children, their parents and teachers for their cooperation.

larly poor at segmenting the spoken words which they hear into constituent syllables and phonemes (Liberman, Shankweiler, Liberman, Fowler, & Fischer, 1977) and also at perceiving similarities in sound
between words which they hear (Bradley & Bryant, 1978). It is plausible to argue that such difficluties in perceiving speech may well
contribute to these children's difficulties in learning to read an
alphabetic language where letters map (if imperfectly) on to the
sounds of speech.

Given these findings two quite different teaching strategies
might be considered. According to the first we should avoid teaching
based on phonic principles, since this would be particularly difficult for these children, and instead perhaps try to teach them to
read using a whole-word strategy (cf. Jorm, 1979). An alternative,
equally reasonable strategy, however, would be to do just the opposite, and try to overcome the difficulties these children experience
with phonics by direct training. Which of these contrasting approaches would be most effective is clearly an emprirical question.

From this it follows that a necessary and complimentary research
strategy, to that of looking at the cognitive deficits associated with
reading retardation, is to examine directly possible methods for teaching these children. Such a strategy is practically useful, and
also holds out the hope of clarifying the nature of the original learning problem. If, for example, certain methods of remedial teaching
can be shown to be particularly successful with retarded readers, who
have failed to learn by conventional methods of instruction, an understanding of this should throw light on the nature of their original learning difficulties. Unfortunately, however, psychologists
have so far paid very little attention to the problem of demonstrating and understanding the effectiveness of various methods of teaching
for retarded readers. The present paper is an attempt to demonstrate,
experimentally, the effectiveness of a certain method of remedial
teaching and at the same time define the features which appear to be
critical to its success.

One of the most consistent and specific suggestions which has
been made about teaching retarded readers concerns the importance of
writing movements (Fernald, 1943; Gillingham & Stillman, 1956; Orton,
1928). The idea behind these methods is that emphasis on the movements made while writing, or sometimes upon the movements made while
manually tracing words as if writing them, may help these children
learn to read and spell.

There are two main variants of these teaching methods which are
both used fairly widely today (Cotterell, 1970; Wolf, 1970). The
first originates with the work of Fernald (1943; Fernald & Keller,
1921). Fernald recommended that children with reading difficulties
be taught to read and spell each word as and when it occurred as
part of their desire to express themselves in written work with their

teacher. Each word is written out by the teacher in large cursive script and the child then traces it with finger contact saying each syllable as it is traced. After each tracing the child tries to write the word without copying it. This procedure is repeated until the word can be written correctly from memory.

A similar but far more systematic method of teaching was developed somewhat later by Gillingham and Stillman (1956). In this method the child is first taught to associate the name and sound of letters with their visual appearance by repeatedly tracing or writing letters while simultaneously saying their name. Following this, the child then goes on to learn to read and spell, beginning with a group of words in which there is a regular spelling to sound correspondence. The method employed in learning these words is similar to that recommended by Fernald, except that in this case the child pronounces the name of each letter as he simultaneously traces or writes it. This procedure is known as simultaneous oral spelling.

These so-called multi-sensory teaching methods are widely used but so far there is no satisfactory evidence from controlled studies as to their effectiveness (Hulme, 1981). From clinical experience it has been found that a variant of the simultaneous oral spelling method, which simply involves having the child name each letter in a word as he writes it, is a highly effective teaching aid for retarded readers (Bradley, 1980). The aim of the present study was to demonstrate the effectiveness of this method of teaching in a controlled experimental setting, and at the same time, by systematically comparing variants of this teaching method, to identify the components which are critical to its success.

If we consider simultaneous oral spelling there would appear to be two possibly critical aspects to the procedure used. The first is that the child writes the word which he is learning to read and spell, and the second is that while writing the child simultaneously says the name of each letter. This could be described as a Visual (seeing the word), Auditory (saying and hearing each letter name) and Motor (writing each letter) method of learning to spell (VAM). It could be either the writing movements, the act of saying each letter name, or the conjunction of both these activities which is critical for the putative success of this method.

In order to examine these possibilities there were two other methods of teaching incorporated into our experimental training study. The second method used was a Visual-Motor (VM) one in which the child wrote the word but only said the word as a whole, not the names of the individual letters. If the writing activity alone is the critical aspect of the VAM method, then performance in the VM and VAM conditions should be equal since both involve the same motor element.

The third condition was a Visual-Auditory (VA) method of teaching.

In this condition the child did not write the word at all. In order
to spell the word the child arranged a series of letters printed on
small cards and simultaneously said the name of each letter as in the
VAM condition. If saying the name of each letter is the critical feature of the VAM method, then learning in the VA and VAM conditions
should be equivalent since both incorporate this element.

As a final condition in the experiment there was an untaught control condition. This was necessary to provide evidence as to whether any of the methods used were effective in teaching the children
to spell.

An additional question which we also considered in this study
was whether the relative effectiveness of these different teaching
methods was the same for retarded readers and children of normal reading ability. We might expect a different pattern of performance
in the two groups, since the VAM method of teaching is claimed to be
of special benefit to retarded readers who have failed to learn with
more conventional teaching methods. Because of this Hulme (1981) compared the effects of tracing movements, as used in the multi-sensory teaching methods considered here, on memory for letter sequences
in normal and retarded readers. The retarded readers were worse at
remembering the letter sequences than the normal readers, but, more
importantly, tracing produced a selective improvement in memory amongst the retarded readers as compared to the normals. This selective
improvement seemed to be a consequence of the retarded readers' poor
verbal memory abilities, since in a comparable experiment using nonverbal letter-like forms, the two groups performed at an equivalent
level, and tracing was of equal benefit to both. These experiments
suggest that methods of remedial teaching which incorporate a motor
element may be especially helpful to retarded readers because they
provide a mnemonic aid which helps to compensate for the retarded reader's verbal memory impairments.

Whether or not this is accepted, it seems reasonable to explore
the relative effectiveness of the teaching methods considered here,
in normal as well as retarded readers. If a certain method of teaching is found to be particularly effective for retarded readers this has both practical and theoretical implications. Practically it
may lead to more effective teaching, and theoretically an understanding of such methods should be relevant to understanding the source
of these children's difficulties in learning to read.

METHOD

Design: There were four conditions in the experiment. The effectiveness of the three different methods of teaching spelling outlined
above were compared with an untaught control condition, for a group
of normal and retarded readers.

On the basis of pre-tests 16 words were selected which none of the children participating in the experiment could spell correctly. The 16 words used were: sew, buy, toe, won, calf, suit, ache, sign, type, tear, soup, cute, laugh, tough, chief, juice.

For each subject these sixteen words were randomly permuted into four groups of four, and the different groups of four words were randomly assigned to one of the four experimental conditions. Each subject was taught three groups of four words, one group in each of the teaching conditions, for four consecutive days from Monday to Thursday. The order of teaching conditions was randomly varied across subjects and each subject received a different random order of conditions on each of the four days of teaching. On the fifth day of the study (Friday) each child was tested for their ability to spell each of the 16 words. This testing was repeated two weeks and four weeks later.

Subjects: Two groups of nine children, one group severely retarded in reading and spelling and a group of children of normal reading and spelling ability were seen in the study.

The details of these two groups are shown in Table 1. The two groups were closely matched for IQ as assessed by the WISC-R and also for spelling ability as assessed by the Schonell Graded Word Spelling Test. A consequence of matching the children on the basis of spelling age is that the normal children, whose spelling ability is appropriate for their age, are considerably younger than the children retarded in reading and spelling. The important point about this matching procedure, however, is that any differences found between the normal and retarded readers cannot be attributed to overall differences in reading and spelling ability.

TABLE 1. Details of the two groups of children seen in the experiment

	Normal Readers	Retarded Readers
Age	6yr 9mth	11yr 0mth
Reading Age (Schonell)	7yr 4mth	7yr 8mth (t= 1.34, N. S.)
Spelling age (Schonell)	6yr 11mth	7yr 1mth (t= 1.08, N. S.)
IQ (WISC-R)	102	100 (t= 0.68, N. S.)

Procedure: The details of the teaching procedures used in the experiment were as follows:

1) Visual-Auditory-Motor (VAM). The word to be learned is presented to the child written on a small card. The experimenter then reads the word to the child, and the child repeats it. The child then writes the word saying the name of each letter as it is written. When the word has been written, the child says the word once more, and the experimenter checks to see that the word has been written correctly. After this, the stimulus word is covered, and the whole process is repeated two more times.

2) Visual-Motor (VM). The procedure here is identical to the VAM method except that the child does not say the letter names as he writes them. He merely says the word, says the word again as he writes it, and then says the word once more when he has written it. As in the VAM method, for each word the procedure is repeated three times.

3) Visual-Auditory (VA). This condition was identical to the VAM condition except that here writing movements were excluded by having the child form the word using letters printed on small cards. In this condition the child says the word, then says the name of each letter as he places it down to form the word, and when the word is formed he says the word once again. This procedure is repeated three times for each word as in the other two conditions.

4) Untaught (UT). No teaching of the words assigned to this condition was undertaken. The child's ability to spell these words was simply assessed at the same times as the words which had been taught. Performance in this condition provides a baseline against which to assess the effectiveness of the teaching received in the other conditions.

RESULTS

The percentage of words correctly spelled by the two groups in each condition and at each of the three times of testing are shown in Table II.

There are several aspects of these results which are of interest. The overall levels of performance in the two groups seem more or less comparable, indicating that the learning task was of roughly equal difficulty for both the normal and retarded readers. All three methods of teaching appear to be effective to some extent as indicated by the higher level of performance in these conditions than in the untaught control condition. Finally, and perhaps most interestingly, the relative effectiveness of the different teaching conditions appears to differ for the retarded and normal readers. For the retarded readers the VAM condition seems by far the most effective, while for the normal readers there is a rather less marked advantage for the VM condition.

The scores for correctly spelled words were subjected to a three=

way (2 X 4 X 3) split plot analysis of variance with groups as a between-subjects variable and conditions and time of testing as within-subjects variables. This analysis revealed a highly significant effect of conditions [F (3,48) = 30.89, p < 0.001] and a highly significant effect of time of testing [F (2,32) = 27.93, p < 0.001]. Overall levels of performance did not differ between the two groups (F < 1.0) but there was a significant interaction between groups and conditions [F (3,48) = 3.13, p < 0.05] confirming that the relative effectiveness of the different methods of teaching was not uniform across the two groups. The only other significant effect was the interaction between time of testing and conditions [F (6,96) = 3.92, p < 0.005].

The nature of these two interactions was further explored using the Tukey HSD test. The interaction between groups and conditions seems attributable to differences in the relative effectiveness of the VAM and VM conditions for the two groups; for the retarded readers the VAM condition was by far the most effective while for normal readers the advantage lies with the VM condition. A Tukey HSD test confirmed this interpretation. For the retarded readers all three methods of teaching produced significant learning as compared to the untaught control condition (p < 0.05 in each case); however, the VAM condition was also significantly better than any other (p < 0.05). For the normal readers once again all three methods produced significant learning as compared to the untaught control condition (p< 0.05) but in this case there was no significant difference between performance on the VM and VAM conditions. Overall then, the pattern of results is most clear-cut for the retarded readers, who learn to spell a significantly greater number of words when taught by the VAM method than by any other. For the normal readers the differences in performance between conditions are less marked, and both methods of teaching involving a motor element (VAM and VM) produce a similar amount of learning.

The interaction between time of testing and conditions seems attributable to the contrast between changes in the three taught conditions over time as compared to the relatively stable level of performance in the untaught control condition. A Tukey HSD test showed that in all three taught conditions there was a significant decline in performance between the first test and the final test four weeks later (p < 0.05 in each case). In the untaught condition, however, there was no significant change in performance between any of the times of testing.

Considering the variations in performance across the times of testing a little more, one might argue that the most critical aspect of a method of teaching spelling is the durability of the learning which it produces. If a method produces learning in the short-term which quickly fades then it may be of limited practical value. In the light of this it was decided that an additional analysis considering

Table 2. Percentage of words correctly spelled in each condition at each test for both groups

Time of Test	Retarded Readers Conditions				Normal Readers Conditions			
	VAM	VM	VA	UT	VAM	VM	VA	UT
1st test	80%	63%	50%	8%	53%	61%	42%	14%
2 week delay	53%	38%	28%	13%	39%	33%	19%	5%
4 week delay	58%	30%	35%	18%	33%	50%	31%	11%

only the results of the last test, four weeks after teaching had end-
ed, might be informative. A two-way (2 X 4) analysis of variance in
which the factors were groups and conditions was run on these data.
This analysis produced a similar pattern of results to the previous
one. Once again there was a significant main effect of conditions
[F (3,48) = 10.30, p < 0.001], a significant interaction between groups and conditions [F (3,48) = 4.40, p < 0.01], and no significant
difference between the groups (F < 1.0).

   This interaction between conditions and groups was once again explored using a Tukey HSD test. The results of this analysis serve to
emphasize the pattern of results obtained in the overall analysis.
For the retarded readers the superiority of the VAM method is even
more clearly in evidence, since only this method produces significantly better performance than the UT condition after a four-week delay
(p < 0.05). The VAM method is again significantly better than the
VM method (p < 0.05) and very nearly significantly better than the
VA method also.

   For the normal readers the differences between the different methods of teaching are once again less clear cut than in the case of
the retarded readers. In their case, after a delay of four weeks, only the VM condition produces significant learning as compared to the
untaught control condition (p < 0.05). However, performance in the
VM condition is not significantly better than performance in either
of the other taught conditions.

DISCUSSION

   The first aspect of our results which deserves consideration is
their practical implications. It has been demonstrated here in a controlled experimental study that the VAM method of teaching spelling
can be effective in teaching children with severe reading and spelling problems. It is in fact likely that in a more realistic remedial
teaching situation this method would be even more effective than it
has been demonstrated to be here. The first factor which may have
served to depress performance in this study is that, because of the
design used, each child experienced three novel teaching methods at
the same time. This made the experiment very demanding, especially
for the retarded readers. If the children had been taught exclusively by the VAM method it is likely that they would have benefitted
even more from it.

   Another aspect of the procedure which may have served to depress learning in the present experimental situation derives from using
the same set of words for all children. This was, of course, necessary in the present study to ensure that no bias existed to make learning in some conditions intrinsically easier than in others . This,
however, ignores a principle which is often put forward as important
in the teaching of retarded readers (e.g., Fernald, 1943; Bradley,

Hulme, & Bryant, 1979) which is that the child should be taught to read and spell words from his own vocabulary which he wishes to learn. Using words from the child's own vocabulary would again be expected to make the VAM method of teaching even more effective for the retarded readers.

It should be stressed that the effectiveness of the VAM method of teaching for retarded readers appears to be an effect of some generality since it has been found in two previous controlled studies involving different groups of retarded readers learning different groups of words (Bradley, in press).

As well as demonstrating the effectiveness of the VAM method of teaching we want to understand the reasons for its success. A Comparison of the different experimental conditions helps to clarify this. Since for the retarded readers the VAM method was significantly more effective than the VM or VA methods, we must conclude that both the motor activity (which is included in the VM condition) and the systematic naming of each letter (which is included in the VA condition) are important to the method's success. The qestion is, how do these two aspects of the method help the retarded reader to overcome his profound difficulties in learning spelling patterns?

Consider first the motor activity involved in writing the word. Previous experiments indicate that the motor activity involved in tracing around letters and graphic forms as if writing them may improve memory for them. This improvement appears to depend upon the generation of a separate motor sensory representation following the tracing activity (Hulme, 1981; Hulme, 1979). If we consider repeatedly writing a word as in the VAM condition it is plausible to suggest that this leads to the establishment in memory of a motor program specifying the movements necessary to write the word. This is an additional form of mnemonic information concerning the spelling pattern of a word. Given that retarded readers often suffer from a verbal memory impairment which would impede storage of spelling patterns in a verbal code, the additional information provided by a motor memory representation of the word may be particularly valuable to them.

Next consider the systematic naming of each letter in the word, which is also important to the success of the VAM method. To learn to read and to spell alphabetic language such as English, the child must learn to use an alphabetic code which maps the constituent phonemes of words onto separate letters. To make things worse, however, this mapping does not take the form of a simple one to one correspondence between letters and sounds, and even if we admit fairly complex rules for relating spellings to sound, there remain 'exception' words which do not appear to conform to any such rules (e.g., Venezky, 1970, Wijk, 1966). As described earlier, Liberman and her colleagues have shown that retarded readers have particular difficulty in segmenting spoken words into their constituent syllables and phonemes and this may plausibly be related to their difficulties in learning to read. More generally, it has been argued that the complex and abstract relationship between alphabetic writing and speech is a major problem in early reading acquisition (Rozin & Gleitman, 1977).

It seems likely that the systematic naming of each letter in the VAM method of teaching helps the retarded reader because it eliminates the need for any explicit analysis of the word into constituent phonemes. Instead, a simple and explicit one-to-one relationship between the written letters and their names is provided. This explicit naming of the letters may enable the retarded reader to code the spelling pattern of the word verbally much more effectively than if he were left to accomplish this alone. It may be that verbal coding is particularly important to the child as a means of remembering the order in which the letters of a word are to be written when it has to be spelled.

It may be relevant that most of the words taught in the present experiment have either complex or totally irregular spelling-to-sound correspondences. In previous experiments with retarded readers the VAM method was found to be equally effective for words with a simple letter-by-letter correspondence between their constituent letters and their pronunciation (Bradley, 1981).

Finally, we must consider the contrast between the results obtained for the retarded readers and those for the normal children who are spelling and reading at the same level. For the normal children learning was best in the VM condition, but performance was not significantly better in this condition than in the VAM condition which also involved writing. It is clear then that the writing activity helped both the normal and the retarded readers to learn to spell.

The real contrast between the two groups, however, concerns the importance of naming the letters. For the retarded readers naming each letter as it was written produced an improvement in learning as compared to just writing the word (VAM was significantly better than VM). For the normal readers, however, in both conditions involving writing performance was roughly equal, and if anything naming each letter in the VAM condition tended to hinder learning. The advantage derived by the retarded readers from naming each letter is, therefore, a selective effect which is specific to this group. It seems likely that the specific benefit afforded to these children by the naming activity relates to their problems in segmenting speech and coding print into verbal memory. For normal readers who do not experience these difficulties, systematically naming each letter in a word seems to be an irrelevant activity which does not help them learn to spell it.

REFERENCES

Bradley, L. Assessing reading difficulties: A diagnostic and reme-
    dial approach. Basingstoke: MacMillan education, 1980.
Bradley, L. The organization of motor patterns for spelling: An ef-
    fective remedial strategy for backward readers. Developmental
    Medicine and Child Neurology, 1981, 23, 83-91.
Bradley, L. and Bryant, P. E. Difficulties in auditory organization
    as a possible cause of reading backwardness. Nature, 1978, 271,
    746-747.
Bradley, L., Hulme, C. and Bryant, P. E. The connexion between diff-
    erent verbal difficulties in a backward reader: A case study.
    Developmental Medicine and Child Neurology, 1979, 21, 790-795.
Clark, M. M. Reading diffiiculties in schools. Harmondsworth: Pen-
    guin, 1970.
Cotterell, G. C. The Fernald auditory-kinesthetic technique. In
    A. W. Franklin and S. Naidoo (Eds.), Assessment and teaching
    of dyslexic children. London: Invalid Children's Aid Associa-
    tion, 1970.
Fernald, G. M. Remedial techniques in basic school subjects. New
    York: McGraw Hill, 1943.
Fernald, G. M., and Keller, H. B. The effect of kinaesthetic factors
    in the development of word recognition in the case of non-read-
    ers. Journal of Educational Research, 1921, 4, 355-377.
Gillingham, A. M. and Stillman, B. U. Remedial teaching for children
    with specific disability in reading, spelling, and penmanship.
    (5th edition). New York: Sackett & Wilhems Litho Corp., 1956.
Hulme, C. The interaction of visual and motor memory for graphic
    forms following tracing. Quarterly Journal of Experimental
    Psychology, 1979, 31. 249-261.
Hulme, C. Reading retardation and multi-sensory teaching: An experi-
    mental study. London: Routledge and Kegan Paul, 1981.
Jorm, A. F. The cognitive and neurological basis of developmental
    dyslexia: A theoretical framework and review. Cognition, 1979,
    7, 19-33.
Liberman, I. Y., Shankweiler, D., Liberman, A. M., Fowler, C., and
    Fischer, F. W. Phonetic segmentation and recoding in the begi-
    nning reader. IN A. S. Reber & D. Scarborough (Eds.), Toward
    a psychology of reading. Hillsdale, N. J. : Lawrence Erlbaum
    Associates, 1977.
Orton, S. T. Specific reading disability - strephosymbolia. Journal
    of the American Medical Association, 1928, 90, 1095-1099.
Rozin, P., & Gleitman, L. The structure and acquisition of reading
    II: The reading process and the acquisition of the alphabetic
    principle. In A. Reber & D. Scarborough (Eds.), Toward a psy-
    chology of reading. Hillsdale, N. J.: Lawrence Erlbaum Asso-
    ciates, 1977.
Rutter, M., Tizard, J. and Whitmore, K. (eds.), Education, health,
    and behavior. London: Longmans, 1970.
Rutter, M., Yule, W. Specific reading retardation. In L. Mann &

D. Sabatino (eds.), The first review of special education. Philadelphia: Buttonwoods Farms, 1973.

Vellutino, F. R. Dyslexia: Theory and research. cambridge, Mass.: MIT press, 1979.

Venezky, R. L. The structure of English orthography. The Hague: Mouton, 1970.

Wijk, A. Rules of pronunciation for the English language. London: Oxford University Press, 1966.

Wolff, A. G. The Gillingham-Stillman Program. In A. W. Franklin & S. Naidoo (Eds.), Assessment and teaching of dyslexic children London: Invalid Children's Aid Association, 1970.

INSTRUCTING LEARNING DISABLED CHILDREN TO MAKE
CONTINUED AND GENERAL USE OF A STRATEGY FOR MEMORIZING INFORMATION[1]

Margaret Jo Shepherd
Department of Special Education
Teachers College, Columbia University
New York, N. Y.

Lynn M. Gelzheiser
Center for Special Education
University of Maine at Farmington
Farmington, Maine

Developmental dyslexia differs from acquired dyslexia in that developmental dyslexia is a reading disorder arising as the child learns to read. Developmental dyslexia can be characterized as failure or inordinate difficulty in the acquisition of normal reading skills, given adequate native ability and adequate instruction (Critchley, 1970). There is evidence that the reading disorder described as developmental dyslexia may co-exist with failures in arithmetic and mathematics achievement (Fleischner, Garnett & Shepherd, 1982; Satz, this volume), spelling failure (Frith, this volume), poor social skills (Bryan, 1981), and poor performance on tasks requiring short-term memory (Torgesen, 1982). This evidence suggests that general difficulty with learning or the acquisition of new skills may be the defining factor in developmental dyslexia. Thus, the terms "learning disability" or "learning disabled" may be used to describe children who might otherwise be called dyslexic (Kirk, 1963).

It is our hypothesis that learning disabled children show performance deficits relative to non-disabled children because of differences in the process of learning. We have employed what is termed "the instructional approach" to developmental cognitive research (Belmont & Butterfield, 1977) to examine differences between learning disabled and non-disabled children. The instructional approach to developmental cognitive research as outlined by Belmont and Butterfield is based on the assumption that the use of instruction in research is required to understand observed developmental differences

1. This work was supported by a contract (300-80-0620) between the Institute for the Study of Learning Disabilities at Teachers College, Columbia University and the Office of Special Education, Department of Education, through Title VI-6 of Public Law 91-230.

in the way children process information. By extension, this approach can be used to describe differences between normal and disabled learning. Experimental tasks which show developmental or normal-disabled differences in performance are appropriate to this method.

With the instructional approach, once an experimental task has been selected, a description of immature and mature, or disabled and normal performance on the task is compiled. From this description, and from current information processing theories, a list of the underlying information processing procedures which could produce the observed performance on the experimental task is proposed. The list should include both the information processing procedures which could produce the poor performance exhibited by immature or disabled subjects, and the information processing procedures which could produce the better performance exhibited by older or normal subjects. It is hypothesized that processes used by mature or normal subjects which are not used by immature or disabled subjects account for the observed performance differences between these subjects.

If the processes suggested to account for developmental or normal-disabled differences are such that measurement can be both direct and reliable, an instructional approach can be employed. Instruction of immature or disabled subjects in the use of the targeted, directly measurable process(es) is instituted.

The results of this instruction confirm or disconfirm hypotheses about the role of the target process(es) in successful performance. If changes in processing and overall performance can be reliably measured, and if the result of instruction is that immature or disabled subjects are observed to use the target process(es) coincident with a performance level that no longer differs from that of mature or normal subjects, then certain inferences follow. It is inferred that the information processing procedures proposed for the experimental task are plausible, and that the instructed, directly measurable process(es) represent a viable conceptualization of the information processing difference that produces performance differences between immature and mature subjects, or disabled and normal subjects.

Belmont and Butterfield (1977) have defined three standards for instructional research to insure that inferences about information processing which are based on instruction are well substantiated. The first dictates how data from instructional research will be analyzed, while the second and third dictate experimental design.

The first standard requires that the size of instructional effect be documented, both with data on the number of children showing improvement and the extent of their improvement. Mature performance is suggested as an adequate standard or criterion to analyze the effect of instruction on immature subjects. Likewise, the performance level of normal or non-disabled subjects is the criterion by which the performance of disabled subjects, before and after instruction is evaluated. In order to substantiate the role of the instructed process, it is not enough to demonstrate significant improvement through instruction. Improvement must eliminate performance differences between groups that previously were different.

The second standard to be met is that the observed improvement and the elimination of differences in performance must be durable findings. The stability over time of changes in processing and performance is required to support the contention that the process is reflected in performance.

The final, most stringent standard is that of transfer or generalization. If the targeted process is responsible for performance changes on the experimental task, then performance changes should also be observed with the use of the target process on tasks with similar information processing demands.

Three studies examining the memory performance of learning disabled children and adolescents are presented as examples of the "instructional approach" to developmental cognitive research. The utility of this research approach with learning disabled children will then be discussed, in light of the hypothesis that these children differ from non-disabled subjects in the way they learn.

The studies addressed these general concerns:
-the performance of learning disabled and non-disabled children from the ages of 9 to 15 on a picture study recall task for which number of pictures recalled was the measure of performance, and the use of a mnemonic strategy of organizing pictures into categories was assumed to be the critical information processing procedure.
-the performance of 9 to 12 year old learning disabled and non-disabled children on the picture recall task after instruction to use the targeted process of organization during study;
-the performance of 12 and 13 year old learning disabled children on a prose recall task with similar processing demands after instruction in the use of sorting with the picture task.

The Experimental Tasks

There is evidence, both empirical and clinical, that children described as learning disabled or dyslexic have difficulty acquiring information for the purpose of immediate recall. The empirical evidence is consistent across a variety of recall tasks which do not have a direct relationship to reading or any other academic skill (Torgesen, 1982). One interpretation of this research is that learning disabled children may have a general memory deficit which is immutable, not subject to change.

Developmental studies of memory conducted with non-disabled children permit a broader and, potentially, more optimistic interpretation of the recall deficits observed among learning disabled children. These studies, influenced by information-processing models of learning and memory, suggest that while some features of memory may be subject to only limited change as a consequence of maturation and experience, others are more flexible, that is, reliable developmental changes are observed. (For a review of this research, see Kail, 19-79). These age-related changes in performance on recall tasks occur because as children mature, they learn to use a variety of strategies for acquiring and retrieving information (Brown, 1982). Furthermore, age-related differences in performance on recall tasks can be eliminated or substantially reduced by teaching younger children to use rehearsal, taxonomic organization, imagery or verbal eleboration when they are asked to acquire and recall information (Pressley, Heisel, McCormick & Nakamura, in press).

Thus, recall tasks are essentially learning tasks, tasks which require learning information and learning how to learn information. The performance differences on these tasks observed between disabled and non-disabled children may result from differences in learning. Differences in performance between the two groups of children may be eliminated or substantially reduced by instructing disabled children to use task-appropriate strategies for learning.

The studies reported here have used free recall tasks which permit taxonomic organization: tasks for which organizing items by category and recalling items in categories are efficient learning strategies. There are two of these tasks, a picture study/recall task which has been used to study the acquisition and use of learning strategies by normally developing children (Moely, Olsen, Halwes & Flavell, 1969; Neimark, Slotnick & Ulrich, 1971) and a study recall task in which chidlren are asked to recall facts from prose.

For the picture recall task, each of 24 pictures is reproduced on a separate card 5 cm. square. The pictures can be grouped into four categories (for example, food, toys, jobs and transportation). Several equivalent sets of 24 items are available (Cort, 1980; Gelzheiser, 1982).

The examiner proceeds through the deck of cards with the child, asking for the names of each picture. Names which are not known are supplied. Children's naming errors (which occur only infrequently) are corrected. The child is told that the task is to memorize the names of the pictures and that he/she will have three minutes to study before being asked to recall the picture names. Children are told that they may use any study procedure which will help them learn and remember the picture names, including moving the pictures. The pictures are placed in front of the child so that no two pictures from the same category are adjacent and the study period begins.

During the study period, the examiner records all observable study behaviors. After three minutes, the cards are covered with a large card board and the child is asked to recall the picture names. Recall is recorded in the exact order in which it is produced. After recall, the final arrangement of the pictures, the arrangement which existed at the close of the study period, is recorded.

Two scores are obtained for each child. The first is a recall score, the number of picture names accurately recalled. The second is a score for organization, sorting the pictures into categories during the study period. Organization, or sorting, is a dichotomous variable. Children either sort all of the pictures into categories or they do not sort at all. Performance is scored "1" if sorting occurs and "0" if it does not occur.

Similar materials and procedures characterize the prose study/ recall task. Two expository passages, one about diamonds and one about pearls, were constructed (Gelzheiser, 1982). Each passage contains 24 facts, grouped by topic into four paragraphs. Each paragraph is preceded by a subheading. The passage about diamonds (adapted from Zim, 1959) will serve as an example.

Diamonds

How diamonds are formed
Diamonds are made from a chemical called carbon. The carbon forms very slowly. Carbon is changed by heat and pressure into crystals. The two kinds of carbon crystals are graphite and diamonds. A little heat and pressure turns carbon into graphite crystals. A great deal of heat and pressure turns carbon into diamond crystals.

Uses of diamonds
Diamonds are useful because they are so hard. In your home, diamonds are used for stereo needles. When they drill for oil, diamonds are used to cut through rocks. Your dentist uses diamond powder when he drills your teeth. Glass is cut using diamond wheels. Wire can be made by pulling metal through a tiny hole in a diamond.

Colors of diamonds
Impurities in some diamonds make them colored. When the color is bright, the diamonds are called fancy. Fancy diamonds can be blue, green or red. Faintly colored diamonds are called off-color diamonds. Off-color diamonds are light yellow or brown. Off-color diamonds are less valuable for jewelry.

The famous Cullinan diamond
The most famous diamond is the Cullinan. This giant

diamond weighed over a pound. The Cullinan was given to
King Edward VII of England. The king had the Cullinan
split into nine large gems and a hundred smaller ones.
These gems are part of the British crown. During World
War II, the British crown gems were hidden in a jar and
buried in a potato field.

The child is given the text and told to follow as it is read to
him/her. The child is then asked to read the text aloud. Errors and
reading time are recorded. The child is then told that the task is
to memorize the facts from the text and that he/she will have ten minutes to study before being asked to recall the facts.

Facts from the story, each printed on a separate strip of card-
board, are placed in front of the child so that no two factors from
the same category are adjacent. Children are told that they may use
any study procedure which will help them learn and remember the facts, including moving the cards on which the facts are printed. During the study period the examiner records all observable study behaviors. After ten minutes, the fact cards are covered and the child is
asked to recall. Recall is recorded in the order in which it is produced. After recall, the final arrangement of the cards, the arrangement which existed at the close of the study period, is recorded.
As with the picture recall task, two scores are obtained for each
child: a recall score and a score for organization during study.

These two tasks conform to the requirements of the "instructional approach". The processing requirements for the picture study/
recall task and age-related changes in the use of the target process
have been documented (Moely et al., 1969; Niemark et al., 1971). The
processing requirements of the prose study/recall tàsk have also be-
en documented (Gelzheiser, Shepherd & Solar, 1982). The use of the
target process with both tasks can be observed during the study period.

SELECTION OF SUBJECTS

Several criteria were used to select subjects for these studies. The learning disabled children had all been classified following procedures used in their respective school districts. From the
pool of children at the appropriate ages classified as learning disabled in each school district, children were selected according to
the following criteria:
  -Full Scale IQ scores between 85 and 125
  -no evidence of primary emotional disturbance (children whose
   records indicated referrals to psychologists or psychiatrists
   were excluded)
  -normal visual acuity (with correction)
  -normal hearing acuity
  -no evidence of seizures, paralysis or any other "hard"

neurological signs
-current placement in a special education program.

The "home" school districts for all subjects (learning disabled and non-disabled) report mean achievement test scores for each grade level at or above the 50th percentile, using national norms. Eighty percent of the subjects came from families where the occupation of the head of the household was rated "manager" or "professional" (U.S. Bureau of the Census, 1981). Ninety percent of the children in the sample were Caucasian, native-born citizens of the United States. English was the native language for all subjects. None of the non-disabled children were receiving any form of special education or related therapy. The ratio of boys to girls in each sample was 4:1. IQ and achievement test scores, as available, are reported separately for each of the three studies.

The Descriptive Study

A descriptive study was conducted to assess the spontaneous study and recall performance of learning disabled and non-disabled children and adolescents on the picture study/recall task. The study addressed three questions:
-How does the recall performance of learning disabled children compare to that of non-disabled children?
-Does the performance of these groups change with age?
-What is the relationship between the observed process used during study and the resultant recall performance in each group?

Subjects

A total of 210 subjects, 30 at each age, from 9 to 15, half classified as learning disabled and half non-disabled, were given the picture recall task. IQ scores were available for 34 of the non-disabled subjects ($\bar{X}$=114.5, SD=9.7) and for 71 of the learning disabled subjects ($\bar{X}$=102, SD=10.8).

Results and Discussions

To describe subject recall, a (2) classification by (7) age two way analysis of variance was computed. The main effect for classification was significant. Learning disabled subjects recalled fewer pictures than non-disabled subjects (LD $\bar{X}$ = 14.1, SD = 3.9; NLD $\bar{X}$ = 15.8; SD = 4.1; F [1,209] = 13.089, p < .001). The interaction between classification and age was non-significant. Figure 1 shows mean recall for each age level and each classification.

A second analysis of variance was computed to assess the effect on recall of organization during the study period. Results of a (2) classification by (2) level of organization two way analysis of variance were: a significant main effect for classification (F[1,209] =

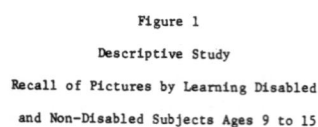

Figure 1

Descriptive Study

Recall of Pictures by Learning Disabled

and Non-Disabled Subjects Ages 9 to 15

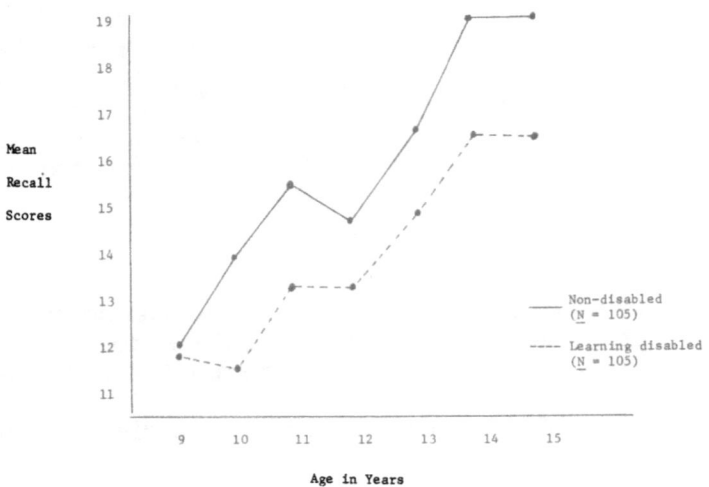

9.69], p < .01), a significant main effect for organization (F[1,209]
= 141.027, p < .001) and a non-significant interaction. The use of
an appropriate strategy during study (sorting the pictures into groups) led to improved recall, and did not have a differential effect
for learning disabled and non-disabled subjects. Figure 2 illustrates the effect of organization on recall for these subjects.

The descriptive study demonstrated that learning disabled subjects exhibited a deficit in recall. This deficit was defined by
comparison of the learning disabled group with a non-disabled group.
Within both groups a relationship between the targeted process of
organization or sorting during study and high recall performance was
observed. The relationship between the target process and recall
performance was tested with an instructional study.

The First Instructional Study:
The Effect of Minimal Instruction on Picture Recall

The first instructional study assessed the effect of instruction in the use of the sorting strategy on the picture recall performance of learning disabled and non-disabled children. A large, representative group of non-disabled subjects were pretested, but not
all of these subjects were included in the instructional phase of

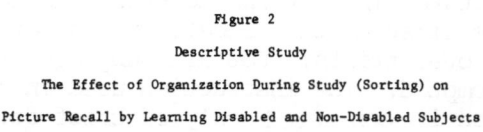

Figure 2

Descriptive Study

The Effect of Organization During Study (Sorting) on

Picture Recall by Learning Disabled and Non-Disabled Subjects

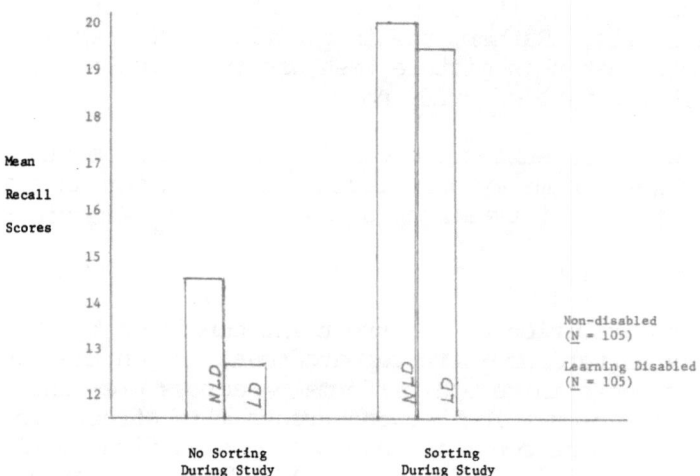

the study. The non-disabled subjects who were included in the study
were selected by "matching" their recall to the recall of the learning disabled subjects. The design in this study was a (2) classification by (2) treatment condition by (2) treatment phase factorial
design.

Subjects

Sixty subjects (30 classified as learning disabled and 30 non-
disabled) participated in this study. The ages of the children were
9-12. Mean IQ for the non-disabled subjects was 114.4 (SD = 9.7)
and for the learning disabled subjects was 103.4 (SD = 9.7). The
mean reading grade equivalent of the non-disabled subjects was 6.5
(SD = 1.8) and for the learning disabled subjects was 3.9 (SD = 1.6).
Mean arithmetic grade eqivalent for the non-disabled subjects was
6.2 (SD = 1.5) and for the learning disabled subjects was 4.6 (SD =
1.8).

Procedure

Subjects were assigned to one of two conditions, practice or
instruction. Children assigned to the practice condition received
6 additional study/recall trials with the pictures. Children

assigned to the instruction condition received brief instruction to organize (sort) the pictures into groups to study and to recall the pictures by group. The first 4 study/recall trials were prompted with the prompts faded over trials. For all subjects, the fifth and sixth trials were unprompted. The instruction used in this study was termed "minimal" because it consisted only of brief directions on how to study and limited opportunity to practice. Because the instruction was so minimal, it is doubtful that its effect was to teach subjects new skills. Rather, the instruction served as an indicator to the subjects that this picture task was one situation that required this particular type of studying.

Retesting of all subjects occured five weeks after intervention. Recall scores were normally distributed, allowing for an evaluation of the effectiveness of treatment using regular parametric statistics.

Results and Discussion

A (2) classification by (2) treatment condition by (2) treatment phase analysis of variance with repeated measures on the last factor assessed differences in recall performance across pre- and post-intervention recall scores. The between groups main effects for classification and treatment condition approached significance (F [1,56] = 3.54, p = .06; F [1,56] = 3.36, p = .07). The within groups main effect for classification was significant (F [1,56] = 37.03, p < .001). The interaction between treatment condition and phase was significant (F = [1,56] = 8.03, p < .01).

There was a significant difference between pretest and posttest scores within the two treatment groups. In this case, the instructional treatment accounts for the significant increase in recall. Both the learning disabled and non-disabled instructed group made significant gains in recall which the practice groups did not. Figure 3 illustrates gains in recall by classification and condition.

To determine if the effect of treatment was greater for the non-disabeld subjects than for the disabled subjects, a Newman-Keuls test of all means pairs was computed using post test mean recall scores. These tests revealed that for each classification the instructed subjects recalled more picture names than the uninstructed subjects (X posttest recall for instructed learning disabled subjects = 14.9, SD = 3.0; X posttest recall for uninstructed (practice) learning disabled subjects = 12.9, SD = p < .05; X posttest recall for instructed non-disabled subjects = 16.9, SD = 3.0; X posttest recall for uninstructed (practice) non-disabled subjects = 14.1, SD = 3.9, p < .01). The recall of the instructed non-disabled subjects was superior to that of the instructed learning disabled subjects (p < .05).

The improvement in recall in the instructed groups coincided

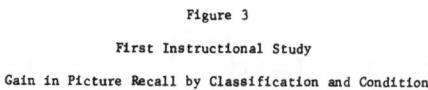

Figure 3

First Instructional Study

Gain in Picture Recall by Classification and Condition

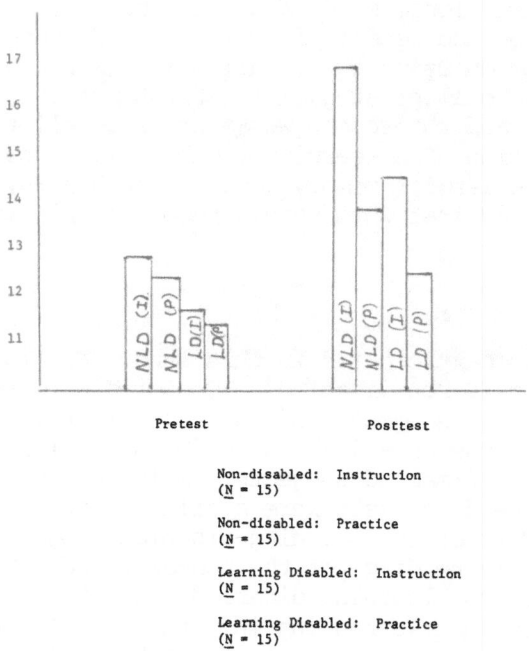

Non-disabled: Instruction
(N = 15)

Non-disabled: Practice
(N = 15)

Learning Disabled: Instruction
(N = 15)

Learning Disabled: Practice
(N = 15)

with retained use of the sorting strategy five weeks after intervention. Twelve of the 15 instructed learning disabled subjects sorted to study at posttest, while only two of the learning disabled subjects in the practice condition used this strategy. Ten instructed non-disabled subjects used this strategy, while only 4 of the practice condition non-disabled subjects sorted.

It would appear that the relationship between organized study and good recall was an important one. Five weeks after intervention, the effects of instruction were still evident in changes in the way the instructed children studied and in improved recall. Both learning disabled and non-disabled children benefited from the instruction and those benefits were maintained over time.

The non-disabled children benefited more from the instruction than the learning disabled children, however. This suggests that other factors besides the target process (sorting) were involved in the performance of the learning disabled children. Once again we turn to instruction to seek a better description of the differences in learning between learning disabled and non-disabled children.

The Second Instructional Study:
The Effect of Extensive Intervention on Picture and Prose Recall

A second instructional study assessed the effect of more extensive intervention on the recall of twelve and thirteen year old learning disabled children using two recall measures which required the use of an organizational strategy. The first measure was the picture study recall task, and the second was a prose recall task. The study addressed the question: Can learning disabled subjects be taught about learning strategies for memory tasks in such a way that they perform well both on the instructed task and on an uninstructed but related memory task?

Subjects

Sixty children participated in this study, 40 classified as learning disabled and 20 non-disabled. IQ scores were available for 18 of the non-disabled subjects and 35 of the learning disabled subjects. Mean IQ for the non-disabled subjects was 115.3 (SD = 8.6) and for the learning disabled subjects was 103.6 (SD = 9.6). Scores from standardized reading tests were available for 15 of the non-disabled subjects and 28 of the learning disabled subjects. The mean percentile ranking in reading for the non-disabled subjects was 74.0 (SD = 25.3) and for the learning disabled subjects was 38.7 (SD = 27.3). The mean percentile ranking in math for the non-disabled subjects for whom scores were available (15 subjects) was 65.1 (SD = 26.8) and for the learning disabled subjects (36 subjects) was 41.7 (SD = 25.2).

Procedure

The design of the study included an instructed learning disabled group, and two no-treatment control groups, one learning disabled and one non-disabled. This design was adopted in anticipation of the high level of performance of the non-disabled group, relative to both ceiling performance for the task, and the performance of the learning disabled subjects. Because, with few exceptions, the non-disabled subjects were performing so well that the demonstration of improvement due to instruction was prohibited by the ceiling effect, no instruction was provided to the non-disabled subjects.

The instruction taught subjects an appropriate way to study for the simpler picture recall task, and did not include any direct statement of how to study for the prose recall task. Children practiced using the instructed study rules with the picture task, but did not practice with the prose task. The instruction was based on a direct instructional model (Becker & Carnine, 1981) and included what has been termed specific generalization training (Brown, 1978). Instruction was provided in a series of 5 lessons spread over a three-week period. Posttesting on the picture recall task and the prose recall task occurred 2 to 3 days after the instructional session.

This intervention was termed extensive through comparison with the thoroughness of instruction provided in generalization studies previously reported (Borkowski & Cavanaugh, 1979). The "minimal instruction" described in Study I illustrates the distinction. Instruction in that study consisted of 5 minutes spent telling the children to use the study rules followed by 6 study/recall trials. The "extensive instruction" in this study included one hour of instruction in when to use the study rules, a rationale for the use of these rules, and feedback on subjects' improved recall due to the use of these rules. Sixteen study/recall trials were included.

Results and Discussion

A 3(treatment condition) by 2 (treatment phase) analysis of variance was computed for picture recall. The between groups main effect for condition was significant (F [2,57] = 3.20, p < .05) and the within groups effect was also significant (F [1,57] = 28.78, p < .001). The interaction between treatment condition and phase effect was significant ([2,57] = 8.58, p < .001).

A Newman-Keuls test of all means pairs was computed. At pretest, the two learning disabled groups did not differ in recall (control group $\overline{X}$ = 16.75, SD = 5.14; instructed group $\overline{X}$ = 15.75, SD = 4.20). Both groups recalled significantly fewer pictures than the non-disabled group at pretest (non-disabled $\overline{X}$ = 19.20, SD = 2.5, p < .05).

At posttest, the instructed learning disabled subjects recalled more pictures than the learning disabled control group (instructed group $\overline{X}$ = 20.65, SD = 3.61; control group $\overline{X}$ = 17.30, SD = 5.51, p < .01). The instructed learning disabled subjects did not differ in recall from the non-disabled control group (non-disabled $\overline{X}$ = 20.30, SD = 3.08). The learning disabled control group continued to recall significantly fewer pictures than the non-disabled group (p < .01). The posttest recall of pictures by the instructed learning disabled subjects was significantly greater than their pretest performance (P < .01). The two no-treatment control groups did not show posttest recall which differed significantly from their pretest recall.

In this study direct and extensive instruction with the picture task produced significant gains in recall by learning disabled subjects. At posttest, these instructed subjects did not show á performance deficit relative to a non-disabled control group who had not received instruction because of their near ceiling level performance.

It is important to be cautious at this point; we have no way of establishing that the mental processing of the learning disabled children instructed to sort was identical to that of the non-disabled children who were spontaneous sorters. What we can conclude is that
instructed performance of the learning disabled children is a reasonable approximation of the spontaneous performance of non-disabled
children in that it produces comparable recall.

The major question addressed in this study was whether learning
disabled subjects would use the instructed sorting strategy with the
uninstructed, but related, transfer task. Would instruction in the
importance of sorting to study with the pictures result in an increase in the number of children who sorted to study with the prose recall task?

At pretest on the prose task, nine of the non-disabled subjects
sorted to study, while five of the learning disabled subjects in the
control group sorted, and three in the instructed group sorted. At
posttest, without any instruction, the non-disabled group gained five additional sorters, while the learning disabled control group gained only one. In contrast, the instruction that learning disabled
subjects received in how to study a related task produced a gain of
eleven sorters. Because of the impressive transfer of use of the
sorting strategy by the instructed learning disabled subjects, the
number of instructed subjects and non-disabled subjects sorting at
posttest was identical (70 percent).

The prose recall data were analyzed in a fashion similar to the
picture recall data. Recall scores were normally distributed, allowing for an evaluation of the effectiveness of treatment using regular parametric statistics. A repeated measures analysis of variance
assessed the differences in recall performance both between the three groups and within groups across the pre- and post-intervention
measures. Significant differences between the three treatment groups were observed (F $[2,57]$ = 12.46, p < .01) and the within groups
test was significant (F $[1,57]$ = 31.21, p < .001). The interaction
was not significant. A series of pairwise comparisons of pretest
and posttest performance were computed.

At pretest, the two groups of learning disabled subjects did
not differ from each other in recall (control $\overline{X}$ = 13.50, SD = 3.76;
instructed $\overline{X}$ = 13.65, SD = 3.00). Both groups of learning disabled
subjects recalled fewer facts than the non-disabled subjects (non-
disabled $\overline{X}$ = 18.35, SD = 2.91, p < .01).

At posttest, the instructed learning disabled subjects recalled more facts than the learning disabled control subjects (instruc-
ted $\overline{X}$ = 17.85, SD = 3.36; control $\overline{X}$ = 15.45, SD = 4.49, p < .01).
However, the non-disabled subjects still recalled more facts than
the instructed learning disabled subjects (non-disabled $\overline{X}$ = 20.05,

SD = 3.48, $\underline{p}$ < .05) and the learning disabled control subjects ($\underline{p}$ < .01).

In comparing pretest and posttest performance, the instructed learning disabled subjects showed significant gain ($\underline{p}$ < .01), as did the non-disabled subjects ($\underline{p}$ < .05). The learning disabled control subjects' posttest performance did not differ significantly from their pretest performance.

This study thus demonstrated that with extensive intervention, learning disabled subjects could be taught to use a strategy that would improve the level of their recall performance on the instructed task. This improved recall performance did not differ from the recall of an uninstructed, but high performing group of non-disabled subjects. The use of that strategy was observed to transfer to an uninstructed but related task. The transfer of the strategy produced improved recall relative to the learning disabled control subjects, but did not raise their level of recall to that of the non-disabled subjects.

SUMMARY

Findings from these studies add to existing evidence of memory deficits on recall tasks among children described as learning disabled. Deficits were observed in the children's uninstructed performance on the picture recall task and the prose recall task.

The nature of these deficits was described by the use of the instructional method. The use of this method has shown that the recall performance of learning disabled children is not fixed or immutable. Instruction in how to study effectively produces improved recall. Thus, it would appear that the initial poor recall of learning disabled children can be explained in terms of how they learn. Without direct instruction, learning disabled children do not learn to study well. The continued poor performance of the uninstructed learning disabled group adds support to the suggestion that these children do not learn the relationship between organization and recall on their own. This hypothesis is also strengthened by the durability of the effects of instruction: instructed learning disabled subjects showed improved recall 5 weeks after intervention.

Use of the instructional method has shown that learning disabled and non-disabled children matched for pretest recall did not respond equally well to minimal instruction. Although the extent of the use of the sorting strategy was equivalent in the two groups, it did not produce equivalent recall performance. This finding suggests that learning disabled children may need more practice to master a skill than non-disabled children and that mastery influences the extent to which the sorting strategy affects recall. Findings from the second instructional study support this interpretation.

The second instructional study supports the hypothesized relationship between instruction and strategy use and recall performance.
After extensive direct instruction with the picture recall task, learning disabled children showed improved recall on both the instructed picture recall task and an uninstructed task with similar processing requirements, the prose recall task. The learning disabled children who had received instruction did not differ in recall from the
uninstructed, near ceiling level performance of the non-disabled children on the picture recall task; however, their recall of facts on
the prose task was less than that of the non-disabled subjects. Again, the relatively poor recall relative to the non-disabled children
coincident with equivalent strategy use, suggests that the non-disabled children were using the strategy more effectively than the learning disabled children.

Findings from these studies suggest that differences between learning disabled and non-disabled children on recall tasks can be reduced by instruction, and that learning disabled children make greater improvement when they receive extensive rather than minimal instruction. The ability to use the strategy for the instructed task
(pictures) with the same effectiveness as the non-disabled children
and to transfer the strategy to an uninstructed task (prose) are the
benefits of extensive instruction for learning disabled chidlren.

CONCLUSION

The use of the instructional method is not meant to restrict
the description of differences in the memory skills of learning disabled and non-disabled children to learned differences. These two
groups of children may also differ in some fixed or fundamental ways. However, the instructional method does remind us that while we
may conceive of memory as a fixed and stable process which underlies
the learning of complex skills, in fact memory performance is alter-
able and interacts with experience in complex ways. Our data suggest that one reasonable way to separate what is fixed from what is
learned is to observe changes which occur after instruction.

Instructional research with learning disabled children has a
much broader role to play than demonstrating which remedial methods
are most effective. A guiding hypothesis in research with learning
disabled children is that they differ from non-disabled children in
their ability to learn. Our data lend support to that hypothesis.
In fact, the data suggest that even within a group of children called learning disabled, there will be differences in response to instruction which suggest significant differences in learning. Our data
also suggest that the type of instruction used defined the extent
of learning.

It is only by instructing learning disabled children that we
can observe such differences. Our use of the instructional method

suggests that we must go beyond a fixed and static view of what a
learning disabled child knows and does not know. We must also observe how this child comes to know more, in order to describe the learning disability.

REFERENCES

Becker, W. C. & Carnine, D. W. Direct instruction: A behavior theory
    model for comprehensive educational intervention with the disad-
    vantaged. In S. W. Bijou & R. Ruiz (Eds.), Behavior modificati-
    on: Contribution to education. Hillsdale, NJ: Lawrence Erlbaum,
    1981.
Belmont, J. M. & Butterfield, E. C. The instructional approach to
    developmental cognitive research. In R. V. Kail & J. W. Hagen
    (Eds.), Perspectives on the development of memory and cognition.
    Hillsdale, NJ: Lawrence Erlbaum, 1977.
Borkowski, J. G. & Cavanaugh, J. C. Maintenance and generalization
    of skills and strategies by the retarded. In N. R. Ellis (Ed.),
    Handbook of mental deficiency: Psychological theory and resear-
    ch (2nd Ed.). Hillsdale, NJ: Lawrence Erlbaum, 1979.
Brown, A. L. Knowing when, where and how to remember: A problem of
    metacognition. In R. Glaser (Ed.), Advances in instructional
    psychology (Vol. 1). Hillsdale, NJ: Lawrence Erlbaum, 1978.
Brown, A. L. Learning and development: The problems of compatibili-
    ty, access and induction. Human Decelopment, 1982, 25, 89-115.
Bryan, J. H. Social behaviors of learning disabled children. In
    J. Gottlieb & S. S. Strichart (Eds.), Developmental theory and
    research in learning disabilities. Baltimore: University Park
    Press, 1981.
Cort, R. Effects of training on recall and use of organizational
    strategies by learning disabled and non-disabled youngsters.
    Unpublished doctoral dissertation, Teachers College, Columbia
    University, 1980.
Critchley, M. The dyslexic child. London: William Heinemann Medi-
    cal Books, Limited, 1978.
Fleischner, J. E., Garnett, K. & Shepherd, M. J. Proficiency in ar-
    ithmetic basic fact computation of learning disabled and non-
    disabled children. Focus on Learning Problems in Mathematics,
    1982, 4, 47-56.
Gelzheiser, L. M. The effects of direct instruction on learning
    disabled children's ability to generalize study behaviors for
    deliberate memory tasks. Unpublished doctoral dissertation,
    Teachers College, Columbia University, 1982.
Gelzheiser, L. M., Shepherd, M. J. & Solar, R. A. Progress report.
    New York: Institute for the Study of Learning Disabilities,
    Teachers College, Columbia University, January 1982.
Kail, R. The development of memory in children. San Francisco:
    W. H. Freeman & Company, 1979.

Kirk, S. A. Behavioral diagnosis and remediation of learning disab-
    ilities. Proceedings of the annual meeting of the Conference
    on Exploration into the Problems of the Perceptually Handica-
    pped Child (Vol 1), 1963.
Moely, B. E., Olson, F. A., Halwes, T. G. & Flavell, J. H. Produc-
    tion deficiency in young children's clustered recall. Develop-
    mental Psychology, 1969, 1, 26-34.
Neimark, E., Slotnick, N. S. & Ulrich, T. Development of memoriza-
    tion strategies. Developmental Psychology, 1971, 5, 427-432.
Pressley, M., Heisel, B. E., McCormick, C. G. & Nakamura, G. V.
    Memory strategy instruction with chidlren. In C. J. Brainerd
    & M. Pressley (Eds.), Progress in cognitive development resear-
    ch (Vol. 2), Verbal processes in children. New York: Springer-
    Verlag, in press.
Torgesen, J. K. The study of short-term memory in learning disabled
    children: goals, methods and conclusions. In K. Gadow & I. Ba-
    ilar (Eds.), Advances in learning and behavioral disabilities
    (Vol. 1), Greenwich, CT: JAI Press, 1982.
U. S. Bureau of the Census. Household and family characteristics:
    March 1980 (Table 7). In Current Population Reports (Series
    p-20, wo. 366). Washington,D. C. : U. S. Government Printing
    Office, 1981.
Zim, H. S. Diamonds. New York: William Morrow, 1959.

DYSLEXIA - DIAGNOSIS AND TREATMENT
FROM THE PERSPECTIVE OF A READING SPECIALIST

Geraldine Burd
Community College of Philadelphia
Philadelphia, Pennsylvania

What happens in actual remedial instruction with dyslexics has
important implications for the evaluating neuropsychologist, and communication between the educator and the clinical evaluator can be
useful in diagnosing and making recommendations for follow-up from
neurological, psychological, and educational data. Using a case study with a neuropsychological evaluation report and spelling tests,
this paper contrasts the perspectives of the reading teacher and neuropsychologist. Unlike the clinical evaluator, the reading specialist sees the patient over a long period of time in treatment and
becomes familiar with problems and progress in a way the single-se-
ssion evaluator cannot.

Also demonstrated is the diagnostic value of adding a writing
sample and standardized spelling test to the standard test battery.
These tests may be readily used to preliminarily diagnose dyslexia,
identify subtypes, reveal student strengths and weaknesses, and point out directions for patterning instruction and treatment.

Further, this paper explains what the diagnosing clinician should know about what the reading specialist can achieve, and, in particular, which kinds of problems make patients good candidates for
the phonic-based Orton-Gillingham method of remediation. It demonstrates the effectiveness of Orton-Gillingham in treating one 8-year-
old's reading and spelling problems, as well as her small motor and
emotional problems.

CASE STUDY

A. History
    Lara, a left-handed third grader, was taken by her parents,

both college English professors, for a neuropsychological evaluation to assess her cognitive strengths and weaknesses, to determine whether neurologic factors were affecting her school performance, and to assist in educational planning. Eight years and ten months old at the time, she had already repeated a grade (first) yet still had difficulty keeping up with her peers and completing required schoolwork. There was no history of learning disabilities in the family, developmental milestones were accomplished within normal limits, but blood incompatibility necessitated a transfusion shortly after birth.

Lara's WPPSI, administered upon entering school at age 5 years 5 months, gave a Full Scale IQ of 124 (Verbal IQ = 126; Performance IQ = 116), with indications of relative visual-motor integrative weakness.

B.   Neuropsychological Assessment

Procedures administered were:

Halstead-Reitan Neuropsychological Test Battery
Wechsler Intelligence Scale for Children-Revised (WISC - R)
Peabody Picture Vocabulary Test (PPVT, FORM A)
Raven's Coloured Progressive Matrices
Bender Gestalt Test (with recall)
Beery-Buktenica Developmental Test of Visual-Motor Integration (VMI)
Symbol Digit Modalities Test (written and oral versions)
Visual Aural Digit Span Test (VADS)
Detroit Tests of Learning Aptitude (selected memory subtests)
Grooved Pegboard
Rey Auditory-Verbal Learning Test
Wide Range Achievement Test (WRAT)

To summarize the results (a full statistical summary is contained in Appendix A), the testing revealed trouble on the Digit Span, in Arithmetic, and deficits in General Knowledge, with some tracking and fine motor problems as well. Reading recognition on the WRAT gave a 4.0 grade equivalent, although word attack skills showed poor development. Her PIAT reading comprehension grade equivalent was 2.8. WRAT spelling was 3.3 grade level, and WRAT Arithmetic skills were at the 2.7 grade level. Throughout testing, the evaluator noted that Lara was highly distractable and had difficulty sustaining attention on tasks as they proceeded. This was interpreted as most likely due to anxiety and lack of self-confidence.

Strengths were found on measures of expressive and receptive word knowledge, verbal abstract reasoning, auditory discrimination, visual, tactile, and spatial recall.

The WISC-R Full Scale IQ of 99 (Verbal IQ of 101; Performance IQ of 96) was significantly lower than previous intelligence tests

(WPPSI Full Scale IQ of 124; Verbal IQ of126; Performance IQ of 116) and was primarily explained by performance anxiety.

Considerable intersubtest scatter was noted, and it was hypothesized that social-emotional factors interfered to give these inconsistencies. Her parents were told that she was probably not dyslexic, and special instruction for her reading and spelling problems was not recommended.

What was recommended, on the basis of these results, was for Lara to remain in a regular educational grouping and take advantage of whatever reading and math support services the school offered in order "to provide her with individual attention, to reinforce classroom learning, and to provide emotional support." Family counselling and assessment of her emotional problems were also suggested.

C. Reading Specialist's Evaluation and Treatment

The family rejected the suggestion of counselling, decided to continue mainstreaming Lara, as recommended, but sought additional private help by a specialist in learning disabilities for Lara's spelling and reading difficulties.

When first seen, Lara was evaluated by the reading specialist using direct diagnosis through analysis of reading and spelling performance. The above quantitative findings were more or less confirmed. Lara did spell and read below her age or grade level and did have attentional problems.

Reading comprehension was on grade level, and Gray Oral Reading gave a 3.5 grade equivalent score, although on the Iota Test of words in isolation Lara scored at Grade 2 and showed little word-attack skill. She either knew the words on sight or produced the sound of the first letter or two and guessed at the rest. Her spelling on both the Ayres-Buckingham Standardized Spelling Test and on the New Stanford Achievement Test (sentence dictation) placed Lara at a 2.4-2.5 grade level, respectively, slightly below her school grade, but considering her age-peers were in 4th grade and her family background and socio-economic level, the performance was considerably below grade level.

SIGNS OF DYSLEXIA

More dramatic, however, and more revealing of what reading specialists would consider dyslexia, were the less quantifiable findings. Lara's handwriting was immature, closer to that of a first-grader than to a child who should have been in 4th grade. Lower-case words were printed in large letters that took up two lines rather than one, and her efforts at writing were extremely labored. She was exhausted by the time she had written twenty primary words and

had to take a break before continuing. On the sentence dictation,
Lara could not keep sentences lined up one below the other in a margin and she showed, along with reversals (ꓤfor 'c'; 'd' for 'b'),
visual errors, phonetic errors, and no familiarity with the conventions of capitalization. Again, the writing was difficult and time-
consuming.

An analysis of the kinds of errors Lara made, along with her
performance style, indicated that she was not simply a child of average intelligence performing slightly below grade level. Her 'problems were severe and her patterns of reading and spelling atypical.
These are signs of dyslexia that cannot be seen from the neuropsychological test battery - only from hearing her read and watching her
spell, then analyzing the error patterns.

The figures 1 and 2 show Lara's initial tests before beginning
one-hour weekly instruction for the next seven and a half months.

ANALYSIS OF SPELLING TESTS

Lara's initial tests reveal, according to Boder's system of sub-
classification, that she is a dysphonetic and dyseidetic dyslexic
(Boder and Jarrico, 1982).

Dysphonetic spellers respond to words "globally", spelling to
try to duplicate the visual configuration of their sight vocabulary.
Lara's 'belog' for 'belong', 'boll' for 'ball', 'wha' for 'way' (probably recalling part of the gestalt of the word 'what' here), 'bla-
ch' for 'black', 'thee' for 'three', 'tab' for 'took', 'wome' for
'women', 'you' for 'yellow'. 'roder' for 'rubber', and 'chs' for
'church' - all patterns approximating the way the word looks, but
not phonetically spelled - are dysphonetic spellings. These are
patterns of spelling not found in normal readers and spellers, only
in dyslexics (Boder and Jarrico, 1982).

The other pattern alerting a reading specialist to the presence
of dyslexia is dyseidetic spelling, spelling that uses a process of
sounding out words "as if they were being encountered for the first
time". Lara's remaining errors were of this variety. These errors
are phonetic and intelligible, but clearly show a deficit in sight
vocabulary and lack of internalization of phonic rules on what should be familiar words and patterns by third grade. Lara's 'dor' for
'door', 'soot' for 'suit', 'tel' for 'tell', 'cach' for 'catch',
'aplss' for 'apples', 'bushis' for 'bushes', and 'ahad' for 'ahead'
are all examples of dyseidetic spelling. Again, these are not the
kinds of errors typically found in normal third and fourth grade
readers and spellers. (Lara's reading miscue patterns were similar;
she usually got the sound of the first one or two letters of a word
and guessed at the rest, using some configurational clues. However,
this paper focusses on the more demonstrable errors of spelling

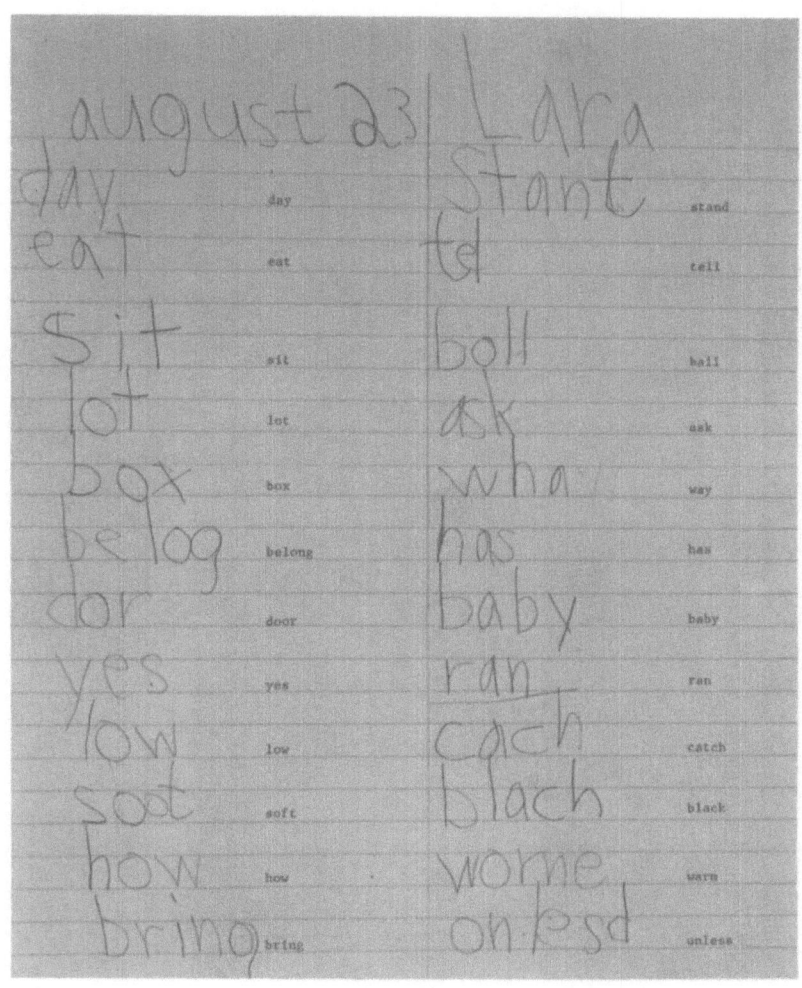

FIGURE 1.   Lara's initial Ayres-Buckingham Spelling Test.   Grade
equivalent score of 2.4

G. Burd

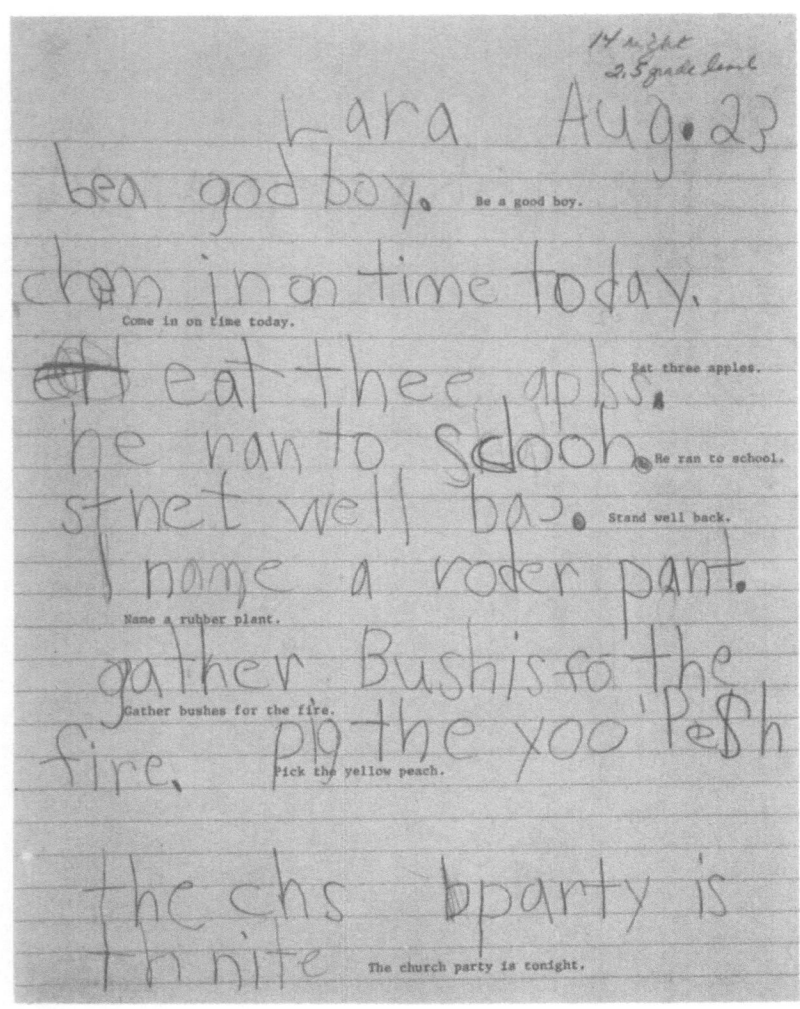

FIGURE 2. Lara's initial New Stanford Achievement Sentence
Dictation Test. Grade equivalent score of 2.5.

rather than addressing reading).

Using these test results and the most widely-accepted definition of dyslexia, "A disorder in children who, despite conventional class-room experience, fail to attain the language skills of reading, wri-ting, and spelling commensurate with their intentional abilities", the reading specialist could readily diagnose the problem and begin appropriate treatment.

ORTON-GILLINGHAM REMEDIAL WORK WITH LARA

Remedial work was begun using the Orton-Gillingham method, a multi-sensory approach that emphasizes phonic instruction through a system of linguistic rules and patterns for spelling and word attack. (It thus adds to the Fernald method of word tracing and its attenti-on to visual configurations another channel of isntruction, the inte-llectual use of logic, often a strength of dyslexics).

The Orton-Gillingham method teaches the 48 English phonemes and the graphemes which represent them and presents rules governing the-ir use in a systematic, structured system. The main teaching prin-ciple in the method is to point out the regularities of English spe-lling. Normal spellers seem to subconsciously absorb these regula-rities, while dyslexics need them pointed out. Instruction at the lowest level begins with teaching letter-sound correspondence of co-nsonants and vowels, especially of the short vowels which most ale-xics (people who have trouble reading and spelling) are unsure of. Beyond that, Orton-Gillingham shows, from the beginning, that, for example, when there is a short vowel sound in English, something di-fferent happens to the spelling. After a short vowel, for instance, the 'ch' sound is spelled 'tch' (which would correct Lara's 'cach'), after a short vowel a 'k' sound is spelled 'ck', (Lara's 'bac'), after a short vowel, 'l's, 'f's, 's's, and 'z's at the end of one-syllable words must be doubled (Lara's 'tel'), as do consonants in multi-syllable words. The rules are structured and presented in or-der of sophistication. At the upper end, for example, Lara was tau-ght that "tion", at the end of a word is the first choice for the "shun" sound; "sion" is used primarily when the root word ends in 's' as in 'tension' and 'television'.

LARA - SEVEN AND A HALF MONTHS AFTER INSTRUCTION BEGAN

Lara learned the rules very quickly (more the behavior of a child with an IQ of 124 than 99), and was able to apply them easily. What seems like a complicated system for normal spellers who are not consciously aware of these patterns is readily absorbed by the dy-slexic child or adult, perhaps because motivation and need is grea-ter and because they see the logic in tasks previously perceived as chaotic. After years of frustration with attempts to spell, some-thing none of the other children seem to have, they now feel some confidence for the first time.

Lara's spelling improvement is most significant. On the Ayres-
Buckingham she gained more than two grade levels, from 2.4 to 4.8.
She showed similar gains on the New Stanford Sentence Dictation, fr-
om 2.5 to 4.4 grade level.

The kinds of errors Lara was making after seven and a half months are again important to note, and these too are periodically analyzed by the reading specialist to assess progress and shape future
instruction (see figures 3 and 4).

Lara's second spelling tests are almost completely free of dyseidetic errors. She has learned the phonetic concepts and usually
spells phonetically now. 'Stanned' for 'stand' is an understable
error and shows she needs some grammatical instruction to choose between homophonic spellings. (It is also encouraging to see her use
of the double 'n' to keep the 'a' in that word short). 'Watch' is
spelled 'wach' but this confusion is probably due to the strange so-
und of the vowel there. (She probably couldn't identify it as a short 'a' but had some sense of the word's visual configuration). That word has to be taught, along with other nonphonetic words, like
her 'clouthing' as a sight word, using Fernald techniques. Note the
other word in the same pattern, 'catch', is now spelled correctly.
'Ankul' is also a phonetic spelling of a nonphonetic word, and the
rules for spelling that one had not yet been taught (consonant - le
as the first choice for the 'ul' sound at the end of a word).

On the New Stanford sentences, too, the pre- and post-testing
differences are remarkable and Lara's spelling is now nearly completely phonetic and rule-structured here as well. It is clear that
Lara by this time has a clear sense of the way English spelling normally works. 'Ahed' for 'ahead', 'helth' for 'health', 'awfir' for
'offer', 'odjechtion,' for 'objection', 'jujj' for 'judge', 'avoied'
for 'avoid', and 'merchunt' for 'merchant' are all phonetically spelled using patterns not yet taught, but all are fairly readable and
logical spellings that reveal which additional rules she needs to be
taught, and that some words may need to be taught as sight words.
The overall sense, now, is of a child who can spell, who has changed
her conception of what spelling requires. (In reading, word attack
improved similarly).

Equally striking and another factor most likely to be missed
even if further neuropsychological testing were done, are the changes in handwriting and coordination.

Lara, during the months of instruction, gradually became more
comfortable holding her pencil and with the physical act of writing.

Her handwriting, too, is markedly improved, despite the fact

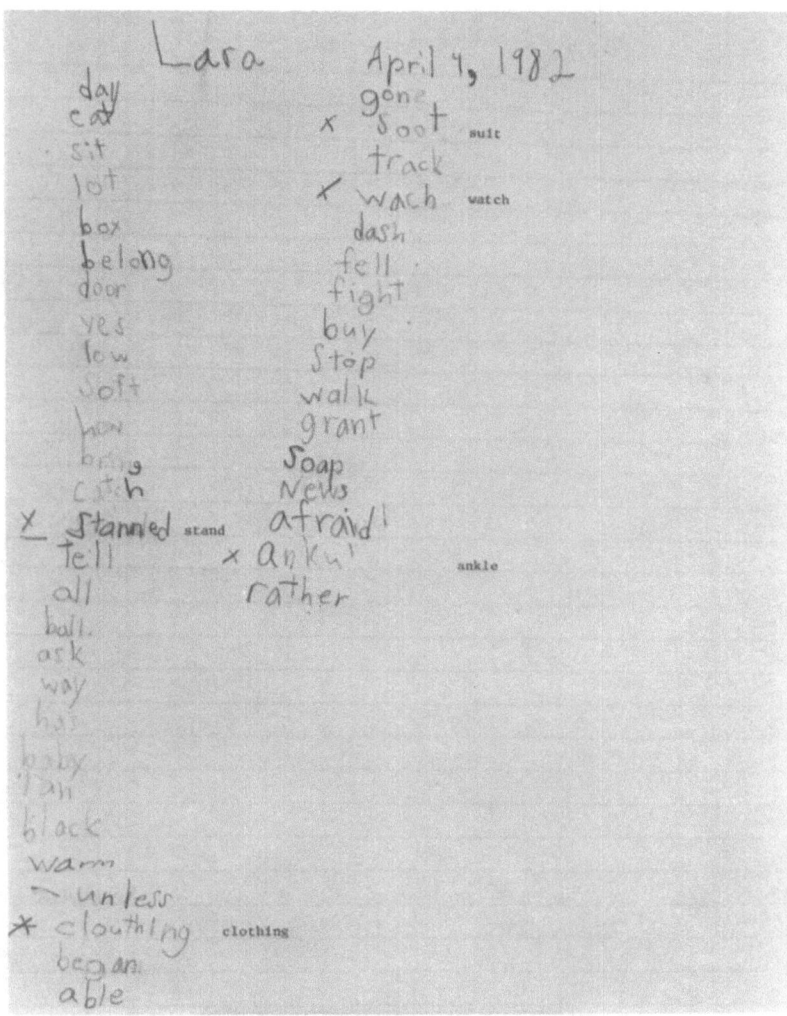

FIGURE 3. Lara's Ayres-Buckingham Spelling Test 7½ months after
           beginning instruction. Grade equivalent score of 4.8.

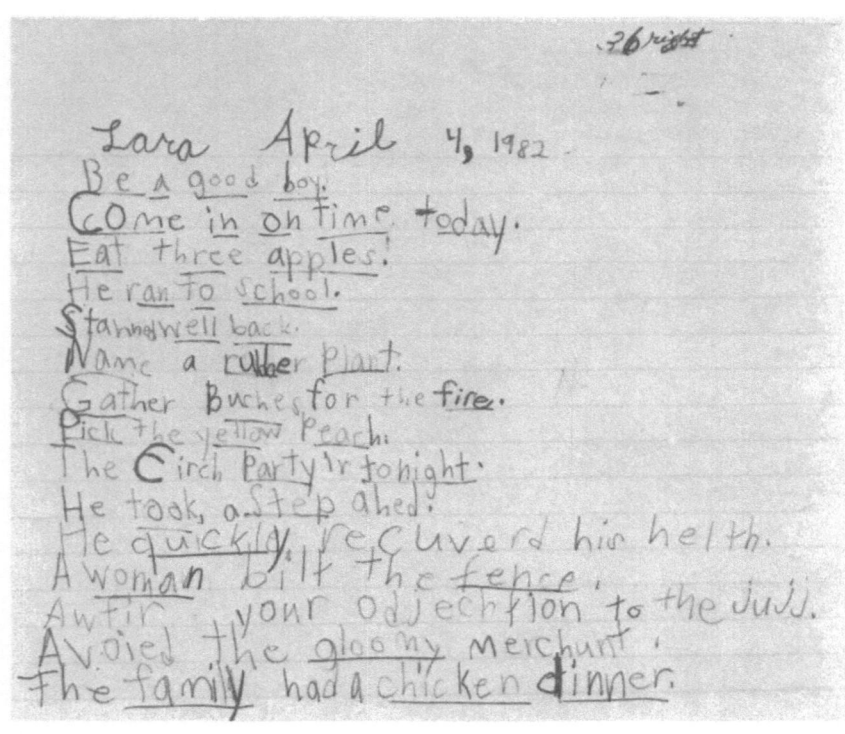

FIGURE   4.   Lara's New Stanford Achievement Sentence Dictation Test
              after 7½ months of instruction.   Grade equivalent score
              of 4.4.

that no handwriting instruction was given; the reading specialist
focused only on reading and spelling deficits. After 7 months of
work, Lara wrote with relative ease and was able, without any direction, to write within the confines of standardly ruled and margined
paper. Although not effortless, her writing was more automatic, less labored, less time-consuming, and capitalization and punctuation
conformed to the conventions.

This kind of spontaneous handwriting improvement is something
Orton-Gillingham teachers typically report. Arlene Sonday, a prominent teacher in Minneapolis, explains it as resulting from the reduction in the number of tasks the dyslexic child has to attend closely to once she has learned to spell by logical phonetic rules. If
a child uses a great deal of energy to try to recall the spelling of
each word, knowing the likelihood of misspelling it is high, she has
little resources to attend to the distracting task of forming letters. After the student learns a logical approach to spelling and is
more certain of that aspect of writing, she is freed to look more
closely at the other elements, namely the appearance of her work.
This hypothesis accounts for the change in handwriting and in capitalization and punctuation, skills that were also never taught in
tutoring sessions. (One might argue that these were skills taught
in school, but they no doubt were taught before this year as well
and were not internalized. The question of why Lara could absorb
these correctly at <u>this</u> point would still need to be addressed, and
gaining some degree of mastery over spelling so that she can go on
to other concerns might explain Lara's improvement).

Her emotional problems also decreased. Lara's parents and teacher reported less anxiety about schoolwork. In tutoring sessions,
Lara was far less distractable as instruction progressed, far more
confident about her ability to spell and read, less anxious about
attacking new words. Again, it is hypothesized that when a child
feels more in control of her academic environment, she becomes less
anxious. Improvement in skills directly affects feelings of self-
worth, and dyslexic children almost inevitably have to question their own intelligence when they see themselves functioning so much below their peers. Teaching them to spell with some degree of preci-
sion is psychologically therapeutic.

Of course, there is more to reading and writing than coding and
encoding, and it is not recommended that Orton-Gillingham be the only type of reading instruction the student receives. However, it
is a valuable component of the dyslexic's total program. The child
who cannot read the words on a page cannot go on to the more sophisticated tasks of comprehension.

CONCLUSIONS

A wealth of information is available from an analysis of reading

and spelling tests, not just from the scores - in both diagnosing
dyslexia and in treating it. The neuropsychologist serves an important function in determing what, if any, neurological and psychological problems are interfering with a subject's efforts to learn to
read and spell, but to get a fuller sense of the disability in these
areas, reading and spelling should be observed more directly and more closely.

There are demonstrably effective techniques to teach the dyseidetic and dysphonetic speller - but they cannot be helped within the
confines of traditional classroom instruction alone. Nor can they
be helped unless the diagnostician is aware of the problem and can
recommend appropriate remediation. The help of a reading specialist,
from the initial evaluation, would be most useful here.

It is true, as the neuropsychological report pointed out, that
Lara had emotional problems, but instead of seeing them as the cause
of her reading and spelling problems, the reading specialist views
them as one of the results of inadequate skills. Improvement of these skills is often more beneficial than counseling.

Dyslexic children almost certainly develop emotional problems,
but they are not necessarily responsive to traditional psychological
counseling or therapy. Providing situations where the dyslexic can
feel and actually be successful makes the child feel more normal.
When Lara could see that her logical effort at spelling, reading,
and thinking could put her in closer proximity to her peers' skills,
she felt better about herself. Reducing the handicap is not through
instruction alone; in many cases counseling is also needed. What I
am advocating is that the diagnosis of dyslexia be made as quickly
and accurately as possible, through the most direct means, and that
the clinical evaluator be aware of what can be done to improve reading and spelling so that he can make more valuable recommendations
to the patient. Traditionally, the clinical evaluator and reading
specialist have had little communication. A closer relationship is
needed.

REFERENCES

Boder, E., and Jarrico, S. Boder test of reading - spelling patterns.
    New York : Grune and Stratton, 1982.

APPENDIX A

Neuropsychological Report Summary Sheet

```
TRAILS A      22"                    WISC-R              CATEGORY - CHILD
TRAILS B     214"            VIQ    101                    INTERMEDIATE   X
TRAILS TOTAL 236"            PIQ     96              1  4  2  2  3 34  4 17  5 24
                             F-S IQ  99                              6  11
SENSORY TEST                 VIS                          TOTAL  42 errors
TACT:  L O R O  B:L 4 R O    PMS
AUD:   L O R O  B:L O R O    TOT WS                   TPT - 6 blocks - CHILD
VIS:   L O R O  B:L O R O    INF      8               LH 3.0      TIME 7.15  Total
                             SIMIL   13               RH 1.7      MEM  5
F. AGNOSIA:  L  O R (1)      ARITH    7               BH 2.45     LOC  5
                             VOCAB (106) 11
F. SYMBOL WRITING:  L O R O  COMP    12               SEASHORE RHYTHM  7 errors
                             DIGIT SP  7
TACT FORM:                   P COMP  10               SPEECH PERCEP   12 errors
ERRORS:  L  1    R  0        P ARR   11
TIME:    L 24,30 R 30.6      BL DES  10               TAPPING: LH 30    RH 32
                             OBJ ASSEM 10          WRAT      GEq.   %ile   S.S
VISUAL FIELDS:               CODING   7           R        4.0     55    102
    Unremarkable            MAZES                  A       2.7     18     86
                                                   S       3.3     39     96
APHASIA FINDINGS:
                             McCARTHY SCALES
                             PICT. MEM            PIAT
                             TAPPING              R.REC
                             VERB-MEM I           R.COMP   2.8      27     91
PPVT IQ 108  MA  10-2  % 67  VERB-MEM II
RAVENS PERCENTILE 25<x<50 MA 8-8½  R-L ORIENT  6½-7½
BENDER MA 7-0 to 7-5 RECALL 4  NUM. MEM I        SYMBOL DIGIT MODALITIES TEST
BEERY-BUKTENICA VMI  6-7 /4, 8-9  NUM. MEM II    W 23(1 error)   O 19(2 errors)
                             MEM SCALE INDEX
LATERAL DOMINANCE
    HAND  L X R
    EYE   L X R              DETROIT TESTS OF LEARNING APTITUDE
    FOOT  L     R X          #6    AUD ATTEN SP UNREL WORD   MA=  6-2
                             #7    ORAL COMMISSIONS          MA=  9-5
HAND DYNAMOMETER             #9    VIS ATTEN SP OBJ          MA=
    L  11 kg.   R  11 kg.    #10   ORIENTATION               MA=
                             #13   AUD ATTEN SP REL SYLL     MA=  8-0
HAND WRITING                 #16   VIS ATTEN SP LET          MA=  8-0
    L  14      R  21         #18   ORAL DIRECTIONS           MA=  8-3

GROOVED PEGBOARD             VADS   Aural-Oral      5
    L  32     R  33  R↓             Visual-Oral     5
                                    Aural-Written   4
REY AUDITORY-VERBAL LEARNING TEST   Visual-Written  5
I  6 II  7 III 11 IV 10 V  8

B  5 VI  8 REC 11 (2 errors)
```

DYSLEXIA IN BILINGUALS[1]

Loraine K. Obler
Aphasia Research Center, Department of Neurology
Boston University School of Medicine
and
Boston Veterans Administration Medical Center

I. INTRODUCTION

Bilingualism as an Experimental Tool

Bilingualism may be viewed as an experiment of nature given to the neurolinguist, not unlike agenesis of the corpus callosum, in order to clarify questions of brain-language correlations. Thus I approach the study of alexia in bilinguals with the assumption that it will tell about how the brain handles reading, in monolinguals as well as bilinguals. For example, using monolingual subjects it has proven impossible so far to determine whether, in the early stages of reading, at the letter identification stage, there is phonological processing going on in addition to letter name labeling. If one studies bilingual subjects who read two alphabets which share phonemes, but not graphic representations of them, as Shanon and Balzano (1980) have done with Hebrew-English readers, one can determine whether the phonological or the naming characteristics are primary, and the extent to which they interact.

In the case which Coltheart, Byng, Masterson, Pryor and Riddoch (in press) describe, bilingualism serves a somewhat different

1. Thanks are due to Linda Manganaro for help in sorting through the literature on polyglot aphasia in order to locate cases with reading impairment. Particular thanks are due to Eva Baharav for her help in coding these materials, researching additional ones, and providing many contributions in the course of drafting this paper. Thanks also to Howard Gardner and Norman Geschwind for directing me to pertinent cases and literature and to Michel Paradis for sharing Hiroko Hagiwara's Masters dissertation with me.

function. In this case, a Nepalese-English bilingual manifested deep dyslexia when reading aloud in Nepalese. Because the patient was
able to give the English translations for Nepalese words, however,
the authors are able to deduce that his reading for comprehension
was intact. In such instances, the special skill bilinguals may have, translation, permits an alternate route to assessing what language competence they have when they are aphasic. So bilingual phenomena may highlight for us issues in the psycholinguistics of reading
and reading disability in general; at the same time, of course, bilingual dyslexics stimulate questions about the nature of brain-language interaction in bilingualism itself. For example, with bilingual subjects one may study the relative organization of the two or
more languages both within and across the hemispheres, (e.g. Obler
et al. 1982, Rapport et al. 1983) and the neurological substrate for
a mechanism to permit a monitor for switching between two languages.
(Obler and Albert, 1978; Kolers, 1966).

Language Phenomena Specific to Bilingualism

    Certain phenomena may be seen as specific to alexia in the bi-
lingual or polyglot. Interference of characteristics of one orthography with another, for example, or confusion of orthographic elements in one script with another, can only occur in the bilingual.
The ability to perform on a language labeling task, that is, to determine which language a letter is in, with no other reading ability
spared, can only occur in the person who has learned to read a second language. Systematic bias in reading words which are homographic
across language (e.g. Pain in English and French) can only occur in
the bilingual. And, most prominently in the literature, a whole range of dissociations between or among writing systems that are deficited, may occur in the bilingual.

    These dissociations in abilities, presumably different from th-
ose existent premorbidly, may take a number of configurations. For
example, the patient may simply read one language better than another, while prior to the aphasia both languages were read equally well; this may occur for reading aloud, for reading comprehension or
for translation of written materials, or for some combination of
those skills. Or, the patient may do better in one language for reading, and in the other for writing. Or, the patient may present
with different types of alexia in each of the two or more languages.
Or, the same alexia type may manifest itself differently in each of
the two languages, due to differences in the orthographic systems
involved (e.g., a letter by letter reader in both languages would
present differently in English and in Chinese). Or the bilingual
may demonstrate antagonistic recovery; as in other language skills,
in this condition the patient recovers reading better in a certain
language at first, then the patient starts to recover reading abilities in the second language which soon overtakes the first language
to recover, which actually gets worse. Finally, there are a number

of cases in which, while reading has recovered in two or more languages, the patient reports that, again contrary to the premorbid
situation, reading in one language "feels" harder than in another.

Explanations for Dissociation in Polyglot Dyslexia

    Several classes of explanation can be drawn on in order to un-
derstand the dissociations which may obtain in bilingual dyslexia.
The first set of explanations draws on structural characteristics
of the language system which is represented orthographically. For
example it is generally believed that the great number of homophones
in Chinese as compared to English is intimately linked to some necessity for an ideographic orthography in order to distinguish them.
In other languages, whether vowels function crucially for distinguishing lexical items interacts with whether or not they are represented in the orthography at all, and if so how they are. For example, Gelb (1963) and others after him, have maintained that Hebrew
and Arabic did not need to represent vowels, but Greek did, and so
the Greeks developed them when borrowing the Semitic script. Whether a language is structured analytically or synthetically (that
is, whether the bulk of the syntax is handled by independent words
or by affixes) may also presumably make a difference in how the orthographic system develops. And differences in the structure of
other semiotic systems such as music presumably underlie the differences between how these systems and languages are represented orthographically, as well as in the brain.

    The second class of explanations for dissociations which have
been proposed revolves around characteristics of the orthographic
system, considered independent of the languages which they represent. Direction of reading is one such characteristic which we will
refer to. A second which is standardly considered in discussions
of bilingual alexia, is whether an orthography is ideographic or
 phonologic. I maintain that a further division needs to be made within the phonologic systems between syllabic and predominantly phonemic systems. And within the phonemic systems, one may
expect, and indeed find, different reading abilities in systems
which are transparent, (like Spanish) with no irregular spellings,
and systems which reflect the history and the morphology of the
language (like English), which therefore contain many irregularities
in the phoneme to grapheme conversion system.

    The third class of factors which may be called upon to explain
differential impairment in bilingual aphasia generally, and bilingual alexia in particular, involves factors in the course of acquisition of a second language. When both languages are not learned
concurrently from infancy, we may ask whether the age at which the
second language was learned, or the manner in which it was learned,
(whether by an oral method, or through writing, or translation),
has influenced the way it is represented in the brain. Differential

representation might then interact with how the second language would be deficited in brain damage. Also one might consider the relative order of acquisition of two languages; for instance, it might make a difference in the eventual representation of the two languages in the brain if an analytic language like Chinese was learned first, followed by a synthetic language like Finnish, or if conversely Finnish was learned first and Chinese second. And even in
the bilingual who learns both languages from infancy, explanations
concerned with the attitude towards each of the languages have been
invoked in order to explain differential recovery. The psychiatrists, such as Krapf (1955 and 1957), have argued that the "mother's"
tongue may bear a special status (and Wolfson (1979) in his Le Schizo et les langues, concurs). Others such as Minkowski (1965) have
maintained that the language in which a love affair was conducted
may recover first, even if that language was neither the first learned, nor the best learned, nor the most recently learned at the
time of stroke.

     Also invoked in order to explain dissociations in recovery of
language ability in aphasia and alexia are factors in how the two
or more languages of the polyglot have been used. Thus it should
be standard practice in research on bilinguals to determine what levels of proficiency were achieved and maintained in each of the languages premorbidly. Pitres (1895) long ago argued that the language which is being used predominantly in the premorbid period is most likely to recover best after an aphasia-producing incident, and
we have demonstrated (Obler and Albert, 1977) that his assertion is
correct, unlike that of Ribot (1892) who argued that the first learned language would most predictably return first. It has also been
argued, and should be studied scientifically, that the language which is used predominantly in the environment of the post-morbid patient (Geschwind, personal communication), or in speech therapy (Coltheart et al.) is the one which will recover best.

Scope of this Paper

     Rather than present a comprehensive synopsis of all the cases
of polyglot alexia in the literature, this paper will focus on two
of the explanatory factors mentioned above: the various characteristics of the orthographic system, and how these interact with manner of acquisition. I choose these two foci because there is a reasonable number of substantially detailed cases to demonstrate the
points I want to make on each of them, and because the former speaks primarily to universal issues of reading while the second speaks
to issues of the neurolinguistics of bilingualism. Having covered
these two topics which involve dissociations in alexia type across
two or more languages, I will briefly describe several important
cases of alexia in which dissociations did not obtain, in order to
remind us that the dissociations in bilingual aphasia and alexia,
while most interesting, are probably not the most frequent form of

impairment or recovery. In conclusion I will mention what little
we know of developmental dyslexia in bilinguals, and refer only in
passing to cases of dissociation between orthographic systems which
do not involve standard languages, in particular music and code systems, since even the alleged monolinguals among us may be considered to have mastered dual systems, whether they be music and writing, or shorthand and writing, and even capital and small letters.

II. ORTHOGRAPHIC SYSTEMS AND THE BILINGUAL ALEXIC

Direction of Reading : Left to Right or Right to Left

First let us consider the cases in which reading direction seems to make a difference. In passing we may note the case of differential reading abilities which Dessoff (1957) reports, which did
not involve aphasia or alexia. This is the case of a 64 year old
white man who came in complaining that he was unable to read. It
turns out that he was only able to read in English through a letter
by letter analysis, but when tested in Yiddish his reading was unimpaired. Since he had no other aphasic symptoms, Dessoff's explanation for his case was that a right inferior quadrant homonymous
scotoma interfered with his scanning to the right, but not, of course, to the left.

A more complex case in which reading direction seems to cause
differential reading abilities after brain damage is that recorded
by Streifler and Hofman (1976). It is the case of a 47 year old
business woman who was right handed, although there was some left
handedness in her family background. After a car accident which
resulted in a slight brain concussion, the patient was in a mild
confusional state and had problems distinguishing left from right.
She had no explicit aphasia, but had a flat, monotonous intonation
after the accident. Her first language had been Polish, but the
first language she learned in the written modalities was Hebrew,
presumably as a language for religious purposes. Her third language then had been German which she read primarily in a Latin (not
Gothic) script.

After the accident the patient was suddenly unable to read
Hebrew except when it was mirror reversed. Likewise when she wrote
in Hebrew, her writing was mirror reversed. Individual letters were mirror reversed as well as words; when shown words in which the
order of the letters was reversed, but the individual letters were
not reversed, the patient could not read them. In Polish and German, by contrast, the patient could only read given standard presentations, and could not read mirror reversed materials. Analogously, she could only write these languages in standard fashion. Unfortunately we do not know more about the manner in which the patient learned the several languages. Presumably she had not practi-
sed mirror writing or reading in any of them. The best explanation

for her differentially spared abilities, then, appears to relate to
the fact that Hebrew is read in a different direction from Polish
and German.

Ideographic versus Phonologic Scripts

In comparing ideographic to phonemic scripts, the classic case
among bilingual aphasics is that of Lyman, Kwan, and Chao (1938).
This is the case of the 42 year old businessman in Shanghai whose
first language was Chinese. His second language, English, he learned in childhood, and continued to use when he went to the University of Glasgow in his adolescence. When first tested, he was suffering from a subcortical parietal occipital tumor which resulted in
a right hemianopia, and no explicit aphasia, although he was a deep
dyslexic in Chinese and a letter by letter reader in English. That
is, in reading aloud in Chinese he was able to read two out of twenty words correctly, and the errors he made were semantically motivated. His English reading aloud was much better (nineteen out of
twenty words) and he could even read abbreviations. We are told that he often read English letter by letter, and indeed it would appear that he was more successful using this "phonological" decoding
mode, which could not work in Chinese due to the ideographic nature
of the system. Two errors are recorded in English, which lead one
to see the strategy the patient was using. He misread <u>day</u> as <u>dry</u>,
and <u>raise</u> he read as <u>rings, no, r-a-i-raise</u>. Again, such a guessing
strategy in a language which one reads phonologically will result
in different sorts of errors, in this case more phonologically motivated paralexias, whereas in Chinese they are more likely to result in semantically motivated paraphasias. As to his writing at
the first testing, it matched his reading abilities. His writing
in Chinese was poor. When asked to copy words, he omitted strokes
and ordered them randomly, contrary to the standard Chinese practice
which prescribes a certain ordering of strokes in any given word.
In addition to the omissions, he would make errors within parts of
characters. In English, by contrast, he made paragraphias which were more phonologically (or morphologically) motivated. To dictation, for example, he wrote <u>intervals</u> as <u>tin teveeds</u> and when asked
to copy the word, he wrote <u>interved</u>.

The patient was operated on and his tumor excised. Two months
after the operation he was tested again. At this time his lesion
was documented to be in the left occipital region going forward to
the angular gyrus. At that time the patient appears to have extended his letter by letter strategy in English to an analagous strategy in Chinese: tracing the characters. Nevertheless he was still
more successful in English, correctly reading 7 out of 11 multiple
word commands, whereas in Chinese he was only able to read 3 out of
11. In English, the authors noted that reading of long words was
particularly impaired as it is regularly in letter by letter reading in alexics, and irregular words were particularly impaired,

again as one would predict given the patient's phonologic decoding
strategy.   In Chinese, somewhat by contrast, the authors note there
was no correlation between the readability of the given word and
the number of strokes it was composed of.   It is worth noting that
calculation has been made of the readability of Chinese characters
in developmental reading studies and it turns out that number of
strokes is not linearly correlated with difficulty of symbol acquisition (Leong, 1973).   This being the case, one may suspect that
Lyman et al.'s calculations looked for a linear correlation rather
than a U-curve correlation and so found no correlation at all.

As to writing, in Chinese the patient was making semantic substitutions, which he never made in English.   In addition, however,
he was also making phonologically related substitutions in Chinese.
The authors noted that his ability to write abstract characters was
particularly impaired.   In some cases he would omit strokes, in others he would have only one correct radical out of two or more, and
in some instances he demonstrated right-left shift of elements within a character.   In English, the authors report that the patient
made "primarily spelling errors".   The examples they give, however,
suggest only one regularization (nursing as nersing).   In another
case two graphically similar letters were confused (be as de).   In
other cases letters were omitted or added (crowded as croed, exci-
tement as exciptement and persecution as percisution).

This patient, then, is of note because he appears to have manifested a different type of dyslexia in each of his two languages,
and this difference appears to be motivated by structural differences in the orthographies of the two languages.   Since even the operation did not change the character of the alexia, for all his impairments were less severe, we may be justified in concluding that
the two languages were organized differently for reading in the brain of this patient, because of the differences in their orthographic systems.

Bisystemic Alexia: Kana and Kanji

While not strictly bilingual of course in a standard sense,
all educated Japanese are at least orthographically bisystemic.
Since it is comprised of two structurally different scripts, the
Japanese writing system provides numerous opportunities for dissociation in alexia. The Kanji script goes back historically to the
Chinese ideographic system, and the Kana scripts are phonologic, of
the syllabic type.   Each child learning the language learns first
the Kana syllabic scripts consisting of 47 basic signs.   Then starting in first grade, the student learns 50 to 100 Kanji characters
each year.   Dissociations in ability with aphasia whereby the Kana
or Kanji scripts are retained have been reported previously (see
Sasanuma, 1980 and review therein).   In standard writing of the
language, Kanji characters are used to represent lexical morphemes,

while the syllabic Kana symbols are used for marking the rich inflectional system of the language. One syllabic system known as Katakana, is generally reserved for foreign loan words, and the other -
Hiragana - is used for grammatical formatives. Thus one might assume that readers have greater familiarity with the Hiragana syllabary.
This is not unlike in English where we are more likely to experience
as familiar whole words in the lower case letters, as compared to u-
pper case letters, although any word can be written and recognized
in either system. All words could be written in Kana, although one
does not see such sentences in Kana, whereas not all words and affixes could be written in Kanji.

   Hagiwara has written a Master's thesis under the direction of
Paradis which reports all cases of alexia in the Japanese literature,
(Paradis et al. in press) . Since simple cases of dissociation in
which either Kana or Kanji scripts are differentially spared have be-
en treated previously (Sasanuma et al.), we will focus on lesser known and more complex dissociations. First let us consider some three
way dissociations. Fukuda (1924, see Paradis et al. in press) reported the case of a 51 year old farmer who had had 4 years of education, apparently enough to have mastered the Kanji and Kana systems.
He suffered encephalitis pursuant to a serpent bite, and manifested
both alexia and right homonymous hemianopia. In reading the patient
skipped the right half of the page. On the left half of the page it
was discovered that Katakana was the hardest for him to read, whereas Kanji reading was nearly perfect. His reading of Hiragana was
intermediate. The errors he made, we are told, were both visually
motivated and semantically motivated. Unfortunately it is unclear
what is meant by semantic here. That is, he may have made errors
which were semantically related to the target, thus suggesting a deep dyslexia, or he may merely have made verbal paralexias. His writing was analogous to his reading, that is, it was like the writing
of an agrammatic, consisting largely or entirely of Kanji words, without the inflections and functors which mastery of the Kana systems
should have added.

   In contrast is the second case, of a 69 year old small business owner, who had had 11 years of education. His embolism resulted
in a pure alexia. By the authors' testing his reading of Kanji symbols was only 40% correct, his reading of Hiragana was 50% correct
while his reading of words in Katakana was 80% correct. It is worth
noting that despite his severe reading disability, the patient was
good at classifying characters into one of the three systems, much
as some bilinguals in European languages can tell whether a letter
belongs to one of their languages without being able to read it. Also it is asserted that this patient could correct "spelling errors".

   By way of further contrast is the case reported by Kurachi and
colleagues (1978 see Paradis et al. in press) in which Kana was better for writing while Kanji was better for reading, a sort of

dissociation reported rarely in polyglot aphasics. This is the case of a 70 year old right handed executive who had a stroke nine months prior to his testing. This stroke resulted in a fluent aphasia with severe anomia and much perseveration. (Lesion localization was unknown). In both reading aloud and reading for comprehension, the patient was good with Kanji characters, but poor with Hiragana characters. In reading aloud in Hiragana, the patient committed paralexic errors. When asked to write, by contrast, the patient was grossly impaired in writing Kanji characters, and less impaired in writing the Hiragana characters.

One must assume that the phonologic versus ideographic nature of Kana versus Kanji scripts interacts with the different familiarity and function of two kana scripts, and of course, lesion localization, to account for the several sorts of alexic dissociation described in this section.

Dissociations between two Phonologic Scripts

One further case reported in the Paradis et al. corpus must be mentioned, since it deals with a patient who had mastered the several Japanese systems, as well as a Latin system. It is the case reported by Inasaka and Kurachi in 1972. A 56 year old right handed man had learned Japanese as his native language, and then had learned German well enough that he was a professor of German in a Japanese university. Although we do not know at what age he learned the language, we do know that he kept a diary in it daily before his accident. A thrombosis to his left cerebral artery one month prior to testing had resulted in visual disturbances, finger agnosia, mild anomia and calculation disturbances (components of the Gerstmann syndrome) as well as hemiparesis of the right extremities, mild color naming deficit, (that is, he named 5 out of 7 colors correctly in Japanese) and mild color agnosia. The patient was a pure alexic: his writing in both languages was intact, and his reading of numbers was fine. When tested in reading at three months post onset the patient read best in the two Kana systems, making a few visual and semantic errors. His reading in German was worst, despite the fact that German has a phonological orthography, as do the Kana systems. His reading in Kanji was intermediate, and there he made semantic errors only. Thus we may again conclude that the phonological versus ideographic dichotomy alone of an orthographic system is not sufficient to explain all alexic dissociations. Yet in this case it is hard to argue that it was his lesser familiarity with reading German which explains his worse reading in that language. It is of interest to note that at 21 months post onset the patient was tested and he read well in all systems. He did however complain that his reading of German was diminished for comprehension.

A second case in which two phonologic systems are differentially impaired is that reported by Karanth, 1981. She tells of a

57 year old right handed man who had been the superintendent in a
customs office in India, a job which required using English. The
patient's first language had been Telugu; his second language, which had been the first he learned to read and write, was Kannada, a
language whose orthography is syllabic, in different ways than is
that of Japanese, it should be noted. That is, in Kannada a separate grapheme is provided for each consonant -vowel combination, a-
nd there are no individual graphemes which represent pure consonants. However each consonant has only a slightly different grapheme
shape depending upon the vowel with which it combines. Thus one can
visually distinguish consonants and vowels. Thus in Kannada pa and
pu will share a gross similarity, whereas in Japanese ba and bu look
no more alike than ba and mo. However it is worth noting that Kannada orthography is learned as if the syllables were each distinct
from each other, and students are drilled to this day in series of
syllabic units.

The third language of this patient was English. When he had a
stroke at the age of 57, it resulted in a right visual field defect,
mild anomia, and a pure alexia, with no other aphasia nor writing
disturbance. His reading of numbers was unimpaired. The patient's
strategy in reading was letter by letter in English and syllable by
syllable in Kannada. Unfortunately for the neurolinguist, the patient made no errors, but his reading was extremely slow. The patient, like that of Inasaka and Kurachi, reported that he experienced Kannada to be harder to read than English. Karanth speculates
that it is the much greater number of orthographic elements in Kannada, the syllables, which rendered that language harder to read,
but we cannot know whether readers of Kannada standardly dissociate
the phonemic elements within a syllable, which would mean that they
have no more elements to recognize than does the reader of English.
Such psycholinguistic experimentation remains to be done.

To conclude, characteristics of an orthographic system, such
as the direction of reading it, or its ideographic versus phonologic nature, or the number of elements to be learned, have all been
called in to explain differential recovery in alexia. Most compelling are the set of cases collected in Japanese, because we have
evidence that the dissociation may work both ways, that is, one or
the other of the two general types of system may be spared. And as
the case of the Japanese professor of German indicates, there may
well be an interaction of orthographic effects with familiarity or
language learning effects which we will now consider.

III. LANGUAGE ACQUISITION FACTORS IN BILINGUAL DYSLEXIA

Differential Proficiency Type in Two Languages

In the second series of cases, discussed here, the authors have convincingly invoked an explanation for differential alexia

which relies on how each of two languages was learned. In some cases, it is, however, difficult to dissociate these explanations from
those relying on differences in the orthographies, particularly as
a number involve bilingualism of Hebrew and a European language.
One such case is reported by Stevens (1957). While not a simple case of alexia, it is instructive. It is the case of a woman with reading epilepsy. In her case the seizures were triggered by reading
Hebrew and music, much more severely than by reading English. The
woman was observed at the age of 24, because of spells in which her
jaw began to twitch. This happened when reading Hebrew, a language
which she used for her prayers as an observant orthodox Jew. (Note
that the patient read the language aloud but could not translate or
otherwise comprehend it). Reading of new music, it appears, was more
likely to precipitate an attack than was reading of familiar music.
By contrast, the patient was able to continue reading of English for
much longer than Hebrew or music before the attacks were triggered.
Stevens's explanation invokes a greater effort involved in reading
Hebrew, although he also refers to the different eye movement patterns which are necessary, - both the right to left scanning, and the
reading of Hebrew vowels which may require vertical movements. I
submit that it is the differential knowledge of the two languages
which contributed to the dissociation. English was a more profici-
ent language, used for comprehension, whereas Hebrew was read by phonological route, and music similarly with sound divorced from explicit meaning, which contributed to the differential impact of reading on the epilepsy.

Halpern (1941) reports a case of alexia in a 23 year old German
man who had learned Yiddish as his first language, and had learned
Hebrew for religious purposes as a child. Only around the age of 20
when he immigrated to Palestine did the patient learn spoken Hebrew.
Soon thereafter he suffered a gunshot wound to the left temporal area which resulted in a right homonymous hemianopia. For five days
he was comatose, and then his language began to recover slowly; at
first he spoke only a stereotypy in German. His reading was tested
four months after the accident, by which time his spoken Hebrew was
somewhat better than his spoken German. This same discrepancy held
true for his reading and writing. In German reading, both aloud and
for comprehension, the patient made numerous paralexias, whereas his
reading in Hebrew was good. Also his writing of German was worse
than his writing of Hebrew. Of course it is difficult to claim that
any particular fact of the patient's language learning history accounts for his differential recovery from alexia, but it is hard not to
point to the gross discrepancies between the manner of acquiring the
two languages which may result in the differential alexia.

Learning One Language Through the Visual Modality

Minkowski (1927 and 1963) reports a similar case. It is the
case of a mechanic who was also a great reader of books. His first

language was Swiss-German, his second language was literary German
which he learned in school, presumably learning it from the writing
modality from early on, and his third and fourth languages were French and Italian. Minkowski also reports "that he was a visual type,
with a vivid visual perception of colors and forms". At the age of
32 the patient suffered a motorcycle accident which resulted in right
hemiparesis and hemihypoesthesia, as well as a global aphasia which
evolved into a Broca's aphasia after several days. After the accident the patient spoke only literary German, to the surprise of his
physicians and his landlady who came to visit him, since the environment in the hospital was that of spoken Swiss-German. From a fair
poverty of speech in literary German in the initial stages, he began
using more words and evidenced some dysarthria, then later paraphasias and agrammatism. His comprehension of both literary German and
Swiss German was good. In addition the patient chose to read German
illustrated papers and he spoke literary German with his landlady who
came to visit him even more than his family did. Five months post
onset the patient began to speak Swiss-German again, but even 12 months post onset he was not speaking it as fluently as he was speaking
literary German and he mixed literary German words and idioms into
Swiss-German, but not conversely. As to French and Italian, in the
16 months during which Minkowski tested him he was never able to speak or understand either of those two languages although he could
read French words phonetically, without comprehension. Unfortunately, it is not made clear what strategy the patient was using in reading German.

     What is of interest is that Minkowski inquired how it was that
the patient was speaking literary German and the patient "himself
explained to us that when speaking literary German he had internal
visual images of printed words, while such images were completely absent with regard to the Swiss dialect". Minkowski points out that
in addition to this, it was the literary German that the patient was
practising for most of the first half year post onset. Minkowski's
bias it should be noted is to find a psychological "affect explanation for recovery of language in a polyglot aphasia" and indeed it
turns out that a young Swiss woman had bitterly disappointed the patient in love several years prior to his accident. On top of this,
his landlady, although addressing him in Swiss-German in her early
visits, was prepared to drill him in literary German when that was
his preference for the first six months, and then in Swiss-German
later. Minkowski's explanation, like that of Halpern in the previous case, was that the patient had "internal visual images of printed words (in literary German) while such images were completely absent with regard to the Swiss dialect".

     The classic case in which we suspect that having learned a se-
cond language primarily through a visual modality enhanced access to
that language after an alexia producing accident is the case of Hinshelwood (1902). His case 1 is the case of a 34 year old man

suffering from tertiary syphilis. At age 31 the patient had had a
transient attack of left hemiplegia; at age 34 he came in with the
complaint that he could not read. The patient's first language was
English; as an educated man he had learned French, then Latin, then
Greek. When tested by the ophthalmologist Hinshelwood, it turned out
that the patient's reading in English was indeed poor, while his ability to read in French was somewhat better. His Latin was better than his French, and his ability to read Greek (Xenophone and New Testa-
ment, for example) and music was quite good.

     In English the patient could read only functors by sight; other-
wise he used a letter by letter strategy. In the other languages he
could "read by sight"; one assumes this means he could recognize many
more words without decoding them letter by letter. This patient is
another case of a patient who when tested at 2½ months post onset evidenced no obvious problems in reading any of his languages, nevertheless he continued to observe that reading of English required of him
the "greatest mental effort" of all languages.

     This series of cases, then, provides the strongest support th-
at different modes of learning orthographic systems may make one system or the other more susceptible to alexia after brain damage. One
assumes that the different modes of acquisition result in (partially)
different systems of organization and/or processing. Specific lesions then render one or another access route less available than it
was pre-morbidly, and reading in that language is thus more severely
impaired.

IV. CASES IN WHICH DIFFERENTIAL ALEXIA DOES NOT OBTAIN

     Lest we are impressed that all cases of bilingual alexia demon-
strate dissociations, let us consider two cases in which the alexia
was similar in type and severity in all the languages the patient
knew before the brain damage. We may consider the case of Sroka et
al (1973), a case in which the patient was a letter by letter dyslexic, and the case of Weisenburg and McBride, (1935) in which the patient was a phonological alexic in all languages. Finally we must
report the case of Pitres (1895) in which the patient was a deep dyslexic in the only language (out of six) he could read at all.

A Case of Letter by Letter Alexia

     The patient of Sroka et al (1973) is a patient whose first lan-
guage was slavic, her second language was German, and her third lang
age was Hebrew. This patient had not had a religious education, and
learned Hebrew when she immigrated to Israel after high school. She
learned Hebrew with no difficulty, it should be noted, and learned t
read all her languages although she had had no formal education in H
brew and so was not particularly good at spelling in the language.
arterovenous malformation in the left posterior cerebral artery

resulted in a lesion to the left occipital subcortical region of the lingual and fusiform gyri. The patient evidenced no aphasia in any of her languages, but initially was unable to read in any of her three languages. Writing however, was intact. We are told that the patient had a color agnosia, although there are no details on this. Reading in all languages was letter by letter. The patient made some misnamings of letters, as letter by letter dyslexics are wont to do, and performed worse on long words.

Her only agnosia was for colors, not for objects nor for faces. Over the course of 2 months the right hemianopsia which had followed the accident, reduced to an upper right quadrant hemianopsia. As she was followed outside of the hospital after the first two and one half months in the hospital, the regression of her color agnosia was documented, at a somewhat slower pace than the regression of her alexia.

In the early stages as the languages began to return for reading it became clear that there was no difference among any of the three languages, nor was there any difference whether the patient was asked to read aloud or to read silently. At one point print was easier to read than handwriting, two substantially different scripts in Hebrew as in English. Both letter blindness and word blindness errors were reported. Thus as she was recovering the patient evidenced particular difficulty with consonants which can be written in opposite directions such as p and q or b and d in English. Neither reading words nor letters could be said to be better. On one day she read the capital letter R as P (perhaps due to the Cyrillic capital P standing for R); on that same day she read the word Rome with no difficulty. Two days subsequent she could not read the word Roam but was able to label the capital letter R. Moreover she made errors of the same sort in Hebrew.

Word length did interact with her abilities to read in all her languages, that is, words of few letters were better read than words of more letters. In Hebrew, it would appear from the examples that are given, the patient could recognize the first three letters of six letter words, that is to say she could read the right hand most half of the word histadrut. The authors tried adding voweling to the Hebrew text, which did not help the patient at all.

The patient developed a strategy which permitted her to get the letter information in. What she did was to move her finger around the outline of letters, at first; then later she drew letters onto the palm of her left hand and finally she drew them into the air. Of course this strategy was easier for short as compared to long words. Early on in the course of her recovery, if she was not permitted to use this strategy to make the movements with her right hand onto her left palm, she could not recognize words and letters. Over the course of her recovery it became clear that she only needed to

make partial movements of the forms of the letters in order to identify them and eventually she appeared to ignore the movements which
she was making in the air. Indeed the patient expressed some concern to the examiners that she might become addicted to the habit. At
this point it was noted that the patient would move her lips in reading to herself, although she did not actually vocalize. This lip
movement was the last gesture remaining, even when her reading had
apparently returned to normal.

     Sroka and her colleagues point out that the fact that the ale-
xia recovered entirely is quite unusual. Their explanation is that
the persistent damage in the angular gyrus as documented by the right hemianopsia which apparently did not recover, was "only functional" and that is why the alexia was reversible. I would propose that
the patient developed alternate strategies to get the information
into the language area, in particular the use of gestures, and perhaps that her being a trilingual had provided more optional routes
for her ability to read.

A Case of Phonological Alexia

     The fourth case of Weisenburg and McBride (1935) is a case of
phonological alexia in all five of the patient's languages, proportional to the extent of his previous proficiency in them. The case
is that of a 49 year old white male professor, who had taught Romance languages. Unfortunately we do not have substantial information
on the order and way in which he acquired the languages; we are told,
however, that English was his first language. The patient suffered
a subcortical thrombosis to his left middle cerebral artery which
resulted in what the authors term an expressive aphasia in both oral
and written modalities. In a marvelous example of early 20th century American scientism, the patient was timed reading 150 words aloud
in each of his 5 languages. The correlation between the amount of
time taken to read the words and the number of errors the patient
made was exact. In English it took him 75 seconds to read the words,
and he made 6 errors; in Spanish it took him 138 seconds to read the
words and he made 11 errors; in French it took him 150 seconds to
read the words and he made 15 errors, in Italian it took him 205
seconds to read the words and he made 19 errors; and in German it
took him 225 seconds to read the words and he made 25 errors. On
more extensive testing of the patient's English, it was discovered
that he could read 93 out of 100 words correctly. He could not label individual letters correctly all the time however, and he either
could not read nonsense words or read them poorly. When reading
paragraphs, the patient read slowly and with what are called "mis-
pronunciations". Interestingly enough these all appear to be off
by only one phonological distinctive feature. Thus the patient read ch as sh, br as pr, ap as ab, pran as pram, plin as pling. The
only example listed which is off by more than one distinctive feature, and that by two features, is ot read as ob.

In writing the patient was able to spell nonsense words, although he made some paragraphias when asked to write real words. Also, he would mix Romance spellings into English, spelling independence with an 'a' or an 'e', a difficulty I cannot ascribe to brain damage, since I make the error myself which I like to attribute to my having learned French.

A Case of Deep Dyslexia

One further case must be mentioned because it is the earliest case of deep dyslexia reported to date. Pitres was clever enough to test the patient in a variety of ways, so we can confirm that his case looked like current cases of deep dyslexia. As the patient was only able to read at all in his first language after his stroke, one cannot presume he would have evidenced deep dyslexia in all his languages. The seventh case of Pitres (1895) is that of a 37 year old man who had been born in Gascony and spoke Patois at home, later he learned standard French, and presumably read that language first. He taught himself English at the age of 15 years, and then learned Spanish and Arabic in the military in North Africa. His sixth language was Italian which he learned at the age of 25 as a resident in Cairo, needing it for his business.

A stroke suffered in Cairo led to global aphasia and a hemiplegia. By six months post onset when the patient returned to his home, his spoken French had returned, but he was anomic. Daily testing provided extensive information which we may summarize. When the patient read French aloud he made semantic errors. His reading of functors was impaired, while his reading of "simple and familiar nouns" was best. When presented with nonsense words the patient performed abysmally; Pitres chose a neurological jargon term as one which would be nonsense for the patient: hemiopie was read as miotais. However his reading of unorthodox spellings of recognizable words was not bad. Thus given Pary, the patient read Paris; given dessaint, the patient recognized dessin, (but given Thunyz, the patient was unable to read Tunis).

As to reading for comprehension in French, the patient's performance was not so impaired as it was in reading aloud. Interestingly, he could catch misspellings. So Pitres composed a test in which beauté was substituted for bonté, and facilement was substituted for aisement, both of which the patient caught.

The patient had great difficulty reading Spanish and Italian, even when he tried a letter by letter strategy. The only words he could read were ones which had French cognates such as assassination, caballero, finestra, and porta. Likewise his reading of English and Arabic was minimal, and it was impossible for him to read music. His reading of numbers, however, as in most alexias, was intact.

V.   CHILDHOOD DYSLEXIA IN BILINGUALS

Unfortunately there is virtually no literature on childhood dyslexia in bilinguals. Critchley (1970) mentions several cases, and gives examples of the children's handwriting, but not detailed analysis. We note in his examples of materials on an Arabic-English dyslexic child, that there may be more visually motivated errors in Arabic, the first language, than there are in English which has a variety of standard dyslexic errors, few of which are motivated by visual similarity between letters. The other cases he presents, a second Arabic-English dyslexic, and a Hebrew-English dyslexic, make analogous errors in writing in both their languages. What additional information we have on individual subjects, entirely anecdotal by clinicians who worked with them, suggests that if a child is dyslexic in learning to read one language, then he or she is <u>as a rule</u> dyslexic in learning to read the next. However the possibility exists that reading of an ideographic language would be easier for a dyslexic child than reading of a phonological one, as reported in the limited study of Rozin (1971). Dyslexia in a first language may improve with the study of a second language whose orthography is greatly different (Spector, 1980). Learning to read at a later age rather than an earlier one, or learning to read a language which one did not know in the oral mode, might be easier or more difficult. Such possibilities remain entirely unstudied until we can discover some cases of dissociation. Boder (personal communication) does report that language specific factors in the orthography seem to effect the types of childhood dyslexia seen across populations. In particular she notes that in an English speaking population, given the irregular phoneme to grapheme rules in that language, she sees substantially more dyseidetic dyslexics, (that is patients who make errors because they cannot recognize words by sight) than in Spanish with its phonologically transparent orthography, where she sees primarily dysphonetic dyslexics (that is, children who cannot decode words phonologically).

VI.   CONCLUSION

The relatively high proportion of differential alexia in cases of brain damage in adult polyglots, as compared to childhood dyslexia, should not go unnoticed; it well may reflect differential brain mechanisms underlying alexia and developmental dyslexia. In our review of the various alexic dissociations which may ensue upon brain damage in adult bilinguals and polyglots, we have focussed on explanations by orthographic structure, and explanations by mode of acquisition language learning. It should be not be forgotten however that there are many other possible explanations, as indicated in the introduction, and further observation of adult alexics will elucidate these. Experimental cross-language work on monolingual adult aphasics would also be desirable to resolve such questions as whether certain languages habitually encourage certain alexic phenomena.

Naturally in all studies of bilinguals all factors relating to the type and experience of bilingualism should be recorded (Obler et al. 1981) and of course it should not be assumed that the bilingual has a similar alexia type in all languages. As Hinshelwood said in 1902

How is it that there are so few recorded cases of these partial forms of word blindness, that is, cases of dissociation in polyglots? I think the reason is simply that the patient is not thoroughly examined by testing his power of reading all the characters and all the languages with which he is familiar....It has been taken for granted that if a patient was unable to read one language, he would therefore be unable to read any language, and that there was no necessity for applying further tests.

Moreover there is an entire literature of bisystematic dyslexia which is beyond the scope of this paper, but which bears study. These are the cases in which a reader of music or a decoder of a signlanguage or code becomes brain-damaged in ways which differentially impair their ability to appreciate written language and written music or visually presented code. An excellent review of the music cases can be found in Judd, Gardner, and Geschwind (1983); the only mention we have found of acquired and developmental dyslexia in codeusers is by Critchley (1942).

What I propose in conclusion, then, is a multi-dimensional approach to the understanding of alexia in bilinguals.

REFERENCES

Albert, M. and Obler, L. The Bilingual Brain: Neurolinguistic and Neuropsychological Aspects of Bilingualism. New York: Academic Press, 1978.

Coltheart, M. The psycholinguistic analysis of acquired dyslexias: some illustrations. Philosophical Translations. Royal Society of London. 1982, B 298, 151-164

Coltheart, M., Byng, S., Masterson, J., Prior, M. and Riddoch, J. Bilingual biscriptal deep dyslexia, (in press).

Coltheart, M., Patterson, K. and Marshall, J. Deep Dyslexia. London: Routledge & Kegan Paul, 1980.

Critchley, M. The Dyslexic Child, Charles C. Thomas, Springfield, III: 1970.

Critchley, M. Aphasic disorders of signalling (constitutional and acquired) occurring in naval signalmen. Journal of the Mt. Sinai Hospital, 1942, 9, 363-375.

Dessoff, M.D. Paracentral Homonymous Hemianopic Scotoma. Archives of Ophthalmology, 1957, 58, 452-454

Gelb, I. J. A Study of Writing (2nd edition), Chicago: University of Chicago Press, 1963.

Halpern, L. Beitrag Zur Restitution der Aphasie bei Polyglotten
    im Hinblick auf das Hebraeische. Schweizer Archiv Fuer Neu-
    rologie und Psychiatire, 1941, 47, 150-154

Hinshelwood, J. Four cases of word-blindness, Lancet, 1902, 1,
    358-363.
Judd, T., Gardner, H., and Geschwind, N.: Alexia without agraphia
    in a composer, Brain, 1983.
Karanth, P. Pure alexia in a Kannada-English bilingual, Cortex,
    1981, 17, 187-198.
Krapf, E. The choice of language in polyglot psychoanalysis.
    The Psychoanalytic Quarterly, 1955, 24, 343-357
Kolers, P. Reading and talking bilingually. American Journal of
    Psychology, 79, 357-376.
Krapf, E. A Propos des aphasies chez les polyglottes. Encéphale,
    1957, 46, 623-629.
Leong, C. K.: Hong Kong. (chapter 18) in Downing, J. (Ed).
    Comparative Reading: Cross National Studies of Behaviour and
    Processes in Reading and Writing. New York: McMillan, 1973.
Lyman R., Kwan, S. & Chao, W. Observations on alexia and agraphia
    in Chinese and in English. Chinese Medical Journal, 1938,
    54, 491-516.
Minkowski, M. Klinischer Beitrag Zur Aphasie bei Polyglotten,
    speziell im Hinblick auf das Schweizerdeutsche. Schweizer
    Archiv fuer Neurologie und Psychiatrie, 1927, 21, 43-72.
Minkowski, M. On aphasia in polyglots in L. Halpern (Ed).
    Problems of Dynamic Neurology. Jerusalem: Hebrew University,
    1963.
Obler, L. and Albert, M. Influence of aging in recovery from apha-
    sia in polyglots. Brain and Language, 1977, 4, 460-463.
Obler, L. and Albert, M. A monitor system for bilingual language
    processing, in M. Paradis, (ed.), Aspects of Bilingualism,
    Columbia, S.C.: Hornbeam Press, 1978.
Paradis, M. The language switch in bilinguals: Psycholinguistic
    and neurolinguistic perspectives. Zeirschrift für Dialekto-
    logie und Linguistik Beihefte. 1980, 32, 501-506.
Paradis, M., Hagiwara, H., and Hildebrandt, N., Dissociations bet-
    ween syllabic and ideographic script processing in Japanese
    brain-damaged patients., manuscript, forthcoming.
Pitres, A. Etude sur l'aphasie chez les polyglottes, Revue de
    Médicine. 1895, 15, 873-897.
Ribot, T. Diseases of Memory; An essay in the positive psychology.
    London: Paul, 1882.
Rozin, P., Poritsley, S. and Sotsky, R. American children with rea-
    ding problems can easily learn to read English represented by
    Chinese characters. Science 1971, 171, 1264-1267.
Sasanuma, S. Acquired dyslexia in Japanese: clinical features and
    underlying mechanisms. In Coltheart M., Patterson, K. and
    Marshall, J. (Eds.), Deep Dyslexia. London: Routledge and
    Kegan Paul, 1980.

Shanon, B. & Balzano, G.: Identification and classification of cha-
    racters in two alphabets. Journal of Psycholinguistic Resear-
    ch, 1980, 9, 261-274.
Spector, N. The effect of instruction in reading, writing and pro-
    nouncing Hebrew on reading, writing and spelling English,
    among children who are slow. Unpublished Ph. D. dissertation,
    Univ. of Minnesota, 1980.
Sroka, H., Solsi, P., & Bornstein, B. Alexia without agraphia with
    complete recovery, Confina Neurologia, 1973, 35, 167-176.
Stevens, H. Reading epilepsy. New England Journal of Medicine,
    1957, 257, 165-170.
Streifler, M. & Hofman S. Sinistrad mirror writing and reading
    after brain concussion in a bi-systemic (Oriento-occidental)
    Polyglot. Cortex, 1976, 12, 356-364.
Weisenburg, T. & McBride, K. Aphasia: A Clinical and Psychological
    Study N.Y.: Commonwealth Fund, 1935, (Case #4, pp. 160-182).
Wolfson, L. Le Schizo et Les Langues. Paris: Gallimard 1970.

SUPPLEMENTARY CASES OF BILINGUAL ALEXIA

April, R. S. and Tse, P. C. Crossed aphasia in a Chinese bilingual
    dextral. Archives of Neurology. 1977, 34, 366-770.
Bychowsky, Z. Ueber die Restitution der nach einem Schaedelschuss
    verlorengegangenen Sprachen bei einem Polyglotten. Monatssch-
    rift fuer Psychiatrie und Neurologie, 1919, Bd 45. Heft, 4,
    183-201.
Chelnov, L. Ob afazil u poliglotow, Izvestiia Akademii Pedagogi-
    cheskikh Nauk RSFSR., 1948, 15, 783-790.
Dreifuss, F. Observations on aphasia in a polyglot poet. Acta
    Psychiatrica et Neurologica Scandinavica, 1961, 36, 91-97.
Gloning, I. and Gloning, K. Aphasien bei Polyglotten. Wiener
    Zeitschrift fuer Nervenheilkunde, 1965, 22, 362-397.
Halpern, L. Observations on sensory aphasia and its restitution in
    a Hebrew polyglot. Monatschrift fuer Psychiatrie und Neuro-
    logie, 1950, 119, 156-173.
Kauders, O. Ueber Polyglotte Reaktionen bei einer sensorischnen
    Aphasie. Zeitschrift fuer die gesamte Neurologie, 1929, 122,
    651-666.
Leichner, A. Ueber die Aphasie der Mehrsprachigen. Archiv fuer
    Psychiatrie und Nervenkrankheiten, 1948, 180, 118-180, 731-775.
Ovcharova, P., Raichev, R., and Geleva, T. Afeziya u Poligloti
    (Bulg.). Neurohirurgiia, 1968, 7, 183-190.
Paradis, M. Aspects of the Japanese writing system relevant to psy-
    cho-and neurolinguistic studies. paper presented at the 9th
    LACUS forum, Northwestern Univ. Evanston, 6 August, 1982.
Nair, K.R. and Virmani, V. Speech and language disturbances in he-
    miplegics. Indian Journal of Medical Research, 1973, 61,
    1395-1403.
Wechsler, A. Dissociative alexia. Archives of Neurology.
    1977, 34, 257.

HEMISPHERIC SPECIALIZATION AND DUAL CODING OF ALPHABET

Carlo Umiltà
Istituto di Fisiologia Umana
Università di Parma,
Via S. Gramsci 14,
43100 Parma
Italy

THE HYPOTHESIS OF THE DUAL ROUTE ACCESS TO THE LEXICON IN READING

The research about the processes involved in reading has led to what is called the dual route hypothesis for explaining lexical access (see a recent review in McCusker, Hillinger and Bias, 1981). The internal lexicon, where the semantic information concerning a given word is stored, would be accessed either through a visual or a phonological code. The visual code of a word consists of representations that are based upon the form of the constituent letters and their interrelations. The phonological code is a representation based upon the phonemes corresponding to the constituent letters. While both codes can be utilized for processing written words, skilled readers usually employ the visual code.

Empirical evidence in support of the dual access comes from the results of those speeded lexical decision tasks that have shown a homophony effect only for nonwords. Typically the subject is shown a visual string of letters and is asked to decide whether it constitutes a word or not by pressing one of two buttons as fast as possible. The fact that the presented word has a corresponding homophone does not affect speed or accuracy of "yes" responses as compared to control words. By contrast, for "no" responses speed and accuracy are lower when the presented string of letters has a corresponding real word than when it has none. This pattern or results can be explained as follows. In the case of words, the lexicon is accessed visually and an entry is found before any effect of homophony becomes apparent. In the case of nonwords, the visual search of the lexicon cannot locate an entry and this allows enough time for the phonological code to build up and show the effect of homophony. As a matter of fact, "yes" responses have always proved faster than "no" responses.

The functional independence of the internal codes arising from
the same word renders it likely that their neural representations reside in different brain structures. Since it is generally accepted
(see e.g., Milner, 1971) that the right and left cerebral hemispheres
are, in the large majority of human beings, specialized for visuospatial and verbal processing, respectively, it seems reasonable to locate accordingly in the brain the two coding systems. The phonological code would be available in the left hemisphere whereas the visual
code would be available in the right hemisphere.

In principle this hypothesis should be easily testable by presenting the strings of letters to the two visual fields, that is by the
so-called divided visual field procedure (see e.g., Young, 1982 and
the third section of the present paper). While the logic of that procedure is no doubt simple, the problems that attach to putting it into effect for reading letter strings are quite complex. The difficulties are both methodological and theoretical. Those of the first
type pertain to the way stimuli are presented. Peripheral presentations are mandatory and exposure time must be less than the latency
of a saccadic eye movement. Most investigators have kept within the
limits of 5-6 degrees from fixation and 100-150 msec of duration.
In these conditions, a post-exposural left-to-right scanning due to
reading habits can become prevalent in yielding an advantage for the
right visual field, thus mimicking a left hemispheric specialization
even when the visual code is involved. This is very likely to be the
case for unilateral presentations. In an attempt to minimize lateral
scanning patterns, words have been presented in a vertical orientation in a few experiments. However, it can be argued that processing
vertical words disrupts usual reading strategies and favors a phonological encoding of letter strings irrespective of whether they are
words or nonwords.

Even if one disregards such technical difficulties, there is a
further problem that hinders the use of the divided visual field procedure in differentiating the role of the two hemispheres in reading
words. It is quite possible that the internal lexicon is located
in only one hemisphere, the left appearing a more likely candidate
than the right. If this is true, those lexical decision tasks which
have allowed the differentiation of the visual and phonological access should always demonstrate a specialization of the left hemisphere
for the required word-nonword discrimination, independently of the
code through which the lexicon is actually accessed.

The above-mentioned factors may have played an important role in
many studies which have shown a reliable left hemispheric specialization for processing words. It is, indeed, hard to find studies that
have employed words as stimuli and have not produced, at least in some conditions, a significant asymmetry in favor of the right visual
field/left hemisphere (see Beaumont, 1982, for a review).

VISUAL AND PHONOLOGICAL REPRESENTATIONS OF SINGLE LETTERS

From the preceding discussion emerges that simpler verbal stimuli and tasks different from reading should be preferred in assessing the relative role of the two hemispheres in processing visual and phonological codes. Obviously, such evidence can have implications for the processes by which one reads words.

In a series of chronometric studies Posner and his associates (see reviews in Posner, 1969; 1978) have demonstrated that even a verbal stimulus as simple as a single alphabetical letter gives rise to two different internal codes. One code is modality-dependent, that is, it is visual when the letter is presented visually, it is acoustic for auditory presentations and somesthetic for tactile presentations. The other code is modality-independent and represents the phonological encoding of the letter, irrespetive of the modality in which it is shown.

This view is based on the temporal hierarchy observed in a letter matching paradigm. Basically, Posner found that reaction times to decide whether two visually presented letters are the same or not are faster when the two letters are physically identical (e.g., AA) than when they share only the same name, that is they are the lower- and upper-case versions of the same character (e.g., Aa). When the two letters have the same shape but differ in size (e.g., Cc), the latencies for matching them are longer than those for physical identity matches but shorter than those for name identity matches. This finding has proved extremely stable and has been replicated in a number of studies.

The temporal hierarchy of response latencies is attributed to the different codes by which the matching operation can be executed. When the two letters are physically identical they can be correctly classified as same on the basis of the visual code. Matches for pairs of letters that have identical shapes but different sizes are based on the visual code but require a time-consuming operation of normalization. In other words, the existence of a size difference extends the time for the visual match because the size of the visual representation of at least one of the letters must be changed. Matches for pairs of letters that have different shapes occur on the basis of the modality-independent phonological code. In this case it is assumed that the visual codes of the two letters contact the phonological information stored in long-term memory, thus extracting the corresponding phonemes. Then the comparison process takes place on the two phonemes retrieved from memory but response latencies reflect the time necessary for this additional operation.

In his first papers Posner (1969) adapted the levels of processing approach to the speeded comparison of letter pairs and proposed

a strictly serial stage model. It is assumed that the letters are
first compared through the visual code and then the successive stages occur only if no match is obtained at this level. At the next higher level the visual representations undergo a process of visual
transformation concerning orientation, if they are disoriented, or
size, if they differ in size. This operation, which requires a measurable amount of time, can yield a match only when the two letters,
though not identical, have the same shape. The highest level of the
hierarchy of stages is that at which the comparison involves the phonological codes. This level is reached only when the two letters share solely their name or when they are different.

A slightly modified version of the serial stage model applied
when the two letters to be compared are shown one after another. It
was assumed that, following the presentation of the first letter, the
temporary visual code is rapidly superseded by the relatively durable
phonological code. Therefore, this version of the model maintained
that, even when the two letters are identical, the comparison involves the phonological code if the inter-stimulus interval is long enough to allow the vanishing of the visual code produced by the first
letter.

More recently, Posner (1978) has given preference to a different
view; that is, the so-called horse race model. The new model maintains that the presentation of the letter gives rise simultaneously
to both the visual and phonological codes. These two codes yield
two isolable processing systems which can be utilized independently
in the comparison. The time courses of the two systems are thought
to be different, thus producing the observed temporal hierarchy of
response latencies. In other words, according to the horse race
model, the visual and phonological codes are used in parallel to
achieve matches but the operations based on the visual code are
usually faster than those based on the phonological code. However,
the notion of the independence of the two systems implies that,
depending on the parameters chosen in a given experiment, the operations based on the visual code may be uniformly faster than those
based on the phonological code, they may overlap, or even the phonological code may be available for yielding a match earlier than the
visual one.

Many studies (see review in Posner, 1978) have supported the
parallel model of letter matching. The critical empirical evidence
corroborating such model concerns the possibility of finding experimental variables which can affect the time course of the operations
based on one code while preserving the time course of those based
on the other. Manipulations of such physical variables as intensity,
size, color, contrast and orientation have usually led to strong effects on visual matches with weaker or no effects at all on phonological matches. Similarly, it has been found that the degree of visual
confusability of the letter set employed and the length of the time

delay between the two comparison letters affect mainly, if not only, physical matches. In contrast, the degree of phonological confusability of the letters which constitute the stimulus set, the number of possible alternatives and the amount of verbal memory load affect only phonological matches.

Even though the evidence in favor of the parallel model seems rather compelling, the notion according to which visually presented letters are matched on the basis of two codes, one visual and the other phonological, whose time courses can be manipulated independently, has recently been challenged. According to Proctor (1981) the two letters are always compared on the basis of the phonological code but the time to extract such code is less for two identical letters than for two letters that have no physical similarity. The advantage of visual over phonological matches would be an instance of the well known priming effect. The visual processing of the first letter favors the visual processing and the retrieval of the phonological code for an identical successive letter, whereas it slows down the same operations for a different letter. As a matter of fact, this model seems well suited for explaining the visual match advantage in the case of successive presentations of the comparison letters but it is difficult to understand how it can account for the same effect in the case of simultaneous presentations.

The tenability of the notion of two independent and isolable systems has also been questioned. Crist (1981) showed that the visual similarity of the letters in the stimulus set had a comparable adverse effect on the speed of both visual and phonological matches. This finding seems simply to suggest that the two systems are less independent than previously thought.

In summary, it can be safely concluded that a visually presented letter yields both a visual and a phonological internal representation and such representations a sufficiently separate to allow a relatively independent manipulation of the time courses of the processes concerning each of them. Hence, the letter matching paradigm introduced by Posner appears to be the best procedure for testing, through the divided visual field method, whether the visual and the phonological codes, and/or the operations based on them, are located in different parts of the brain.

THE STUDY OF HEMISPHERIC SPECIALIZATION THROUGH THE DIVIDED VISUAL FIELD METHOD

Even though there are several more direct methods for studying the functional specializations of the two cerebral hemispheres of the human brain (e. g., the neurospychological testing of brain-damaged and commissurotomy patients; the observation of asymmetries contingent upon cognitive processes in the cerebral blood flow or the electrical cortical activity in normals), the method of channe-

lling sensory information directly to a single hemisphere in normal
subjects is by far the most popular. This method comprises, besides
the divided visual field procedure, the dichotic listening procedure
in the auditory modality (Berlin, 1977; Krashen, 1976), a similar
procedure in the tactile modality (Gardner & Ward, 1979), and also
a slightly different procedure that requires the recording of lateral
eye movements during the execution of cognitive tasks (Ehrlichman
& Weinberger, 1978).

As already pointed out the logic of the divided visual field
procedure is very simple (see, e.g., Young, 1982). It exploits the
arrangement of the human visual system in order to confine visual
stimulation to one single hemisphere, at least initially. Visual
stimuli received at the two right hemiretinae of both eyes are transmitted along the visual pathways directly to the left hemisphere, whereas visual stimuli received at the left hemiretinae are transmitted
directly to the right hemisphere. In other words, stimuli shown to
the right of the current point of fixation reach the cortex of the
left hemisphere, whereas those to the left of fixation reach the right hemisphere. Visual information thus confined initially to one
hemisphere is then conveyed to the other hemisphere along the forebrain commissures, of which the corpus callosum is the most notable
one. Of course, we can be certain that the stimulus is initially
sent to only one hemisphere on condition that fixation is controlled
properly and exposure time does not exceed the latency of a saccadic
eye movement. Critical to the divided visual field method is the
assumption that, when information is effectively restricted to one
visual field, subsequent responses can be referred to the activity
of the contralateral hemisphere.

Although the tendency to attribute any asymmetry, in terms of
speed and/or accuracy of response, between the two visual fields to
an underlying hemispheric specialization is unjustified (White, 1969;
1972), it must be stressed that such basic assumption has proved tenable in the vast majority of the studies. Hence, it is now generally held that an asymmetry in favor of the right field points to a
left hemispheric specialization, whereas a left field advantage points to a right hemispheric specialization. By saying that the above-
mentioned relationship between visual field asymmetries and hemispheric specialization has gained wide acceptance, I do not mean to imply
that there is also an adequate model for explaining it. It is worth
stressing that, in fact, we observe differences in speed and accuracy
of response between the visual fields and from them we make inferences concerning hemispheric specialization. The divided visual field
method, as any other purely behavioral method, does not allow a direct assessment of hemispheric specialization.

The models proposed in order to explain how hemispheric specialization yields visual asymmetries fall mainly into two classes. There are structural and attentional models and of both classes exist

several versions. Since they have been discussed in detail by Cohen (1982) here only the three most widely accepted among them will be outlined.

All structural models assume that performance is superior when the hemisphere directly accessed through the contralateral field is the locus of the neural structures specialized for the kind of processing required by the task. The absolute specialization version makes the further assumption that lateralization of a given function is complete. That is, only the hemisphere specialized for that function can perform it. Hence, the difference in speed of response between the two visual fields represents the time taken for information to be transmitted across the forebrain commissures when the stimulus is presented to the field corresponding to the nonspecialized hemisphere. This model has been challenged on the ground that the observed differences are too large if compared with the estimates of interhemispheric transmission time obtained by neurophysiological and behavioral methods (Berlucchi, 1972). Furthermore, the field asymmetries are not limited to response latency but concern also accuracy. However, as Berlucchi (1972) has convincingly argued, the interhemispheric crossing postulated by the absolute specialization model is likely to affect negatively the quality of the transmitted information, thus yielding longer transmission times and differences in accuracy between the visual fields.

The relative specialization version of the structural model maintains that cognitive functions are not wholly lateralized to one hemisphere. Both hemispheres can perform a given function but one is more efficient (faster and/or more accurate) than the other. According to this model, a stimulus is always processed by the hemisphere directly accessed through the contralateral field and the differences in speed and/or accuracy beteen the two fields are attributable to a difference in information processing capability between the two hemispheres. In other words, field asymmetries are not due to interhemispheric transmission time but to a difference in the level of efficiency between the specialized and the nonspecialized hemisphere.

The attentional models differ from the structural ones because they postulate that it is the allocation of attention to the sensory domain of one hemisphere that increases the efficiency of information processing within that hemisphere. A very popular version of the attentional model has been proposed by Kinsbourne (1970; 1975). It assumes that expectancy for verbal stimuli yields a greater activation of the left hemisphere, whereas expectancy for visuospatial stimuli yields a greater activation of the right hemisphere. Such unbalanced activation of the specialized hemisphere induces an attentional shift and a perceptual bias in favor of the stimuli presented to the corresponding visual field, thus optimizing processing efficiency in that field. In some sense, Kinsbourne's model locates field asymmetries at a more peripheral stage than other models do.

Even if the role of hemispheric specialization in bringing about the
differences in speed and/or accuracy between the two visual fields is
not denied, those differences are attributed to a bias in the orientation of attention which favors the stimuli shown in the field connected directly to the specialized hemisphere.

The foregoing sketchy presentation no doubt fail to do justice
to the complexity of the three models which have gone some distance
in linking field assymmetries to hemispheric specialization. However-
er, the kind of summary that has been attempted had the main purpose
of stressing the fact that, when a difference between the visual fields is obtained, a great deal of caution is required before jumping
to conclusions about hemispheric specialization. What is important
is to keep in mind that the divided visual field method provides a
quite indirect assessment of the lateralization of cognitive functions and any theory based solely on it is likely to go well beyond
the evidence which is at present available.

THE ROLE OF HEMISPHERIC SPECIALIZATION IN PROCESSING THE VISUAL AND
THE PHONOLOGICAL CODES

The following general conclusions seem to be justified in view
of what has been said so far.

1) The different functional specializations of the two cerebral hemispheres of the human brain are interpretable in terms of a verbal/
visuospatial dichotomy. That is, in right-handed people the left hemisphere carries out the analysis of verbal stimuli better (i.e.,
faster and more accurate responses) than the right, whereas the right hemisphere has better performances than the left for visuospatial
processing. Within the framework of this dichotomy it has been established that phonological encoding and processing are likely to be
the most lateralized among the functions that characterize the specialized activity of the left hemisphere (see, E.g., Moscovitch,1979).
There is also a tendency to describe the left hemisphere as a sequential,serial, temporal or analytic processor and the right hemisphere as
a parallel, gestalt or holistic processor (see Bradshaw & Nettleton,
1981, for a comprehensive review). While those dichotomies are consistent with some of evidence existing in the literature, the verbal/
visuospatial one is still the most accepted. Moreover, none of the
proposed alternative dichotomies denies the superiority of the left
hemisphere for verbal processing and the superiority of the right hemisphere for visuospatial processing. Their main aim is to give a
more basic account than that allowed by the well established verbal/
spatial distinction of the way the two hemispheres process information.

2) A visually presented letter gives rise to both a visual code and
a relatively independent phonological code. These two codes yield
two different and isolable systems which can be utilized for processing the letter. In a letter classification task, two identical

letters take less time to be matched than two letters that have the
same shape but differ in size or orientation, which in turn are matched faster than two letters that share only the same name. It is
assumed that in the first case (physical matches) the letters are compared on the basis of the visual code. In the second case (analogue
matches) they are compared on the basis of the visual code after a
time-consuming operation of normalization. In the third case (name
matches) the process of comparison involves the phonological code
whose retrieval from memory takes a measurable amount of time.

3) Although a note of caution is in order, it seems well established
that the divided visual field method allows a reliable assessment of
the side of hemispheric specialization in normal subjects. In choice
reaction time tasks, faster and/or more accurate performance for stimuli shown in the right visual field indicates a left hemispheric specialization, whereas an asymmetry in favor of the left visual field
indicates a right hemispheric specialization.

    Assuming that the three preceding points depict correctly the
available evidence, we should expect an advantage of the right visual
field for letter matches based on the phonological code and an advantage of the left visual field when the letters are matched through
the visual code. The results of those studies that have employed the
divided visual field method in speeded letter matching tasks, where
physical, analogue and name matches could occur, will be summarized
in the last part of the present paper.

A) Name Matches: When the two letters have different shapes and
thus can be correctly classified as same solely on the basis of their
common phonological code a right visual field superiority has almost
always been reported (Cohen, 1972; Davis & Schmit, 1973; Geffen, Bradshaw & Nettleton, 1972; Hellige, 1976; Hellige, Cox & Litvac, 1979;
Ledlow, Swanson & Kinsbourne, 1978; Niederbhul & Springer, 1979; Segalowitz & Stewart, 1979; Simion, Bagnara,Bisiacchi, Roncato & Umiltà, 1980; Umiltà, Sava & Salmaso, 1980). This was true even when vertical presentations were employed in order to avoid the effect of
post-exposural scanning strategies. The only study that apparently
stands against this general agreement (Salmaso & Umiltà, 1982) can
in fact be considered confirmatory of the phonological nature of name
matches. In that study only vowels were used and no visual field asymmetry was found in one experiment, while a left visual field advantage was found in the other in which script-like visually rather complex characters were shown. These findings were explained by assuming that, as suggested by dichotic listening studies (see reviews
in Krashen, 1976; Springer, 1977), the phonological features of vowel
sounds, as opposed to those of other speech sounds like stops and fri-
catives, are amenable both to right and left hemispheric processing.
In the case of script-like stimuli, the better ability of the right
hemisphere to process complex visuospatial material emerged at the
level of visual encoding and then produced an advantage for the right

hemisphere also at the successive stage of phonological processing, which per se was not lateralized (for a discussion of the notion of transmitted lateralization see Moscovitch, 1979).

When there is a sufficiently long delay between the two letters of the pair, the visual code is replaced by the phonological code and thus the comparison is thought to take place through the latter even if the two letters are identical. Accordingly, in this condition a right field advantage has been reported (Kirsner, 1979; Wilkins & Stewart, 1974). Converging evidence comes also from studies that required phonological processing in the framework of a different experimental paradigm (Moscovitch, 1973; Umiltà, Frost & Hyman, 1972). For example, when the letters to be discriminated differed, when pronounced only in the consonant sound there was a right field superiority, whereas the asymmetry reversed if the letters could be discriminated only by the vowel sound.

In conclusion, all the existing evidence points clearly to a preferential involvement of the left hemisphere in processing the phonological code. However, even in this case a note of caution does not seem out of place. According to the dual coding model two different letters, that is two letters with a different name, can be correctly classified solely on the basis of the phonological code (Posner, 1969; 1978). In spite of this, the predicted advantage of the right visual field for "different" responses has proved elusive and some studies have found no lateral asymmetry (Hellige, 1976) or even a left field superiority (Davis & Schmit, 1973; Geffen et al., 1972). No explanation is presently available for such discrepancies.

B) Physical matches: When the two letters are identical they are matched by the visual code. The results of such physical matches were much less reliable than those for name matches and every possible outcome is reported in the literature. Some studies have shown a superior performance in the left visual field (Cohen, 1972; Davis & Schmit, 1973; Geffen et al., 1972), while others have found no asymmetry (Ledlow et al., 1978; Segalowitz & Stewart, 1979; Simion et al., 1980; Umiltà et al., 1980) or a right field superiority (Simion et al., 1980). When a very short delay was introduced between the two letters, and thus the visual code was still available for performing the match, Wilkins and Stewart (1974) found no asymmetry and Kirsner (1979) an advantage for the left field.

The failure to demonstrate a reliable right hemisphere superiority for matches based on the visual code is in agreement with Moscovitch's (1979) hypothesis of an equal ability of the two hemispheres to conduct simple visuospatial processing. The right hemispheric specialization could manifest itself, according to this notion, only when the task requires higher-order spatial processing capabilities. This seems quite reasonable since both hemispheres are no doubt equally involved in the early stages of visual analysis, whereas it is well established that the right hemisphere plays a preponderant role in analysing complex spatial material. Some indication that the superiority of the left visual field depends on the visual complexity of the stimuli can be found in two studies (Umiltà et al., 1980; Salmaso & Umiltà, 1982) in which physical matches were obtained with both simple print-like letters and complex script-like letters. The former showed no field asymmetry, whereas the latter yielded a clear-cut superiority for the left visual field. On the other hand, in a recent review Davidoff (1982) has aptly pointed out that, even if for simple visual tasks reliability is not common, when asymmetry is observed it is usually in favor of the left field.

To sum up, the safest conclusion to date seems to be that the visual code is processed equally easily by both hemispheres. However, much additional evidence is required before such notion can rest on a firmer ground.

c) Analogue matches: Only one study (Simion et al., 1980) has dealt with the lateralization of the normalization processes performed on the visual code when the two letters have the same shape but differ in either size or orientation. The hypothesis was that the three operations involving the visual code (i.e., rotation, size normalization and visual comparison) should have brought about an advantage for the left visual field. This view is usually held on the basis of the results of two studies (Bradshaw, Bradley & Patterson, 1976; Cohen, 1975) that have presented some evidence indicating a left field superiority for mental rotations. However, there seems to be no theoretical or empirical justification for likening mental rotations, which involve the generation of a visual image, to the operations of normalization that take place automatically on the visual code (see Simion, Bagnara, Roncato & Umiltà, 1982, for a discussion of this distinction). In fact, the Simion et al's (1980) study did not show any laterality effect for analogue matches which required a transformation of both size and orientation. When the two letters differed only in size, there was a right field superiority in one experiment and no asymmetry in another.

In conclusion, it would seem that visual normalization processes pertain to the domain of those simple, lower-order visuospatial functions for which, according to Moscovitch's (1979) suggestion, no hemispheric specialization exists. It is apparent, however, that this is a very tentative conclusion since a few experiments do not allow to go any distance toward a sound assessment of laterality effects.

REFERENCES

Beaumont, J. G. Studies with verbal stimuli. In J. G. Beaumont

(Ed.), Divided visual field studies of cerebral organization.
    London: Academic Press, 1982.
Berlin, C. I. Hemispheric asymmetry in auditory tasks. In S. Harnard
    et al. (Eds.), Lateralization in the nervous system. London:
    Academic Press, 1977.
Berlucchi, G. Anatomical and physiological aspects of visual funct-
    ions of the corpus callosum. Brain Research, 1972, 37, 371-392.
Bradshaw, J. L. and Nettleton, N. C. The nature of hemispheric spe-
    cialization in man. The Behavioral and Brain sciences, 1981,
    4, 51-93.
Bradshaw, J. L., Bradley, D. and Patterson, K. The perception and
    identification of mirror reversed patterns. Quarterly Journal
    of Experimental Psychology, 1976, 28, 221-246.
Cohen, G. Hemisphere differences in a letter classification task.
    Perception and Psychophysics, 1972, 11, 139-142.
Cohen, G. Hemispheric differences in the utilization of advance in-
    formation. IN P. M. A. Rabbitt and S. Dornic (Eds.), Attention
    and performance V. London: Academic Press, 1975.
Cohen, G. Theoretical interpretations of lateral asymmetries. In
    J. G. Beaumont (Ed.), Divided visual field studies of cerebral
    organization. London: Academic Press, 1982.
Crist, W. B. Matching performance and the similarity structure of
    the stimulus set. Journal of Experimental Psychology: General,
    1981, 10, 269-295.
Davidoff, J. Studies with non-verbal stimuli. In J. G. Beaumont
    (Ed.), Divided visual field studies of cerebral organization.
    London: Academic Press, 1982.
Davis, R. and Schmit, V. Visual and verbal coding in the interhemi-
    spheric transfer of information. Acta Psychologica, 1973, 37,
    229-240.
Ehrlichman, H. and Weinberger, A. Lateral eye movements and hemis-
    pheric asymmetry: A critical review. Psychological Bulletin,
    1978, 85, 1080-1101.
Gardner, E. B. and Ward, A. W. Spatial compatibility in tactile-vis-
    ual discrimination. Neuropsychologia, 1979, 17, 421-425.
Geffen, G., Bradshaw, J. L. and Nettleton, N. C. Hemispheric asymme-
    try: verbal and spatial encoding of visual stimuli. Journal
    of Experimental Psychology, 1972, 95, 25-31.
Hellige, J. B. Changes in same-different laterality patterns as a
    function of practice and stimulus quality. Perception and
    Psychophysics, 1976, 20, 267-273.
Hellige, J. B., Cox, P. J. and Litvac, L. Information processing in
    the cerebral hemispheres: Selective hemispheric activation and
    capacity limitations. Journal of Experimental Psychology: Gene-
    ral, 1979, 108, 251-279.
Kinsbourne, M. The cerebral basis of lateral asymmetries in atten-
    tion. Acta Psychologica, 1970, 33, 193-201.
Kinsbourne, M. The mechanism of hemispheric control of the lateral
    gradient of attention. In P.M.A. Rabbitt and S. Dornic (Eds.),
    Attention and Performance V, London: Academic Press, 1975

Kirsner, K. Hemispheric differences in recognition memory for lett-
    ers. Bulletin of the Psychonomic Society, 1979, 13, 2-4.
Krashen, S. D. Cerebral asymmetry. IN H. Whitaker and H. A. Whita-
    ker (Eds.), Studies in Neurolinguistics Vol. 2. New York:
    Academic Press, 1976.
Ledlow, A., Swanson, J. M. and Kinsbourne, M. Reaction times and
    evoked potentials as indicators of hemispheric differences for
    laterally presented name and physical matches. Journal of Ex-
    perimental Psychology: Human Perception and Performance, 1978,
    4, 440-454.
McCusker, L. X., Hillinger, M. L. and Bias, R. G. Phonological reco-
    ding and reading. Psychological Bulletin, 1981, 89, 217-245.
Milner, B. Interhemispheric differences in the location of psycholo-
    gical processes in man. British Medical Bulletin, 1971, 27,
    272-277.
Moscovitch, M. Language and the cerebral hemispheres: Reaction time
    studies and their implications for models of cerebral dominance.
    In P. Pliner et al. (Eds.), Communication and Affect: Language
    and thought London: Acadmeic Press, 1973.
Moscovitch, M. Information processing and the cerebral hemispheres.
    In M. S. Gazzaniga (Ed.), Handbook of Behavioral Neurobiology,
    Vol. 2: Neuropsychology. New York: Plenum Press, 1979.
Niederbuhl, J. and Springer, S. P. Task requirements and hemisphere
    asymmetry for the processing of single letters. Neuropsycholo-
    gia, 1979, 17, 689-692.
Posner, M. I. Abstraction and the process of recognition. In G.
    Bower and J. T. Spence (Eds.), The psychology of learning and
    motivation, Vol. 3. London: Academic Press, 1969.
Posner, M. I. Chronometric exploration of mind. Hillsdale, N. J.:
    Erlbaum, 1978.
Proctor, R. W. A unified theory for matching-task phenomena. Psy-
    chological Review, 1981, 88, 291-326.
Salmaso, D. and Umiltà, C. Vowel processing in the left and right
    visual fields. Brain and Language, 1982, 16, 147-157.
Segalowitz, S. J. and Stewart, C. Left and right lataralization for
    letter matching: Strategy and sex differences. Neuropsycholo-
    gia, 1979, 17, 521-525.
Simion, F., Bagnara, S., Bisiacchi, P., Roncato, S. Umiltà, C. Late-
    rality effects, levels of processing, and stimulus properties.
    Journal of Experimental Psychology: Human perception and Perfo-
    rmance, 1980, 6, 184-195.
Simion, F., Bagnara, S., Roncato, S. and Umiltà, C. Transformation
    processes upon the visual code. Perception and Psychophysics,
    1982, 31, 13-25.
Springer, S. P. Tachistoscopic and dichotic listening investigations
    of laterality in normal human subjects. In S. Harnard et al.
    (Eds.), Lateralization in the nervous system, New York: Acade-
    mic press, 1977.
Umiltà, C., Frost, N. and Hyman, R. Interhemispheric effects on ch-
    oice reaction time in one-, two- and three-letter displays.

    Journal of Experimental Psychology, 1972, 93, 198-204.

Umiltà, C., Sava, D. and Salmaso, D. Hemispheric asymmetries in a
    letter classification task with different typefaces. Brain and
    Language, 1980, 9, 171-181.

White, M. J. Laterality differences in perception: A review. Psycho-
    logical Bulletin, 1969, 72, 387-405.

White, M. J. Hemispheric asymmetries in tachistoscopic information
    processing. British Journal of Psychology, 1972, 63, 497-508.

Wilkins, A. and Stewart, A. The time course of lateral asymmetries
    in visual perception of letters. Journal of Experimental Psycho-
    logy, 1974, 102, 905-908.

Young, A. W. Methodological and theoretical bases of visual hemifield
    studies. IN J. G. Beaumont (ed.), Divided visual field studies
    of cerebral organization. London: Academic Press, 1982.

THE IMPORTANCE OF GRAPHEME - TO - PHONEME
CONVERSION RULES IN BEGINNING READERS

Francisco Valle Arroyo
Dept. of Psychology
University of Oviedo
Oviedo, Spain

This paper is an attempt at studying reading processes from a developmental point of view. It might very well be the case that the reading processes used by beginning readers are completely different from those of adult and experienced readers.

Historically three types of reading models have been propounded: phonological, mediated and non-phonological (Massaro, 1975). The first type of model, on the one hand, assumes that adult readers should necessarily convert visual stimuli (letters and words) into phonological codes prior to lexical (semantic) access, while the third argues that good readers never need such a translation; on the other hand, mediated models of reading maintain that adults should have and use both pathways, the difference between the various mediated models being the importance each assigns to these two routes. Coltheart (1980), among many others, based on rational grounds as well as on empirical evidence, assumes that good adult readers must have three different routes for reading, which he call: routes A, B and C, route A being the normal and consequently the most important one in experienced readers, though routes B and C, if less important are still necessary in some situations, for example, reading unknown words and non-words, and solving semantic decision tasks with pseudohomophones. (See Coltheart (1980) for a more detailed account of this standpoint). But the relative importance of these three routes might vary with age and my suspicion is that children who learn to read rely more on grapheme-to-phoneme conversion rules than adults. In other words, children might begin by a necessary translation of visual into acoustic codes (route B) and only at the end of their learning process accomplish reading aloud by a direct route without necessitating such grapheme-to-phoneme conversion (route A). (Route C is out of question here, since we are dealing with real words).

My suspicion is based on theoretical considerations as well as
on empirical findings. The theoretical intuition - as a matter of
fact, Tomatis's (1979) intuition - is that perhaps writing is the
first tape-recording device ever used in the word, the first method
of making speech permanent in time. What I mean is that speech is
earlier in time than writing. When a child begins to read, he already knows how to listen and how to speak. In other words, he
possesses considerable phonological and semantic representations and
knows how to relate them (sound and meaning). What he must learn
when he begins to read is a new representation - the visual one- and
a new system of relating this new code with the pre-existing representations. The relation between the new code and the other two
can theoretically be established in two different ways; either by
connecting the visual representation to the phonological one which
is already connected to the semantic code (route B) or by relating
the visual code with the semantic one, already in connection with
the acoustic code (route A). The view defended here is that the first pathway might be the normal one for beginning readers even when
for adults the other could be - and this seems to be the case - the
most effective and operative. And the reason is this: we spend so
much time learning the correspondences between letters and syllables
and their sounds that the habits acquired during this process should
be operative for some time, at least. As Massaro (1975) puts it,
summarizing the phonological model point of view:

> If somehow the printed symbols on the page could be made to
> speak, all that the young reader would have to do is just
> listen. So why teach him that this particular sequence of
> symbols means one thing and not another if he can learn that
> the sequence of symbols sounds one way and not another ?
> Once he recognizes the sound, the meaning will follow direct-
> ly based on what he already knows. More appealing is the po-
> ssibility that there are fewer printed symbol-sound corres-
> pondences to learn than printed symbol-meaning corresponden-
> ces, (p. 260)

at least in those languages which are almost perfectly phonetic
like Italian, and probably also in such languages as English where
the grapheme-to-phoneme correspondence is not biunivocal, since it
is still possible to formulate a limited set of pronunciation rules
(Wijk, 1966).

The empirical findings come from two different sources of information: 1) from confusion matrices in readers and non-readers
with single letters shown tachistoscopically, and 2) from some copying errors made by eleven children who, according to their teachers, were dyslexic - in fact, they were the worst readers and writers in their classes.

A. CONFUSION MATRIX EXPERIMENT

Here the hypothesis was formulated as follows: if reading consists of learning an acoustic code for a visual representation and if the grapheme-to-phoneme conversion rules are used systematically, then non-readers should make only, or, at least, mainly visual errors, whereas readers would be more prone to make phonetic confusions.

METHOD

Subjects: Three groups of children were used: the Non-reader (NR) group (children of 3 and 4 years of age), the Transition (T) group (5 and 6), and the Reader (R) group (7 and 8 year olds). (Schooling in Spain can begin anywhere from 5:8 to 6:9, depending on which month of the year the child was born). There were ten children in each group, who had been selected - within each group - from a sample of 20 if and only if they had an above-average score in the Frostig test of development of visual perception.

Procedure: Each subject was shown tachistoscopically 2, 3 or 4 letters for a period of time which ranged from 700 msec to 4 sec. The number of letters shown as well as the presentation time were determined in a pilot study. The child had to report the letters shown by writing them down. The idea was that the number of letters to be written outnumbered the child's memory span by one so that confusion errors could be obtained. Even when he/she could not remember the entire set of letters shown he/she required to guess the letter or letters not recalled. The letters reported were compared with the letters shown in the tachistoscope and the result entered in the appropriate cell of the confusion matrix. The criterion used to decide the error type (visual or phonological) was the number of visual (graphic) or phonological (acoustic) features shared by the letters shown and the reported ones. As a matter of fact, for the phonological confusion a composite criterion was employed in which these three factors were taken into account: the phonological features of the letter reported, the number of syllables of the letter name, and the phonological features of the other components of the name of the letter reported; that is, we considered the phonological representation of the letter name instead of the phonological representation of the letter itself. The reason for doing this was that the only possible way to read single letters is by saying their names.

RESULTS

Table 1 shows a summary of the percentage of visual, phonological and mixed errors made by each group. The T group performed in a way not significantly different from the NR group, although there was a decrease in the visual errors and an increase in the phonological confusions as predicted. An analysis of variance was made with the NR and the R groups only, and, at the same time, the

TABLE 1. Percentage of Errors in the three Groups

Error Type	NR	T	R
Visual	78.43	78.20	50.00
Phonetic	7.18	10.25	36.61
Mixed (Visual & Phonetic)	14.37	11.53	15.38

mixed errors were excluded from the analysis, first because of their own problematic nature, and second, because there was no difference whatsoever in the performance of the three groups.

The interaction between the reading level and the type of errors (visual or phonological) made, which constituted the central point of the hypothesis, was statistically significant, $F(1,36)=55.01$, $p < .001$. However, still in the R group the percentage of visual errors was higher than the phonological confusions which might perhaps be explained by the fact that the reading level of the R group was relatively low. Had we had a group with a higher reading efficiency, an inversion in the patterns of results might have been obtained, i.e., a number of phonological errors higher than the visual confusions, as happened in Conrad's [1964] study.

B.   COPYING ERRORS IN CHILDREN

Method and Results: The errors made by eleven children aged from 6:6 to 9:4 have been analyzed, too. These children were the worst readers in their classes, as stated above. They were asked to perform a copying task. The originals presented consisted of: a. the single letters of the Spanish alphabet in random order, b. 22 single words, c. four single sentences, d. a paragraph. As might be expected the error rate was very low; 71 errors in total which represent 3.51% of the total number of words and letters; however, many of these 71 errors, namely 26 (37.14%), resulted in perfect nonsense homophones. Here is a list of some of the errors made. (In parentheses the number of errors made either by the same child or by different children).

NOTES ON SPANISH PHONOLOGY TO EXPLAIN THE COPYING ERRORS

a.   Even though in standard Spanish (Castilian) c, z on the one hand, and s on the other represent different phonemes, in American Spanish and in some parts of spain these letters all represent different graphemes of the same phoneme /s/. In fact, all the errors marked with a were made by the same child who showed the phonological characterstics of American Spanish in his spontaneous speech.
b.   The final "d" in native Spanish speakers tends to be pronounced as "z"/θ/; and therefore those children who copied the original "libertad" as "libertaz" seem to be relying on grapheme-to-phoneme conversion rules more than on a direct lexical access.
c.   The "h" in Spanish is always silent.

Notes	Original	Transcription	Copy	Transcription	Errors
a	cocina	/koˈθina/	cosina	/koˈsina/	(2)
b	libertad	/liberˈtaθ/	libertaz	/liberˈtaθ/	(2)
a	fresa	/ˈfresa/	freza	/ˈfreθa/	(1)
f	cambiar	/kamˈbiar/	canbiar	/kamˈbiar/	(3)
	poco	/ˈpoko/	poquo	/ˈpoko/	(1)
e	devolverlo	/debolˈberlo/	debras-barlo	/debrasˈbarlo/	(1)
f	hombre	/ˈombre/	honbre	/ˈombre/	(2)
f	bombon	/bamˈbon/	bonbon	/bamˈbon/	(3)
q		/k/	qu	/ku/ (letter name)	
	cerca	/ˈθerka/	cerqua	/ˈθerka/	(1)
c, f	hambre	/ˈambre/	ambre	/ˈambre/	(1)
f	temprano	/temˈprano/	tenprano	/temˈprano/	(2)
d	seguir	/seˈgir/	segir	/seˈxir/	(1)
d	protegia	/proteˈxia/	proteguia	/proteˈgia/	(1)
e	devolverlo	/debolˈberlo/	devorbelo	/devorˈbelo/	(1)
	llamaba	/ʎaˈmaba/	llamada	/ʎaˈmada/	(1)
	decidir	/deθiˈdir/	decicir	/deθiˈθir/	(1)
f	cambio	/ˈkambio/	canbio	/ˈkambio/	(1)
g	llevo	/ˈʎebo/	yevo	/ˈdʒebo/	(1)

d.   The writing of "seguir" as "segir" and "protegia" as "proteguia" are the two faces of the same coin. The "g" in Spanish can have two pronunciations, either as /g/ or as /x/. It is pronounced /g/ when followed by "a", "o" or "u", and as /x/ when it precedes "i" or "e", but in this latter case it returns to the occlusive pronunciation if a "u" intervenes; i. e., "seguir" is pronounced as /segir/ but "regir" as /rexir/. So the child who made the error of writing "segir" instead of "seguir", and the one who wrote "proteguia" instead of "protegia" are using the grapheme-to-phoneme conversion rules, but in an inappropriate way; they have not completely mastered the rule.

e.   Spanish-speaking people do not make any difference in the pronunciation of "b" and "v". Both are sounded as /b/.

f.   In Spanish it is compulsory to write "m" - to represent a nasal consonant - before "p" and "b". But if a perfect reader finds "n" before "p" or "b", he/she will pronounce it in exactly the same way

as if "m" had been written, and would know that the writer made an
orthographic error.
g.   For many Spaniards "ll" and "y" may have the same pronunciation
/dʒ/ or something close to it, when they precede a vowel. That is
why writing "llevo" as "yevo" is a pseudohomophone.

DISCUSSION

The results from both studies seem to corroborate the importance grapheme-to-phoneme conversion rules have in the beginning reader. Neither in the confusion matrix experiment nor in the copying
task was route B required; -(remember that the important point, here,
is route B since C is also postulated to account for adults' ability
to read non-words, but this was not the case in these tasks)- the
results, however, are difficult to explain unless one admits that
children are using such a route. In both situations adult readers,
according to Marshall's or Coltheart's models (this volume), are
supposed to use the direct route and, at most, visual errors would
be expected. Of course, there were some graphic confusions, but, as
stated previously, most of them were phonological and, consequently
there is some empirical indication that children might predominantly
use the grapheme-to-phoneme conversion strategy even in those situations in which such a strategy might be useless for adults. This
idea is not completely new. Coltheart (1980), after discussing the
effects of articulatory suppression on reading capacity, concludes
by saying that suppression of articulation has no effect on the reading comprehension of skilled readers and states that "it might be
another story with children or poor readers" (p. 215). The results,
although they might suggest that beginning readers do not use the
direct route as frequently as adults do, do not tell us whether the
grapheme-to-phoneme conversion is pre-lexical or post-lexical. I
believe that this conversion is pre-lexical, but the experimental
design has to be changed if such a question is to be answered.

REFERENCES

Coltheart, M. Reading, phonological reading, and deep dyslexia. In
       M. Coltheart, K. Patterson and J. Marshall (eds.), Deep Dysle-
       xia, London: Routledge and Kegan Paul, 1980.
Conrad, R. Acoustic confusions in immediate memeory. British Jour-
       nal of Psychology, 1964, 55, 75-84
Massaro, D. W. Understanding Language: An Information-Processing
       Analysis of Speech Perception, Reading and Psycholinguistics,
       New York: Academic Press, 1975.
Tomatis, A. A. Educación y Dislexia, Madrid:CEPE, 1979.
Wijk, A. Rules of pronunciation for the English language, London:
       Oxford University Press, 1966

HYPERLEXIA : DEVELOPMENTAL READING WITHOUT MEANING

Dorothy M. Aram   Douglas F. Rose   Samuel J. Horwitz
Departments of Pediatrics and Neurology
Case Western Reserve University
Rainbow Babies and Children Hospital
Cleveland, Ohio

INTRODUCTION

Children with precocious reading ability despite profound cognitive and language disorders have been described at least as early as 1917, referred to as idiot savants (Parker, 1917; Phillips, 1930) or as a variant of developmental psychoses (Cain, 1969; Goodman, 1972). Initially, referred to as "hyperlexia" by Silberberg and Silberberg (1967, 1968, 1971), several reports have appeared within the past fifteen years further documenting these children's atypical cognitive and reading development (deHirsch, 1971; Elliott & Needleman, 1976; Goodman, 1972; Huttenlocher & Huttenlocher, 1973; Mehegan & Dreifus, 1972; and Richman & Kitchell, 1981). Recently Healy, Aram, Horwitz and Kessler (1982) studied a group of 12 hyperlexic children concluding that these children present an identifiable syndrome characterized by early and advanced word recognition skills coupled with serious language disorders, especially in comprehending meaning. Further, a strong family history for reading disorders especially in males was demonstrated.

The present paper provides a detailed study of the reading abilities of a hyperlexic individual who is now an adult, and relates this developmental reading disorder to acquired forms seen in adults. This case study exemplifies a developmental ability to establish grapheme-phoneme correspondence rules, and to a lesser but striking degree, direct print to sound associations despite a marked deficiency with meaningful associations.

CASE HISTORY

MD is a 39 year old white male, predominantly right-handed

although he performs some nonlearned tasks such as wiping dishes
and opening doors with his left hand. He is the only son of a
retired violist with the Cleveland and Pittsburgh Symphony Orchest-
ras and is living currently in a group home for retarded adults.
Repeated WAIS results place his measured IQ in the 60 range, although
functionally he is judged to be somewhat lower. He spends his day
at a sheltered workshop for the retarded, has been an apprentice
to a piano tuner and is an accomplished pianist. Each spring he
gives a recital in a local fine arts school where in 1982 he played
Beethoven's Sonata in E^b Major, Mendelssohn's Rondo-Capriccioso,
and with his piano teacher, Mozart's two-piano Concerto in F Major.
In addition to his highly developed technical accomplishments in
piano, he possesses several "idiot savant-like" skills including
date calculating (i.e., given a specific date he will give the day
of the week on which the date falls) and spelling backwards words
up to 12 letters in length.

His birth history was uncomplicated. Regarding developmental
history, gross motor development was late-normal with sitting at
8 months and walking at $14\frac{1}{2}$ months. He used a few single words at
15 months but these disappeared shortly thereafter. At 2 years,
9 months, he was hospitalised at University Hospitals in Cleveland
with a chief complaint of absent speech. During that admission he
was noted to repeat words, but to use no spontaneous meaningful
speech and no articulated consonants. He was reported in the medical chart to have been able to repeat the alphabet and to sing, without words but with perfect pitch, over 100 songs including 1940's
popular songs (e.g., Ramona), classical passages, and the Star
Spangled Banner. During that hospitalization he was diagnosed as
autistic and then began a long series of special school placements
including an inpatient residential treatment program in Pennsylvania.
By $4\frac{1}{2}$ years, MD was reading license plates and street names but
until $7\frac{1}{2}$ or 8 years, his only meaningful speech consisted of a-a
for mama and a-e for daddy. Not until 8 years of age did MD begin
to articulate consonants.

Medical history is negative including family history for reading and other developmental problems. EEG's have been performed
on at least 3 occasions, in 1945, 1949 and most recently in September of 1982, and all have been normal. A pneumoencephalogram at
$5\frac{1}{2}$ years of age was reported to be normal and a recent CT scan performed in September 1982 likewise was interpreted as normal, although
a mildly dilated left lateral ventricle was noted. Other than the
behavioral manifestations of poor eye contact, some rocking, hyper-
ventilation and repeated smelling of objects, the clinical neurological findings have been negative.

A summary of language testing revealed current performance on
most lexical or syntactic comprehension tests to fall at or below a
4 or 5 year level. For example, the Peabody Picture Vocabulary

Test (Dunn, 1965) resulted in a 5-year, 10-month age equivalent, and syntactic comprehension using the Northwestern Syntax Screening Test : Receptive (Lee, 1969) was at a 4 year level. Token Test (Di Simoni, 1978) results revealed no difficulty with retention of concrete perceptually-based information, as MD correctly completed all 40 items in the first 4 subtests. On Part 5 of the Token Test MD correctly carried out only 6/21 items, falling somewhat below a 4 year level using the Simoni norms for children.

Expressively, MD uses very little spontaneous language and does not sustain conversation. He does, however, answer questions with brief one or two-word responses and also uses a considerable amount of stereotyped connected phrases, such as "You are my teacher; Next time you will know," "Keep these in order," "You must think first," "Cover your mouth when you yawn." On the expressive portion of the Northwestern Syntax Screening Test (Lee, 1969), MD scored at approximately a $3\frac{1}{2}$ year level, although his expressive language would be judged atypical of any stage of normal development. MD is able to repeat sentences with elementary structure but can not repeat most complex syntactic structures, and has almost no ability to identify semantically anomolous sentences or to identify and correct agrammatic sentences (Dennis & Whitaker, 1976). He is able, however, to repeat 6 digits forward and backward consistently and often 7.

Results of formal reading tests demonstrate the marked discrepancy between his ability to read meaningful and non-meaningful words and his very limited comprehension (Table 1). His performance on the Woodcock Reading Mastery Tests (Woodcock, 1973) is as follows. Letter Identification is virtually perfect, failing only to recognise a cursive Q referring to it as a "2". MD was able to correctly read 123 of 150 of meaningful words, scoring at a 5th grade level. Word Attack, in which he was required to read non-meaningful words, was also almost perfect, his only error being reading cigbet as kigbet. In contrast, Word Comprehension in which he was required to read and complete frames such as boy-girl; man-_____, or red-stop, green-_____, was considerably depressed. Finally, Passage Comprehension was almost non-existent except for a few of the initial items where picture cues were provided, (e.g., The duck is swimming in the _____, written next to a picture of a duck swimming in a pond). Results on the Woodcock-Johnson Psycho-Educational Battery (Woodcock, Johnson, 1977) were closely comparable with high ability to read both meaningful and especially non-meaningful words, but very limited ability to comprehend passages.

RESULTS OF EXPERIMENTAL READING TASKS

A series of experimental reading tasks were administered to compare directly MD's ability: (1) to read orally words versus his lexical/semantic knowledge of the same word; (2) to read orally both orthographically regular and exception words; and (3) to use stress

TABLE I. Performance on standardized reading tests

	Number correct	Grade Level
Woodcock Reading Mastery Tests		
Letter Identification	44/45	6.2
Word Identification	123/150	5.0
Word Attack (cigbet-> kigbet)	49/50	12.9
Word Comprehension	24/70	2.8
Passage Comprehension	7/85	1.9
Woodcock Johnson Psycho-Educational Battery		
Letter-Word Identification	38/54	6.5
Word Attack	22/26	11.0
Passage Comprehesnion	9/26	2.0

to mark semantic/syntactic contrasts in his oral reading.

Oral Reading Versus Lexical/Semantic Knowledge

To demonstrate further the discrepancy between oral reading and lexical-semantic comprehension, a number of tasks were administered to compare directly words read versus words understood. The first 100 items of the Peabody Picture Vocabulary Test (PPVT) (Dunn, 1965) were administered in three conditions. First in the standard form, that is, the word was presented auditorily and MD was required to indicate by pointing at the one of four pictures representing the spoken word. A month later the task was repeated having MD orally read the word and then indicate his choice; and finally, on a third session, MD was asked to read orally the 100 items which were simul- taneously transcribed by 2 examiners and taped to resolve any dis- agreements in transcription. Table 2 gives his comparative perfor- mance in these three conditions. For the first 50 items, there was little difference between the conditions. His errors in auditory and reading comprehension were virtually identical, except that he correctly identified eagle when presented with the written word, but not when the word was presented auditorilly. He correctly read all but three of these 50 items, self-correcting all three when asked to "try again." For the second 50 items on the PPVT, notable differ- ences emerged with 17/50 and 19/50 items identified correctly on the auditory and reading comprehension tasks respectively. Only 12 items were correctly selected in both auditory and reading compre- hension tasks. Because of the 25% chance of correctly guessing the right answer on the PPVT, he appeared to have truly comprehended no more than these 12 items. In contrast, he orally read correctly 37/50 items. The words correctly read are listed in Table 2 with

TABLE 2.   PPVT: First 50 Items

	Auditory Comprehension	Reading Comprehension	Oral Reading
Number correct	45/50	46/50	47/50
Errors	kangaroo goggles peacock freckle eagle	kangaroo goggles peacock freckle	tying->trying* weiner->winner* tumble->trouble*

PPVT: Items 51-100

| Number correct | 17/50 | 19/50 | 37/50 |

*self corrected on second attempt

TABLE 3.   PPVT: Items 51-100

Printed Word	Orally Read As	Error
*stadium	-sediəm	/t/ omission
bereavement	-brívmənt	/ə/ omission
excavate	-ɛksɪvaɪt	/k/ omission or c->s
submerge	-sʌbmədʒə	stress error
*hassock	-hæzák	stress; s->z
kayak	-keyɪk	ai->e
canine	-kɛɪnɪn	ai->ɪ
confining	-kənfɪnɪŋ	ai->ɪ
precipitaion	-prəkɪpɪteʃən	c->k/s
ceremony	-kɛrəmonɪ	c->k/s
amphibian	-æmpibiən	ph->p/f
chemist	-ʃəmɪst	ch->tʃ and artic. error
meringue	-mɛrɪndʒu	segmentation; g->dʒ

*correct in both auditory and reading comprehension

an asterisk by those items correctly identified in both the auditory and reading comprehension tasks.

MD's oral reading errors on the last 50 items are listed in Table 3. Some of the errors (stadium->sediəm; bereavement->brivmənt) appear to be errors of consonant or syllable omissions, possibly on an articulatory basis. <u>Excavate</u>, read as ɛksɪvaɪt, could be viewed as either an error of omission in which the /k/ was omitted, or the <u>c</u> may have been read as an /s/. Stress errors frequently

occur in MD's reading and these were noted on submerge->súbmerge and
hassock->hæzák, which also includes an error of voicing of the /s/.
The next three errors were vowel errors. He then produced two errors
in which a soft c was read as /k/, thereby producing prekipitation/
precipitation and keremony/ceremony. Chemist becomes semist in which
he appears to have read ch as /tṣ/ but through an articulatory error
dropped the /t/. Amphibian was read as æmpibiən. Meringue was read
as mɛrɪn dʒu, which appears to be the result of a segmentation error
and reading g as /dʒ/.

To further examine MD's discrepant oral reading and lexical/
semantic knowledge, a task developed by Schwartz, Saffran and Marin
(1980) for thier patient WLP, was administered, expanding their procedures to include a lexical decision task. Schwartz, Saffran and
Marin used a group of high frequency (defined as greater than 30
occurrences per million using Thorndike and Lorge word count) and
low frequency (less than 6 occurrences per million) animal names,
color names and body parts, and asked their subject to read the word
orally and then indicate if the word was an animal, color or body
part. This was followed by a picture identification task.

A lexical decision task was presented first, using the 80 animal, color and body part words as real word stimuli, with 80 parallel
nonword forms constructed by changing the vowel for all items except
bull, which required a vowel addition to form boull, because all
single vowel changes resulted in meaningful words. MD was given the
stack of 160 randomized words and nonwords all typed individually
on index cards and was asked to sort the cards into stacks labeled
word and not word. The results are presented in Table 4. MD was
able to correctly select 60/80 of the real words as words, demonstrating considerably more than chance recognition of words versus non-
words. As can be seen at the bottom of Table 4, his ability to identify "wordness" was clearly a function of word frequency. The only
high frequency word he did not correctly identify as a word was bull,
calling it a nonword. His performance for the low frequency words
appears to be category dependent, having fairly good success with
animals, slightly less success with body parts and much difficulty
with color names.

Next MD was given a randomized stack of cards each printed with
a single animal, body part or color word and was asked to again put
these in stacks labeled animal, body part and color. Results as given
in Table 5 again are frequency-dependent, having only one error for
high frequency words (tongue erroneously placed in the animal category). For low frequency words he was 80% correct for animals, 70%
correct for body parts, but only 10% correct for low frequency
colors.

Finally, MD read orally and selected the picture referent for
all animal, body part and color words. Again, this was highly

TABLE 4.   Lexical Decision

		Non words	Words
Words		20	60
Non-Words		60	20

		Words Correctly	Words Incorrectly
Animals			
high freq.	(N=20)	19	1 (bull)
low freq.	(N=20)	13	7
Body Parts			
high freq.	(N=10)	10	0
low freq.	(N=10)	6	4
Color Names			
high freq.	(N=10)	10	0
low freq.	(N=10)	2	8

TABLE 5.   Matching to Category Label

		Animal	Body Part	Color
Animal Names				
high freq.	(N=20)	20	0	0
low freq.	(N=20)	16	4	0
Body Parts				
high freq.	(N=10)	1	9	0
low freq.	(N=10)	3	7	0
Color Names				
high freq.	(N=10)	0	0	10
low freq.	(N=10)	7	2	1

dependent on word frequency with all high frequency colors matched
to the referent and orally read correctly, all 10 body parts read
correctly with only heel being misidentified, and only one animal
name misread, bi*/bear (refer to Table 6). MD's performance on low
frequency body parts and color words is given in Table 7. All but
2 low frequency body parts were read correctly with torso read as
t*so, and abdómen stressed on the second syllable, an alternate but
acceptable form. The only body parts correct in all three lexical/

TABLE 6. High frequency Animals, Body Parts, and Colors

| | Number Correct | |
	Matching to Picture	Oral Reading
Animals	14/20*	19/20***
Body Parts	9/10**	10/10
Colors	10/10	10/10

*misidentified: bull, deer, dog, eagle, lion, deer
**misidentified: heel
***read bear-> biɤ

TABLE 7. Low Frequency

Body Parts	Lexical Decision	Match to Category Label	Match to Picture	Oral Reading
Abdomen	NW	animal		ӕbdɔ́mən
Ankle			X	
Chin				
Elbow			X	
Hip			X	
Kidney	NW		X	
Thigh	NW	animal	X	
Thumb			X	
Torso	NW	animal	X	tɔ́ɪso
Wrist				
Number correct	6/10	7/10	3/10	8/10

Colors

	Lexical Decision	Match to Category Label	Match to Picture	Oral Reading
Amber	NW	animal		
Auburn	NW	animal		əbɤ́n
Beige		animal		
Crimson	NW	animal	magenta	
Ebony	NW	body part	maroon	ɛbóní
Fuchsia	NW	body part	beige	
Lavender		animal	peach	
Magenta	NW	animal	yellow-orange	magɛntə
Maroon	NW			maɪun
Turqoise	NW	animal	orange	
Number correct	2/10	1/10	4/10	6/10

TABLE 8. Low Frequency Animals: Errors

	Lexical Decision	Match to Category Label	Match to Picture	Oral Reading
Alligator			otter	
Baboon	NW		hyena	
Buzzard		body part	gorilla	
Crocodile			hippo	krovkɪdail
Gazelle	NW	body part	elk	
Giraffe				
Gopher			panther	gafᴙ
Gorilla	NW		penguin	
Hippo	NW		rhinoceros	
Hyena			kangaroo	haina
Kangaroo			otter	
Leopard	NW			liəpard
Llama	NW			
Octopus		body part	gopher	aktɔpʌs
Ostrich		body part		ovstrɪkt
Panther				
Raccoon				
Rhinoceros			crocodile	rɪnoᴙkᴙovs
Tortoise	NW		alligator	tʃtoɪs
Zebra				
Total number correct	13/20	16/20	7/20	12/20

semantic tasks were <u>chin</u> and <u>wrist</u>. For the color names, all of
his oral reading errors were errors of stress except <u>magenta</u> which
he read as <u>magenta</u>. Although he indicated the correct referent for
5 of 10 color names, only one of these, <u>maroon</u>, was categorized
correctly as a color. Table 8 demonstrates MD's difficulty identifying pictorial referents for low frequency animal names. MD correctly matched 7 of 20 words to their pictured referrent, being correct
on all 3 lexical/semantic tasks for only 3 animals (giraffe, panther
and raccoon). He misread 8 of 20 with vowel changes on all but two
which represented stress errors, octəpʌs and tʃtois.

Regular Versus Exception Words

     MD's reading of orthographically regular versus exception words
was examined, through use of the set of regular and exception words
used by Schwartz, Saffran and Marin (1980) and adapted from Baron
(1977). Results are as follows: MD correctly read 31 of 39 pairs
of word contrasts given in Table 9. Table 10 lists errors, 3 of
which involved regular words (all vowel errors), and only 5 exception
words, all of which were regularized.

TABLE 9.   Baron's Regular and Exception Words
           31/39 Correctly Read Pairs

Regular		Exception	Regular		Exception
tooth	-	blood	suck	-	sure
maker	-	water	tone	-	gone
along	-	among	crew	-	sew
soft	-	both	liquid	-	liquor
float	-	broad	honey	-	hour
open	-	once	pinch	-	pint
whip	-	whom	advice	-	police
motor	-	woman	holder	-	dollar
goes	-	does	toes	-	shoe
boost	-	flood	sink	-	ninth
corn	-	word	match	-	watch
divine	-	marine	hand	-	want
summit	-	sugar	fuse	-	busy
couch	-	touch	wheel	-	whole
hose	-	lose	bone	-	gone
			treat	-	great

TABLE 10. Baron's Regular and Exception Words
           Incorrect Items

Regular	Irregular
cape	cafe -> kerf
swoop	sword -> sward
hunter	honest -> hangs
cheap	sweat -> swit
toll -> tall	doll
holy -> holly	honor
alike	elite -> ilait
foul -> fvl	tour
Errors : 3/39	5/39

Table 11 summarizes by printed letter MD's oral reading responses on standardized reading tests, the PPVT and the animal body
part and color tasks for several of the exceptional consonants and
consonant combinations. An asterisk indicates if MD had indicated
comprehension for the word and a cross if he had failed a comprehension task for the word. Oral reading from standardized reading
tests did not test directly the meaning of the words and thus are
not followed by an asterisk or cross. For /c/ he clearly has the
rule of hard c as in coast, the only instance listed here, but
observed repeatedly. Soft c before /i/ or /e/ is variable as sometimes this is observed as in cent and even when he does not know
the meaning of the word as in descend. At other times the soft
c before e or i is pronounced as /k/, as in keremony, prekipitation,

TABLE 11.

Printed Letter	Regular Words	Exception Words
c	coast+	unsociable
	descend+	ocean
	cent	
	ceremony - kɛrəmonɪ+	
	precipitation - prəkɪpɪteʃən+	
	rhinoceros - rɪnovkɹovs+	
	cythe - kaiʔə	
ch	chicken*	ache
	chin*	stomach*
	archer+	machine
		chemist - ʃmɹst+
g	gable+	submerge+
		urgent
		magenta-> magɛnta+
		frigid-> frɪgɪd
h	hunter	honor
	honey	hour
		honest-> hanes
ph	sulphuric	
	gopher-> gafer+	
	sapphire-> sɹfir	
	amphibian-> æmpibiən+	
	physician-> pəziʃən	
qu	liquid	liquor
	banquet	
s	summit	sugar
	suck	sure
sw	swoop	sword-> sward
	sweat-> swit	
wh	whip*	whom
	wheel	whole

+ - demonstrated not to comprehend meaning
* - demonstrated to comprehend meaning

TABLE 12.   Other Exception Words

Read Correctly	Read Incorrectly
aisle	debt-> dɛbt
enough	depot-> débot
gazelle	opossum-> apasʌm
guess	psalm-> pasəm
know	yacht-> yakt
once	
one	
soldier	

rhinovkerous, and <u>kaithe</u>. On the other hand, he read the exception
words <u>unsociable</u> and <u>ocean</u> with no difficulty. Regular <u>ch</u> as /tʃ/
was almost always observed; but as well he has learned to pronounce
correctly the irregular <u>ch</u> in <u>ache</u>, <u>stomach</u> and <u>machine</u>, although
<u>chemist</u> became ₅mist. Regular <u>g</u> as in <u>gable</u> is pronounced with no
difficulty as are irregular <u>submerge</u> (except for stressing the wrong
syllable) and <u>urgent</u>. As we have seen magenta-> magɛnta and
frigid-> frɪgrd. Further examples of reading exception words are
given in Table 12.

MD's ability to read exception words as exemplified in these
last several slides, while not perfect, does appear to demonstrate
considerable ability to form direct print to sound associations,
often in the absence of meaningful interpretation.

CONTRASTIVE STRESS IN ORAL READING

MD's frequent errors of stress in words of more than one
syllable has been demonstrated above. Although for MD's level of
cognitive and language ability he has achieved a surprising degree
of competence in applying segmental reading rules, he has not achieved an equal degree of competence in the use of stress, evidencing
further his lack of semantic and syntactic comprehension. To test
his contrastive use of stress, MD was asked to read 40 sentences
developed by Whitaker (1976). Twenty sentences contained noun
forms of 2-syllable words, such as <u>detail</u>, <u>content</u>, <u>subject</u>, in which
the first syllable would be stressed. The other 20 sentences contai-
ned the same words used as verbs in which the stress should fall
on the second syllable. MD appeared to incorporate stress as an
inherent part of the word, having one stress pattern irrespective
of the use of the word as a noun or verb. His typical pattern was
to stress the second syllable for both verb and noun forms in sentences (Table 13). He did, however, have exceptions to the stress-
the-2nd-syllable rule for <u>present</u>, <u>record</u>, and <u>rebel</u>, in which the
1st syllable was stressed for both forms. He does use one contrast
correctly, <u>suspect</u>, in "The police questioned the suspect for five
hours," and "I suspect you are not telling the truth." He maintained
the contrastive stress for suspect on two trials.

DISCUSSION

Interpreted within the models of acquired dyslexias presented
by Marshall (this volume) and Coltheart (this volume), MD is adept
at grapheme-phoneme correspondences (Route C), has developed word
specific print to sound associations to a lesser but impressive
degree (Route B), but utilizes lexical/semantic representation
(Route A) minimally.

The parallels between this case of hyperlexia, a developmental
reading disorder, and several reports of acquired dyslexia are

TABLE 13. Contrastive Stress

First syllable stress for both noun and verb forms	Second syllable stress for both noun and verb forms		
present	combat	content	object
record	compact	contrast	progress
rebel	compress	contract	project
	console	convict	subject
	conduct	desert	
	contest	detail	

Contrasting stress for noun and verb forms

The police questioned the súspect for five hours.

I suspéct you are not telling the truth.

striking. MD's reading dissociations appear to most closely mimic
the acquired surface dyslexic patient, MP, reported by Bub (in Press),
who likewise demonstrated very poor ability on several lexical decision and semantic categorization/identification tasks, yet demonstrated an exceptional ability to read orally both regular and exception
words. As with our patient, MP's reading of exception words was imperfect and was found to be related to the predictability of the
orthographic rule. MD also shares characterstics in common with
reading disorders secondary to dementia, particularly Schwartz,
Saffran and Marin's patient, WLP (1979, 1980), although WLP's semantic and ultimately grapheme-phoneme correspondence routes were impaired to a greater degree than for MD, resulting in WLP's principal
use of the direct print to sound association route.

In summary, MD represents a case of developmental hyperlexia
maintaining into adulthood, in which a very high degree of competence in forming grapheme-phoneme correspondences has been developed
as exemplified in reading of both real words and nonwords. Further,
he appears to have established a considerable store of word-specific
print to sound associations as exemplified in his reading of exception words. Much of this oral reading, however, appears to be accomplished without meaning, bypassing lexical/semantic representation.

REFERENCES

Baron, J. Mechanisms for pronouncing printed words: Use and acquisition. In D. LaBerge and S. J. Samuels (Eds.), Basic Process

in Reading: Perception and Comprehension. Hillsdale, N. J.:
Lawrence Erlabaum, 1977.

Bub, D. N. The nature of the non-semantic reading route - evidence
for whole-word and algorithmic print-to-sound mapping. In M.
Coltheart, K. Patterson, and J. C. Marshall (Eds.), Surface
Dyslexia. London: Routledge and Kegan Paul, In Press.

Cain, A. C. Specific "isolated" abilities in severly psychotic
young children. Psychiatry, 1969, 32, 137-149.

de Hirsch, K. Are hyperlexics dyslexics? Journal of Special Education, 1971, 5, 243-246.

Dennis, M. and Whitaker, H. A. Language acquisition following hemi-
decortication: Linguistic superiority of the left over the right
hemisphere. Brain and Language, 1976, 3, 404-433.

DiSimoni, F. The Token Test for Children. Boston: Teaching Resources
corporation, 1978.

Dunn, L. M. Peabody Picture Vocabulary Test, (Rev. Ed.), Circle
Pines, Minn.: American Guidance Service, Inc., 1965.

Elliott, D. E. and Needleman, R. M. The syndrome of hyperlexia.
Brain and Language, 1976, 3, 339-349.

Goodman, J. A case study of an "autistic savant": Mental function
in the psychotic child with markedly discrepant abilities.
Journal of Child Psychology and Psychiatry, 1972, 13, 267-273.

Healy, J. M., Aram, D. M., Horwitz, S. J., Kessler, J. A study of
hyperlexia. Brain and Language, 1982, 17, 1-23.

Huttenlocher, R. R. and Huttenlocher, J. A study of children with
hyperlexia. Neurology, 1973, 23, 1107-1116.

Lee, L. L. The Northwestern Syntax Screening Test, Evanston, Ill.:
Northwestern University Press, 1969.

Mehegan, C. C. and Dreifus, R. E. Hyperlexia - exception reading
ability in brain damaged children. Neurology, 1972, 22, 1105-
1111.

Parker, S. W. Pseudo-talent for words. Psychology Clinics, 1917,
11, 1-7.

Phillips, A. Talented imbeciles. Psychology Clinics, 1930, 18,
246-265.

Richman, L. C. and Kitchell, M. M. Hyperlexia as a variant of developmental language disorders. Brain and Language, 1981, 12
203-212.

Schwartz, M. F., Marin, O. S. M., and Saffran, E. M. Dissociations
of language function in dementia: A case study. Brain and
Language, 1979, 7, 277-306.

Schwartz, M. F., Saffran, E. M., and Marin, O. S. M. Fractionating
the reading process in dementia: Evidence for word-specific
print-to-sound associations. In M. Coltheart, K. Patterson,
and J. C. Marshall (Eds.), Deep Dyslexia, London: Routledge
and Kegan Paul, 1980.

Silberberg, N., and Silberberg, M. Hyperlexia: Specific word
recognition skills in young children. Exceptional Children,
1967, 34, 41-42.

Silberberg, N., & Silberberg, M. Case histories of hyperlexia. Journal of School Psychology, 1968, 7, 3-7.

Silberberg, N., & Silberberg, M. Hyperlexia: The other end of the continuum. Journal of Special Education, 1971, 5, 233-242.

Whitaker, H. A. Contrastive Stress. Unpublished test protocol, 1976.

Woodcock, R. W. Woodcock Reading Mastery Tests. Circle Pines, MN: American Guidance Service, Inc., 1973.

Woodcock, R. W. & Johnson, M. B. Woodcock-Johnson Psycho-Educational Battery. Boston: Teaching Resources Corporation, 1977.

INTERHEMISPHERIC INTEGRATION OF CONFLICTING INFORMATION BY A SPLIT-BRAIN MAN [1]

Justine Sergent
Department of Psychology
McGill University
Montreal, Canada

The surgical sectioning of the corpus callosum for the relief of intractable epilepsy has provided a unique research opportunity to study the competence and processing capacities of the cerebral hemispheres. Sperry and Gazzaniga have initiated this type of research in humans, and considerable evidence has now accumulated showing that each isolated hemisphere can perceive, think, memorize, and learn independently and essentially outside the realm of awareness of the other (Gazzaniga, in press; Sperry, 1982). This has been referred to as the disconnection syndrome and has served as a basis for the discussion of brain-mind relationships and the suggestion that splitting the brain results in a state of mental duality. In this chapter, I will not dwell on the specific processing skills of the cerebral hemispheres as such, but I will rather examine a more general aspect of split-brain functioning that bears implications on the issue of mental duality. I must mention at the outset that the experiments reported herein constitute only a preliminary set of studies, and I will not be able to offer an unequivocal account of the data which in fact raise more questions than they answer.

One startling fact about split-brain patients is that, despite their having two independent and different cognitive processors, they behave as unified individuals and they seldom display signs of hesitation, confusion or dissociation in their day-to-day activities.

---

1. I am grateful to Michael Gazzaniga and Jeffrey Holtzman for allowing me to test J. W., and for their support and their suggestions. I am also indebted to Michael Corballis, Peter Milner, and Harry Whitaker for their helpful comments and suggestions.

Were it not for the results from specially designed experiments, cutting the corpus collosum would be regarded as resulting in no neurological and psychological sequels. This was the conclusion reached by Akelaitis (1944) after examining an earlier series of split-brain patients, and, although there are some dramatic examples of interference and rivalry between the two sides of the body (e.g., Geschwind, 1981), they essentially remain exceptions in the normal environment. Thus, while casual observation of split-brain patients suggests that they are capable of, and indeed display, unified purposeful behavior, experimental investigation has usually focussed on hemispheric differences and has less often examined how the two disconnected hemispheres could operate together.

Although the corpus callosum is the major structure linking the two hemispheres, there are subcortical commissures that may provide a route for transfer and exchange of information between the two sides of the brain and allow for integration of some lower-order information (e.g., Trevarthen, 1974). This has been illustrated in recent experiments showing that information received by one hemisphere may interfere with, or facilitate, the performance of the other. For example, Holtzman, Sidtis, Volpe, Wilson, and Gazzaniga (1981) observed that one hemisphere could direct attention to a specific localization in space when a spatial cue had been presented to the other hemisphere: compared to a neutral cue, a valid cue speeded the localization of relevant information while an invalid cue slowed it down. Zaidel (1982) has reported results suggesting transfer of information as he observed interhemispheric semantic facilitation in a lexical decision task. These spatial and semantic priming effects across the hemispheres indicate some communication between the two sides of the brain, but there is as yet no evidence that patterned information can be transferred from one hemisphere to the other.

Another explanation for the apparent absence of the hemisphere disconnection syndrome outside experimental situations has been the suggestion that the same information is projected to both hemispheres through, for instance, head and eye movements, whereas in laboratory settings information can be directed to only one hemisphere. This explanation however may not be sufficient since there is evidence that different decisions may be reached by the two hemispheres after processing the same information. For example, Levy and Trevarthen (1976) showed that the right hemisphere of split-brain patients matched pictures according to visual similarity while the left hemisphere matched the same pictures according to functional association. When the two hemispheres are simultaneously stimulated, one should thus anticipate a behavior of response competition or the taking over of control by one hemisphere with neglect of information received by the other hemisphere.

Much of our knowledge about split-brain functioning comes

from experiments in which a response is requested from each stimulated hemisphere, and the results have been used to support the claim
of mental duality in these patients. It is questionable however
whether the design of these experiments is appropriate to draw such
a conclusion. They mainly consist of either a unilateral presentation followed by one response from the stimulated hemisphere, or a
bilateral simultaneous presentation followed by two responses, one
from each stimulated hemisphere. In the latter condition, double
responses to stimuli in both fields are extremely rare, and patients
generally respond to one field, ignoring the other (e.g., Levy, in
press). Therefore, in these studies, each hemisphere is considered
in isolation, makes a decision on its own, and produces its response.
Such a procedure necessarily requires that the two hemispheres operate separately from stimulus reception to response production, and
it sets the conditions for testing mental duality, but it cannot
provide us with evidence of an absence of mental unity. To further
examine the possibility of unified behavior in split-brain patients
within a laboratory setting, a different approach may be used, one
that would require the subject to produce a single response based
on information simultaneously presented to the two hemispheres. By
projecting at the same time, to the two hemispheres, information
associated with conflicting responses, one may examine the capacity
of the disconnected hemispheres to aim at the same goal and thus to
integrate divergent information before the production of a single
response.

EXPERIMENTS

    The subject was J.W., a 28 year old right-handed split-brain
patient from the Wilson's series. He was operated on 3 years ago,
according to the two-stage procedure of Dr. Wilson. Both the corpus
callosum and hippocampal commissures were sectioned, while the
anterior commissure and massa intermedia were spared. J. W. has
been tested by Gazzaniga and his colleagues and has shown the
typical disconnection syndrome. Although his anterior commissure
was left intact, he has displayed no sign of interhemispheric transfer as some other patients of the Wilson series have (Risse, LeDoux,
Springer, Wilson,& Gazzaniga, 1978); he cannot name words projected
to his right hemisphere but he has a good deal of language comprehension in this hemisphere. He was however one of the two split-
brain patients showing interhemispheric transfer of spatial information for the control of attention, as observed in the forementioned
study by Holtzman et al. (1981). It is not clear how much transfer
was achieved in J. W. in this task, as no individual data were
presented despite an interaction between the subjects (P. S. and
J. W.) and cue type, and in view of the fact that P. S. displays
paracallosal transfer not present in other split-brain patients
(Gazzaniga, Sidtis, Volpe, Smylie, Holtzman, & Wilson, 1982). More
information about J. W. can be found in previous publications
(Holtzman et al., 1981; Sidtis, Volpe, Holtzman, Wilson, &

Gazzaniga, 1981; Wilson, Reeves, & Gazzaniga, 1982).

The experiments were conducted in the mobile laboratory of
Gazzaniga and his colleagues. The stimuli were 8 letters (4 consonants: H, N, R, S, and 4 vowels: A, E, O, U) appearing 2° to the
right and/or left of fixation on a video screen of an Apple II
computer. Each letter subtended a visual angle of .8° and the exposure duration was 100 msec. A response panel with two keys was
placed in front of J. W. who responded by moving one arm to the right
or left of the central resting position and pressing a key. Latency
and accuracy were automatically recorded. The subject responded
with only one arm, and the right arm was always tested first.

J. W. was tested in three stages, each involving a different
experimental condition. The first stage consisted of a unilateral
presentation of one letter, and the task was to press one key if the
letter was a vowel and another key if it was not a vowel. This
condition was run in two sessions of 48 trials, each session with
a different hand. The aim of this first stage was to establish the
skill of each hemisphere to perform this letter-categorization task.
The results are displayed in Table 1, and they show that the two
hemispheres were equally competent in deciding whether or not a
letter was a vowel, in terms of both speed and accuracy. This finding therefore provided a guarantee that any response asymmetry in
the subsequent bilateral presentation condition could not be attributed to a differential hemispheric competence in performing this
letter-categorization task. Had a difference in performance between
the two hemispheres been obtained, a simultaneous presentation would
likely result in the superior hemisphere taking over, and neglect
of the information projected to the inferior hemisphere. It should
be noted however that J. W. responded faster to vowels than to non-
vowels, and this pattern and its consequences will be examined more
thoroughly below.

The second stage of the experiment was the crucial condition
of this investigation. Two letters were simultaneously flashed so
that one letter was projected to the right hemisphere (RH) and the
other to the left hemisphere (LH). Six different combinations of
the two-letter presentation were possible: two identical vowels,
two different vowels, a vowel to the RH and a consonant to the LH,
a vowel to the LH and a consonant to the RH, two identical consonants, two different consonants. J. W. was requested to press one
key if at least one vowel was presented and another key if no vowel
was presented. There were 2 sessions of 96 trials, with a different
hand responding in each session.

Thus, the two important letter combinations were those in which
different categories of letter were projected to the two hemispheres,
which implied that information associated with different responses
had to be processed and the conflict resolved for the production of

TABLE 1. Mean latencies, standard error, and percentage of correct responses by J. W. in the unilateral presentation of **vowels** and non-vowels as a function of the responding hand and the hemisphere stimulated

UNILATERAL PRESENTATION

		VOWEL		NON-VOWEL	
		LVF-RH	RVF-LH	LVF-RH	RVF-LH
RIGHT HAND	Mean (msec)	564	538	640	676
	St. Er.	56	43	29	51
	% correct	92	100	100	100
LEFT HAND	Mean (msec)	578	619	702	731
	St. Er.	32	24	29	35
	% correct	100	100	100	100

Note: Comparisons:

Right hand: Vowel to LVF-RH vs. Non-vowel to RVF-LH: $p > .05$
            Vowel to RVF-LH vs. Non-vowel to LVF-RH: $p > .05$

Left hand: Vowel to LVF-RH vs. Non-vowel to RVF-LH: $p < .05$
            Vowel to RVF-LH vs. Non-vowel to LVF-RH: $p > .05$

TABLE 2. Mean latencies, standard error, and percentage of correct responses by J. W. in the bilateral presentation of vowels and non-vowels as a function of the responding hand

BILATERAL PRESENTATION

		SV	DV	VR	VL	SC	DC
RIGHT HAND	Mean (msec)	574	556	771	739	843	725
	St. Er.	14	25	63	53	67	42
	% correct	100	100	100	100	92	75
LEFT HAND	Mean (msec)	466	442	563	793	713	687
	St. Er.	21	15	33	51	42	59
	% correct	92	100	100	100	83	100

SV: Same vowels   VR: Vowel to right hemisphere
DV: Different vowels   and consonant to left hemisphere
SC: Same consonants   VL: Vowel to left hemisphere
DC: Different consonants and consonant to right hemisphere

a correct response. Current understanding of split-brain functioning would suggest that the conflict condition should result either
in one letter being ignored, presumably that in the visual field
contralateral to the responding hand, or to one hemisphere taking
over, presumably the left in this language related task, or to
response confusion and competition due to opposite decisions reached
by the two hemispheres.

     The results did not conform to any of these predictions. As
shown in Table 2, J. W. was capable of perfectly accurate performance
with either hand in the conflict condition. The hand that was directly controlled by the hemisphere receiving the vowel responded faster than the other hand, but there was no neglect of information,
even by the RH when it received the vowel and when the right (ipsilateral) hand responded. In addition, while latencies to the presentation of two vowels were significantly shorter than those in
the conflict condition (except the condition VR with the left hand
responding p > .05), latencies to the conflict conditions were not
longer than those to the presentation of two consonants. This may
indicate that little, if any, confusion or competition took place
when conflicting information was presented to the two hemispheres.

     It must be noted at this point however that, in the unilateral
conditions, the mean latency of "yes" (vowel) responses was shorter
than that of "no" (consonant) responses. To inquire about the extent
of this difference and its implications for the present results, the
variability of reaction times across trials within each presentation
condition was examined and statistical tests were carried out to
compare performance in each two unilateral conditions that were associated in the bilateral condition. Thus, for both the left and the
right hand responding, unilateral performance for vowels in the RH
was compared to performance for consonants in the LH, as was unilateral performance for vowels in the LH compared to performance
for consonants in the RH. Considering variability across trials as
an estimate of errors of measurement, a t test was applied on these
data (Ferguson, personal communication), and the significance of
each comparison is shown in Table 1. In the right-hand responding
condition, "yes" responses were not significantly faster than "no"
responses (p > .05). In the left-hand responding condition, latencies to vowels in the LH were not significantly different from latencies to consonants in the RH; however, latencies to vowels presented in the RH were significantly shorter than latencies to consonants presented in the LH (p < .05). Thus, except in the latter
condition, "yes" and "no" decisions could be arrived at approximately
simultaneously in the two hemispheres. On the other hand, a "yes"
decision in the RH could be made significantly faster than a "no"
decision in the LH when J. W. responded with his left hand.

     In the bilateral presentation, the only conflicting condition
that did not yield a significant increase in latency from the two

vowel-condition to the conflicting was that involving a vowel to the RH and a consonant to the LH when the left hand was used, that is the condition in which "yes" responses were significantly faster than "no" responses in unilateral presentations. These patterns of results may thus indicate that, at least in three of the four conflicting conditions, some integration of the divergent information had to be achieved for a correct response to be made.

A third experiment was conducted to further examine on what basis interhemispheric communication could be achieved. The letters were again presented bilaterally, but this time J. W. was requested to press one key if the two letters were identical and another key if they were different, independent of their category. J. W. proved unable to match the bilaterally presented letters, and his performance was not significantly different from chance, with 47% of correct responses. His responses were also examined to see if he had kept responding according to letter category, but this was not the case, and he apparently responded at random. Thus, the identity of the letter was known only to the hemisphere that received it, and this suggests that the interhemispheric communication observed in the second part could be achieved only after a decision on the category of the letter had been made within each hemisphere. It may then be the outcome of such independent decisions that was somehow integrated and resolved before the production of a single response.

DISCUSSION

The results of the second experiment do not readily conform to predictions that could be made on the basis of current understanding of split-brain functioning. The forementioned studies that have reported evidence of interhemispheric transfer of spatial and semantic information had used a priming paradigm and successive presentations of the stimuli, with one response based on the information received by the last-stimulated hemisphere. In the present critical experiment, J. W. was perfectly accurate with either hand when his two hemispheres were simultaneously presented with information requiring conflicting responses. It is this perfect accuracy along with the absence of response competition that has to be explained. Several interpretations could account for this performance, and they will be examined in turn.

Although some form of overt or covert cross-cuing may be a strategy to which split-brain patients sometimes resort (eg., Hillyard & Gazzaniga, 1971), this seems an unlikely strategy in a task involving bilateral presentation and with latencies less than one second. Moreover, J. W.'s reaction times were approximately of the same order as those of a group of normal subjects performing exactly the same task (It may be noteworthy that normals showed no increase in latencies from the two-vowel presentation to the conflicting presentation).

540   J. Sergent

It is conceivable that the task could be performed without any
need for integration across the hemispheres. Since the conflict condition always requested a "yes" response and since "yes" responses
in the unilateral conditions were made faster than "no" responses,
the hemisphere receiving the vowel may have initiated the response
earlier than the hemisphere receiving the consonant. The longer
latency in the conflict condition would then be the result of interference by the hemisphere receiving the consonant on the arm which
had already initiated the "yes" response. The results of the conflict
conditions would thus reflect peripheral interaction rather than interhemispheric integration (Gazzaniga, personal communication).
There are however several difficulties with this interpretation.
J. W. did not display overt signs of hesitation in responding, which
should have been present if the "yes" response were first initiated
and later interfered with by a "no" command. In addition, "yes"
responses were significantly shorter in only one unilateral condition
(vowel to the RH and consonant to the LH, and left-hand responding).
In the three other conditions, latencies to vowels and consonants
were not significantly different. An interpretaion in terms of peripheral interaction would require that "yes" responses were always
faster than "no" responses to obtain perfect accuracy in the conflict
conditions. This seems to be unlikely given the absence of significance between "yes" and "no"latencies. Moreover, that J. W. was as
accurate with the arm ipsilateral to the hemisphere receiving the
vowel as he was with the contralateral arm may indicate that some
integration had to be achieved before the execution of the response,
at least to inhibit the response of the contralateral hemisphere
which was unaware of the identity of the letter received by the ipsilateral hemisphere. In fact, the only condition to which the peripheral interaction interpretation could apply (condition VR with the
left-hand responding, see Table 2) indicates that interference from
the hemisphere receiving the consonant produced only a small non-
significant increase in latencies from the two-vowel presentation
condition.

Although this interpretation has inherent difficulties, it
cannot be dismissed. In an attempt to further examine this issue,
Gazzaniga (personal communication) has since then conducted the same
experiments on V. P., a split-brain patient operated on by Rayport
(see Sidtis et al., 1981).

The results of V. P. are presented in Table 3. As is apparent
in the upper part of this table, V. P.'s two hemispheres did not prove
as efficient in performing the unilateral conditions, especially when
the right hand was used. As a consequence, the right-hand bilateral
condition involving a vowel to the RH and a consonant to the LH resulted in the LH taking over the control of the response and in a
failure to respond to the vowel received by the RH. As noted earlier,
unless the two hemispheres can reach a decision about equally fast

TABLE 3. Mean latencies, standard error, and percentage of correct responses by V. P., in the unilateral and bilateral presentations of vowels and non-vowels

UNILATERAL PRESENTATION

		VOWEL		NON-VOWEL	
		LVF-RH	RVF-LH	LVF-RH	RVF-LH
RIGHT HAND	Mean (msec)	1144	788	1218	812
	St. Er.	188	40	90	47
	% correct	100	100	92	100
LEFT HAND	Mean (msec)	952	1089	1506	838
	St. Er.	81	99	105	35
	% correct	92	100	100	92

BILATERAL PRESENTATION

		SV	DV	VR	VL	SC	DC
RIGHT HAND	Mean (msec)	701	672	–	1232	932	1009
	St. Er.	29	10	–	274	71	148
	% correct	100	100	8	92		
LEFT HAND	Mean (msec)	848	705	1544	1148	1824	1661
	St. Er.	73	25	188	176	183	185
	% correct	100	100	92	92	96	96

when tested separately, the bilateral condition cannot provide an appropriate test. The left-hand responding condition offers nonetheless some indication that interference as such may not be sufficient to account for the results. Consonants unilaterally presented to the LH were responded to slightly faster than vowels unilaterally presented to the RH. When these two conditions were simultaneously presented, V. P. proved able of an almost perfect performance even though some "no" decisions must have been made faster than "yes" decisions. This suggests that, provided the two hemispheres reach a decision at about the same time as in this condition for V. P. and as it was the case for J. W., the conflicting decisions can be resolved before a response is made. Thus, although an explanation in terms of peripheral interaction remains a possiblity, other interpretations should be considered.

Another possibility is that interhemispheric integration was achieved through the anterior commissure. It has been reported for example that this commissure could mediate interhemispheric transfer of visual information (Gross, Bender, & Mishkin, 1977), and some split-brain patients have shown a remarkable capacity to name words projected to the RH, presumably due to transfer through the anterior commissure (Risse et al., 1978). However, this finding has not been replicated in other patients whose anterior commissure was intact (McKeever, Sullivan, Ferguson, & Rayport, 1981), and Greenblatt, Saunders, Culver, and Bogdanowicz (1980) have suggested that the splenium of the corpus callosum may not have been entirely sectioned in Risse et al's (1978) patients. In any case, J. W. has never shown such a capacity to name words presented in his right hemisphere.

Much of the belief that the anterior commissure in man could transfer information on which visual discrimination is performed comes from findings obtained with monkeys, but these findings may not directly apply to humans. For example, the area critical in visual discrimination and pattern recognition in monkeys, the infero-temporal cortex, sends efferents to the contralateral hemisphere through the anterior commissure (e. g., Gross et al., 1977). However, Levine (1982) has indicated that the structure whose lesion induces comparable pattern-recognition deficits in the monkey and man may not be located in comparable brain areas. In the monkey's brain, this structure is located in the same coronal plane as the anterior commissure; in man's brain, it is quite posterior and even caudal to the splenium of the corpus callosum. This may make it more probable that interhemispheric connections of this area in man is achieved through the splenium rather than through the anterior commissure.

This is not sufficient however to rule out transfer through the anterior commissure in J. W., since some reorganization of cerebral connections may have taken place. One may thus examine the type of information that could have been exchanged between the hemispheres to perform the integration observed in the second experiment. It is a safe assumption that the identity of the letters was not transfer-red. If it were, J. W. should be able to name letters presented to his right hemisphere and should have succeeded in matching the bi-laterally presented letters. It is also established that the ante-rior commissure cannot mediate the transfer of a motor program needed to carry out a movement (cf. Volpe, Sidtis, Holtzman, Wilson, & Gazza-niga, 1982). Thus the only information that the anterior commissure could transfer was the outcome of the decision on the category of the letter, that is, higher-order non-visual information. This implies that the final decision about the response would be made within either hemisphere. There is however no clear evidence that the anterior commissure can transfer such higher-order information.

To account for the complete absence of errors and competition in J. W.'s response to the conflicting condition, another interpretation may be considered. Information about the outcome of the independently made decisions may be available to some subcortical structure to which each hemisphere is equally linked and in which resolution of the opposite decisions and integration can be achieved. A final decision would be made at such a level before a response was triggered. This explanation is not without difficulty either, and there is no available evidence as to the anatomical basis of such a process, but the brainstem would appear the most likely structure that could mediate such an integration, as already suggested by Trevarthen (1974). This explanation could account for the longer reaction time to the conflict condition compared to the presentation of two vowels, which was observed even when a vowel was projected to the hemisphere contralateral to the responding hand. This latency increment may reflect some further processing which would be useless if this hemisphere could trigger the response directly.

This interpretation suggests that split-brain patients may have the capacity to resolve conflicting decisions made by each hemisphere when a single response has to be produced, and this may be one explanation for their absence of disconnection syndrome in most of their activities in a normal enviornment. Patients whose anterior commissure has been sectioned also display unified behavior, which may indicate that the sparing of the anterior commissure in J. W. was not critical in his performance. Moreoever, the present suggestion that the outcome of a decision made in one hemisphere is accessible to the other hemisphere, at least when few alternatives are involved, allows several predictions. When a task requires a "yes"-"no" binary response, some interhemispheric transfer should take place. For example, matching bilaterally presented stimuli should be possible if only two stimuli are used and if the subject attributes a "yes" response to one of them and a "no" response to the other. Although there is no empirical evidence of this as yet, several experiments in which a binary response was requested have shown that a verbal response could be made after stimulation of the RH. These experiments were conducted on patients of the Vogel-Bogen's series, whose anterior commissure was sectioned. For example, Hillyard and Gazzaniga (1971) showed that these patients could tell whether a "1" or a "0" had been presented to either hemisphere, using a verbal response or a key-pressing response with the right hand. They suggested that this resulted from subcortical transfer of visual information, but the present experiments indicate that a transfer of <u>visual</u> information as such is unlikely. Instead, a binary code associated with the decision on each stimulus may have been accessible to the left hemisphere which could then produce a verbal response. Milner and Taylor (1970) also reported findings that are explainable by the present suggestion. All eight split-brain subjects they tested could say "yes" or "no" in response to whether or not they felt a pressure on their left thumb. Four subjects could tell "one" or "two" in a two-point discrimination on the left hand, and only 2 subjects could tell "up" or "down" in the discrimination of movement on a left finger. From these data, they concluded that the right hemisphere can speak. It would seem more likely that a binary code was transferred from the right to the left hemisphere which could then initiate the verbal response. The reduction in the number of patients able to produce a verbal response may come from the increased difficulty in assigning a "yes"-"no" code to the particular binary sensations. (A large number of these patients are limited intellectually, and transforming an "up" or "down" sensation into a "yes"-"no" code requires some strategy that few split-brain patients may be able to implement on their own.)

This interpretation would thus suggest that rudimentary transfer may take place through some subcortical structure, which allows for integration of simple decisions across the two sides of the brain. The nature of the information that is exchanged remains difficult to determine. It could be simply a yes-no binary code but it may as well be some non-cognitive emotional information associated with the positive or negative nature of the decisions.

CONCLUSION

The present experiments have yielded results showing that a split-brain patient could produce a single response after conflicting information had been projected to the two disconnected hemispheres. This performance was achieved with either hand and when either hemisphere received the information associated with the response, but without transfer of the identity of the letter received by each hemisphere. There was no indication that J. W. could not simultaneously attend to both fields of stimulation in this letter-categorization task at which the two hemispheres were equally competent when separately tested. No hemisphere systematically took over the control of the response in contrast to situations that call for the "specialized" competence of one hemisphere (e.g., Levy, in press).

No definitive interpretation of these results can be offered, and more research is needed to understand the processes underlying such a performance. The fact that vowels and consonants were not responded to equally fast suggests an interpretaion in terms of peripheral interaction. Such an interpretation cannot apply however to all combinations of stimulus presentation and cannot explain the absence of errors and response competition in the conflict conditions. Classes of stimuli that would yield identical latencies would be necessary to further examine the validity of this interpretaion.

The present results may be accounted for by a capacity to integrate information at a subcortical level, at least when a fairly simple decision has to be made and few alternatives present themselves. By requesting a single response from the bilateral stimulation, it was possible to show that J. W.'s two hemispheres were simultaneously aiming at the same goal. Previous experiments had essentially considered the two hemispheres in isolation and had supported the concept of mental duality, but they had established the conditions for such a conclusion. The present experiments suggest that splitting the brain does not necessarily split the mind and that the human brain may be striving to maintain mental unity.

REFERENCES

Akelaitis, A. J. Study of gnosis, praxis and language following section of corpus callosum and anterior commissure. Journal of Neurosurgery, 1944, 1, 94-102.

Gazzaniga, M. S. Right hemisphere language following brain bisection: A twenty-year perspective. American Psychologist, in Press.

Gazzaniga, M. S., Sidtis, J. J., Volpe, B. T., Smylie, C., Holtzman, J., & Wilson, D. H. Evidence for paracallosal transfer after callosal section. Brain, 1982, 105, 53-63.

Geschwind, N. The perverseness of the right hemisphere. The Behavioral and Brain Sciences, 1981, 4, 106-107.

Greenblatt, S. H., Saunders, R. L., Culver, C. M., & Bogdanowicz, W. Normal interhemispheric visual transfer with incomplete section of the splenium. Archives of Neurology, 1980, 37, 567-571.

Gross, C. G., Bender, D. B., & Mishkin, M. Contributions of the corpus callosum and the anterior commissure to visual activation of inferior temporal neurons. Brain Research, 1977, 131, 227-239.

Hillyard, S. & Gazzaniga, M.S. Language and speech capacity of the right hemisphere. Neuropsychologia, 1971, 9, 273-280.

Holtzman, J. D., Sidtis, J. J., Volpe, B. T., Wilson, D. H. & Gazzaniga, M.S. Dissociation of spatial information for stimulus localization and the control of attention. Brain, 1981, 104, 861-872.

Levine, D. N. Visual agnosia in monkey and man. In D. J. Ingle, M. A. Goodale, & R. J. W. Mansfield (Eds.), Analysis of Visual Behavior, Cambridge, MA: MIT Press, 1982.

Levy, J. Language, cognition, and the right hemisphere: A response to Gazzaniga. American Psychologist, In Press.

Levy, J. & Trevarthen, C. Metacontrol of hemispheric function in human split-brain patients. Journal of Experimental Psychology: Human Perception and Performance, 1976, 2, 299-312.

McKeever, W. F., Sullivan, K. F., Ferguson, S. M., & Rayport, M. Typical cerebral hemisphere disconnection deficits following corpus callosum section despite sparing of the anterior commissure. Neuropsychologia, 1981, 19, 745-755.

Milner, B. & Taylor, L. B. Somesthtic thresholds after commissural section in man. Neurology, 1970, 20, 378.

Risse, G., LeDoux, J., Springer, S. P., Wilson, D. H., & Gazzaniga, M. S. The anterior commissure in man: Functional variation in a multi-sensory system. Neuropsychologia, 1978, 16, 23-31.

Sidtis, J. J., Volpe, B. T., Holtzman, J. D., Wilson, D. H., & Gazza-
    niga, M. S. Variability in right hemisphere language function:
    Evidence for a continuum of generative capacity. Journal of
    Neuroscience, 1981, 1, 323-331.
Sperry, R. W. Some effects of disconnecting the cerebral hemispheres.
    Science, 1982, 217, 1223-1226.
Trevarthen, C. Functional relationships of disconnected hemispheres
    with the brain stem and with each other: Monkey and man. In
    M. Kinsbourne & W. L. Smith (Eds.), Hemispheric Disconnection
    and cerebral Functions. Springfield, Ill.: Charles C. Thomas,
    1974.
Volpe, B. T., Sidtis, J. J., Holtzman, J. D., Wilson, D. H., & Gazza-
    niga, M. S. Cortical mechanisms in praxis: Observations follo-
    wing partial and complete section of the corpus callosum in man.
    Neurology, 1982, 32, 645-650.
Wilson, D. H., Reeves, A. G., & Gazzaniga, M. S. "Central" commi-
    ssurotomy for intractable generalized epilepsy: Series two.
    Neurology, 1982, 32, 687-697.
Zaidel, E. Reading by the disconnected right hemisphere: An apha-
    siological perspective. In Y. Zatterman (Ed.), Wenner Gren
    Symposium on Dyslexia. London: Plenum Press, 1982.

THE USE OF ADULT ACQUIRED NEUROPSYCHOLOGICAL SYNDROMES AS MODELS OF CHILDHOOD DEVELOPMENTAL DISORDERS

David Benjamins
Children's Hospital of Michigan
3901, Beaubien Boulevard
Detroit, Michigan

This paper will consider the appropriateness of using adult acquired neuropsychological syndromes as models for childhood developmental disorders. The examination of this idea is important because our usual way of thinking about disorders in children is conditioned to some extent by our experiences with adults. Even the use of words such as dyslexia or aphasia, implies a relationship between the childhood disorder and the adult disorder, even when the labels are modified by such terms as congenital or developmental. Our thinking is conditioned by reference to adult models and we need to review explicitly, whether or not this is appropriate.

In this paper, I want to consider this comparison in a particular sense. That is, whether or not consideration of adult models of acquired disorders, which are similar to childhood disorders, can tell us anything about the brain mechanisms involved in childhood developmental disorders. This particular question is somewhat different than a more general question, about whether comparison of adult acquired disorders with childhood developmental disorders is useful at all. There may be some heuristic value in such comparisons, even though it is not possible to learn directly about brain dysfunctions from such comparisons. It is certainly true that a good analysis and description of various developmental disorders from a phenomenological viewpoint is essential, before consideration of the brain basis for these problems.

Presumably, the function of a neurologist interested in these disorders, is to try to understand the brain behavior relationship involved. It is probably not appropriate, however, to try to employ the traditional neuropsychological way of thinking with regards to these problems. The traditional neuropsychological task, when faced with a patient, was to analyze the behavioral deficits of the patient and then, on the basis of the analysis, to localize a lesion within the brain. It is probably the case that most children with developmental disorders of learning, language and behavior, do not have "lesions" in the sense that adults with specific neuropsychological deficits do. We all believe that these children do have some variety of brain dysfunction. Our problem is whether or not we can make any kind of statement about what way the brain is going wrong in these children. More specifically, we want to know whether examination of adults with the same or similar problems, which they acquired as adults, give us any clues as to what might be wrong with the brain in children with developmental disorders.

On this occasion, I do not want to examine any specific data or any specific study with attempts to do this, but to consider some more general reasons, which we need to examine before we embark upon such study - which will help us to decide whether or not this is a useful approach. And then, after doing that, to consider any possible ways in which we can make a transition, backwards as it were, from adults to children in our thinking about brain-behavior relationships.

One can examine at least four factors in the analysis of this question: first, etiology; secondly, the nature of the systems affected, both from a functional and an anatomical sense; thirdly, the neuro-anatomical substrate of undeveloped versus developed skills; and fourthly, the ability of the system under consideration for recovery and reorganization.

ETIOLOGY

The etiology or cause of developmental disorders in children of language, learning and behavior, is by and large not known. At least in some children, however, it is apparent that this difficulty can be the result of a specific brain insult. For example, intrauterine infection with rubella virus can cause both hearing difficulties and subsequent language difficulties. Also, it is known that children with cerebral palsy, which is secondary to birth trauma or birth anoxia, are at a higher risk for learning disabilities of various sorts than normal children. However, in many children there is no history or evidence on examination of any identifiable specific insult to the nervous system. In these children, we may postulate that the difficulties are the result of a deviation of a specific developmental process in the brain, or perhaps, the result of one extreme of normal variability of the developmental process. These factors may perhaps be under genetic control, since there is some reason to believe that certain developmental disorders run in families.

However, it is apparent that most processes which affect the developing central nervous system, whether these processes occur during intrauterine life, during the birth process, or during early life, are diffuse generalized processes, although they may have focal emphasis.

On the other hand, brain lesions which in adults produce specific neuropsychological syndromes, are usually very focal processes. Most frequently, these are the result of cerebrovascular disease. These cerebrovascular disorders, while they do occur in the developing nervous system in young children, are much less common than in adults.

In summary then, processes which produce specific neuropsychological syndromes in adults are usually specificable and usually produce discrete lesions in specific parts of the brain. In children, on the other hand, we are uncertain as to the cause of the problems. But, the majority of the difficulties which produce brain damage or brain dysfunction in children are diffuse, generalized processes which affect the whole brain.

DIFFERENCES IN SYSTEMS AFFECTED

Regardless of the etiology, the systems affected in children versus adults are very different. This can be considered both from a functional point of view, without regard to the specifics of brain structure, or it may be considered from a neuroanatomical point of view.

From a functional point of view, the mental or cognitive structures or systems which are eventually going to result in mature expression of behavior, learning, language and cognition are still in an immature state and still evolving.

Neuroanatomically of course, the brain is undergoing drastic changes, including myelination, formation of dentritic connections and so on. It is certainly possible to consider these two sorts of processes separately, and perhaps, this is necessary in order not to confuse levels of explanation, however, it is attractive to believe that these two levels are related in some way. More specifically, that the elaboration of cognitive structures depends upon, to some degree, the evolution of a neuroanatomical substrate for their function.

In any event, the results of perturbation of an immature system, whether regarded functionally or anatomically, certainly would be different than the result of the same insult or perturbation applied to a mature developed system.

As an example of that, we might consider the effect of hearing loss or deafness on the speech and language system. Certainly the

speech, and also the language of a congenitally deaf person when he
reaches adulthood is very different than the speech and language system of an adult who becomes deaf as an adult (Northern and Downs,
1974).

BRAIN BEHAVIOR RELATIONSHIPS FOR LEARNED ABILITIES VERSUS BRAIN
BEHAVIOR RELATIONSHIPS NECESSARY FOR LEARNING ABILITIES

The neuroanatomical locus or loci, or the parts of the brain
most intimately involved with specific tasks in the adult may be much different than those used to learn the task in infancy and childhood. This point, of course, is really a subpoint of the previous
notion of developed systems versus undeveloped systems. Brain mechanisms used for specific tasks while they are being acquired, may be
much different than those eventually used when the task is performed
as a practiced skill. For example, on a functional level, one might
consider the role of attention during acquisition of an ability versus the role of attentional factors once the role is highly practiced. When an ability is acquired and easily performed, we say that
it is automatized. By definition then, we mean that the use of this
skill or ability not longer requires much attention. However, during the period of acquisition, attentional factors may be extremely
important. So thus, attentional disorders may interfere with skills
or abilities ·being acquired at the time, but not interfere with the
abilities or skills which are already acquired.

With regard to neuroanatomical locus of the underlying brain
mechanism involved, one might consider some recent studies on musical abilities. Dichotic listening studies using certain musical tasks have demonstrated a left ear advantage in naive subjects for the
task. This implies that the task is mainly performed with right hemisphere processing. However, the same dichotic listening task in
trained musicians reveals a right ear advantage (Bever and Chiarello,
1974). This implies a left hemisphere processing for that particular task.

The implication of these studies is that, as training in a musical skill proceeds, the underlying way that the brain handles the
task changes, perhaps from a holistic approach to a more analytical
one, and thus, the hemispheric locus shifts from the right hemisphere to the left. This sort of change may occur in various kinds of
learning tasks. Thus, it is conceivable that an insult to a particular area of the brain might interfere with acquisition of a particular skill, but not with the performance of that skill once it has
became learned, overlearned or practiced.

RECOVERY AND REORGANIZATION

In general, it is true that the immature nervous system is better at recovery from insult than a mature nervous system. Recent

animal studies have emphasized the importance of experience in bringing about this recovery, and allowed speculations about the properties of the undeveloped nervous system which allow for recovery (Goldman and Lewis, 1978).

Studies of acquired aphasia in children are of particular interest. If an insult to the left hemisphere in a child results in aphasia, the ability of the child to recovery from this insult is better than the ability of an adult to recovery from the same insult. The recovery is limited, however, as shown in the recent studies of Woods (1978). Some children who have sustained this brain damage become epileptic. If seizures from the damaged area are uncontrolled medically, sometimes it is necessary to remove the damaged left hemisphere. If this is done, the left hemispherectomy usually does not produce aphasia. This demonstrates the ability of the intact right hemisphere to take over language function.

In this case, we have some understanding of the mechanisms of recovery. The recovery occurs by means of reorganization and re-distribution of functions within the remaining intact areas.

CONCLUSION

To conclude, there are a number of reasons why brain behavior relationships may not be the same in children as compared to adults. Therefore, it seems reasonable to say that even if the typologies or neuropsychological profiles of disabilities can be demonstrated to be the same in children with developmental disorders as in adults with acquired neuropsychological deficits, this does not necessarily mean that the same brain structures are involved in the two cases.

In order to understand the brain basis of developmental disabilities in children, we need both more direct evidence of brain dysfunction in these children and a better theoretical understanding of the development of specialization of brain regions.

With regard to direct evidence of brain dysfunction, we currently have some evidence of a neuroanatomical sort, both from a few neuropathological studies of children with developmental disabilities and CT Scan, and other neuroanatomic studies. These studies are useful, but they do not give us direct evidence of how brain physiology or function is disordered. It is hoped that newer studies, such as Electroencephalographic Evoked Potential Studies, may give us more direct evidence of disordered brain function in children with developmental disorders.

Our present understanding of the abilities of the brain to recovery from insult, makes it difficult to understand how there can be specific, discrete functional disorders in children. For example, we do see children with specific language deficits and relatively intact functions in other cognitive areas. Given the ability of the right hemisphere to take over for a damaged left hemisphere, how do we account for this specific deficit ?

One explanation, of course, would be bilateral lesions, which do occur occasionally. But this does not explain the situation in most children.

Hopefully, explanation will derive from a better theoretical framework of understanding of the development of hemispheric specialization in children. The notion of competitive interaction between the hemispheres proposed by Galin (1979) may be a beginning in this direction.

REFERENCES

Northern, J. L. and Downs, M. P. Hearing in Children: Baltimore: Williams and Wilkins, 1974.
Bever, T. G. and Chiarello, R. J. Cerebral dominance in musicians and non-musicians. Science, 1974, 185, 537-539.
Goldman, P. S. and Lewis, M. E. Developmental Biology of Brain Damage and Experiences. In Carl Cotman (Ed.) Neuronal Plasticity. Raven Press: New York, 1978.
Woods, B. T. and Teuber, H. L. Changing patterns of Childhood Aphasia. Annals of Neurology, 1978, 3, 273-280.
Galin, D. EEG studies of Lateralization of Verbal Processes in the Neurological Bases of Language Disorder in Children's Methods and Directions for Research. NINCDS Monograph No. 22 Ed. Ludlow, C. L. and DoranQuire, M. E. 1979.

ON THE USE OF WORD AND CONTEXT BASED INFORMATION SOURCES EVALUATED

BY ORAL READING ERROR ANALYSIS[1]

Josephine S. Goldsmith
Graduate School of Education
Rutgers University
New Brunswick, New Jersey

Mark J. Nicholich
Reading Disabilities Research
Institute
Rutgers Medical School
Piscataway, New Jersey

The extent to which children attend to words versus context as they learn to read has not been fully determined. Currently, two conflicting views of the course of normal reading development make quite different predictions on this issue. The first is the view of top-down modellers of the reading process (Goodman, 1969; Smith, 1978). These researchers posit that reading, specifically word perception, is facilitated by the language redundancies of the text. This conceptually driven view is supported by the information processing studies of the late 60's and early 70's which demonstrated a variety of context effects, and sought to establish the psychological reality of various extra-word units from the phrase (Levin & Kaplan, 1970) to the clause (Fodor & Bever, 1965) and the paragraph (Koen, Becker & Young, 1969). The strong version of this position is stated by Goodman (1976) who believes that words derive their meaning from context to the extent that accurate word perception is not crucial to the development of reading skill.

Recently the notion that word perception can be speeded through the use of prior context has been called into question by Stanovich (1980) who makes a distinction between two types of contextual facilitation: facilitation of comprehension and facilitation of word perception. He states that his reanalysis of a large body of data supports the existence of the first type of context facilitation, but he concludes that facilitation of the second type is not a usual part of normal reading. He goes on to state that the use of context to speed word perception would be useful only to poor readers to compensate for their difficulties in decoding. He holds

1. Preparation of this article was supported by NICHHD Grant #HD 12278-04.

that it is more economical for good readers to perceive words in a
data driven fashion, thus saving cognitive capacity for comprehension.

    Stanovich's point of view has been supported by recent studies
which purport to show a context effect for young readers. For example,
Schvaneveldt, Ackerman & Semlear (1977) used a lexical decision task
with second and fourth grade pupils. Although the children's ability to identify a letter string as a word increased with grade and
context, the magnitude of the association effect decreased over
development. While better readers identified words faster, there
was no consistent relationship between good reading and the semantic
association effect. It appeared that the "poor readers use semantic
context at least as much as better readers do" (p. 615). Additionally, Stanovich, West, and Feeman (1981) tested the effects of congru-
ous, incongruous, and neutral context on the time to read to words
for children in second grade. They found that context effects
decrease with predictability, development and practice.

    Therefore, it is unclear whether attention to word or context
based information sources is the pattern in normal reading development. This lack of information is unfortunate since contrastive
study of the use of language systems by normal and disabled readers
has implications for the study of reading disability. If disabled
readers develop the same behavior as normals at a slower rate, we
could conceptualise reading disability as a developmental lag. In
contrast, if disabled readers show different patterns of attention
to words and context, reading disability might be more accurately
characterized as a developmental difference. Following this line
of investigation, it is possible that subtypes of disabled readers
might be characterized according to their use of word and context
based language systems.

    This paper reviews the results of a series of studies on this
topic in which we have been engaged in over the past several years.
These studies have investigated the use of word and context based
information sources in both normally developing and reading disabled
children, using the method of oral reading error analysis.

ORAL READING ERROR ANALYSIS

    The method of oral reading error analysis was developed for
the purposes of psycho-educational diagnosis by Goodman and his
colleagues. These workers developed a research instrument, the
Taxonomy (Goodman, 1969; Goodman & Burke, 1969) and a version designed for classroom use, The Reading miscue inventory (Goodman &
Burke, 1972). The procedure is that each of the child's errors is
compared to the word in the text on various scales designed to
measure similarity of both conceptually driven systems such as
Semantic Similarity and Meaning Change and data driven systems such
as Graphic Similarity and Sound Similarity (Goodman & Burke, 1972).

The technique has several advantages.

1. It permits relatively direct inferences as to the strategies children use when they attempt to read difficult words.

2. Error analysis is of interest as one of few techniques with the potential to measure the relative importance of word and context-based language systems as they are used in concert. With refinement of the procedures, findings could potentially partial the contributions to each error of both word and context based information sources (Goldsmith, Nicolich & Haupt, 1982).

3. It is not a laboratory technique, but closely reflects a natural classroom reading situation, even to the use of typical school reading materials.

4. The technique is appropriate to use with readers of a wide variety of ages and abilities.

Because of limitations found in attempting to apply the clinical instruments developed by Goodman and his colleagues to studies using canonical analyses adaptations of the scales were developed. The resulting eleven scales reported by Goldsmith, et al. (1982) are as follows.

System Categories

1. Utterance Type (Insertion, pause, reversal, substitution omission).

2. Word Type: Degree to which substitution is word-like (Word, morphologically word-like utterance, accidental esoteric utterance, nonsense or phonemic word-part utterance).

3. Form Class of Target Word (A 21 item list based on semantic adjustments to traditional form class distinctions).

4. Phonemic Similarity (Based on a grapheme list derived from Venezky).

5. Graphic Similarity (Incorporates graphic aspects - inflections, length and ascenders).

6. Semantic Network Relationship (Error is synonymous, subordinate, superordinate, or associate to the target word).

7. Syntactic Acceptability (Adaptation of Hood's (1976-77) scale of contextual appropriateness).

8. Semantic Acceptability (As above).

9. Meaning Change (From Goodman & Burke, 1972).

10. Correction (Categories include correction and partial correction as well as stability and worsening of errors).

11. Regression.

The scales measure the similarity of the target word to the child's utterance at an ordinal level. Most scales range from 1 to 4, with rating of 1 indicating the highest degree of similarity. The exception is Phonemic Similarity, a proportional scale, which ranged from 1 to 9.

As reported by Goldsmith et al. (1982) inter-rater reliability for a random sample of 500 errors showed 96 percent agreement within one point and 80 percent exact agreement.

Experiment I - Normal Subjects

Goldsmith (1982) reported a test of the system using a developmental sample. Subjects for this study were 51 average readers, all pupils in three school districts in Central New Jersey. Fourteen children were in grade two, fifteen in grade four and twenty two in grade six. All of the children had a WISC IQ in the normal range and showed at least grade level achievement on the Woodcock Word Identification, Passage Comprehension and Word Attack subtests.

MATERIALS

Each subject read two passages, one of narrative and one of science content. The passages had been pre-tested with a pilot sample of children in the target grades in order to assure that the readers would produce errors at the desired rate of seven to ten percent. This is a low frustration rate: high enough to force all available strategies into use, but not so high as to cause reading to fall apart. The grade levels of the resulting materials were as follows: Children in grade two read materials at fourth grade level, while those in grades four and seven read materials at seventh and tenth grade levels respectively.

Since unexpected differences between passages intended to behave equally have been an irritating confounding effect in verbal learning research (Clark, 1973; Goldsmith & Nicolich, 1977), we took care to attempt to equate the passages on several linguistic dimensions. First, passages for each grade were equated through the agreement of two readability procedures. The Fry (1977) and Spache (1968) procedures were used for second grade passages and the Fry and Dale-Chall (1948) for more difficult passages. Additionally, narrative and science passages at each grade level had closely similar mean word frequencies as measured by the Carroll, Davies and Richman count (1971) and numbers of cohesive ties. Cohesive ties were measured using Fine's (1978) adaptation of the system developed by Halliday and Hasan (1976).

PROCEDURE

Children were tested individually by one of the research team members. Each child read first the narrative and then the science passage. Each passage was followed by a close comprehension test. Before reading the passages, children read a randomized alphabet as a baseline measure of reading speed, and a list of words randomly selected from an alternate passage of equal difficulty. All readings were taped for later analysis.

RESULTS

The data were submitted to several factor analyses based on a varimax rotation of the principal components solution with equal commonalities. These analyses were performed for each subject, for each grade, and for the entire group as shown in Table 1. In all cases, a simple structure emerged with three factors, accounting for 66 to 88% of the variance. The factors were a semantic factor, a correction factor and a decoding factor. These consistent results across all analyses, suggest that the procedures measure three aspects of reading. Two of these: the semantic factor and the decoding factor have received wide attention in the literature. In contrast, the correction factor has not been discussed in the context of word and text based information sources. Factor 3 measures the extent to which a child is successful in self-correction and the degree to which attempts at correction bring the error closer to the target. This factor appears to measure self-monitoring behavior, perhaps a type of metacognitive awareness.

Although the importance and effects of metacognitive strategies have received substantial attention as a separate area of inquiry, we are not aware of other research in which the relative role of this kind of monitoring behavior has been examined as contrasted to the importance of decoding (or data driven) and context (or conceptually driven) aspects of reading. The importance of correction is underscored by its emerging as the second factor in the analysis and accounting for 22 to 26% of the variance.

DEVELOPMENTAL FINDINGS

Having tested our procedures for reliability and appearance of an interpretable factor structure, we next examined the developmental trends, displayed in Table 2.

We found that four scales showed significant differences over development. These were Phonemic Similarity (F(2,50)=7.16, p<0.001);

J. S. Goldsmith and M. J. Nicholich

TABLE 1. Factor Loadings and Eigenvalues for Pooled Data:
Grades Two, Four, and Six

	Factor 1	Factor 2	Factor 3
Phonemic Similarity	-.067	.929	-.073
Graphic Similarity	.109	.926	-.056
Semantic Network	.749	.256	.087
Syntactic Acceptability	.873	-.136	.004
Semantic Acceptability	.890	.111	-.007
Meaning Change	.834	.167	.035
Correction	-.069	-.099	.874
Regression	.140	-.017	.864
Eigenvalue	2.89	1.93	1.40
% Variability	36	24	18
Cumulative %	36	60	78

TABLE 2. Means and Standard Deviations of Four Scales

Grade	N	Phonemic Similarity	Syntactic Acceptability	Semantic Acceptability	Correction
2	14	4.79 (.77)	2.05 (.46)	2.84 (.67)	1,39 (.23)
4	15	4.61 (.68)	2.23 (.26)	3.07 (.33)	1.47 (.19)
6	22	4.01 (.55)	2.36 (.32)	3.27 (.42)	.41 (.17)
D	7	4.43 (2.48)	2.32 (.78)	3.24 (.96)	1.69 (1.29)

Syntactic Acceptability$(F(2,50)=3.21, p<0.05]$; Semantic Acceptability $(F(2,50)=3.47, p<0.05)$; and Correction$(F(2,50)=171.93, p<0.001)$.

Using Duncan's Multiple Range Test, it was found that for
Phonemic Similarity grades 2 and 4 were similar but grade 6 was lower
(and with our scales therefore closer to the target word). In
contrast, Syntactic Acceptability and Semantic Acceptability showed
no differences on adjacent grades, but a difference from grades 2
to grade 6. Therefore, we reported a developmental trend with the
younger children using more meaning loaded, semantic strategies

while older children show more decoding strategies when encountering difficult words. These findings are in conflict with those of top down modellers (Goodman, 1962; Smith, 1978) who suggest that semantically loaded errors are "better" errors. If we define the strategies used by more skillful readers as, by definition, "better", we find that more mature sixth grade average readers show fewer semantic and more decoding strategies in their error patterns. This finding supports the interactive compensatory view of Stanovich, who has suggested that reliance on decoding may be more typical of good readers since such a strategy is more time efficient than hypothesis testing or attempting to guess ahead to identify upcoming words in text.

Experiment II - Disabled Readers

Based on the developmental data outlined above, a similar test was made with a group of severely disabled readers.

SUBJECTS

Subjects for this study were ten reading disabled children, six in grade five, two in grade six and one in each of grades seven and eight. Like the normal achievers, these subjects had a WISC IQ in the normal range. However, their reading ability was approximately two years below grade level on at least one of the Woodcock subtests.

METHOD

Materials, procedures, and data analysis were the same as for the normally achieving subjects. In order to match for error rate, the disabled children read passages which had been used with younger normal readers so that both samples read at a low frustration rate with a mean of seven to ten percent errors.

RESULTS

The factor analysis for the disabled readers showed the simple structure with three factors as found for the normal group. Since the results are similar to the developmental patterns, no separate table is presented. The means for the disabled readers on the four scales which showed developmental differences are incorporated into Table 2. On these scales the disabled readers behave overall like fourth grade students. Their scores on Phonemic Similarity and Syntactic and Semantic Acceptability fall between those of fourth and sixth graders with no significant differences. The one scale which shows a significant difference is the Correction scale. As may be seen in Table 2, disabled readers are clearly much less effective at correction than are the normals of any grade tested.

TABLE 3.   Length and Frequency of Words in Error:
Normals Versus Disabled Readers

Group	Syllables	SFI Frequency
2N	1.64 (.29)	57.44 (4.15)
2S	1.78 (.62)	63.05 (4.27)
4N	1.91 (.31)	62.58 (4.75)
4S	2.39 (.32)	57.37 (3.82)
6N	2.56 (.36)	56.73 (5.58)
6S	2.12 (.32)	57.63 (4.22)
DN (5)	1.57 (.07)	67.45 (1.22)
DS (5)	1.51 (.15)	63.69 (.28)

TABLE 4.   Time Measures in Seconds for Average and Disabled Readers

Group	Random Words	Oral Narrative	Oral Science	Oral Alphabet
2	38.25 (10.60)	314. 79 (94.61)	324.07 (106.19)	18.59 (5.43)
4	39.69 (14.87)	251.37 (79.90)	335.81 (99.63)	13.53 (3.77)
6	35.95 (8.55)	259.27 (63.23)	260.20 (62.83)	12.98 (3.89)
d	43.35 (24.28)	317.57 (102.8)	320.84 (110.07)	14.3 (8.47)

We also examined differences between the disabled and average readers on frequency in printed text of words in error and on several timed measures. Frequency was measured by the Standard Frequency Index (SFI) (Carroll, Davies and Richman, 1971). Table 3 shows the frequency of words in error for the normals at each grade and for the disabled readers. From these data it appears that disabled readers consistently err on both shorter words and higher frequency words than do their normal peers. This trend is demonstrated less in terms of statistical than educational importance. Statistically significant differences are found in two situations. In the science passages the disabled readers are significantly lower in the syllable length of words in error relative to all grades of normal readers. Additionally, on the word frequency measure the same difference appears in the narrative passages. Since these two measures are highly correlated, the pattern suggests that disabled readers have more difficulty with the more frequent words, hence the structure words. This influence is supported by the much lower variance found for the number of syllables and the frequency of the words in error for the disabled readers. As opposed to average readers, even in the second grade, the disabled readers consistently have more difficulty with high frequency, shorter words.

The time data in Table 4 show some suggestive differences. In no case were the differences significantly differed statistically; yet the disabled fifth grade readers read at speeds closer to those of second graders. The differences for the per-item speed were larger for the words in isolation as opposed to the words in context supporting the finding that poor readers have particular difficulty with words in isolation (Biemiller, 1977-78).

CONCLUSIONS

Analysis of this small sample of disabled readers can at best reveal the proverbial directions for future research. Overall these children perform like lagging developmental readers with the exception of some patterns which bear attention for continued work. The difficulties in correction, in reading higher frequency words and implied time problems should be validated not only with much larger samples but with subpopulations more selectively defined. From present findings it is quite likely that developmental lag readers are most prevalent, that true dyslexics are rarer than predicted and that a search for the dyslexics will require constant refinement of measures and techniques.

REFERENCES

Biemiller, A. Relationships between oral reading rates for letters, words and simple text in the development of reading achievement. Reading Research Quarterly, 1977-78, 13, 223-253.

562   J. S. Goldsmith and M. J. Nicholich

Carroll, J., Davies, P., and Richmond, B. Word frequency book. New York: Houghton Mifflin, 1971.

Clark, H. A. The language-as-fixed effect fallacy: A critique of statistics in psychological research. Journal of Verbal Learning and Verbal Behavior, 1973, 12, 335-359.

Dale, E. and Chall, J. S. A formula for predicting readability. Columbus: Ohio State University, Bureau of Educational Research, 1948.

Fine, J. Conversation, cohesive and thematic patterning in children's dialogues. Discourse Processes, 1978, 1, 247-266.

Fodor, J. A. and Bever, T. G. The psychological reality of linguistic segments. Journal of Verbal Learning and Verbal Behavior, 1965, 4, 414-420.

Fry, E. B. Fry readability graph: Clarification, validation and extension to level 17. Journal of Reading, 1977, 21, 242-252.

Goldsmith, J. Word and context in developmental reading. Paper submitted for publication, Reading Disabilities Research Institute: University of Medicine and Dentistry of New Jersey, 1982.

Goldsmith, J. S. and Nicholich, M. J. Word boundaries revisited: A first grade study. In P. D. Pearson and J. Hansen (Eds.), Reading: Theory, research and practice. Clemsen, S. C.: National Reading conference, 1977.

Goldsmith, J. S., Nicolich, M. J. and Haupt, E. J. A system for the analysis of word and context-based factors in reading. National Reading Conference Yearbook, 1982, In press

Goodman, K. S. Analysis of oral reading miscues: Applied psycholinguistics. Reading Research Quarterly, 1969, 5, 9-30.

Goodman, K. S. Words and morphemes in reading. In Psycholinguistics and the teaching of reading. K. S. Goodman and J. T. Fleming (Eds.), Newark, Delaware: International Reading Association, 1976, 497-508.

Goodman, K. S. and Burke, C. L. Study of children's behavior while reading orally. Final report, Office of Education - Bureau of research, 1969. ERIC Document ED 021698.

Goodman, Y. M. and Burke, C. L. Reading miscue inventory. New York: MacMillan, 1972.

Halliday, M. A. K. and Hasan, R. Cohesion in English. Lengman, 1976.

Hood, J. Qualitative analyses of oral reading errors: The interjudge reliability of scores. Reading Research Quarterly, 1976-77, 11(4), 557-598.

Koen, F., Becker, A. and Young, R. The psychological reality of the paragraph. Journal of Verbal Learning and Verbal Behavior, 1969, 8, 41-53.

Levin, H. and Kaplan, E. J. Grammatical structure and reading. In H. Levin and J. Williams (Eds.), Basic Studies on Reading. New York: Basic books, 1970.

Schvaneveldt, R., Ackerman, B. P., and Semlear, T. The effect of semantic context on children's word recognition. Child Development, 1977, 48, 612-616.

Smith, F. Understanding Reading (second edition). New York: Holt,

Rinehart and Winston, 1978.

Spache, G. D. Good Reading for Poor Readers. Champaign, Ill.: Garrard, 1968.

Stanovich, K. E. Toward an interactive-compensatory model of individual differences in the development of reading fluency. Reading Research Quarterly, 1980, 16, 32-71.

Stanovich, K. E., West, R. F. and Feeman, D. J. A longitudinal study of sentence context effects in second-grade children: Tests of an interactive-compensatory model. Journal of Experimental Child Psychology, 1981, 32, 185-199.

DIFFERENCES IN LEVELS OF PROCESSING RELATED TO AGE

Francesca Simion   and   Beatrice Benelli
Istituto di Psicologia dell'Età Evolutiva
Piazza Capitaniato, 5
35100 Padova
Italy

Many experimental studies have been carried out to demonstrate
that a multicomponent complex skill as reading can be described through a series of processing stages (LaBerge & Jay Samuels, 1974).
A visual word activates different codes: visual, phonological, semantic and some operations take place within each code. Consequently
reading disabilities could be due either to the inability to deal
with the different internal codes produced by a word (Posner, 1978;
Snowling, 1980) or to the difficulties to operate within each code.
While theories differ about the relationship between letter processing and word processing, almost all acknowledge that children must
identify and discriminate among letters in order to read fluently
(Gibson, 1969). Posner (1978) reviewed some studies to show that
separable codes are activated when a visual word is presented. These include the physical (visual) and the phonetic codes found for individual letters. Thus many of the question to which the reading
process has been subjected can benefit from studies on matching of
letters. To trace the nature of the codes activated and the time
course of the efficiency of letter processing could help reading researchers to a better understanding of the early letter processing
skills. The general aim of the present study is to define the codes
upon which different operations take place and to isolate the stages
of visual information processing both with alphanumeric and nonalphanumeric material. More specifically the study is aimed to clarify
if 1) the nature of the stimuli affects the type of codes activated;
2) the time course of the efficiency in the activation of the codes
depends on age; 3) children at different age levels can perform operations within each code with the same proficiency. These questions
give rise from those studies that have shown differences in response
latencies related to stimulus material (see Proctor, 1981 for a review) and to age (Reitsma, 1978; Mc Farland, Frey, Landreth, 1978).

Posner's technique seems very suitable to test these hypotheses. His
approach rested on the temporal hierarchy found in response latencies. Reaction times (RTs) are faster when the two letters are physically identical (PI matches: AA) than when they have the same shape
but are different in size (Analogue Identity matches: A**A**). RTs are
even slower when the two letters share only the same name (Name Identity matches: Aa).

The concept of processing levels was applied to this hierarchy
where each successive level serves to produce a more abstract code.
When an alphabetical letter is visually presented to a subject, two
independent systems, each capable of extracting a correct code
(one visual and the other phonetic) are active in parallel and process the letters. If the task requires to compare two physically
identical letters they are classified as same on the basis of the
visual code whereas when they share only the same name they are matched on the basis of the phonetic code. The analogue match take place on the basis of the visual code after an operation of normalization of one of the two letters.

Experiment 1 tests whether the time to operate transformations
upon the visual code varies as a function of age and the time to retrieve information from long term memory correlates with the increasing ability to deal with verbal material. Experiment 2 verifies if
the nature of the two codes depends on the type of stimulus material.
Our assumption is that with nonalphanumeric material there are physical properties that can be used in the classification task and that the operations to abstract these rules are carried out upon a higher order spatial code. In contrast the only rule that join two letters not physically identical is their name. Therefore the two codes for matching alphanumeric and nonalphanumeric material are likely to be different.

EXPERIMENT 1: The hypothesis predicts that since the visual code is
present from the beginning of the life while the phonetic is only later acquired no age related differences have to be found when children compare the stimuli on the basis of the visual code. On the contrary such differences could appear at the name level because this
process requires to retrieve information from long term memory.

Method: Subjects were 24 children, 12 (6 males and 6 females) of
mean age 6.7 and 12 (6 males and 6 females) of mean age 10.7. They
performed a same-different classification task with 80 pairs of pri-
ntlike letters formed with A and E. Same responses could be given
to PI matches (AA), to AI matches (A**A**) and to NI matches (Aa). Different responses were given to letters differing in name. The stimuli were tachistoscopically presented for 200 msec. Subjects judged same or different by pressing one of the two keys on the response panel in front of them (see Figure 1).

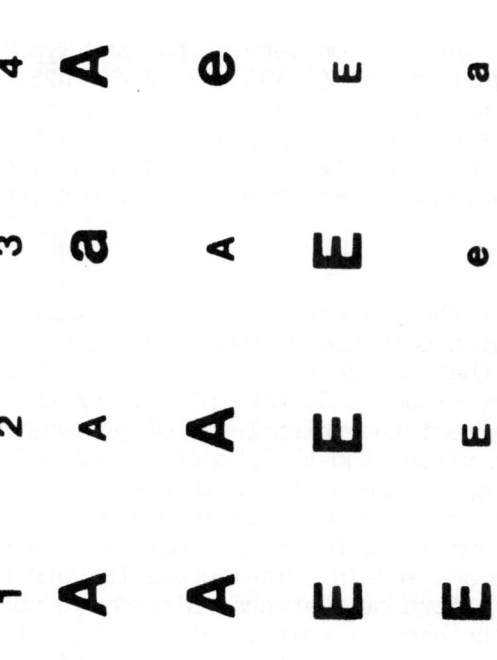

FIGURE 1. Examples of the letters employed: 1) Physical identity matches; 2) analogue identity matches; 3) Name identity matches; 4) Different pairs.

Results: A 2x2x2x3 mixed ANOVA was performed on the mean RTs for
same responses only, where Sex and Age were between subjects factors
and Type of Match was within subjects factors. The significant main
effects were: Age F(1,20) + 26.91, p < .001. Younger children responded slower than older (1091 msec vs 808 msec). Stimuli F(1,20) =
23.45, p < .001. Subjects were faster in processing As than Es (915
msec vs 983 msec). Type of match F(2,40) = 36.86, p < .001 PI matches were 83 msec faster than AI matches (837 msec vs 920 msec) and
253 msec faster than NI matches (837 msec vs 1090 msec).

The same analysis of variance carried out on errors showed two
significant main effects: Age F(1,20) = 10.18 p< .005. Accuracy increased with age. Older children made less errors than younger (4.8%
vs 9.8%). Type of match F(2,40) = 34.29 p < .001. The percentage
of errors increases as a function of the level of processing (PI =
1.25%; AI = 4.3%; NI = 16%).

Also a first order interaction between Age and Type of match
reached statistical significance F(2,40) = 5.02 p< .025. The percentage of errors does not significantly differ at the first two levels of processing for the two age groups, while at the third level
younger children make significantly more errors than older. This
result demonstrates a speed accuracy trade off effect (see Figure 2).

Discussion

The main finding of the present experiment is that Posner's paradigm was replicated with both age groups. Furthermore the results
support the hypothesis that no age related differences are present
when operations upon the visual code take place. On the contrary
practice and learning affect the third level of processing. Both
groups can activate the visual and the phonetic code and they can
retrieve with the same speed the phonetic information related to the
grapheme but the cost is a lower level of accuracy for younger subjects. Both codes are available to and automatically activated by
the children of the two age levels. The access to both codes does
not require attention, effort or awareness already in the first grade for most children (Guttentag & Haith, 1978; 1979). Practice and
learning do not seem to affect the automatic activation of the two
codes but they affect the accuracy in retrieving the information from long term memory.

EXPERIMENT 2: Previous studies have demonstrated that the three levels of processing identified with letters are present also with nonalphanumeric material (Bagnara, Roncato, Simion & Umiltà, 1978).
However objects share not only the "name" but also some physical properties that can be utilized as a "classification rule". Two triangles of different shape and size can be judged as same on the basis of some spatial relationships that are not present when an upper-
case and a lowercase letter are considered. Letters can be compared

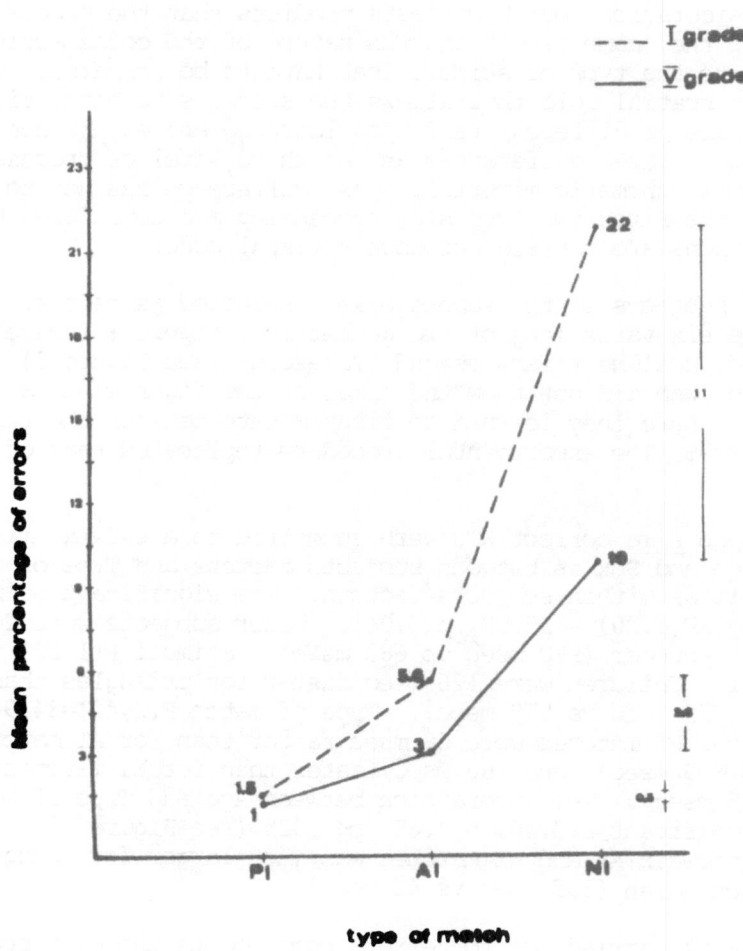

FIGURE 2. Mean percentage of errors as a function of age and type
of match.

only on the basis of the phonetic code, pictures can be compared through operations carried out upon a higher order spatial code. Following these considerations our hypothesis predicts that the process
of comparison at the "name level" and the nature of the codes activated are related to the type of stimuli that have to be compared. The
abstraction of a spatial rule that allows the subjects to categorize
two objects as same or different rely upon learning and experience.
So we predict age related differences at the third level of processing even for nonalphanumeric material. This difference has not to
be present when the first two levels of processing are considered because the operations are carried out upon a visual code.

Method:" 24 new subjects of the same age were selected as before.
The stimuli were six variations of two geometrical figures: isoscel-
es, right-angled, scalene triangles and trapezoids (see Figure 3).
Younger children, who did not know the names of the figures had a
training session where they learned to discriminate between the two
classes of figures. The experimental procedure replicated that of
Experiment 1.

Results: The mean same correct RTs were submitted to a 2x2x2x3 mixed ANOVA with Age and Sex as between subjects factors and Type of
Match and Stimuli as within subjects factors. The significant main
effects were: Age $F(1,20) = 29.99$, $p< .001$. Older subjects were 268
msec faster than younger (950 msec vs 682 msec). Stimuli $F(1,20) =
20.65$, $p< .001$. Children were 126 msec faster for triangles than
for trapezoids (753 msec vs 879 msec). Type of match $F(2,40)=34.94$,
$p < .001$. RTs for PI matches were 68 msec faster than for AI matches (737 msec vs 805 msec), and 168 msec faster than for NI matches
(737 msec vs 905 msec). The interaction between Age and Type of Match was also significant $F(2,40) = 4.65$, $p< .025$ (see Figure 4).
The difference between AI and NI matches was much larger for younger
than for older children (155 msec vs 45 msec).

        The same ANOVA carried out for errors complements the correspo-
nding effects present in RTs data. Accuracy increases as a function
of age and decreases as a function of the type of match.

Discussion and Conclusion

        The hypothesis of no age related differences for the operations
upon the visual code is confirmed also with geometrical figures.
The interval between physical and analogue identity matches does not
differ in the two age groups. On the contrary when operations upon
a higher order spatial code are required age related differences are
present. This finding confirms our hypothesis of an experience and
practice effect upon this level of processing. Older children can
utilize the spatial rule more proficiently than younger.

        To summarize the results of the two experiments support the

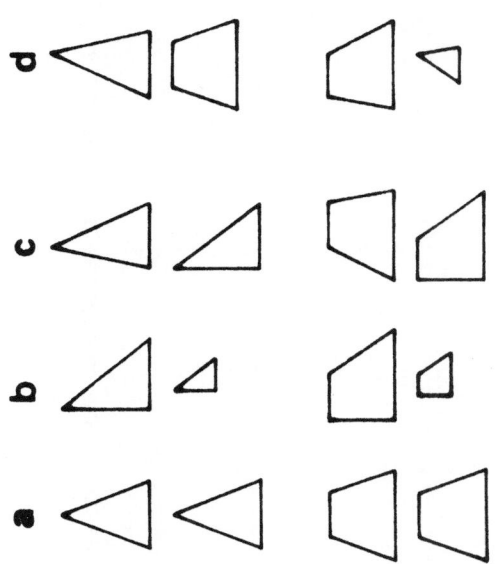

FIGURE 3. Examples of the geometrical figures employed: a) Physical identity matches;
b) Analogue identity matches; c) Name identity matches; d) Different pairs.

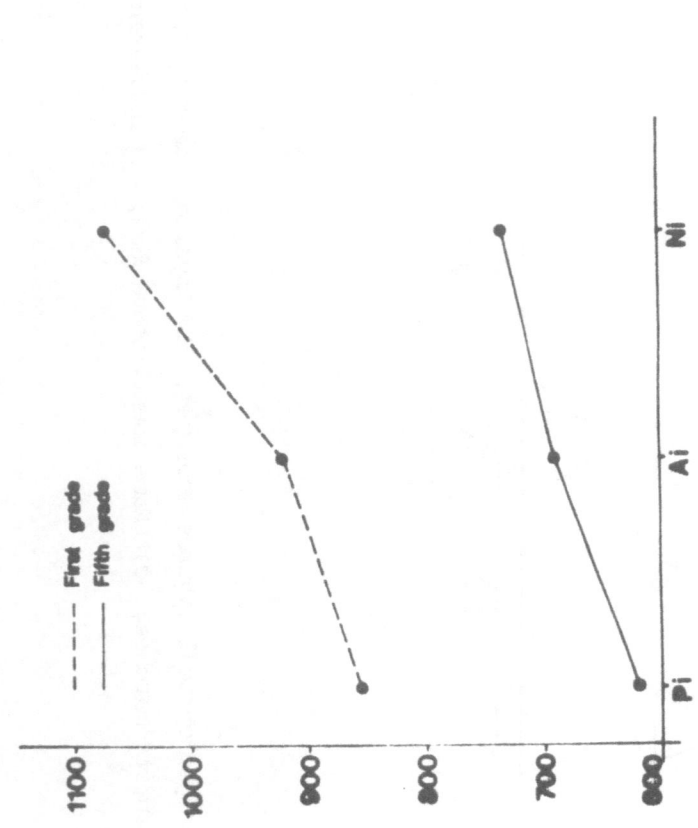

FIGURE 4.   Mean reaction times for same responses as a function of age and type of match.

hypotheses that children perform operations upon the visual code with the same proficiency at different age levels. The time course of these operations is not affected by age and by stimulus material. On the contrary when a higher order level of processing is required to compare the stimuli and a more abstract code has to be activated, age related differences are present depending on experience with that code. Experience affects differently the two types of material: for letters it affects accuracy, for figures it affects speed and accuracy. A possible explanation of these findings could be that different operation take place upon different codes. For letters the grapheme-phoneme correspondence requires to shift from the visual to the phonetic code. For figures the comparison can be performed through operations that rely upon the abstraction of visually available features. The lack of speed differences between the two age groups in experiment 1 at the third level of processing could be due to the already developed automaticity in letters processing for first graders (Guttentag & Haith, 1978; 1979). The presence of this difference in experiment 2 could be due to the higher level of the familiarity that older chidlren have with the spatial rule.

REFERENCES

Bagnara, S., Roncato, S., Simion, F. & Umilta, C. Different levels in processing simple geometrical figures. Perceptual and Motor Skills, 1978, 47, 511-514.

Gibson, E. J.. Principles of perceptual learning and development. New York: Appleton-Century-Crofts, 1969.

Guttentag, R. E. & Haith, M. M. A developmental study of automatic word processing in a picture classification task. Child Development, 1979, 50, 894-896.

Guttentag, R. E. & Haith, M. M. Automatic processing as a function of age and reading ability. Child Development, 1978, 49, 707-716.

Laberge, D. & Jay Samuels, S. Toward a theory of Information Processing in Reading. Cognitive Psychology, 1974, 6, 293-323.

Mc Farland, C. E. Jr., Frey, T. J., Landreth, J. M. The acquisition of abstract letter codes, Journal of Experimental Child Psychology, 1978, 25, 437-466.

Posner, M. I. Chronometric exploration of mind. Hillsdale, New Jersey: Lawrence Erlbaum Associates, 1978.

Proctor, R. W. A unified theory for matching-task phenomena. Psychological Review, 1981, 88, 291-326.

Reitsma, P. Changes in letter processing in beginning readers. Journal of Experimental Child Psychology, 1978, 25, 315-325.

Snowling, J. M. The development of grapheme-phoneme correspondence in normal and dyslexic readers. Journal of Experimental Child Development, 1980, 29, 294-305.

INFORMATION VALUE OF
PRINT SIZE ON READING PERFORMANCE

Pentti Laurinen   and   Göte Nyman
University of Helsinki
Department of Psychology
Ritarikatu 5
00170 Helsinki 17
Finland

Reading can be considered as an information processing task in which the subject uses his visual and cognitive processing resources to act on the data he receives in the form of a written text. The visual text information is usually highly redundant and the individual features of the letters are relatively clear and free from noise. Furthermore, because of the knowledge of the language rules and the context of the task, the reader does not need all the visual information he receives to grasp the message mediated by the letters and the words. For example, it is possible to drop out a large amount of separate letters and words of a text without making it impossible for the reader to understand its meaning (cf. Haber & Hershenson, 1980). In other words, the quality of the visual system of a normal reader is not the critical factor determining his performance in reading.

However, when the processing capacities of the higher cognitive stages are abnormally limited because of a damage to the brain or because of underdevelopment, the role of the visual functions may become critically important for fluent and accurate reading. This can be realized by considering some of the very basic processes that the visual pattern information must undergo during its transmission along the visual pathways towards the higher brain centers. Firstly, the interfering visual noise in the letters must be removed so that their essential features become recognizable. Possible sources of such a noise are, for example, the quality of the print, effects of the room lighting and the reflectance of the paper, extraneous markings in the text etc. Secondly, unique and correct representation of the letters and words must be created so that their processing at various cognitive stages becomes fast and reliable.

If the noise in the visual patterns is not removed in an appropriate way, the formation of the representations becomes difficult
and requires considerable processing load from the brain. For example, if the early input stages of the visual system are defective,
then even some minor noisy details in the text may increase the processing load at other stages that are involved in the reading. An
increase in such a load is always deteriorating for the reading performance because it also increases the time needed for the process
and makes the reading slower and inaccurate. An extreme example of
such a phenomenon is the symptom of a severe visual agnosia in which
the patient is unable to recognize a familiar form or a pattern if
extra lines or other noise details are superimposed on it (Wolpert,
1924).

There are many possible ways that can be used to improve the
reception of the visual information available in the written text,
but basically it is always a question of how to make the text as noise free and redundant as possible. The most simple and trivial way
to improve both of these factors is to increase the print size and
the contrast of the text. This is physically straightforward, but
is it useful for the reader?

Perception of visual patterns and reading

Spatial pattern perception - and also perception of letters -
is often considered in terms of the Fourier theory as it has been
fruitfully applied in the study of human spatial vision (cf. Campbell & Robson, 1968; Cornsweet, 1970). According to this approach,
any spatial pattern can be described in terms of its spatial frequency spectrum analogously to the way a complex tone is described by
its tonal frequency components. A low voice for example, consists
of mainly low tone frequencies, while a high-pitched voice contains
high tone frequencies. In the case of visual patterns, large patterns can be represented by a set of low spatial frequency (cycles
per degree of a visual angle) sinusoidal gratings and small details
by the higher frequencies (for a general introduction to the topic,
see Cornsweet, 1970).

Without going into the details of the Fourier approach to vision, it can be generally stated that the spatial information content
of a visual pattern is determined by the distribution of the spatial
frequency energy among the different spatial frequencies of its spectrum. Increasing or decreasing the size of a pattern corresponds
to a shift of its total spectrum along the spatial frequency axis
without changing the form of the spectral energy distribution. For
example, when the size of a letter is decreased, its spectrum is
shifted towards higher frequencies. However, because of the limited
resolution of the eye optics and the neural structures of the visual
system, the highest frequency components may be filtered out as a

result of the decrease in the letter size. At recognition threshold, only the most critical spatial frequency components of the letter contribute to its visibility.

In the following, we will describe some of our studies concerning the effects of print size on the reading performance of both normal and dyslectic children. The results are interpreted in terms of the factors that in general affect the performance of any capacity limited processor. Furthermore, an alternative view to the visual effects of print size is offered based on the application of the sampling theory as it is known in the theory of signal processing.

METHOD

Experiment I

Subjects: A total of 28 children participated in the reading experiment where the effects of print size to the reading performance were studied. They were divided into three age groups (7, 8, and 12 years) corresponding to the school grades of 1, 2, and 6 respectively. In each group there were 8 normal children with no reading difficulties. An additional fourth group was formed of 4 dyslectic chidlren (3 boys, 1 girl), each at the 6th grade. The type of the dyslexia in all of them can be considered as developmental in nature; they all had at least a normal intelligence and no behavior problems or a history of neurological disorders; their progress at school was otherwise normal except for the difficulties encountered in reading. The visual functions of all the children were normal or normal after correction.

Materials: The reading task was a simple word matching task in which the subject decided whether the two words in a word pair were identical or not. The four letter words were selected from a collection of list of the 300 most common 4-letter finnish words (Mikkonen & Strömnes, 1969). The presented words in a pair could differ from each other only by one letter. Five letter sizes were studied: .1, .25, .5, 1 and 2 deg. They were presented as lists of word pairs and each list consisted always of word pairs of which 50% were identical and 50% were different.

The letters were black and they were presented against a white background. Only block letters were studied and the number of different word pairs used was 100 for each letter size. The space between the words in a pair was four spaces so that the total space occupied by the pair was 12 spaces.

Procedure: Blocks of different word pairs and different sizes were presented in a random order to the subjects. The viewing distance was held constant (30 cm) by having the subjects lean the back of their heads on a prop and by setting the word list on a stand in

front of them. The responses 'same' or 'different' were recorded
on tape with accompanying code of the list presented. The subjects
were instructed to read the word pairs silently and as accurately as
possible to decide whether the words presented were identical or not.
The accuracy of the performance was especially stressed. The inspection time of the word pairs was not limited. Before the experiment
was started, some practice trials were conducted until the experimenter was convinced that the subject had understood the task correctly.

EXPERIMENT II

Subjects: Three adult subjects participated in the experiments where the effect of spatial sampling density to the recognition of letters was studied. One of the subjects did not know the purpose of
the experiment. Two of the subjects were emmetropic and one had a
corrected visual acuity better than 1.0. None of them had a history
of reading or writing difficulties.

Materials: The stimulus letters were digitized by scanning letter
transparencies with a flying spot that was formed on an oscilloscope
screen under computer control. The area scanned had the size of 32
x 32 points that were rectangularly spaced. The digitized letters
were stored in the computer and then transformed into binary versions in which the character and the background had their own luminance
values.

     The sampled versions of the binary letters were generated by
setting every 2nd, 3rd, 4th etc. point in the original binary matrix
to the background value to obtain a series of sampled letters. Examples of the binary images and the sampled ones are shown in Figure
1. 12 different letters were studied (A, B, C, D, E, F, G, K, L, O,
P, AND Y). The sampled letters were presented under computer control on a Tektronix 5103 N oscilloscope display that had a white (P4)
phosphor. The frame frequency used was 50 Hz and the luminance of
the background was about 20 cd/m^2 that corresponds rather well to
the normal room illuminance. The sample points were shown against
this background and they were seen as clearly visible bright spots
of light. The exposure duration was always 100 msec.

     The letter heights studied were .25, .5, 1, and 2 deg. These
values were obtained by viewing the letters from different distances
that varied from 57 cm to 485 cm. The stimuli were viewed binocula-
rly and with natural pupils. Between the stimulus presentations a
dim fixation point was seen on the display. A chin rest aided the
subject in keeping a good fixation.

Procedure: The sampled letters were presented one at a time and the
subject indicated the name of the letter. If he could not recognize
the letter, he was instructed to make the best possible guess. The
order of letter presentation was randomized for the 12 different   ‑

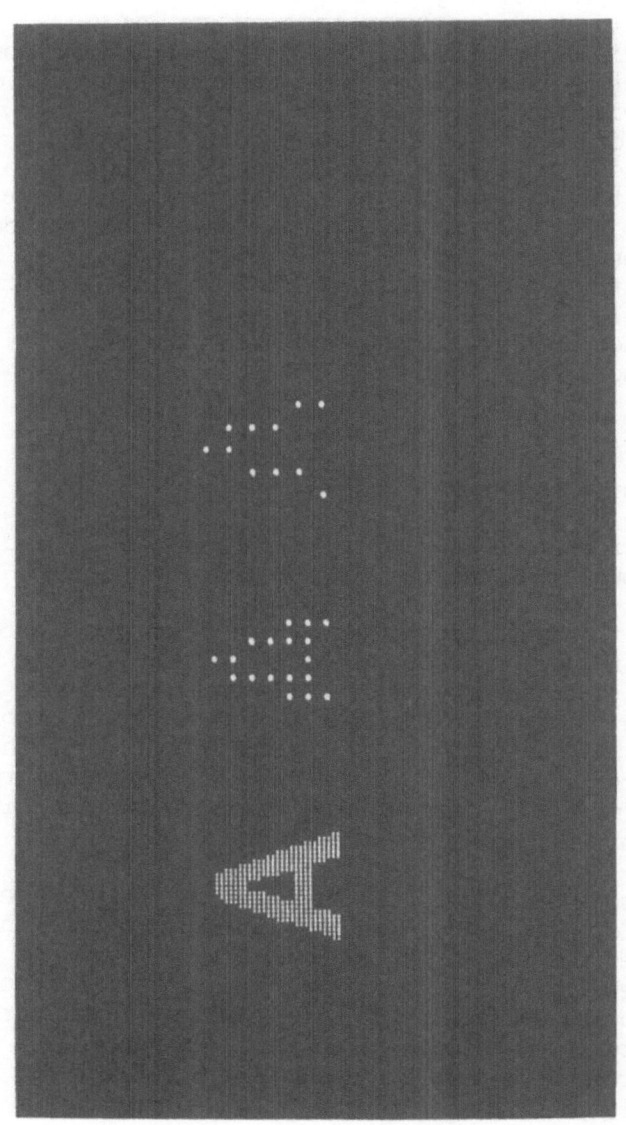

FIGURE 1. Examples of the binary letters used in Experiment II. The original letter 'A' as it was recorded through the scanning is shown to the left. Its two different sampled versions are also shown to demonstrate the kind of sampled letters that were used during the experiments. The sampling lattice was rectangular and it was produced by setting regularly spaced points to a constant luminance value and by giving all the other points a background value.

letters studied and the 20 sampling densities used. The procedure
was repeated at each viewing distance. The sampling density at which the first misnaming occured was taken as the threshold. To guarantee that the subject was attentive and fixated his gaze correctly
at the stimulus presentation, he was instructed to tell if he was not
adequately prepared when the stimulus was shown. In such cases the
presentation was repeated. The order of letter presentation was co-
unterbalanced at different viewing distances.

When eccentric vision was studied the experimental conditions
were otherwise similar to those described above with the exception
that only monocular viewing (the nasal field of the right eye) was
studied. Only three different letters were studied (K, L, O) but
other letters from the 12 different letters were also shown in a random fashion so that the subject did not know which letters were actually of interest to the experimenter. The responses to the 'dummy'
characters were not analyzed. The threshold sampling densities for
the letter identification were examined at four different eccentricities in the nasal field (0, 2, 4, and 8 deg). The eccentricity was
defined as the distance of the fixation point from the center of the
stimulus matrix on the display.

RESULTS

Experiment I: Print size and reading errors.

The number of errors made at each print size was calculated for
each experimental group. The results are shown in Figure 2.

It is seen that the dyslectic children in the 6th grade group
made almost the same number of errors at each print size as the normal children in the 1st grade group did. The normal children of the
6th grade and the 2nd grade did not differ in the number of errors
made. Furthermore, they made only a few errors (0 - 4%). On the
basis of these results it can be estimated that the dyslectic group
is at least 3 years (mean 4.5 years) behind their normal group in
the performance of this simple word match task.

When the print size increases, the number of errors made decreases for all the children studied. The most prominent reduction in
the error rate occured for the normal beginners in reading (1st grade) and for the dyslectics. In fact they reached almost an error
free performance with the largest print size. For the other normal
groups the results are not meaningful with this respect because they
did not make many errors. We have later confirmed the findings in
a study where 41 dyslectics from a 3rd grade were examined.

The results of experiment I demonstrated the improving effects
that the increased print size has in the cases where reading difficulties are considerable. However, it is not a simple matter to

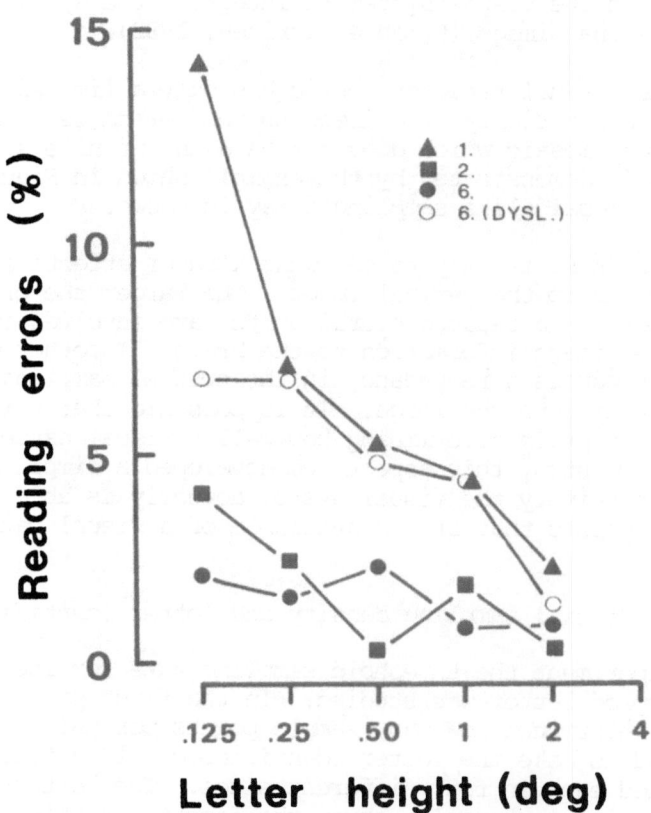

FIGURE 2. The effect of letter size to the number of errors made
in a word match task. Each function represents the performance
of pupils in one school grade. Filled symbols indicate the normal readers at different grades and the open symbols denote the
dyslectics of the 6th grade. Eight pupils in each normal group
were studied. The size of the dyslexia group was four.

explain why the increase in print size has such an improving
effect upon reading. In another context we have been interested in
the visual system's capacity to use spatial sample information to recognize the visual patterns of which only sample points are visible
to the subject. This problem is interesting because it is inherent
in many pattern vision theories that concern the capacity of the neural structures in the visual system to integrate the spatial information in the retinal image (Nyman & Laurinen, 1982).

Because the retinal receptor mosaic has only a limited sampling
density at each eccentricity, the image on the retina is always sampled by a discrete mosaic which does not have an infinite spatial resolution. This is demonstrated by the example shown in Figure 3A
where a receptor mosaic-like sampling array is shown.

From Figure 3A it is easy to see what kind of effects an increased print size has to the retinal image. The larger the print size,
the more receptors, and related neural units, are involved in the transmission of the image information to the brain. In other words,
the increase introduces a redundancy in the spatial sampling that is
applied by the retina to the image. It is possible that this redundancy is a key factor in determining how well a visual pattern can
be recognized. To study this aspect, we developed a simple method
to study how effectively the visual system actually is able to utilize the sample points that it has available of a visual pattern to
recognize it.

Experiment II: Spatial sampling density and letter identification

In this experiment the threshold sampling rate for identifying
a spatially sampled letter was studied. In the first part of the
experiment, we determined how many sample points per unit visual
angle are needed to make the letter identifiable. 12 different letters were studied each in four different sizes. The letters were
sampled by a regular rectangular array the density of which was varied to obtain the different sampling rates. The results are seen
in Figure 4.

It is evident that for each letter studied, the threshold sampling rate for correct identification increases with decreasing size. The slope of the function in Figure 4 is nearly one suggesting
a rather simple relationship between the threshold sampling rate and
the letter size. This indicates also a rather trivial result, namely that for different letter sizes the critical measure describing
the identifiability of a letter is the number of sample points per
letter width (or other letter related measure), not per unit visual
angle. Only for the smallest letters the number of samples needed
for recognition was relatively higher than that obtained for other
large letters.

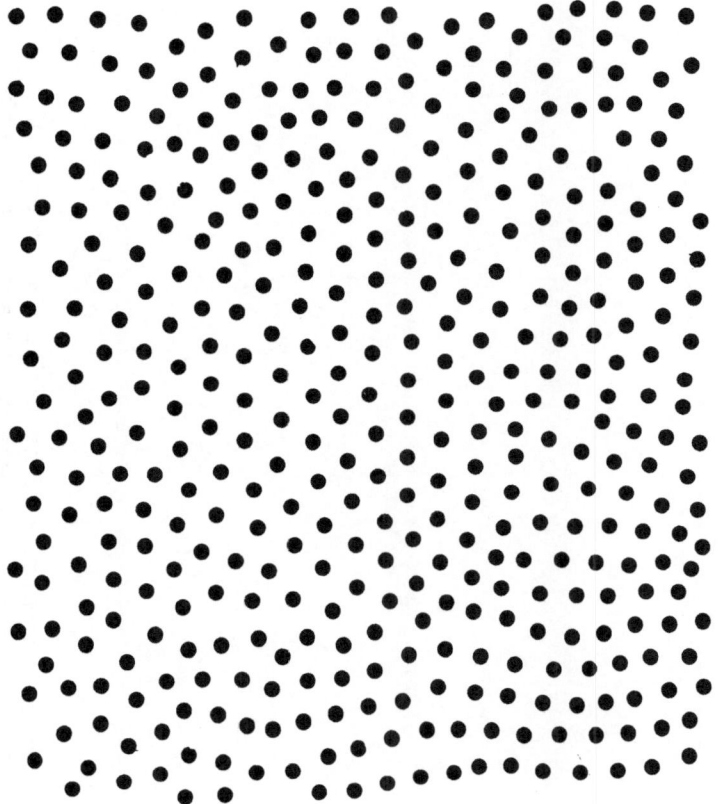

FIGURE 3A. A schematic description of the distribution of the retinal cones in the fovea. The figure has been prepared according to a photograph from Polyak (1957) and it represents an approximate area of .2 x .2 deg. Thus a letter of normal print size
just fills the area shown in the figure. Increasing the print
size increases also the number of cones activated by the letter.

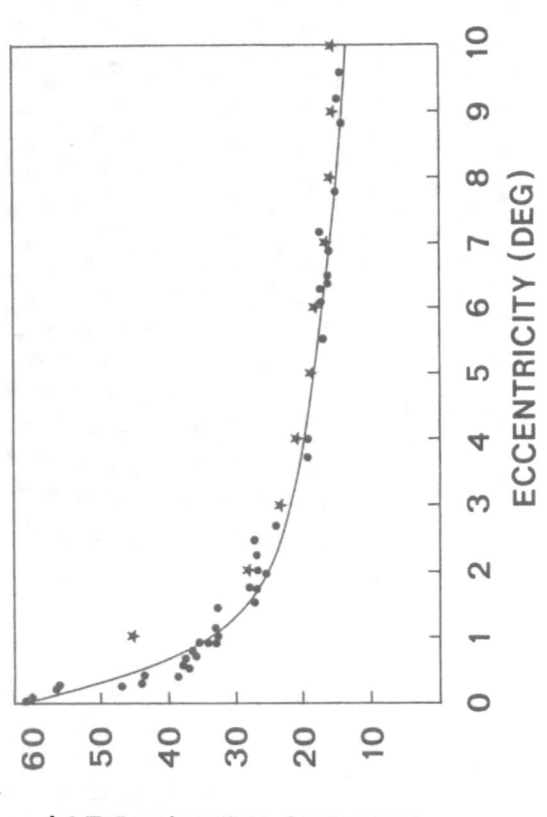

FIGURE 3B.   Resolution of the cone mosaic as calculated by taking the inverse of the intercone distance as a measure of resolution. The data points are from Österberg (1935) (filled dots) and Polyak (1957) (stars). The continuous line has been fitted by eye to the data from Österberg.

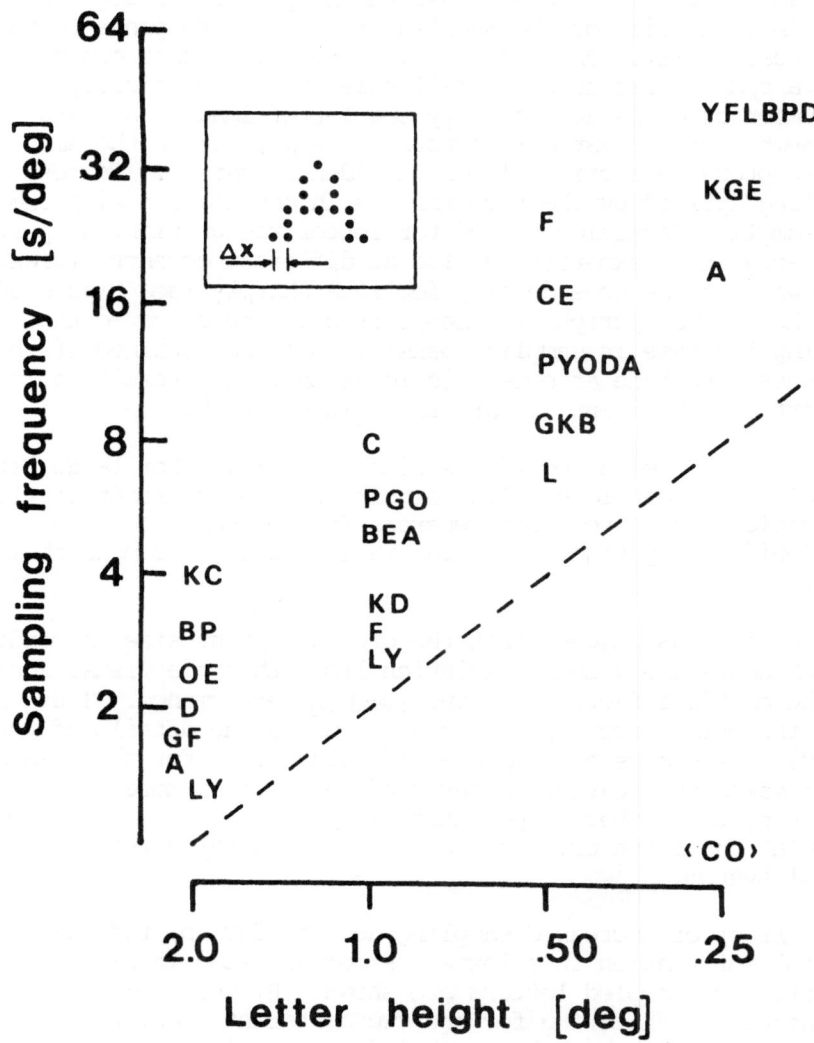

FIGURE 4. Threshold sampling densities for letter recognition as
a function of letter size. The sampling density is expressed
in terms of the sampling rate applied in the horizontal and
vertical dimensions of the rectangular sampling lattice. 12
different letters were used in the study and the result for each
letter is indicated by its position in the figure. The two letters in the brackets could not be recognized at all at the specified size. The dashed line indicates the minimum sampling
rate that must be applied in order to make it theoretically possible to reconstruct a sampled sinusoidal grating waveform having the spatial period length equal to the letter height indicated at the abscissa. The results represent the means of three
settings from one subject (S. K.).

P. Laurinen and G. Nyman

   The smallest letter we used had the height of .25 deg that is
about 5 times the size of the Snellen 'E' that corresponds to the
normal visual acuity. Thus the actual information that can be obtained from a sampled letter of a small size is also critically limited
by the number of cones activated by the letter image. At larger sizes the number of activated receptors increase, making the sampling
by the receptors less critical for the identification. To test if
the sampling applied by the receptors is in correlation with the threshold sampling densities needed for letter recognition, we performed the recognition experiments also at different eccentricities.
It is known that the cone density declines sharply (see Figure 3B)
towards the retinal periphery. Hence it could be expected that a corresponding increase in sampling density would be obtained if the
measurements were made at eccentric locations. The results of this
second part of experiment II are shown in Figure 5.

   The results are in accordance with this view. For large letters (2 deg) the threshold sampling density remains constant at all
eccentricities from 0 to 8 deg, whereas for the small letters (.5
deg) a significantly higher sampling rate is needed to make them recognizable.

   These findings suggest that the ordinary print size in reading
is so much above the visual resolution limit that the visual acuity
is not the critical factor limiting reading performance. Thus, increasing the print size - even though it makes the details of the
letters visible - does not improve the readability for this reason.
Rather it makes the spatial features of the letters more redundant
by increasing the number of potential sample points available for
the stimulation of the critical receptors or neural structures in
the visual system.

   The effect of increased sampling density for the redundancy of
the spatial information in a letter is demonstrated in Figure 6 where two different sampled letters are shown. By performing a so-called reconstruction filtering for the two different sampling rate cases shown, it can be shown how much information is gained by increasing the sampling rate.

   It is possible that the visual system performs some kind of a
reconstruction filtering for the sampled letters to make them visually identifiable. In fact, such a filtering process can be considered as a noise removal process in which only the essential features
of the letters are preserved to make the formation of a good representation possible.

DISCUSSION

   The main goal of the experiments described here was to analyze
the effects of print size to the readability of written text. It

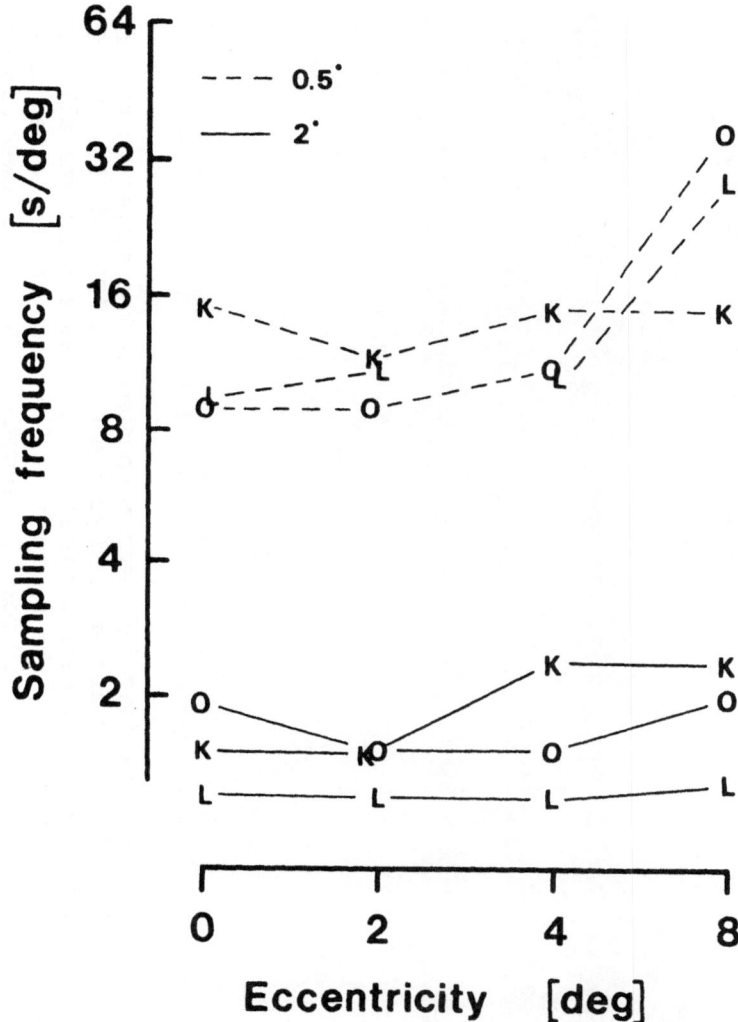

FIGURE 5. Threshold sampling densities for letter recognition as
a function of the eccentricity of viewing. Two different letter
sizes (.5 deg and 2 deg) were studied. The eccentricity is expressed in degrees and it indicates the angular distance of the
fixation point from the center of the stimulus matrix.

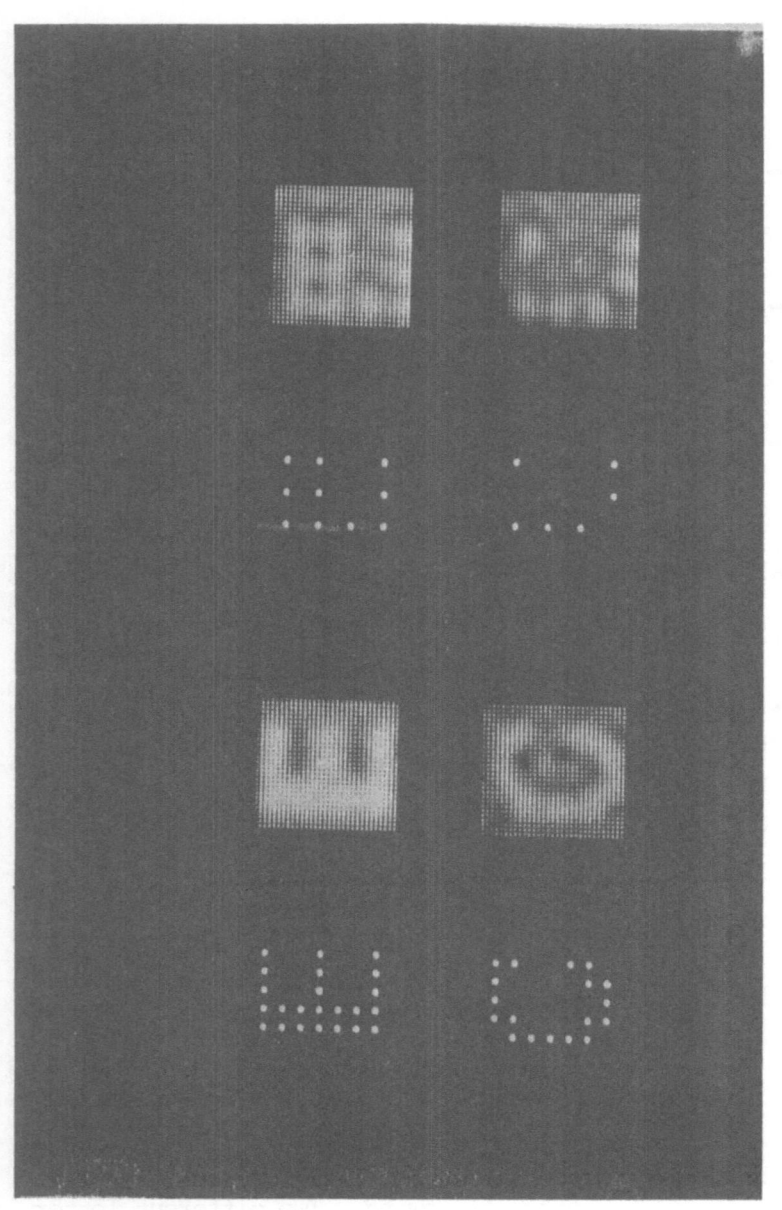

FIGURE 6. Demonstration of the form specific information carried by the sample points of a letter. Two different sampling densities are applied to the letters 'E' and 'C'. The form information was recovered by a low-pass filtering operation that was similar for all cases. A. When a dense sampling density is applied, the reconstructed version of the letter is still easily recognized, i. e. the letter specific form is recovered. B. At a lower sampling density the form of the reconstructed letter becomes noisy and not easily recognizable. In other words, form information is lost in the coarse sampling.

was found that within the range of letter heights studied (.25 - 2 deg), an increase in print size improved the reading performance of the beginning readers of the first school grade and the dyslectics of a higher grade. In other words, it was demonstrated that poor readers gained equally from the simple manipulation of the text size.

Even though the size manipulation applied was a simple one, it is not well known why the increased print size was so effective in improving the reading performance. It could be suggested that the reading difficulties are somehow connected with weak visual functions and the increase in print size simply makes the letter and word features easier to recognize. Of course this explanation is not in accordance with our results because both the normal beginning readers and the dyslectics gained equally from the increased print size. Furthermore, no visual deficits were found in the children participating in our study.

An alternative explanation to the results of experiment I is that by increasing the letter size also the spatial redundancy of the letter pattern is increased. Hence, also the letter features become better accessible for the spatial sampling processes applied by the visual system. To find out if this is the case, we conducted experiments with normal readers to whom we presented spatially sampled letters. The results suggest that a critical measure describing how well spatially sampled letters are recognized is the number of sample points available per letter area, not per some unit retinal area. In other words, the density of the retinal sampling in normal vision is not the critical factor limiting the visual recognition of letters.

However, our results suggest that when a letter is near its recognition threshold because of its small size or because it is presented at the outer fovea, an increased sampling rate can improve its recognition. It must be remembered that for the letters that were presented eccentrically at 0 - 4 deg, a constant angular sampling density was required for recognition even though the retinal receptor density and visual resolution at those eccentricities varies considerably. Thus, letter recognition is not critically dependent on the visual acuity of the subject.

Our results emphasize that one must not overestimate the role of pure visual functions (e.g. visual acuity, contrast sensitivity etc.) in reading because reading is a complex task that requires the operation of many cognitive and sensory function. However, when the quality of the receiving visual apparatus is not appropriate for the task, an additional processing load is imposed on the cognitive resources of the reader. In normal persons this can be demonstrated by applying the technique of eccentric viewing in which case the performance in letter recognition is weak because of a limited sensory processing capacity. It is possible that an analogous situation occurs for the dyslectics who gain from the increase of the print size also in the case of foveal vision. In other words, to them the spatial redundancy introduced by increasing the print size, increases the functional sampling density that their visual systems can apply to the visual patterns. Hence, the letters and words became easier to recognize and the poor visual reception of the signals does not cause an unnecessary load to the higher cognitive processes.

REFERENCES

Campbell, F. W. & Robson, J. G. Application of Fourier analysis to the visibility of gratings. J. Physiol. (Lond.) 197, 551-566, 1968.
Cornsweet, T. N. Visual perception. New York: Academic Press, 1970.
Haber, R. N. & Hershenson, M. The Psychology of Visual Perception. New York: Holt, Rinehart & Winston, 1980.
Mikkonen, V. & Stromnes, F. Association values of one thousand language characteristic items for finnish students. Rep. Inst. Psychol., 33, University of Turku, Finland, 1969.
Nyman, G. & Laurinen, P. Reconstruction of spatial information in the human visual system. Nature 297, 324-325, 1982.
Polyak, S. The Vertebrate Visual System. Chicago & London: The University of Chicago Press, 1957.
Österberg, G. A. Topography of the layers of rods and cones in the human retina. Acta Ophth., suppl. 6., 1935.
Wolpert, I. Simultanagnosia. Z. Gez. Neurol. Psychiat., 93, 1924.